THE
NURSING
EXPERIENCE

Notice

Medicine is an ever-changing science. As new research and clinical experience broaden our knowledge, changes in treatment and drug therapy are required. The author and the publisher of this work have checked with sources believed to be reliable in their efforts to provide information that is complete and generally in accord with the standards accepted at the time of publication. However, in view of the possiblity of human error or changes in medical sciences, neither the author nor the publisher nor any other party who has been involved in the preparation or publication of this work warrants that the information contained herein is in every respect accurate or complete, and they are not responsible for any errors or omissions or for the results obtained from use of such information. Readers are encouraged to confirm the information contained herein with other sources. For example and in particular, readers are advised to check the product information sheet included in the package of each drug they plan to administer to be certain that the information contained in this book is accurate and that changes have not been made in the recommended dose or in the contraindications for administration. This recommendation is of particular importance in connection with new or infrequently used drugs.

SECOND EDITION

THE NURSING EXPERIENCE

TRENDS, CHALLENGES, AND TRANSITIONS

Lucie Young Kelly, R.N., Ph.D., F.A.A.N.

PROFESSOR EMERITUS OF PUBLIC HEALTH AND NURSING
Columbia University
New York, New York

CONTRIBUTING AUTHOR
Sally Solomon Cohen, R.N., M.S., F.A.A.N.
Columbia University
New York, New York

McGRAW-HILL, INC.
Health Professions Division
New York   St. Louis   San Francisco   Auckland
Bogotá   Caracas   Lisbon   London   Madrid
Mexico   Milan   Montreal   New Delhi   Paris
San Juan   Singapore   Sydney   Tokyo   Toronto

THE NURSING EXPERIENCE

1234567890 DOC DOC 9876543210

ISBN 0-07-105390-5

This book was set in Times Roman by J.M. Post Graphics, Corp.

The editors were Gail Gavert and Mariapaz Ramos Englis.

The production supervisor was Richard Ruzycka.

Cover photos by Anita Jones Horner.

The text and cover were designed and the project
was supervised by M 'N O Production Services, Inc.

R.R. Donnelley/Crawfordsville was the printer and binder.

Library of Congress Cataloging-in-Publication Data

Kelly, Lucie Young.
    The nursing experience: trends, challenges, and transitions
Lucie Young Kelly; contributing author, Sally Solomon Cohen.—
2nd ed.
      p. cm.
    Includes bibliographical references and index.
    ISBN 0-07-105390-5
    1. Nursing—Vocational guidance. 2. Nursing. I. Cohen, Sally
Solomon. II. Title.
    [DNLM: 1. Nursing—trends. WY 16 K292n]
RT82.K43 1992
610.73—dc20
DNLM/DLC
for Library of Congress   91-43536
                                        CIP

CONTENTS

PART II
NURSING IN THE HEALTH CARE SCENE

PREFACE

The most exciting part of nursing may well be that it is such a big and important part of a rapidly changing health care scene. As I wrote this second edition, it was again impressive to see how many of those changes have occurred in a relatively short time and the increasing impact of nursing. Moreover, as I meet my colleagues around the country, I am more than ever convinced that nurses and our new breed of students expect to take part in this action. Students recognize the need to know what is going on in society and health care and what they can do about it as much as they want information about their career options and what to expect as they enter the world of nursing. Needless to say, their teachers want to prepare them in the best possible way, both for their clinical and their professional roles. This book has been structured to meet the needs of both.

The first edition of *The Nursing Experience* was written at the request of teachers, who asked for "something like *Dimensions of Professional Nursing*, but shorter." Then, as now, they faced the problem of cramming more and more clinical content into the curriculum without neglecting the trends and issues, history, legal aspects, and nursing theories that were once separate courses. All these and more are found in these pages. Moreover, this edition is set up in a format similar to that of the more comprehensive sixth edition of *Dimensions*, which was published in 1991, so that the latter can easily be used to enlarge on the topics discussed. Again, the easily read exhibits, tables, and appendixes consolidate many facts in a brief, visual, organized format. For instance, the new Appendix 1 summarizes the major studies and reports about nursing, from 1912 to 1991. The updated Appendix 2 presents not only data about other health personnel, but the major issues and trends in the fields. Appendix 3, also updated, allows the reader to compare nursing competencies at graduation, as well as basic information about all the nursing programs. Other popular features, such as the overview of parliamentary procedures, the legislative process, the exhibit on theories, (enlarged), and information about the major nursing organizations are again provided. The objectives and key points in each chapter, which teachers and students say are quite helpful, are continued.

Needless to say, every chapter has been updated, except the history chapters, which people have told me to leave alone. However, I've added many new references. The extensive references and bibliography for all chapters are new, with the exception of some classics. They are from diverse sources, so that interested students may research a topic more thoroughly.

There is considerably more information about nursing supply and demand, the dilemmas in health care delivery, ethics, all facets of law, and various other emerging issues that nurses face in practice today. The predictions for the future, a unique part of this book, are often a source of lively discussion.

The Nursing Experience is intended to give a large amount of important information in a compact, visual format that will have continuing value as the nurse becomes educated and practices. Most of all, it is intended to stimulate thinking and discussion, to pique curiosity, and to encourage involvement in nursing. Knowledgeable nurses will create the future of nursing, and I hope that this book will help them.

ACKNOWLEDGMENTS

It is almost impossible to list all those who have contributed in some way to this book. Some have written or commented to me personally about what they liked, needed, or wanted more of in relation to the first edition of *The Nursing Experience*; I listened and followed through. Many of those acknowledged in *Dimensions of Professional Nursing* deserve a second thanks because much of what they provided in one way or another was the basis of this edition of *The Nursing Experience*.

I also wish to thank the organizations and individuals who allowed me to use their materials, all of which are credited throughout the book.

For major assistance in obtaining photos, I acknowledge Dr. Maryann Fralic, Robert Wood Johnson University Hospital, New Jersey; Margaret Harrington RN and Ranete Koster, Jewish Home and Hospital for Aged, New York; Barry Waldman, New York State Nurses' Association; Lyle Churchill, Visiting Nurse Service of New York; Dr. Robert Piemonte and Caroline Jaffe, National Student Nurses' Association; Lt. Col. Carolyn Feller, U.S. Army Nurse Corps; Capt. Jerry Herbel, U.S. Air Force Recruiting Service; Dr. Joan Trofino, Riverview Medical Center, New Jersey.

For her contribution to the theory exhibit, I would like to thank Dr. Josephine Ryan, University of Massachusetts School of Nursing at Amherst. A very special person, Sally Solomon Cohen of Columbia University, who was the contributing author of *Dimensions of Professional Nursing,* is also named contributing author of *The Nursing Experience.* She revised Chapter 10 and has been helpful in many other ways with information, advice, and collegial support.

This book might still be handwritten if it were not for Faith Smalls, assistant to the editors at *Nursing Outlook,* who always gave me back a nearly perfect typed manuscript in a remarkably short time. I couldn't have managed without her and give her my special thanks.

Finally, my appreciation to Patricia Casey, previously the Macmillan/Pergamon editor with whom I worked, who was unfailingly helpful and cheerful. I have been fortunate in the support and interest of my colleagues. To them, the teachers and the students of nursing, this is for you.

THE
NURSING
EXPERIENCE

PART I
THE
EVOLUTION OF
NURSING

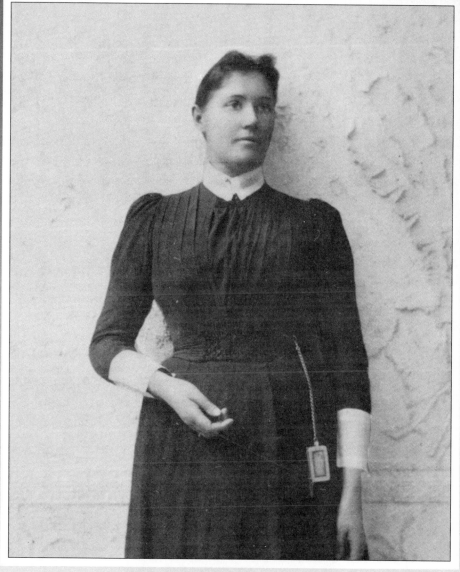

Isabel Hampton Robb, nursing leader and
first president of ANA.

CHAPTER 1

CARE OF THE SICK
HOW NURSING BEGAN

OBJECTIVES

After studying this chapter, you will be able to:

1. Recognize the contributions of early civilizations to care of the sick.
2. Discuss how various nursing orders influenced the evolution of nursing.
3. Describe at least three ways in which Florence Nightingale influenced the development of nursing.

What does it matter whether or not we know anything about nursing history? A lot. Nursing today was formed by its history. Its development since ancient times, within the social contexts of those times, explains many things: its power or lack of power, its educational confusion, and the makeup of its practitioners. The changing relationships between nursing and other health care professions, nursing and other disciplines, and nursing and the public can be traced and better understood with the knowledge of past history. The impact of social and scientific changes on nursing and nursing's impact on society are ongoing processes that need to be studied; nursing does not exist in a vacuum.

Sometimes there is a repetition of history. For instance, a 100 years ago, there were many arguments within and without the nursing profession about nursing education; this scenario is being repeated today. Seventy-five years ago, the question of nursing licensure was hotly debated; today, it is again a major concern. For 50 years, studies have documented reasons for nurses' discontentment with their jobs; only now are some changes being made. These issues affect the practice of every nurse; in some cases, they are a factor in determining whether the nurse even chooses to stay in the profession. Understanding the past can be very useful in making decisions that shape the future.

CARE OF THE SICK IN EARLY CIVILIZATIONS

Undoubtedly, some form of nursing activity has existed since earliest civilization. Although for thousands of years concepts of health and illness were closely related to belief in the supernatural, there is evidence that plants were used as medicine, as well as heat, cold, and even some types of primitive surgery. In primitive times there were medicine men and women, but nursing care probably fell to the women of the family unit.

Records of the early known civilizations were sometimes written by the physicians of the time and provide interesting information on the care of the sick. There were also occasional references to nurses. In *Babylonia* for instance, one of the great civilizations that lay between the eastern Mediterranean and the Persian Gulf, a legalized medical system existed. There were even laws that punished physicians for malpractice. Some of the treatments included diet, rest, enemas, bandaging, and massaging (with or without incantations), and care was given by some type of lay nurse.

Although the ancient *Hebrews* attributed their illnesses to God's wrath, under the leadership of Moses they developed principles and practices of hygiene and sanitation. They performed various kinds of surgery and dressed wounds, using sutures and bandages. Nurses are mentioned in the *Old Testament,* but other than visiting and possibly caring for the sick in the home, their role is not clear.

Ancient *Egypt,* located along the Nile, also was noted for its laws on health and sanitation, which included regulations about diet and personal hygiene. There were medical schools and at least one school of midwifery for women, whose graduates taught physicians about "women's conditions." Excavated medical papyri have descriptions of nursing procedures, such as dressing wounds, but again, the nurses' duties are not clear.

The first hospitals were probably established in pre-Christian *India.* Records identify the first special nursing group: men who staffed the hospitals

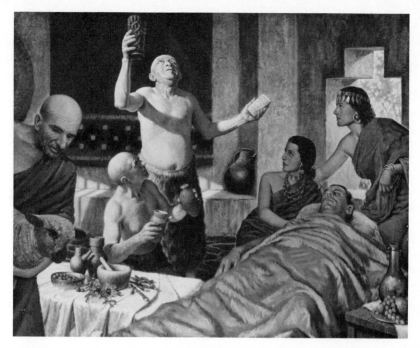

Physicians in ancient Babylonia treated the sick with a mixture of medicine and charms; nurses were probably the women in the family. (*Courtesy of Parke, Davis and Company.*)

and performed some nursing functions. Actually, they may have been more like physicians' assistants. The Indian physicians were exceptionally skilled in surgery and used many drugs in their treatments, although, as in other civilizations, magic and evil spirits were part of medical belief.

In ancient *China,* both acupuncture and drug therapy were used. These were incorporated into the theory of yang and yin. Yang, the male principle, is light, positive, and full of life; yin, the female principle, is dark, cold, and lifeless. When the two are in harmony, the patient is in good health. The Chinese also refined ancient measures of hydrotherapy, massage, and other physical techniques, and promoted systematic exercise to maintain physical and mental well-being. Many of these treatments are still used effectively today.

Greece, too, had its demons, spirits, and gods related to illness, with Asclepios (Roman version: Aesculapius), the classic god of medicine, honored by the founding of temples for the sick, which were actually more like health spas. The staff of Asclepios, intertwined with the snakes or serpents of wisdom and immortality, are thought to be the basis of today's medical caduceus. The greatest name in Greek medicine is *Hippocrates* (about 400

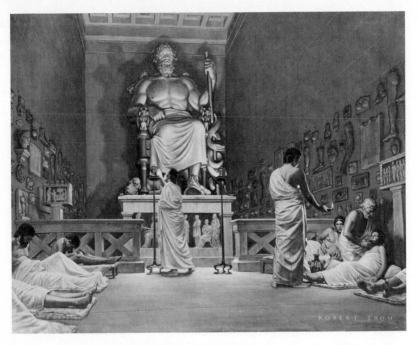

In the Greek temple of Asclepios, (Aesculapius) the god of medicine, priests combined prayer and rituals with various treatments. (*Courtesy of Parke, Davis and Company.*)

B.C.), who developed patient assessment and recording and rejected the supernatural origins of disease. His establishment of high ethical standards is reflected in the Hippocratic oath still taken in many medical schools. For centuries after his death, the medical books he had written were the basis of medical knowledge. There is no account of nurses.

Rome's most lasting contribution to medicine may have been the founding of hospitals, at first primarily for the military as they conquered new territories. Both male and female attendants (nurses?) were used. Medical care was in the hands of the Greeks, like the great *Galen* (about 200 to 130 B.C.), who lived in Rome.

CHRISTIANITY'S IMPACT ON NURSING

In the early Christian era, bishops were given responsibility for the sick, the poor, widows, and children, but the deacons and deaconesses carried out the services. It appears that there was a group of specially designated women (deaconesses, widows, virgins, and matrons) who cared for the sick. *Phoebe,* mentioned in the Bible by Paul, was the first deaconess actually identified as giving nursing care. There were other noted women in the first centuries of Christianity, frequently designated as saints later. *Olympias,* a rich aristocratic widow of Constantinople, erected a convent and with 40 deaconesses cared for the sick. *Marcella,* a wealthy Roman, converted her palace into a monastery and, among other things, taught the care of the sick to her followers. *Fabiola* was one of Marcella's group and became a Christian convert. Also wealthy, she founded the first free hospital for the poor and personally nursed the sickest and filthiest people who came to her. St. Jerome wrote letters of praise about both women.

The Middle Ages (about 500 to 1500 A.D.) has a mixed record in sick care. During the first half, called the *Dark Ages,* medical and nursing care, though needed, was barely available as wars, ignorance, famine, and disease flourished. The Christian church was obsessed with its belief that the main purpose of human beings on earth was to prepare for a future life and thus saw little need for science and philosophy. The teachings of hygiene and sanitation from earlier civilizations were discarded. Except for the eastern Roman and Moslem empires, medical knowledge stagnated.

During the Middle Ages, the deaconesses, suppressed by the Western churches in particular, gradually declined and became almost extinct. As the deaconesses declined, the religious orders grew stronger. Known as *monastic orders* and composed of monks and nuns (though not in the same orders), they controlled the hospitals, running them as institutions concerned more with the patients' religious problems than with their physical ailments. However, monks and some nuns were better educated than most people in those times, and their liberal education may well have included some of the medical writings of Galen.

Lay citizens banded together to form *secular orders.* Their work was similar to that of the monastic orders in that it was concerned with the sick and needy, but they lived in their own homes, were allowed to marry, and took no vows of the church. They usually adopted a uniform, or habit. Nursing was often their main work.

The *military nursing orders,* known as the *Knights Hospitallers,* were the outcome of the Crusades, the military expeditions undertaken by Christians in the eleventh, twelfth, and thirteenth centuries to recover the Holy Land from the Moslems.

The most prominent of these three types of orders—religious, military, and secular—were the Order of St. Benedict, Knights Hospitallers, Hospital Brothers of St. Anthony, Third Order of St. Francis, Beguines of Flanders, Order of the Holy Ghost (Santo Spirito), Grey Sisters, and Alexian Brotherhood.

NURSING CARE IN EARLY HOSPITALS

Gradually, more hospitals in which the sick received care were established as the need increased. At the close of the Middle Ages, there were hospitals all over Europe, particularly in larger cities such as Paris and Rome. In England, too, several hundred were established, some of which still remain. Hospitals in England during the Middle Ages differed from those on the Continent in that they were never completely church controlled, although they were founded on Christian principles and accepted responsibility for the sick and injured. The oldest and best-known English hospitals from a historical point of view are St. Bartholomew's, founded in 1123; St. Thomas's, founded in 1213; and Bethlehem Hospital, founded in 1247, originally as a general hospital, which later became famous as a mental institution, referred to frequently as *Bedlam*.

The Hotel Dieu of Paris, founded about 650, had an unfavorable record as far as nursing is concerned. Staffed by Augustinian nuns who did the cooking and laundry as well as the nursing, and who had neither intellectual nor professional stimulation, the hospital was not distinguished for its care of patients. The records of nursing kept by this hospital were well done, however, and have been a source of enlightenment for historians.

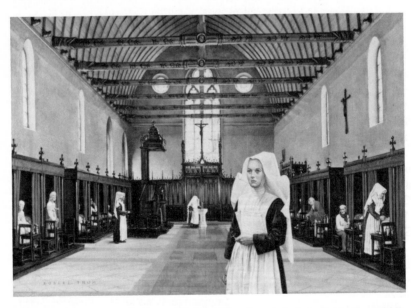

The Hotel Dieu of Paris was one of the earliest hospitals founded in the Middle Ages. (*Courtesy of Parke, Davis and Company.*)

The nursing care in most early hospitals was essentially basic: bathing, feeding, giving medicines, making beds, and so on. It was rarely of high quality, however, largely because of the retarded progress of nearly all civilization and the shortsighted attitude toward women that was typical of the Dark Ages. Even after the Renaissance (1400 to 1550), during which Paracelsus, Vesalius, and Paré made major contributions in pharmaceutical chemistry, anatomy, and surgery, hospital nursing remained at the same basic level.

During the Reformation (beginning about 1500), which resulted in the formation of various Protestant churches, the Protestant leaders saw the vacuum in the care of the sick and urged the hiring of nurse deaconesses and elderly women to do nursing. By the end of the eighteenth century, nurses of some kind functioned in hospitals. Conditions were not attractive, and much has been written about the drunken, thieving women who tended patients. However, some hospitals made real efforts to set standards. Already a hierarchy of nursing personnel had begun, with helpers and watchers assigned to help the *sisters,* as the early English nurses were called.

In other parts of Europe, nursing was becoming recognized as an important service. Diderot, whose *Encyclopedia* attempted to sum up all human knowledge, said that nursing "is as important for humanity as its functions are low and repugnant." Urging care in selection, since "all persons are not adapted to it," he described the nurse as "patient, mild, and compassionate. She should console the sick, foresee their needs, and relieve their tedium."[1]

The dreary picture of secular nursing is not totally unexpected, given the times. Because proper young women did not work outside the home, nursing had no acceptance, much less prestige. Even those nurses not in the Dickens's Sairy Gamp mold or those desiring to nurse found themselves in competition with workhouse inmates, who were cheaper workers for hospital administrations. (Actually, most care was still given at home by wives and mothers.) It was acceptable to nurse as a member of a religious order, when the motivation was, of course, religious and the cost to the hospital was little or nothing.

A startling development during the Reformation was the disappearance of male nurses. The Protestant nursing orders were female, and except for a few male orders like the Brothers Hospitallers of St. John of God, the Catholic nursing orders after 1500 were primarily made up of women. Among the most noted were the Sisters of Charity (France) and the Irish Sisters of Charity and the Sisters of Mercy.

During the nineteenth century, several nursing orders were revived or originated that had substantial influence on modern nursing. In most instances, these orders cared for patients in hospitals that were already established, in contrast to the orders of earlier times, which had founded the hospitals in which they worked. Among the most influential orders was the Church Order of Deaconesses, an ancient order revived by Theodor Fliedner, pastor of a small parish in Kaiserswerth, Germany. (Florence Nightingale later obtained her only formal training there.) The Protestant Sisters of Charity, under Sister Elizabeth Fry, worked among prisoners and the physically and mentally ill.

Of the nursing orders established by the Church of England, the most noted were the Sisters of Mercy in the Church of England and St. Margarets of East Grinstead, both of whom were involved with "district" or home nursing. The Anglican order that did the most for hospital nursing in this period was St. John's House, founded in 1848 in London, whose purpose was to train members of the church "to act as nurses and visitors to the sick and poor."[2] The original plan required the order to be associated with a hospital in which women under training or those already educated could gain experience and exercise their calling. The program was very successful.

Exhibit 1-1

Three Centuries of Scientific Landmarks

William Harvey (1578–1657), England	First to describe completely (except for the capillary system) and accurately the circulatory system.
Thomas Sydenham (1624–1689), England	Revived the Hippocratic methods of observation and reasoning and in other ways restored clinical medicine to a sound basis.
Antonj van Leeuwenhoek (1632–1723), Holland	Improved on Galileo's microscope and produced one that permitted the examination of body cells and bacteria.
William Hunter (1718–1783) and his brother John (1728–1793), Scotland	Founded the science of pathology.
William Tuke (1732–1822), England	Reformed the care of the mentally ill.
Edward Jenner (1749–1823), England	Originated vaccination against smallpox.
René Laennec (1781–1826), France	Invented the stethoscope.

Many of the Catholic and Protestant orders went to the New World, founding hospitals in Canada, the United States, and Mexico. Cortez is credited with founding the first hospital in the New World, located in Mexico City, and within 20 years, most major Spanish towns had one. Hospitals in the New World were no better than those in Europe, and given the hard living conditions, there were numerous health problems.

Progress in medicine and science during these centuries (Exhibit 1-1) was accompanied by accelerated interest in better nursing service and nurses' training. Neither was achieved to a significant degree, however, despite the fine work of dedicated men and women who belonged to the nursing orders of the time. Limited in number and inadequately prepared for their nursing functions, the members of these orders could not begin to meet the need for their services. Such care as patients received in the majority of institutions was grossly inadequate.

Oliver Wendell Holmes (1809–1894), United States	Furthered safe obstetric practice, pointing out the dangers of infection.
Crawford W. Long (1815–1878), United States	Excised a tumor of the neck under ether anesthesia in 1832 but did not make his discovery public until after Dr. William T. Morton announced his in 1846.
Ignaz P. Semmelweis (1818–1865), Austria-Hungary	Recognized that infection was carried from patient to patient by physicians and instituted preventive measures for puerperal fever in new mothers.
Louis Pasteur (1822–1895), France	Founder of microbiology and developer of pasteurization; developed preventive inoculations against anthrax, chicken cholera, and rabies.
Lord Joseph Lister (1827–1912), England	Developed and proved the theory of bacterial infection of wounds.
Robert Koch (1843–1910), Germany	Founded modern bacteriology. identified the tubercle bacillus.
Wilhelm Röntgen (1845–1923), Germany	Discovered x-rays in 1895 and laid the foundation for the science of roentgenology and radiology.
Pierre Curie (1859–1906), France, and his Polish wife, Marie (1867–1934)	Discovered radium in 1898.

In the mid-nineteenth century, therefore, the time was right—perhaps overdue—for the revolution in nursing education that originated under the leadership of Florence Nightingale and that influenced so greatly and so quickly (from a historical point of view) the nursing care of patients and, indeed, the health of the world.

THE INFLUENCE OF FLORENCE NIGHTINGALE

It has been said that Florence Nightingale, an extraordinary woman in any century, is the most written-about woman in history. Through her own numerous publications, her letters, the writings of her contemporaries, including newspaper reports, and the numerous biographies and studies of her life, there emerges the picture of a sometimes contradictory, frequently controversial, but undeniably powerful woman who probably had a greater influence on the care of the sick than any other single individual.

Called the founder of modern nursing, Nightingale was a strong-willed, intelligent woman who used her considerable knowledge of statistics, sanitation, logistics, administration, nutrition, and public health not only to develop a new system of nursing education and health care but also to improve the social welfare systems of the time. The gentle, caring lady of the lamp, full of compassion for the soldiers of the Crimea, is an accurate image, but no more so than that of the hard-headed administrator and planner who forced changes in the intolerable social conditions of the time, including the care of the sick poor. Nightingale knew that tender touch alone would not bring health to the sick or prevent illness, so she set her intelligence, her administrative skills, her political acumen, and her incredible drive to achieve her self-defined missions. In the Victorian age when women were almost totally dominated by men—fathers, husbands, brothers—and it was undesirable for them to show intelligence or profess interest in anything but household arts, this indomitable woman accomplished the following:

1. Improved and reformed laws affecting health, morals, and the poor.
2. Reformed hospitals and improved workhouses and infirmaries.
3. Improved medicine by instituting an army medical school and reorganizing the army medical department.
4. Improved the health of natives and British citizens in India and other colonies.
5. Established nursing as a profession with two missions: sick nursing and health nursing.[3]

The new nurse and the new image of the nurse that she created, in part through the nursing schools she founded, in part through her writings, and in part through her international influence, became the model that persisted for almost 100 years. Today, some of her tenets about the "good" nurse seem terribly restrictive, but it should be remembered that in those times not only the image but also the reality of much of secular nursing was based on the untutored, uncouth workhouse inmates for whom drunkenness and thievery were a way of life. It was small wonder that each Nightingale student had to exemplify a new image above reproach.

Early Life

Florence Nightingale was born on May 12, 1820, in Florence, Italy, during her English parents' travels there. The family was wealthy and well educated, with a high social standing and influential friends, all of which later would be useful to Nightingale. Primarily under her father's tutelage, she learned Greek, Latin, French, German, and Italian, and studied history, philosophy, science, music, art, and classical literature. She traveled widely with her family and friends. The breadth of her education, almost unheard of for women of the times, was also considerably more extensive than that of most men, including physicians. Her intelligence and education were recognized by scholars, as indicated in her correspondence with them.

Nightingale was not only bright but, according to early portraits and descriptions, slender, attractive, and fun-loving, enjoying the social life of her class. She differed from other young women in her determination to do something "toward lifting the load of suffering from the helpless and miserable."[4] Apparently, the encouragement of Dr. Samuel Gridley Howe and his wife, Julia Ward Howe (who wrote "The Battle Hymn of the Republic"), during a visit to the Nightingale family home in 1844 helped to crystallize Florence's interest in hospitals and nursing. Nevertheless, her intent to train in a hospital was strongly opposed by her family, and she limited herself to nursing family members.

Although remaining the obedient daughter, Nightingale found her own way to expand her knowledge of sick care. She studied hospital and sanitary reports and books on public health. Having received information on Kaiserswerth in Germany, she determined to receive training there—which was more acceptable because of its religious auspices. On one of her trips to the Continent, she made a brief visit and was impressed enough to spend three months in training and observation there in 1851. Her later efforts to study with various Catholic orders were frustrated. However, she got permission to inspect the hospitals in various cities during her tours. She examined the general layout of the hospital, as well as ward construction, sanitation, general administration, and the work of the surgeons and physicians. Apparently, these observational techniques and her analytical abilities then and later were the basis of her unrivaled knowledge of hospitals in the next decade. Few of her contemporaries ever had such knowledge.

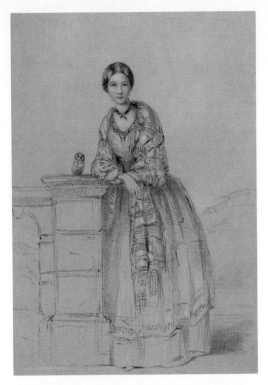

Florence Nightingale with her owl Athena.

In 1853, Nightingale assumed the position of superintendent of a charity hospital (probably more of a nursing home) for ill governesses run by titled ladies. Although she had difficulties with her intolerant governing board, she did make changes considered revolutionary for the day and, even with the lack of trained nurses, improved the patients' care. And she continued to visit hospitals. Just as Nightingale was negotiating for a superintendency in the newly reorganized and rebuilt King's College Hospital in London, England and France, in support of Turkey, declared war on Russia in March 1854.

Crimea: The Turning Point

The Crimean War was a low point for England. Ill-prepared and disorganized in general, the army and the bureaucracy were even less prepared to care for the thousands of soldiers both wounded in battle and prostrated by the cholera epidemics brought on by worse than primitive conditions. Not even the most basic equipment or drugs were available, and, as casualties mounted,

Turkey turned over the enormous but bare and filthy barracks at Scutari, across from Constantinople, to be used as a hospital. The conditions remained abominable. The soldiers lay on the floor in filth, untended, frequently without food or water because there was no equipment to prepare or distribute either. Rats and other vermin came from the sewers underneath the building. There were no beds, furniture, basins, soap, towels, or eating utensils, and few provisions. There were only orderlies, and none of these at night. The death rate was said to be 60 percent.

In previous wars, the situation had not been much different, and there was little interest on the battle sites, for ordinary soldiers were accorded no decencies. But now, for the first time, civilian war correspondents were present and sent back the news of these horrors to an England with a newly aroused social conscience. The reformers were in an uproar; newspapers demanded to know why England did not have nurses like the French Sisters of Charity to care for its soldiers, and Parliament trembled. In October 1854, Sidney Herbert, Secretary of War and an old friend of Florence Nightingale, wrote, begging her to lead a group of nurses to the Crimea under government authority and at government expense. Nightingale had already decided to offer her services, and the two letters crossed. In less than a week, she had assembled 38 nurses, the most she could find who met her standards— Roman Catholic and Anglican sisters and lay nurses from various hospitals— and embarked for Scutari. Even under the miserable circumstances found there, Nightingale and her contingent were not welcomed by the army doctors and surgeons, who refused the nurses' services.

Nightingale chose to wait to be asked to help. To the anger of her nurses, she allowed none of them to give care until one week later, when scurvy, starvation, dysentery, exposure, and more fighting almost brought about the collapse of the British army. Then the doctors, desperate for any kind of assistance, turned to the eager nurses.

Modern criticisms of Florence Nightingale frequently refer to her insistence on the physician's overall authority and her own authoritarian approach to nursing. The first criticism may have originated with her situation in the Crimean War. In mid-century England her appointment created a furor; she was the first woman ever to be given such authority. Yet, despite the high-sounding title that Herbert insisted she have—General Superintendent of the Female Nursing Establishment of the Military Hospitals of the Army—her orders required that she have the approval of the Principal Medical Officer "in her exercise of the responsibilities thus vested in her."[5] Although no "lady, sister, or nurse" could be transferred from one hospital to another without her approval, she had no authority over anyone else, even orderlies and cooks. What she accomplished had to be done through sheer force of will or persuasion. Her overt deference to physicians was probably the beginning of the doctor-nurse game.

Whatever the limitations of her power, Florence Nightingale literally accomplished miracles at Scutari. Even in the week of waiting, she moved into the kitchen area and began to cook extras from her own supplies to create a diet kitchen, which for five months was the only source of food for the sick.

Nightingale had powerful friends and control over a large amount of contributed funds—a situation that gained her some cooperation from most physicians after a while. Through persuasion and the use of good managerial techniques, she cleaned up the hospital: the orderlies scrubbed and emptied slops regularly; soldiers' wives and camp followers washed clothes; and the vermin were brought under some control. Before the end of the war, the mortality rate at Scutari declined to 1 percent.

When the hospital care improved, Nightingale began a program of social welfare among the soldiers—among other things, seeing to it that they got sick pay. The patients adored her. She cared about them, and the doctors and officers reproached her for "spoiling the brutes." News correspondents wrote reports about the "ministering angel" and "lady with the lamp" making late rounds after the medical officers had retired—which inspired Longfellow later to write his famous poem "Santa Filomena." England and America were enthralled, and she was awarded decorations by Queen Victoria and the Sultan of Turkey.

But all did not go well. The military doctors continued in their resentment and tried to undermine her. There were problems in her own ranks, dissension among the religious and secular nurses, and problems of incompetence and immorality. No doubt Nightingale was high-handed at times. Despite praise of her leadership, she was also called "quick, violent-tempered, positive, obstinate, and stubborn."[6] Certainly she drove herself in all she did.

When the situation at Scutari was improved, she crossed the Black Sea to the battle sites and worked on the reorganization of the few hospitals there—with no better support from physicians and superior officers. There she contracted Crimean fever (probably typhoid or typhus) and nearly died. However, she refused a leave of absence to recuperate and stayed in Scutari to work until the end of the war. She supervised 125 nurses and forced the military to recognize the place of nurses.

On her return from the Crimea, Nightingale took to her bed, or at least to her rooms, and emerged only on rare occasions. There is much speculation on this illness—whether it was a result of the Crimea fever, neurasthenia, a bit of both, or whether she simply found it useful to avoid wasting time with people she did not want to see. For she was famous now and had been given discretion over the so-called Nightingale Fund, to which almost everyone in England had subscribed, including many of the troops.

From her experiences, and to support her recommendations for reform, Nightingale wrote a massive report entitled *Notes on Matters Affecting the Health, Efficiency, and Hospital Administration of the British Army,* crammed with facts, figures, and statistical comparison. On the basis of this and her later well-researched and well-documented papers, she is often credited with being the first nurse researcher. Reforms were slow in coming but extended even to the United States when the Union consulted her about organizing hospitals. In 1859 she wrote a small book, *Notes on Nursing: What It Is and What It Is Not,* intended for the average housewife and printed cheaply so that it would be affordable. These and other Nightingale works are still amazingly readable today—brisk, down-to-earth, and laced with many a pithy comment. For instance, in *Notes on Hospitals,* written in the same year, she compared the administration of the various types of hospitals and characterized the management of secular hospitals under the sole command of the male hospital authorities as "all but crazy."[7]

Her knowledge was certainly respected, and she was consulted by many, including the Royal Sanitary Commission on the Health of the Army in India.

The Nightingale Nurse

In 1860, Nightingale utilized some of the 45,000 English pounds of the Nightingale Fund to establish a training school for nurses. She selected St. Thomas's Hospital because of her respect for its matron, Mrs. S. E. Wardroper. The two converted the resident medical officers to their plan, although apparently most other physicians objected to the school. The students were chosen; the first class in the desired age range of 25 to 35 years and with impeccable character references numbered only 15. It was to be a one-year training program, and the students were presented with what could be called terminal behavioral objectives that they had to reach satisfactorily. Students could be dismissed by the matron for misconduct, inefficiency, or negligence. However, if they passed the courses of instruction and training satisfactorily, they were entered in the "Register" as certified nurses. The Committee of the Nightingale Fund then recommended them for employment; in the early years, they were obligated to work as hospital nurses for at least five years (for which they were paid).

The students' time was carefully structured, beginning at 6 A.M. and ending with a 9 P.M. bedtime, which included a semimandatory two-hour exercise period (walking abroad had to be done in twos and threes, not alone). Within that time there was actually about a nine-hour work and training day (a vast difference from future American schools). This included bedside teaching by a teaching sister or the Resident Medical Officer and elementary instruction in "Chemistry, with reference to air, water, food, etc.; Physiology, with reference to a knowledge of the leading functions of the body, and general instruction on medical and surgical topics"[8] by professors of the medical school attached to St. Thomas's, given voluntarily and without payment.

The Nightingale school was not under the control of the hospital and had education as its purpose. The Nightingale Fund paid the medical officers, head nurses, and matron for teaching students, beyond whatever they earned from the hospital in carrying out their other duties. Both the head nurses and the matron kept records on each student, evaluating how she met the stated objectives of the program. The students were expected to keep notes from the lectures and records of patient observation and care, all of which were checked by the nurse-teachers. At King's College Hospital, run by the Society of St. John's House, an Anglican religious community, midwifery was taught in similar style and with similar regulations, again under the auspices of the Nightingale Fund Committee. And, at the Royal Liverpool Infirmary, nurses were trained for home nursing of the sick poor under a Nightingale protocol but were personally funded by a Liverpool merchant-philanthropist. As Nightingale said in 1863, "We have had to introduce an entirely new system to which the older systems of nursing bear but slight resemblance. . . . It exists neither in Scotland nor in Ireland at the present time."[9]

The demand for the Nightingale nurses was overwhelming. In the next few years, requests also came for them to improve the workhouse (poor-house) infirmaries and to reform both civilian and military nursing in India. In response to these demands, Nightingale wrote many reports, detailing to the last item the system for educating these nurses and for improving patient care, including such points as general hygiene and sanitation, nutrition, equipment, supplies, and the nurses' housing conditions, holidays, salaries, and retirement benefits. (For India, she suggested that they had better pay good salaries and provide satisfactory working and living conditions, or the nurses might opt for marriage, because the opportunities there were even greater than in England.) She constantly reiterated that she could not supply enough nurses but, when possible, she would send a matron and some other nurses, who would train new Nightingale nurses.

Maintaining standards was a constant struggle. Even St. Thomas's Hospital slipped, and Nightingale, who had been immersed in the Indian reforms, had to take time to reorganize the program. What evolved over the years, from the first program, was one of preparation for two kinds of nursing practitioners: the educated middle- and upper-class ladies who paid their own tuition and the still carefully selected poor women who were subsidized by the Nightingale Fund. The first were given an extra year or two of education to prepare them to become teachers or superintendents; a third choice was district nursing. "This nurse must be of a yet higher class and of a yet fuller training than a hospital nurse, because she has not the doctor always at hand and because she has no hospital appliances at hand."[10] The special probationers were expected to enter the profession permanently. The second group were prepared to be hospital ward nurses.

In Nightingale's later years, she came into conflict with the very nurses who had been trained for leadership. In 1886, some of these nurses, now superintendents of other training schools, wanted to establish an organization that would provide a central examination and registration center, the forerunner of licensure. Nightingale opposed this movement for several reasons: nursing was still too young and disorganized; national criteria would not be as high as those of individual schools; and the all-important aspect of character could not be tested. She fought the concept with every weapon at her disposal, including her powerful contacts, and succeeded in limiting the fledgling Royal British Nurses' Association to maintaining a "list" instead of a "register."

Nightingale's prolific writings on nursing have survived, and some of them are still surprisingly apt. Often they reflected her concern about the character of nurses and her own determination that their main focus be on nursing. One principle from which Nightingale did not swerve was that nurses were to nurse, not to do heavy cleaning ("if you want a charwoman, hire one"); not to do laundry ("it makes their hands coarse and hard and less able to attend to the delicate manipulation which they may be called on to execute"); and not to fetch ("to save the time of nurses; all diets and ward requisites should be brought into the wards"). Then, as in many places now, status and promotion came through assumption of administrative roles, but Nightingale recognized that "many are valuable as nurses, who are yet unfit for promotion to head nurses." Her alternative, however, would not be greeted favorably today—a raise after 10 years of good service!

Nightingale also commented on other issues considered pertinent today. Continuing education was a must, for she saw nursing as a progressive art, in which to stand still was to go back. "A woman who thinks of herself, 'Now I am a full nurse, a skilled nurse. I have learnt all there is to be learned,' take my word for it, she does not know what a nurse is, and she will never know: she has gone back already."[11] Although there is no evidence that she took any action to help end discrimination against women, Nightingale believed that women should be accepted into all the professions, but she warned them, "qualify yourselves for it as a man does for his work." She believed that women should be paid as highly as men, but that equal pay meant equal responsibility. In a profession with as much responsibility as nursing, she said, it was particularly important to have adequate compensation, or intelligent, independent women would not be attracted to it.

Until the end of her life, she was firm on the need for nurses to obey physicians in medical matters. However, she stressed the importance of nurse observation and reporting because the physician was not constantly at the patient's bedside, as the nurse was. She was adamant that a nurse (and woman) be in charge of nursing, with no other administrative figure having authority over nurses, including physicians. She knew the importance of a work setting that gave job satisfaction. In words that are a far-off echo of nurses' complaints today, she wrote:

Besides, a thing very little understood, a good nurse has her professional pride in results of her Nursing quite as much as a Medical Officer in the results of his treatment. There are defective buildings, defective administrations, defective appliances, which make all good Nursing impossible. A good Nurse does not like to waste herself, and the better the Nurse, the stronger this feeling in her.[12]

Planner, administrator, educator, researcher, reformer, Florence Nightingale never lost her interest in nursing. At age 74, in her last major publication on nursing, she differentiated between sick nursing and health nursing, and emphasized the primary need for prevention of illness, for which a lay "Health Missioner" (today's health educator?) would be trained.

When Nightingale died on August 13, 1910, she was to be honored by burial in Westminster Abbey. However, she had chosen instead to be buried in the family plot in Hampshire, with a simple inscription: "F.N. Born 1820, Died 1910."

KEY POINTS

1. A certain amount of the ritualistic mystique and belief in spirits or gods pervaded care of the sick in early civilizations.

2. Records of early civilizations emphasize treatment given by those designated as physicians, but there appear to have been men and women fulfilling nursing roles of some sort.

3. In early Egypt, India, China, Greece, and Rome, as well as in the lands of the Hebrews, setting rules of hygiene and sanitation, using herbs, and performing surgery were part of the care of the sick.

4. The Romans are generally credited with building the first hospitals, but in the Christian period, "houses for the sick" were available for the sick poor, often tended by men or women in religious and secular orders.

5. In 1860, Florence Nightingale founded modern nursing at St. Thomas's Hospital in London with organized training programs that included both theory and practice, careful selection of students, and freedom from hospital control.

6. In her careful observations and recording and her use of statistics in matters affecting health care and administration in the British army, in hospitals throughout Europe, and in the community, Nightingale is often credited with being the first nurse researcher.

7. Nightingale made many pertinent observations and recommendations on nurses and nursing practice, such as the need for nurses to be free from other duties so that they could concentrate on nursing, as well as

the need for holistic care, for home care, for continuing education, for adequate compensation, and for a satisfactory working environment.

REFERENCES

1. Bullough B, Bullough V. *The care of the sick: The emergence of modern nursing*. New York: Prodist, 1978, p. 69.
2. Moore J. *A zeal for responsibility: The struggle for professional nursing in Victorian England, 1868–1883*. Athens, GA: The University of Georgia Press, 1983, p. 3.
3. Barritt ER. Florence Nightingale's values and modern nursing education. *Nurs Forum,* 12(4):7–47 (1973).
4. Bullough and Bullough, op. cit., p. 86.
5. Seymer LR. *Selected writings of Florence Nightingale*. New York: Macmillan Publishing Company, 1954, p. 28.
6. Barritt, op. cit., p. 8.
7. Seymer, op. cit., pp. 222–223.
8. Ibid., p. 244.
9. Ibid., p. 234.
10. Ibid., p. 316.
11. Pavey AE. *The story of the growth of nursing*. London: Farber and Farber, 1938, p. 296.
12. Seymer, op. cit., p. 276.

CHAPTER 2

NURSING IN THE UNITED STATES

AMERICAN REVOLUTION TO NURSING REVOLUTION

OBJECTIVES

After studying this chapter, you will be able to:

1. Explain how early nursing schools in the United States were established and functioned.
2. Name at least five early nursing leaders and their contributions to nursing.
3. Identify factors that influenced major changes in the education of nurses in the period between 1900 and 1965.
4. Describe how major changes in the practice of nursing in the period between 1900 and 1965 were influenced.
5. Identify the key findings of major studies and reports about nursing before 1965.

The first 100 years of American nursing show an interesting pattern. At the close of the nineteenth century and the dawn of the twentieth, there was rapid establishment and expansion of the new training schools for nurses. Many exciting developments that included breakthroughs unheard of for a woman's occupation occurred just as rapidly, thanks to the intelligence, initiative, and risk taking of an extraordinary group of women. Then for most of the next 50 years, progress seemed slow, with a patient chipping away at the many obstacles to quality education and practice. However, after World War II, another rapid series of changes moved nursing into a new era, a revolution that created both opportunities and risks for the emerging profession.

THE VOLUNTEERS

Just as the Crimean War spotlighted the activities of Florence Nightingale and the importance of nursing, the Civil War was an impetus for the development of training programs for nursing in the United States. There had never been an organized system for the care of the sick and wounded in wartime. During the American Revolution, some basic care was given by camp followers, wives, women in the neighborhood and "surgeon's mates" who may have been employed by the army.[1]

When the Civil War began in 1861, untrained women quickly volunteered to become nurses. Dorothea Dix, well known by then, was appointed by the Secretary of War to supervise these new "nurses." Meanwhile, members of religious orders also volunteered, and nursing in some of the larger

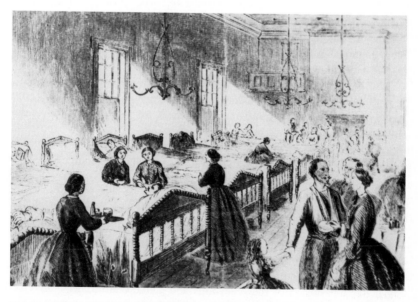

Nurses at the U.S. General Hospital in Georgetown. Most of the nurses were volunteers without any nursing training.

government hospitals was eventually assigned to them because of the in-
experience of the lay volunteers.

Except for that group, almost none of the thousands of Northern women
who served as nurses during the war had any kind of training or hospital
experience. They can be categorized as follows:

1. The nurses appointed by Miss Dix or other officials as legal employees
    of the army for 40 cents and one ration a day.
2. The sisters or nuns of the various orders.
3. Those employed for short periods of time for menial chores.
4. Black women employed under general orders of the War Department
    for $10 a month.
5. Uncompensated volunteers.
6. Women camp followers.
7. Women employed by the various relief organizations.[2]

Because of the prejudice against the idea of Southern women as nurses in
the terrible conditions in Confederate hospitals, only about 1,000 served,
mostly as volunteers. As in the North, many nuns did the nursing.

Some of the information on what the Civil War nurses did comes from
the diaries of Northern and Southern women and the writings of Louisa May
Alcott and Walt Whitman, both Northern volunteers. In her journal, Alcott
described her working day, which began at six. After opening the windows,
because of the bad air in the makeshift base hospital, she spent her time
"giving out rations, cutting up food for helpless boys, washing faces, teaching my attendants how beds are made or floors are swept, dressing wounds,
dusting tables, sewing bandages, keeping my tray tidy, rushing up and down
after pillows, bed linens, sponges, and directions. . . . "[3] Volunteers also
read to the patients, wrote letters, and comforted them. Apparently, even
the hired nurses did little more except, perhaps, give medicines. But so did
the volunteers, sometimes giving the medicine and food of their choice to
the patient, instead of what the doctor ordered. However, many of these
women were very strong, and were outspoken about incompetence and
corruption; sometimes one carried her complaints to the Secretary of War
and got action.

By 1862, enormous military hospitals, some with as many as 3,000 beds,
were being built, although there were still some makeshift hospitals—former
hotels, churches, factories, and almost anything else available. Floating
hospitals were also inaugurated and served as transport units, with nurses
attending the wounded. According to one army hospital edict, the nurses,
under the supervision of the "Stewards and Chief Wardmaster," were responsible for the administration of the wards, but many of their duties
appeared to be related more to keeping the nonmedical records of patients

and reporting their misbehavior than to nursing care. If the patient needed medical or surgical attendance, the doctor was to be called.

Georgeanna Woolsey wrote that the often incompetent contract surgeons treated the nurses without even common courtesy because they did not want them and tried to make their lives so unbearable that they would leave. The formidable nurse Mary Ann (Mother) Bickerdyke attacked the surgeons and officers who were drunk, refused to attend the wounded, or injured them further because of their incompetence. She managed to have a number of them dismissed (in part because of her friendship with General Grant and General Sherman). Another fighter was Clara Barton. One story told about her is that while supervising the delivery of a wagonload of supplies for soldiers, she neatly removed an ox from a herd intended for the Union Army, so that some starving Confederate wounded would have food.[4]

Only in recent years has attention been given to the black nurses of the Civil War or before. (Actually, a black Jamaican woman also volunteered in the Crimean War.) Harriet Tubman, the "Moses of her people," not only led many black slaves to freedom in her underground railroad activities before the war but also nursed the wounded when she joined the Union army. Similarly, Sojourner Truth, abolitionist speaker and activist in the women's movement, also cared for the sick and wounded. Susie King Taylor, born to slavery and secretly taught to read and write, met and married a Union soldier and served as a battlefront nurse for more than four years, although she received no salary or pension from the Union army.[5]

There were other heroines, untrained women from the North and South, caring for the sick and wounded with few skills but much kindness, and, as in the Crimea, the soldiers were sentimentally appreciative, if not discriminating. On the other hand, given the circumstances, what they accomplished was amazing.[6]

Even when paid, Civil War nurses had little status and no rank. An investigative report by the United States Sanitary Commission noted that nurses had not been well treated or wisely used. Nevertheless, the Civil War opened hospitals to massive numbers of women, well-bred "ladies," who would otherwise probably not even have thought of nursing. Some of these, such as Abby, Jane, and Georgeanna Woolsey, later helped lead the movement to establish training schools for nurses.

NURSING EDUCATION: THE FIRST 60 YEARS

The nursing role of women in the Civil War, however unsophisticated, and the fame of Florence Nightingale brought to the attention of the American public the need for nurses and the desirability of some organized programs of training.

More physicians became interested in the training of nurses and, at a meeting of the American Medical Association (AMA) in 1869, a committee to study the matter stated that it was "just as necessary to have well-trained, well-instructed nurses as to have intelligent and skillful physicians." The committee recommended that nursing schools be placed under the guardianship of county medical societies, although under the immediate supervision of lady superintendents; that every lay hospital should have a school; and that nurses should be trained not only for the hospital but for private duty in the home.[7]

Although a number of training programs for nurses and midwives existed before the Civil War, what is considered the first American school to offer a graded course in scientific nursing, based on guidelines set by Florence Nightingale, began in 1872 at the New England Hospital for Women and Children. Women physicians gave the twelve lectures that comprised the formal education of the 12-month course. The students who received a small allowance after three months worked from 5:30 A.M. to 9:00 P.M. and slept in rooms near the ward so that they were available when needed. One of the first graduates was Melinda Ann (Linda) Richards, thereafter called America's first trained nurse (probably because, of all of the nurses who graduated from this primitive early program, she moved on to be a key figure in the development of nursing education). Richards, like some of the other students in the schools that evolved, had already been a nurse in a hospital. Some schools would not accept these students because they wanted to set a new image. Another outstanding graduate of the New England Hospital for Women and Children (1879) was Mary Mahoney, the first trained black nurse.

In 1873, three schools were established that were supposedly based on the Nightingale model. The Bellevue Training School in New York City was founded through the influence of several society ladies who had been involved in Civil War nursing, including Abby Woolsey. Although the school attempted to follow Nightingale principles and reported that it was attracting educated women, its overall purpose was to improve conditions in a great charity hospital, and much of the learning occurred on a trial-and-error basis. Nevertheless, Bellevue had a lot of interesting firsts: interdisciplinary rounds where nurses reported on the nursing plan of care; patient record keeping and writing of orders, initiated by Linda Richards, who became night superintendent; and the first uniform, by stylish and aristocratic Euphemia Van Rensselaer, which started a trend.

The Connecticut Training School was started through the influence of another Woolsey, Georgeanna, and her husband, Dr. Francis Bacon. Through negotiation with the hospital, the superintendent of nurses was designated as separate from, and not responsible to, the steward (administrator) of the hospital, and teaching outside the wards was permitted. Good intentions notwithstanding, the students soon were sent to give care in the homes of sick families, with the money going to the School Fund—and the school could boast that for 33 years it was not financed or directed by the hospital.

The Boston Training School was the last of that first famous trio. Again, a group of women associated with other educational and philanthropic endeavors spearheaded its organization, but this time their goal was to offer a desirable occupation for self-supporting women and to provide good private nurses for the community. After prolonged negotiations that allowed the director of the school rather than the hospital to maintain control, the Massachusetts General Hospital assigned "The Brick" building to the school because it (The Brick) "stands by itself; represents both medical and surgical departments; and offers the hard labor desirable for the training of nurses."[8] Apparently, there was rather poor leadership, and nurses continued to do menial tasks, with little attention given to training. When Linda Richards became the third director, she reorganized the work, started classes, and set out to prove that trained nurses were better than untrained ones.

Other major training schools that were to endure into the next century were founded in the next few years, somewhat patterned after Nightingale's precepts. Their success and the popularity of their graduates resulted in a massive proliferation of training schools. In 1880, there were 15; by 1900, 432; by 1909, 1105 hospital-based diploma schools. Hospitals with as few as 20 beds opened schools, and the students provided almost totally free labor. Usually the only graduate nurses were the superintendent and perhaps the operating room supervisor and night supervisor. Students earned money for the hospital, for after a short period they were frequently sent to do private nursing in the home, with the money reverting to the hospital, not the school. Except for the few outstanding schools, all Nightingale principles were forgotten: the students were under the control of the hospital and worked from 12 to 15 hours a day—24 if they were on a private case in a home. Lessons, if any, were scheduled for an hour late in the evening when someone was available to teach. (It wasn't necessary for all students to be available.) Moreover, if the "pupils" lost time because of sickness, which was almost always contracted from patients or caused by sheer overwork, the time had to be totally made up before they could graduate.

Why then did training schools draw so many applicants? Because the occupational opportunities for untrained women were limited to domestic service, factory work, retail clerking, or prostitution. Higher education for women was limited to typewriting or teaching, but these were seldom taught in universities. Those colleges and universities that did admit women rarely prepared them for professions. Even with the strict discipline, hard work, long hours, and almost no time off, after a year or two of training (the second year consisting of unabashedly free labor to the hospitals), the trained nurse could do private duty at a salary ranging from $10 a week to the vague possibility of $20 (if she could collect it), a far cry from the $4 to $6 average of other women workers. Of course, on these cases, she was a 24-hour servant to the family and patient, lucky to have time off for a walk. And because there were necessarily months with no employment, even an excellent nurse was lucky to gross $600 a year.[9]

The more famous hospital schools, in particular, had hundreds and even thousands of applicants a year. On the other hand, there were a multitude of hospitals and sanitoriums of all kinds that were looking for students to meet their staffing needs, and for these, high-quality applicants were frequently lacking. Consequently, application standards were lowered rapidly. Apparently, most schools admitted a class of 30 to 35[10] (in some cases determined by their staffing and financial needs). Attrition, caused in part by the extremely high rate of student illness and the unpleasant working and living conditions, was often 75 percent.

Student admission requirements varied, but all nurse applicants were female. Some hospitals accepted men in programs but gave them only a short course and frequently called them *attendants*. In 1888, at Bellevue Hospital, the Mills School was established with a two-year course, but for a long time its graduates were also called *attendants*. Other schools admitting men followed. Blacks were also generally silently excluded. Over the years, training schools for black nurses were founded, the first organized in 1891 at the Provident Hospital in Chicago.

The minimum age for all students was generally 21 years. Eight or fewer years of schooling were common, but usually good health and good character were absolute prerequisites. Obedience in training was essential, and a student could be dismissed as a troublemaker if the overworked girl grumbled, talked too much, was too familiar with men, criticized head nurses or doctors, or could not get along wherever placed. Married women and those over 30 were frequently excluded because they could not "fall in with the life successfully." And, of course, if they were divorced, they were totally unacceptable.

In the 1890s, only 12 percent of nurse training was theory, consisting of some anatomy and physiology, materia medica, perhaps some chemistry, bacteriology, hygiene, and lectures on certain diseases. The leading schools developed their own institutional manuals, but a few pioneering texts were also written by nurses before 1900.[11]

Even into the twentieth century, students continued to live a slavelike existence, without outward complaint, and were poorly housed, overworked, underfed ("rations of a kind and quality only a remove better than what we might place before a beggar," said a popular journal), and unprotected from life-threatening illness (80 percent of the students in the average hospital graduated with positive tuberculin tests). If they survived all this, it was no wonder that they were expected to graduate as "respectful, obedient, cheerful, submissive, hard-working, loyal, pacific, and religious."[12] It was not professional education; it was not even a respectably run apprenticeship, because learning was not derived from skilled masters, but rather from their own peers, who were but a step ahead of them.

These principles of sacrifice, service, obedience to the physician, and ethical orientation are embodied in the Nightingale Pledge, written in 1893 by Lystra E. Gretter, superintendent of the school at Harper Hospital in Detroit, a pledge still frequently recited by students today.

> I solemnly pledge myself before God and in the presence of this assembly;
>
> To pass my life in purity and to practice my profession faithfully;
>
> I will abstain from whatever is deleterious and mischievous and will not take or knowingly administer any harmful drug; I will do all in my power to maintain and elevate the standard of my profession, and will hold in confidence all personal matters committed to my keeping and all family affairs coming to my knowledge in the practice of my calling;
>
> With loyalty will I endeavor to aid the physician in his work, and devote myself to the welfare of those committed to my care.[13]

Although the passage of the first licensure laws in 1903 (discussed later) set standards for nursing education, there was little improvement. The laws were not mandatory. Most training schools remained under the control of hospitals, and the needs of the hospital took priority over those of the school. For instance, it was not until 1912 that an occasional nurse received time from hospital responsibilities in order to organize and teach basic nursing, and superintendents were warned not to "neglect" patient care in favor of the school or they would face punishment. The hours were still long, and the students continued to give free service, with "book learning" as an afterthought. Only in California, where an Eight-Hour Law for Women was passed in 1911, was there any movement to include student nurses (not even graduate nurses). Yet, when the bill was introduced in 1913, it was fought bitterly not only by hospitals, as might be expected, but also by physicians and nurses.[14]

While the Flexner Report of 1910 was bringing about reform in medical schools, eliminating the correspondence courses and the weaker and poorer schools, Adelaide Nutting and other leaders were agitating for reform in nursing education. In 1911, the American Society of Superintendents of Training Schools for Nurses presented a proposal for a similar survey of nursing schools to the Carnegie Foundation. Ignoring nursing, the foundation directed a considerable amount of its funds to such studies in dental, legal, and teacher education.

Although women were having a little more success in being accepted in colleges and universities, there was only limited movement to make basic nursing programs an option in academic settings. The University of Minnesota program, founded in 1909 by Dr. Richard Olding Beard, a physician who was dedicated to the concept of higher education for nurses, became the first enduring baccalaureate program in nursing. Even this was more similar to good diploma programs than to other university programs. Although eventually the students had to meet university admission standards and took some specialized courses, they also worked a 56-hour week in the hospital and were awarded a diploma instead of a degree after three years. Similar programs were started by other universities that took over hospitals or started new ones, in part to obtain student services for their hospitals. Just before World War I, several hospitals and universities, such as Presbyterian Hospital of New York and Teachers College, Columbia University, offered degree options. These developed into five-year programs with two years of college work and three years in a diploma school. This became a common pattern that lasted throughout the 1940s.

One of the more daring experiments of the times was the Vassar Training Camp. In the summer of 1918 a preparatory course in nursing was established at Vassar from which the students would move to selected schools of nursing to complete the program in little more than two additional years. A large percentage of the women completed the program and entered the nursing

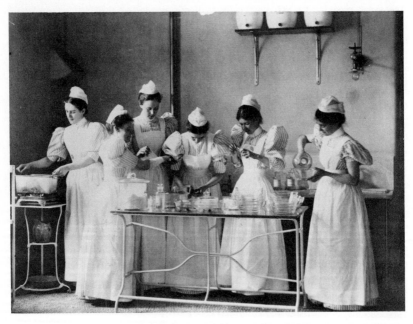

Nursing students, Class of 1897, in a treatment room in the early days of the Presbyterian Hospital Training School for Nurses, which became the Columbia University School of Nursing. (*Courtesy of Columbia University School of Nursing.*)

schools they had selected. Many of nursing's leaders arose from this group. Because this and similar programs were generally of considerably higher quality than those of the training schools, the movement of nursing education toward an academic setting received another nudge.

By the end of World War I, nursing had serious problems. There was a shortage of nurses, because many who had switched careers "for the duration" returned to their own field, and others appeared not to be attracted. In part, it was an image problem, one that was to continue to haunt nursing, but another important factor was that nursing education was in trouble. As Isabel Stewart said, "The plain facts are that nursing schools are being starved and always have been starved for lack of funds to build up any kind of substantial educational structure."[15] Later, this problem was clearly pinpointed by prestigious study committees (see Appendix 1).

In 1918, Adelaide Nutting had approached the Rockefeller Foundation to seek endowment for the Johns Hopkins School of Nursing, stressing the need for improvement in the education of public health nurses. The meeting resulted in a committee to investigate the "proper training" of public health nurses, an investigation that quickly concluded that the problem was nursing education in general. The finding of the 1923 Goldmark Report concluded that schools of nursing needed to be recognized and supported as separate educational components with not just training in nursing, but also a liberal education. Moreover, "Superintendents, supervisors, instructors, and public health nurses should in all cases receive special additional training beyond the basic nursing course."[16]

Although the report had little immediate impact, it did result in Rockefeller Foundation support for the founding of the Yale School of Nursing (1924), the first in the world to be established as a separate university department with its own dean, Annie Goodrich. Although a few other such programs followed, progress lagged, for many powerful physicians reached the public media with their notions that nurses needed only technical skills, manual dexterity, and quick obedience to the physician. Charles Mayo, for instance, deciding that city-trained nurses were too difficult to handle, too expensive, and spent too much time getting educated, wanted to recruit 100,000 country girls.[17]

This attitude was not new. Almost from the beginning, there were physicians who objected to so much education for nurses and devoted considerable medical journal space to raging about the "overtrained nurse." One physician even suggested a correspondence course for training nurses to care for the "poor folks," and a New York newspaper editorial proclaimed, "What we want in nurses is less theory and more practice."[18] But then, this was at a time when a leading Harvard physician insisted that serious mental exercise would damage a woman's brain or cause other severe trauma, such as the narrowing of the pelvic area, which would make her unable to deliver children.[19]

However, there was also farsighted physicians who supported not "teaching a trade, but preparing for a profession," as Dr. Richard Cabot noted in 1901. But even popular journals recognized that student nurses were being exploited by hospitals and that the kind of student being encouraged into nursing by school principals was one seen as not too bright, not attractive enough to marry, and too poor to be supported at home.

A study following close on the heels of the Goldmark Report soon reaffirmed the inadequacy of nursing schools and practicing nurses. *Nurses, Patients, and Pocketbooks*[20] pointed out that the hasty postwar nurse-recruiting efforts had not improved the lot of the patient or the nurse. In 1928, problems included an oversupply of nurses, geographic maldistribution, low educational standards, poor working conditions, and some critically unsatisfactory levels of care.

NURSING'S EARLY LEADERS

In many ways, early nursing education and nursing leaders were intertwined. After graduating from one of the better training programs, these nurses often assumed dual positions as both superintendent of nursing in hospitals and superintendent of the training school. Since students provided almost all of the nursing service, with the exception of a few supervisors, the training school received much of the leaders' attention. They took the responsibility seriously. They were concerned with the quality of the students and the program, and much of what they did was directed at improving nursing education. In a male-dominated society, working in what was barely becoming an accepted, respectable occupation, these unusual women were not only talented but were also determined risk takers.

Before the new century was far along, they were responsible for setting nursing standards, improving curricula, writing textbooks, starting two enduring professional organizations and a nursing journal, inaugurating a teacher training program in a university, and initiating nursing licensure. They were a mixed group, but with certain commonalities: usually unmarried but, except for Lavinia Dock, not feminist. Almost all were involved in the early nursing organizations. Fortunately, most were also great letter writers and letter savers as well as authors, so that there are many fascinating insights into their lives. (See, in particular, the Christy series in *Nursing Outlook,* mentioned in the Bibliography.) Some highlights follow.

America's first trained nurse, Linda Richards, had a continuing impact on the training schools because she spent much of her career moving from hospital to hospital in what seems to have been an improvement campaign. In those earliest days, almost any graduate was considered a prime candidate for starting another program. Some undoubtedly lacked the intellectual and leadership qualities needed, so that the new schools, if not actual disasters, were frequently of poor quality. Linda Richards apparently had the skill and authority to upgrade both the school and the nursing service, which were, after all, almost inseparable. However, she seemed willing to accept school management that tied the economics of the hospital to student education, usually to the detriment of the latter.

One of the most noted nursing figures was Isabelle Hampton, who left teaching to enter Bellevue Training School in 1881. Not only was she attractive and charming, but she was "in every sense of the word a leader, by nature, by capacity, by personal attributes and qualities, by choice, and probably to some extent by inheritance and training; a follower she never was."[21] In her two major superintendencies, she made a number of then radical changes—cutting down the students' workday to 10 hours and eliminating their free private duty services. For the Johns Hopkins program, which she founded, she recruited feisty Lavinia Dock, who was still at Bellevue, to be her assistant. They must have made an interesting pair, for Lavinia, also a "lady," was outspoken and frequently tactless, particularly with physicians.

Adelaide Nutting graduated in that first Hopkins class, and the three became friends.[22] Nutting followed Hampton as principal of the school when in 1894 Isabel married one of her admirers, Dr. Hunter Robb, and, as was the custom, retired from active nursing. (Letters of the time reveal the anger, dismay, and even sadness of her colleagues at her marriage. They were sure Dr. Robb was not nearly good enough for her; besides, she was betraying nursing by robbing the profession of her talents.) Nevertheless, Isabel Hampton Robb maintained her interest in nursing and continued to be active in the development of the profession. In 1893, she had been appointed chairman of a committee to arrange a congress of nurses under the auspices of the International Congress of Charities, Correction, and Philanthropy at the World's Fair (Columbian Exposition) in Chicago. There, before an international audience of nurses, she voiced her concern about poor nursing education and stated that the term *trained nurse* meant "anything, everything, or next to nothing" in the absence of educational standards. At the same time, Lavinia Dock pointed out that the teaching, training, and discipline of nurses should not be provided at the discretion of doctors. Similar themes were repeated in other papers, as well as the notion that there ought to be an organization of nurses. Shortly after the Congress, 18 superintendents organized the American Society of Superintendents of Training School for Nursing, which was to become the National League of Nursing Education, (NLNE) in 1912. Its purpose was to promote the fellowship of members, establish and maintain a universal standard of training, and further the best interests of the nursing profession. The first convention of the society elected Linda Richards president.[23]

Another attendee at those early meetings was Sophia Palmer, descendant of John and Priscilla Alden and a graduate of the Boston Training School, who, after a variety of experiences, organized a training school in Washington, D.C., over the concerted opposition of local physicians who wanted to control nursing education. She approved the actions that were taken by her colleagues but was impatient with what seemed to be the blind acceptance of hospital control of schools. "She had a very intense nature and, like all those who are born crusaders, had little patience with the slower methods of persuasion. . . . She was like a spirited racehorse held by the reins of tradition."[24]

Within a short time, Palmer and some of the others in the Society, including Dock and Isabel Hampton Robb, recognized the need for another organization for all nurses. Although some of the training schools had alumnae associations, they were restrictive; in some cases, their own graduates could not be members, and any "outsider" could not participate. Therefore, if a nurse left the immediate vicinity of her own school, there was no way in which she had any organized contact with other nurses. In a paper given in 1895, Palmer stressed that the power of the nursing profession depended on its ability to organize individuals who could influence public opinion. Dock also made recommendations for a national organization. In 1896, delegates representing the oldest training school alumnae associations and members of an organizing committee of the Society selected a name for the proposed organization: Nurses' Associated Alumnae of the United States and Canada (which became the American Nurses' Association in 1911). They also set a time and place for the first meeting (February 1897 in Baltimore) and drafted a constitution. At the end of that February meeting, held in conjunction with the fourth annual Society convention, the constitution and by-laws were adopted, and Isabel Hampton Robb was elected president. Among the problems discussed at those early meetings were nursing licensure and the creation of an official nursing publication.

There were a number of nursing journals: the *British Journal of Nursing,* established by one of England's nursing leaders, Ethel Gordon Fenwick; and, in the United States, the short-lived *The Nightingale,* started by a Bellevue graduate; *The Nursing Record* and *The Nursing World,* also short-lived; and *The Trained Nurse and Hospital Review,* which Palmer edited for a time and which continued for 70 years. But the leaders of the new organizations wanted a magazine that would promote nursing, owned and controlled by nursing.

For several years there was discussion, but no action, until another committee on the ways and means of producing a magazine was formed. In January 1900, they organized a stock company and sold $100 shares only to nurses and nurses' alumnae associations. By May, they had a promise of $2400 in shares, and almost 500 nurses had promised to subscribe. Admittedly, they had overstepped their mandate, they reported to the third annual convention of the Nurses' Associated Alumnae, but they were given approval to establish the magazine along the lines formulated. The J. B. Lippincott Company was selected as publisher, and Sophia Palmer became editor, which she did on an unpaid basis for the first nine months. (She had become director of the Rochester City Hospital in New York.) As the first issues went for mailing in October, it was discovered that the post office rules prevented its being mailed because the journal's stockholders were not incorporated. M. E. P. Davis and Sophia Palmer assumed personal responsibility for all liabilities of the new *American Journal of Nursing,* and it went out. The *Journal* was considered the official organ of the nursing profession, but the stock was still held by alumnae associations and individual nurses. It was Lavinia Dock who donated the first share of stock to the association, and by 1912 the renamed American Nurses' Association (ANA) had gained ownership of all the stock of the American Journal of Nursing Company, which it still retains.[25]

One other major organization, the American Red Cross, was established by a nurse, Clara Barton, the schoolteacher who had volunteered as a nurse and directed relief operations during the Civil War and served with the German Red Cross during the Franco-Prussian War in 1870. (The establishment of the International Red Cross as a permanent international relief agency that could take immediate action in time of war had occurred in Geneva in 1864 with the signing of the Geneva Convention guidelines). After her return to the United States, Barton organized the American Red Cross and persuaded Congress in 1882 to ratify the Treaty of Geneva so that the Red Cross could carry on its humanitarian efforts in peacetime. Clara Barton, however, was not an active part of the nursing leadership that was molding the profession.[26]

That group had another immediate aim. The Society recognized that the nurses were at a disadvantage because they had no postgraduate training in administration or teaching, so a committee consisting of Robb, Nutting, Richards, Mary Agnes Snively, and Lucy Drown was formed to investigate the possibilities. At the sixth Society convention, they reported their success. James Russell, the farsighted dean of Teachers College, Columbia University, in New York, had agreed to start a course for nurses if they could guarantee the enrollment of 12 nurses, or $1000 a year. The Society agreed. Members of the Society screened the candidates, contributed $1000 a year, and taught the course—hospital economics. Later, the students were also allowed to enroll in psychology, science, household economics, and biology. Anna Alline, one of the two graduates of the first class, then took over the total administration of the course.

There was one more major goal to be reached: licensure of nurses. Not only did the hundreds of hospital-based schools vary greatly in quality, but the market was also flooded with "nurses" who had been dismissed from schools without graduating, "nurses" from six-week private and correspondence courses, and a vast number of those who simply called themselves nurses. It was inevitable that people became confused, for when they hired nurses for private duty in their homes, the "nurse" could present one of the elaborate diplomas from a $13 correspondence course that guaranteed that anyone could become a nurse, a real or forged reference, or a genuine diploma from a top-quality school. How could they judge? Therefore, because of the dreadful care given by individuals representing themselves as nurses, the public was once more disenchanted with nurses. Nursing's leaders were determined that there must be legal regulation, both to protect the public from unscrupulous and incompetent nurses and to protect the young profession by establishing a minimum level of competence, limiting all or some of the professional functions to those who qualified. Medicine already had licensing in some states, and many aspiring professions were also moving in that direction.

In September 1901, at the first meeting of the newly formed International Council of Nurses, which was held in Buffalo, a resolution was passed, stating that "it is the duty of the nursing profession of every country to work for suitable legislative enactment regulating the education of nurses and protecting the interests of the public, by securing State examinations and public registration, with the proper penalities for enforcing the same."[27]

Despite considerable opposition to nurse licensure from untrained nurses, managers, and proprietors of poor training programs, and some physicians, licensure was achieved and basic educational standards were set. In 1903, North Carolina, New Jersey, Virginia, and New York passed laws. However, New York's law was the strongest. For instance, New Jersey's law omitted a board of any kind; North Carolina had a mixed board of nurses and doctors and allowed a nurse to be licensed without attending a training school if vouched for by a doctor. It should be remembered, though, that all nurse licensure laws in those times were permissive, not mandatory. That is, only the registered nurse (RN) title was protected. Untrained nurses could continue to work as nurses as long as they did not call themselves RNs.

One of the key figures in community health nursing was Lillian Wald. After graduating from the New York Hospital School of Nursing and working a short time, she decided to enter the Women's Medical College. When she and another nurse, Mary Brewster, were sent to the Lower East Side to lecture to immigrant mothers on the care of the sick, they were shocked at what they saw; neither had known that such abject poverty could exist. Wald left medical school, moved with Mary Brewster to a top-floor tenement on Jefferson Street, and began to offer nursing care to the poor. After a short while, the calls came by the hundreds from families, hospitals, and physicians. People were cared for, whether or not they could afford to pay. The concern of these nurses was not just giving nursing care but seeing what other services could be made available to meet the many social needs of the poor.

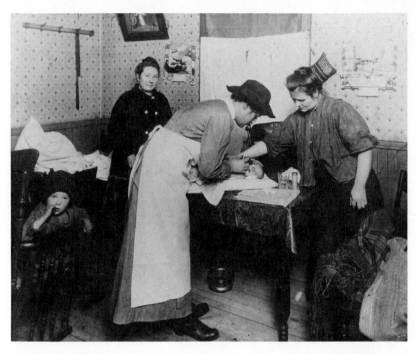

The visiting nurses from Henry Street cared for many poor families, often immigrants in New York City. (*Courtesy of the Visiting Nurse Service of New York.*)

After two years of such success, larger facilities, more nurses, and social workers were needed. In 1895, Wald, Brewster, Lavinia Dock, and other nurses moved to what was eventually called the Henry Street Settlement, a house bought by philanthropist Jacob H. Schiff. By 1909, the Henry Street staff had 37 nurses, all but 5 providing direct nursing service. Each nurse was carefully oriented to the customs of the immigrants she served and was able to demonstrate the value of understanding the family and the environment in giving good nursing care. Each nurse kept two sets of records, one for the physician and another recording the major points of the nurse's work. School nursing was also started by Lillian Wald, who suggested that placing nurses in schools might help solve the problem of the schools having to send home so many ill children.[28]

Another outstanding public health nurse was Margaret Higgins Sanger. She became interested in the plight of the poorly paid industrial workers, particularly the women. She herself was married and had three children when she decided to return to work in public health. She was assigned to maternity cases on the Lower East Side of New York, where she found that pregnancy, often unwanted, was a chronic condition. In 1912, one of her

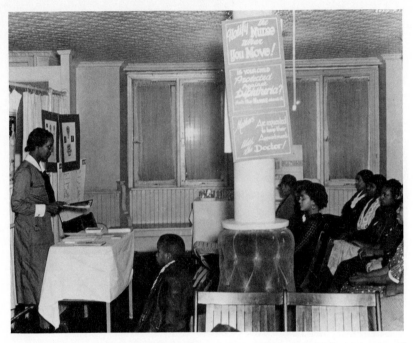

Visiting nurses taught families how to stay as healthy as possible (*Courtesy of the Visiting Nurse Service of New York.*)

patients died from a repeated self-abortion after begging doctors and nurses for information on how to avoid pregnancy. That was apparently a turning point for Sanger. After learning everything she could about contraception, she and her sister, also a nurse, opened the first birth control clinic in America in Brooklyn. She was arrested and spent 30 days in the workhouse but continued her crusade. She fought the battle for free dissemination of birth control information for decades, against all types of opposition, until today, birth control education is generally accepted as the right of women and as one nursing role.[29]

In the 23 years between World Wars I and II, nursing was affected by the Great Depression and by adoption of the Nineteenth Amendment to the Constitution in August 1920, granting women the right to vote. Of the two, the latter had less immediate impact. Nurses showed relatively little interest in fighting for women's rights, and only one, Lavinia Dock, can be called an active feminist. "Dockie" was a maverick of the times. A tiny woman who loved music and was an accomplished pianist and organist, she also seemed to take on the whole world in her battle for the underdog. Early on, she decided that nurses could have no power unless they had the vote. Her speeches and writings were brilliant, but she did not move her colleagues. Nevertheless, she devoted a good part of her life to working for women's rights. In England, she joined the Pankhursts and landed in jail. Back in the United States, she picketed the White House. Her colleague, Isabel Stewart, wrote, "They all went into the cooler for the night. I think it just pleased her no end."[30]

For all her devotion to women's rights, Dock remained committed to nursing. She was editor of the *Journal*'s Foreign Department from 1900 to 1923, during which she quarreled regularly with editor Sophia Palmer and managed to ignore World War I because she was a pacifist. She was also involved with the International Council of Nurses and was the author of a number of books, including *Health and Morality,* published in 1910, in which she discussed venereal disease. She was equally outspoken on this forbidden subject in open meetings. A number of nurses had become infected because physicians frequently refused to tell nurses when patients had the disease. Dock also regularly criticized her profession for withholding its interest, sympathy, and moral support from "the great, urgent throbbing, pressing social claims of our day and generation."[31]

There were other nurses who put their mark on nursing in its first 60 years. Anne Goodrich reported on the poor nursing conditions in military camps during World War I, which resulted in the establishment of the Army School of Nursing. She became its first dean, and the high quality of the educational program, with only six to eight duty hours (unlike civilian hospitals), made it an overwhelming success. Isabel Stewart, who succeeded Adelaide Nutting (the first nurse ever to receive a professorship at Columbia University), in her 39 years at Teachers College set up a respected graduate program. Mary Breckenridge founded the Frontier Nursing Service in 1925; its staff was a mixture of British and British-trained American midwives.[32] And in 1922, six nursing students at Indiana University founded Sigma Theta Tau, nursing's honor society, now an international organization.

Little is known about either black or male nurses. However, after the Civil War, recognized black nurse leaders included Mary Mahoney, the first black nurse to graduate from a training program; Jessie Scales, the first district nurse; and Martha Franklin, founder of the National Association of Colored Graduate Nurses (NACGN). Adah Thomas led the fight to gain acceptance of black nurses by the army. She had corresponded extensively with Jane Delano, chairman of the national committee of the American Red Cross through which army nurses were enrolled at the time, and urged black nurses to enroll in the American Red Cross. Finally, a month after the armistice was signed in 1918 and in the midst of the flu epidemic, the first black nurses were assigned to army camps in Ohio and Illinois, with other assignments following. (However, it was not until World War II that black nurses were accepted into the military service.)[33]

THE NURSE IN PRACTICE

In the late nineteenth and early twentieth centuries, the graduate trained nurse had two major career options; she could do private duty in homes or, if she was exceptional (or particularly favored), gain one of the rare positions as head nurse, operating room supervisor, night supervisor, or even superintendent. The latter positions were, of course, much more available before the flood of nurses reached the market. Even so, in private duty, trained nurses often competed with untrained nurses who were not restrained from practicing in many states until the middle of the twentieth century. And, given the long hours and taxing physical work in home nursing, most private nurses found themselves unwanted at 40, with younger, stronger nurses being hired instead. Some of the more ambitious and perhaps braver nurses chose to go west to pioneer in new and sometimes primitive hospitals.

The practice of nursing was scarcely limited to clinical care of the patient. Job descriptions of the time appear to have given major priority to scrubbing floors, dusting, keeping the stove stoked and the kerosene lamps trimmed and filled, controlling insects, washing clothes, making and rolling bandages, and other unskilled housekeeping tasks, as well as edicts for personal behavior (see the accompanying ad). Nursing care responsibilities included, in addition to carrying out the orders of the physician,

> making beds, giving baths, preventing and dressing bedsores, applying friction to the body and extremities, giving enemas, inserting catheters, bandaging, dressing blisters, burns, sores, and wounds, and observing secretions, expectorations, pulse, skin, appetite, body temperature, consciousness, respiration, sleep, condition of wounds, skin eruptions, elimination, and the effect of diet, stimulants, and medications.[34]

At the end of the nineteenth century, there was a marked growth of large cities in the United States. Although the cities had their beautiful public buildings, parks, and mansions, they also had their seamy sides—the festering slums where the tremendous flow of immigrants huddled. Between 1820 and 1910, nearly 30 million immigrants entered the United States, with a shift in numbers from Northern European to Southern European by the early 1900s. Health and social problems multiplied in the slum areas. Somehow, Americans did not seem to feel a great need to serve the sick poor in their homes; after all, there were public dispensaries and charity hospitals. Some visiting nurse groups were formed, but by 1900 it was estimated that only 200 nurses were engaged in public health nursing.

In 1912, the Red Cross established the Rural Nursing Service. Lillian Wald, at a major meeting on infant mortality, had cited the horrible health conditions of rural America, the high infant and maternal mortality rates, the prevalence of tuberculosis, and other serious health problems and suggested that the Red Cross operate a national service, similar to that of Great Britain. (Red Cross involvement gradually decreased until, with increased government involvement in public health, it discontinued the program altogether in 1947.)

However, in 1915, it is estimated that no more than 10 percent of the sick received care in the hospitals, and the majority of people could not afford private duty nurses. From this need, a public health movement emerged that increased the demand for nurses. At first most of these nurses concentrated on bedside care, but others, like those coming from the settlement houses, took broader responsibilities. Nevertheless, there were no recognized

Wanted: A Very Special Nurse to Care for 50 Patients at a Local Hospital

Duties and requirements:

- Daily sweep and mop the floors of your ward. Dust the patients' furniture and windowsills.
- Maintain an even temperature in your ward by bringing in a scuttle of coal for the day's business.
- Light is important to observe the patient's condition. Therefore, each day fill kerosene lamps, clean chimneys and trim wicks. Wash the windows once a week.
- The Nurses' notes are important in aiding the physician's work. Make your pens carefully. You may whittle nibs to your individual taste.
- Each nurse on duty will report every day at 7:00 A.M. and leave at 8:00 P.M. except on the Sabbath on which you will be off from 12:00 noon to 2:00 P.M.
- Graduates in good standing with the Superintendent of Nurses will be given an evening off each week for courting purposes, or two evenings a week if you go to church regularly.
- Each nurse should lay aside from each pay day a goodly sum of her earnings for her benefit in her declining years, so that she will not become a burden. For example, if you earn $30 a month, you should set aside $15.
- Any nurse who smokes, uses liquor in any form, gets her hair done at a beauty shop, or frequents dance halls will give the Superintendent of Nurses a good reason to suspect her worth, intentions and integrity.
- The nurse who performs her labors, serves her patients and doctors faithfully without fault for a period of five years will be given an increase by the Hospital Administration of five cents a day, providing there are no hospital debts that are outstanding.

Source: Reportedly an ad in a western newspaper in 1887.

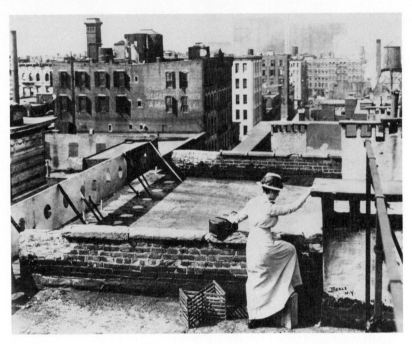

A turn of the century public health nurse climbing over the rooftops of the tenements to visit patients on the lower East Side of New York. (*Courtesy of the Visiting Nurse Service of New York.*)

standards or requirements for visiting nurses. Therefore, in June 1912, a small group of visiting nurses, representing unofficially some 900 agencies and almost four times that many colleagues, founded the National Organization for Public Health Nursing (NOPHN), with Lillian Wald as the first president. It was an organization of nurses and lay people engaged in public health nursing and in the organization, management, and support of such work. The leaders of the group selected the term *public health nursing* as more inclusive than *visiting nursing;* it was also reminiscent of Nightingale's health nursing, which had focused on prevention. One of its first goals was to extend the services to working- and middle-class people, as well as to the poor.

By 1916, public health nurses were being called on to be welfare workers, sanitarians, housing inspectors, and health teachers as well. A number of universities began offering courses to help prepare nurses to fulfill this multifaceted role, and Mary Gardner, one of the founders of NOPHN and an interim director of the Rural Nursing Service, authored the first book in the field, *Public Health Nursing*. One of the observations she made was that although broad-minded physicians recognized that public health nurses helped them produce results that would not have been possible alone, the more conservative feared interference by nurses and were resentful of them. She noted that a service had a better chance of success if it was started with the cooperation of the medical profession, and pointed out ways nurses could avoid friction with physicians and still be protected from the incompetents.

Gradually various other nursing specialties developed, such as anesthesia, industrial nursing, and nurse midwifery. However, it was the Great Depression, which followed the stock market crash in 1929, that helped alter nursing practice drastically. This was a period of high unemployment for nurses. As financial crises hit their clientele, private duty nurses found that there was little demand for their services. The situation worsened as nurses who were laid off in offices and industry, as well as married nurses, also looked for private duty cases. Both the Goldmark Report and *Nurses, Patients, and Pocketbooks* (Appendix 1) had warned that the overproduction and maldistribution of nurses would soon cause a problem, but no action had been taken. Now a reevaluation of nursing and nursing education was imperative. The result was the closing of many small schools and an increased concern for high standards, the setting of an eight-hour day for private duty nurses, and the employment of graduate nurses in hospitals. Unfortunately, the last also had long-lasting bad effects. By 1933, some nurses worked in hospitals for little more than room and board. It took many years for nurses to earn reasonable wages and to gain some autonomy in their practice.

Some help finally came with the Roosevelt Administration, when relief funds were allocated for bedside care of the indigent and nurses were employed as visiting nurses under the Federal Emergency Relief Administration (FERA). Ten thousand unemployed nurses were put to work in numerous settings under the Civil Works Administration (CWA) in public hospitals, clinics, public health agencies, and other health services. The follow-up Works Progress Administration (WPA) then continued to provide funds for nurses in community health activities.[35]

Of all the entrants into nursing, two groups got particularly short shrift— men and blacks. The prejudice against men was specially related to nursing and has persisted to some extent (see Chapter 4). As the distorted image of the female nurse evolved, men did not seem to fit the concepts held by powerful figures in and out of nursing. Therefore, although men graduated from acceptable, usually totally male nursing schools and attempted to become active members of the ANA, even forming a men's section, their numbers and influence remained small until the post–World War II era.

Black nurses were caught in the overall common prejudice against their race. Individual black nurses, as noted earlier, broke down barriers in various nursing fields. As early as 1908, they organized the National Association of Colored Graduate Nurses (NACGN), both to fight against discriminatory practices and to foster leadership among black nurses. Although the ANA had a nondiscriminatory policy, some state organizations did not, and a rule that the nurse must have graduated from a state-approved school to be an

ANA member eliminated even more black nurses. Finally, in 1951, the NACGN was absorbed into the ANA, which required nondiscrimination for all state associations as a prerequisite for ANA affiliation.

In 1924, it was reported that only 58 state-accredited schools admitted blacks, and most of these were located in black hospitals or in departments caring for black patients in municipal hospitals. Of these schools, 77 percent were located in the South. Twenty-eight states offered no opportunities in nursing education for black women. Most of the southern "schools" that trained black nurses were totally unacceptable, and many of those approved barely met standards. Moreover, there were some 23,000 untrained black midwives in the South, but no one made the effort to combine training in nursing and midwifery, which would have been a distinct service. In 1930, there were fewer than 6000 graduate black nurses, most of whom worked in black hospitals or public health agencies that served black patients. Opportunities in other fields either were not open to them or could not admit them because they did not, understandably, have the advanced preparation necessary. Middle-class black women were usually not attracted to nursing, because teaching and other available fields offered more prestige and better opportunities.

It was not until a 1941 executive order and the corresponding follow-through that any part of the federal government made any effort to investigate the grievances and deal with the complaints of blacks. Later, the Bolton Act opened the doors of participating nursing schools to blacks. Yet, overt and covert methods were used in both the North and the South to prevent the more able black nurses from assuming leadership positions—some as simple as advancing the least aggressive. And for all the desperate need for nurses, the armed forces balked at accepting and integrating black nurses. Not until the end of World War II and after some aggressive action by the NACGN and the National Nursing Council for War Service did this situation change.

WARTIME NURSING

Another influence on nursing was nurses' participation in American wars. Ironically, although the military was not prepared to care for its sick and wounded in the short but deadly Spanish-American War, once more the military physicians objected to the presence of women nurses. Finally, when men lay dying of malaria, dysentery, and typhoid, women from the training schools took over. Their letters and journals relate the horrible conditions under which they worked. Some literally worked themselves to death in the army hospitals in the South. One of the most serious diseases that nurses

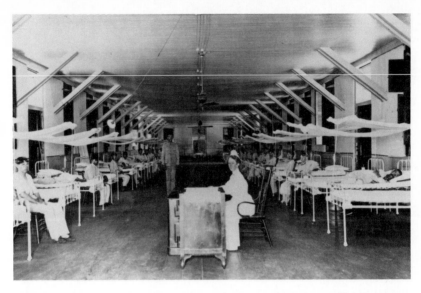

Spanish-American War (1898)—Army contract nurse on a ward at the First Reserve Hospital, Manila, P.I. (*Courtesy of the Center of Military History, Department of the Army.*)

contended with was yellow fever, about which little was known. In testing the theory that the disease was caused by a certain type of mosquito, nursing gained its first martyr. Twenty-five-year-old Clara Maas of East Orange, New Jersey, volunteered to be bitten by a carrier mosquito. After being bitten several times, she died of yellow fever and is still considered a heroine in helping to prove the source of the disease.

The value of nurses in wartime was clear after the Spanish-American War, and recommendations were made that a regular corps of nurses ready for wartime duty be formed. Yet some military authorities were still hostile. So, although the number of women army nurses had reached 1158 by September 1898, by the next July there were only 202. Despite this setback, a group of influential women, including some prominent nurses, eventually lobbied through a bill, and the Army Nurse Corps was established on February 2, 1901.[36]

It took longer for the Congress to act on a Navy Nurse Corps, although it had the support of the Navy's Surgeon General, but finally it, too, became a reality in 1908. World War I was different from other wars the United States had fought, both because of its international dimensions and the kinds of weapons that were used. The service of the nurse in the nightmarish battle conditions of World War I, coping with the mass casualties, dealing with injuries caused by the previously unknown sharpnel and gas, and then battling influenza at home and abroad, is a fascinating and proud piece of history.[37]

Both the Army and Navy Nurse Corps were expanded during this time, but not enough nurses were available and recruitment standards dropped. (Even though there were male nurses who volunteered, they, like black nurses, were not accepted in the nurse corps.) Nursing leaders then formed a committee to devise methods of dealing with the problems related to care of the sick in the military, in hospitals, and in homes. Later the committee was given governmental status and very limited funding. The members found once more what had been true before and would be again: in wartime there are not enough nurses to meet the need. While efforts were made to recruit and produce nurses more rapidly, and they succeeded to some extent for the duration, there was inevitably a shortage afterward. When patriotic fervor faded away, the unpleasant conditions while "in training" and afterward, at a time when other working conditions were improving, made nursing a less desirable occupational choice. The high quality of students in the Rainbow

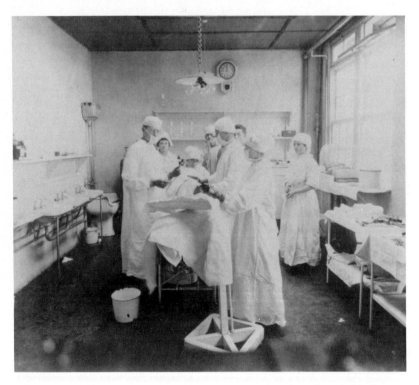

Army nurses are part of the operating room team in a base hospital in France, 1919. (*Courtesy of the Center of Military History, Department of the Army.*)

Division of the Vassar Training Camp mentioned earlier was more the exception than the rule. The Army School of Nursing that emerged from World War I was also highly unusual.

In World War II, the role of nurses was even more extensive and perhaps even more dangerous. Once more nurses proved themselves able and brave in military situations.[38] Many were in battle zones, and some became Japanese prisoners of war.[39] Their stories have been told in films, books, plays, and historical nursing research and are well worth reading (see Bibliography). The war created opportunities, freedom, and also problems for nurses that proved to be long-lasting in both nursing education and practice. Some related to the nursing shortage that was again critical. There were not enough nurses for both the home front and the battlefield, even with stepped-up efforts to encourage women to enter nursing programs.

Finally, legislation was passed in 1943 establishing the Cadet Nurse

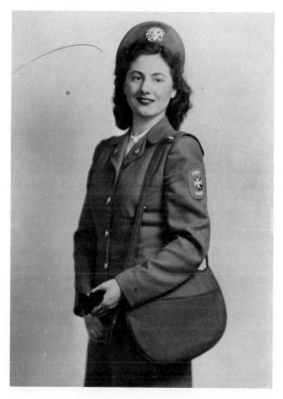

The Cadet Nurse program during World War II, which provided federal money to train nurses, was responsible for major changes in nursing education.

Corps. The Bolton Act, the first federal program to subsidize nursing education for schools and students, was a forerunner of future federal aid to nursing. For payment of their tuition and a stipend, students committed themselves to engage in essential military or civilian nursing for the duration of the war. The students had to be between 17 and 35 years old, in good health, and with a good academic record in an accredited high school. This new law brought about several changes in nursing. For instance, it forbade discrimination on the basis of race and marital status and set minimum educational standards. The first standard, theoretically accepted, was not always implemented in good faith. The second, combined with the requirement that nursing programs be reduced from the traditional 36 months to 30, forced nursing schools to reassess and revise their curricula.[40]

Two other major efforts to relieve the nursing shortage had long-range effects in the practice setting. One was the recruitment of inactive nurses back into the field. For the first time, married women and others who could work only on a part-time basis became acceptable to employers and later became part of the labor pool. The other change was the training of volunteer nurse's aides. Although such training was initiated by the Red Cross in 1919, it was discouraged later by nurses, particularly during the Depression. During World War II, both the Red Cross and the Office of Civilian Defense trained more than 20,000 aides. At first, they were used only for nonnursing tasks, but the increasing nurse shortage forced them to take on basic nursing functions. After the war, with a continued shortage, trained aides were hired as a necessary part of the nursing service department. Their perceived cost effectiveness stimulated the growth of both aide and practical nurse training programs and eventually increased federal funding for both.

Finally, major changes occurred within the armed forces. Nurses had held only relative rank, meaning that they carried officers' titles but had less power and pay than their male counterparts. In 1947, full commissioned status was granted, giving them the right to manage nursing care. At the same time, as noted previously, discrimination against black nurses ended but, oddly enough, in the male-controlled armed services, it was not until 1954 that male nurses were admitted to full rank as officers.

When the Korean War broke out in 1950, the army again drew nurses from civilian hospitals, this time from their reserve corps. War nursing on the battlefront was centered to an extent on the Mobile Army Surgical Hospitals (MASH), located as close to the front lines as possible. Flight nurses, who helped to evacuate the wounded from the battlefront to military hospitals, also achieved recognition. When that war was over and nurse reservists returned to their civilian jobs, it is possible that their experiences increased their discontent with working situations at home. (For further readings on nursing during the Vietnam War, which is beyond this time period, see the Bibliography sources for Chapter 7.)

TOWARD A NEW ERA: STUDIES AND ACTION

The usual postwar nurse shortage occurred after World War II, but this time for different reasons. Only one of six army nurses planned to return to her civilian job, finding more satisfaction in the service. Poor pay and unpleasant working conditions discouraged civilian nurses as well. In 1946, the salary for a staff nurse was about $36 for a 48-hour work week, less than that for typists or seamstresses (much less men). Salaries were supposed to be kept secret, and hospitals, in particular, held wages at a minimum, with such peculiarities as a staff nurse earning more than a head nurse. Split shifts were common, with nurses scheduled to work from seven to eleven and from three to seven, with time off between the two shifts. The work was especially difficult, because staffing was short and nurses worked under rigid discipline. Small wonder then that in one survey only about 12 percent of the nurses queried planned to make nursing a career; more than 75 percent saw it as a pin-money job after marriage or planned to retire altogether as soon as possible. Unions were beginning to organize nurses, so in 1949 the ANA approved state associations as collective bargaining agents for nurses. However, because the Taft-Hartley Act excluded nonprofit institutions from collective bargaining, hospitals and agencies did not need to deal with nurses. In addition, the ANA no-strike pledge took away another powerful weapon. As noted previously, one answer that administrators saw was the hiring of nurse's aides. The use of volunteers and auxiliary help—that is, anyone other than licensed or trained nurses, practical nurses, aides, or orderlies—increased tremendously.

One group of workers that proliferated in the postwar era was practical nurses, defined by ANA, NLNE, and NOPHN as those trained to care for subacute, convalescent, and chronic patients under the direction of a physician or nurse. Thousands who designated themselves as practical nurses had no such skills, and their training was simply in caring for their own families or, at most, aide work. Although the first school for training practical nurses appeared in 1897, by 1930 there were only 11, and in 1947 there were still only 36. With the new demand for nurse substitutes, 260 more practical nurse schools opened by 1954, mostly in hospitals or long-term care institutions and a few in vocational schools. Aiding the movement was funding under federal vocational education acts. There were, unfortunately, also a number of correspondence courses and other commercialized programs that did little more than expose the student to some books and manuals and present her with a diploma. By 1950, there were 144,000 practical nurses, 95 percent of them women, and, although their educational programs varied, their on-the-job activities expanded greatly—to doing whatever nurses had no time to do. By 1952, some 56 percent of the nursing personnel were

nonprofessionals, and some nurses began to fear that they were being replaced by less expensive, minimally trained workers.

Nevertheless, with working and financial conditions not improving, the
nursing shortage persisted. Soon, a team plan was developed with a nurse
as a team leader, primarily responsible for planning patient care, perhaps
caring for patients with more complex problems, and less prepared workers
carrying out the care plan for other patients. Although the team plan has
persisted for years, it has done little to improve patient care, since generally
it has not been carried out as originally conceived. Rather, it has kept the
nurse mired in paperwork, away from the patient or required to make constant
medication rounds. Often practical nurses have carried the primary responsibilities for patient units on the evening and night shift, with the few nurses
available stretched thin, "supervising" these workers.

There were more nurses than ever at mid-century, but there were also
tremendously expanded health services, a greater population to be served,
growth of various insurance plans that paid for hospital care, a postwar baby
boom with in-hospital deliveries, new medical discoveries that kept patients
alive longer, and a proliferation of nurses into other areas of health care.
Hospitals still weren't the most desirable places to work, and economic
benefits were slow in coming. Moreover there were now more married nurses
who chose to stay home to raise families. Studies done in 1941, 1948, and
1958 (Appendix 1), all of which pointed out some of the economic and
status problems of nurses, particularly in hospitals, went largely ignored by
administrators.

Nursing for the Future was a study conducted by Esther Lucile Brown,
a social anthropologist, and related to both nursing education and nursing
service. The report received mixed reviews. Many nurses felt threatened,
and some physicians and hospital administrators considered it a subversive
document, fearing that it had economic security implications for nurses.
(Nor did they appreciate the fact that the authoritarianism of hospitals was
pinpointed, as was the dilemma of the nurse caught between the demands
of physicians and administrators.)

In the 1950s, Frances Reiter began to write about the *nurse clinician,* a
nurse who gave skilled nursing care on an advanced level. This concept
developed into that of the clinical specialist, a nurse with a graduate degree
and specialized knowledge of nursing care, who worked as a colleague of
physicians. At the same time, the development of coronary and other intensive care units called for nurses with equally specialized technical knowledge, formerly the sole province of medical practice. In Colorado in 1965,
a physician, in collaboration with a school of nursing, was pioneering another
new role for nurses in ambulatory care. As the nurses easily assumed responsibility for well-child care and minor illnesses, they called upon their
nursing knowledge and skills, as well as a medical component. What emerged
was the *nurse practitioner.* (These roles are described in Chapter 7.)

Nursing education was also going through a transition period in those decades. In the years immediately after World War II, the quality of nursing education was under severe criticism. There was no question that in the diploma schools, where most nurses were educated, there was frequently poor teaching, inadequately prepared teachers, and major dependence on students for services; often two-thirds of the hours of care were given by students. There were also the findings of Esther Lucile Brown, who had gathered her data by visiting nursing schools and health care facilities and consulting with many key people in the health care field, including nurses. Her findings were not much different from those in earlier reports, and 22 years later, in another national study, *An Abstract for Action,* the author noted that many of the recommendations in *Nursing for the Future* were still valid but unfulfilled. Brown particularly cited the poor quality of many schools and the fact that many diploma schools were operated for the staffing benefit of the hospital. (Even in the years of the Great Depression, when hospital administrators complained bitterly about the cost of nursing programs, their economic benefit was clear and most were kept.) One strong recommendation of the Brown report was "that effort be directed to building basic schools of nursing in universities and colleges, comparable in number to existing medical schools, that are sound in organizational and financial structure, adequate in facilities and faculty, and well-distributed to serve the needs of the entire country."[41]

The slow rate of growth of collegiate programs, even into the next decade, resulted in part from the uncertainty of nurses about what these programs should be and how they should differ from diploma education. Another factor was the anticollegiate faction in nursing that saw no point in higher education—a faction that was cheered and nurtured by a large number of physicians and administrators. While the Brown report did result in a reexamination of beliefs and attitudes about educational practices, it was also viewed as a threat to the comfortable status quo by hospital administrators, some doctors, and diploma nurses. However, both this report and the 1950 report *Nursing Schools at the Mid-Century,* a follow-up report sponsored by six nursing organizations, are credited with being the impetus for an established process of accreditation in nursing. Those schools that chose to go through the voluntary process and that met the standards were placed on a published list, which for the first time gave the public, guidance counselors, and potential students some notion of the quality of one school compared with another (Appendix 1).

Eventually, accreditation proved a significant force in improving good schools and closing poor ones (although it has also been accused of rigidity throughout the years). Actually the NLNE, which, as the National League for Nursing (NLN), later assumed responsibility for accreditation, had been involved in curriculum study and development since the publication of its 1917 *Standard Curriculum for Schools of Nursing* and its 1929 *A Curriculum for Schools of Nursing.* By 1937, these works were considered extremely helpful to those responsible for nursing programs, but their curricula were perhaps too inflexible. Out of this came *A Curriculum Guide for Schools of Nursing,* which was greatly influenced by a study directed by Isabel Stewart that had looked at "the most progressive idea and practices" in basic nursing education. The new guide, intended, according to Stewart, for students of professional caliber preparing themselves for a profession, placed much greater emphasis on application of the sciences. The role of the clinical instructor was stressed, and all faculty members were encouraged to use newer and more creative methods of teaching. The guide was never revised again, but it was used in many schools for another quarter-century.

The study that probably changed nursing education more dramatically than any other was the doctoral research of Mildred Montag at Teachers College in New York. *Community College Education for Nursing,* published in 1959, was the report of a five-year project based on her dissertation. In this "action research" project, seven junior community colleges cooperated by establishing two-year associate degree (AD) programs for nursing. It was the right time for such programs with the rapid growth of community colleges and the availability of new types of students—mature men and women and the less affluent, who seized this opportunity for a college degree and a career. The project evaluation, including follow-up of the 811 graduates, presented persuasive arguments for the development of more such programs. (Chapter 5 discusses in more detail the original Montag dissertation and its effect on nursing education.) Twenty-five years later, associate degree programs made up the largest segment preparing nurses for RN licensure. AD education also had an effect on other nursing programs. It was probably partially the influence of the AD programs, which were nondiscriminatory and generally nonpaternalistic in their relations with students, that helped loosen the tight restrictions on nursing students' personal lives in both diploma and some baccalaureate programs. Still, even into the late 1960s, some diploma schools excluded married students and men. The growth of AD programs ultimately outran all others in nursing except practical nurse programs.

Federal funding of nursing education also had a major impact on nursing education. As noted earlier, nursing education was first subsidized during World War II with enactment of the Bolton Act in 1943. However, it was in effect only for the duration of the war, since its intent was to overcome the serious nursing shortage. There was no further funding of nursing education until the Health Amendments Act of 1956 provided traineeships, which did not have to be paid back, to prepare nurses for administration, teaching, supervision, and public health through both short-term and full-time study. However, useful as this was, even more far-reaching was the 1963 report *Toward Quality in Nursing, Needs and Goals.* It was prepared by a group of nurses, other health professionals, and members of the public appointed by the Surgeon General of the U.S. Public Health Service to advise him on nursing needs and the role the government should take in providing adequate nursing service for the public. The report, which cited major deficits in the number of nurses adequately prepared to meet the health needs of the future, had great influence. An obvious problem was the lack of qualified teachers; even in so-called university programs, nurses did not meet the usual requirements for teaching. Another was the almost total lack of educational background in management by nurses who held administrative and managerial positions. The enactment of the *Nurse Training Act of 1964* not only provided funding for students and schools for the next five years, but in its later forms, continued to provide a varied amount of support to nursing education and research until today.[42]

Such federal assistance was particularly important in the development of graduate programs in nursing education. Few such programs existed, and often nurses who sought graduate degrees turned to other disciplines such as education. However, even with the growth of graduate nursing programs, it was not until the 1960s that graduate education in clinical nursing was more readily available. This may have been due to the forms of federal funding. In fact, one outcome of such funding was the tendency for schools to develop educational programs according to the funding available—a great problem for the continuity of programs for minorities, continuing education, and clinical specialties when this "soft money" later diminished or evaporated altogether.

Nursing research also tended to make slow progress. Although there were studies of nursing service, nursing education, and nursing personality, most were done with or by social scientists. When nurses assisted physicians and others in medical research, it was just that—assisting. Nursing leaders realized that nursing could not develop as a profession unless clinical research focusing on nursing evolved. One of the first major steps in that direction was the 1952 publication of *Nursing Research,* a scholarly journal that reported and encouraged nursing research. The other was the ANA's establishment of the American Nurses' Foundation in 1955 for charitable, educational, and scientific purposes. Of course, federal funding also had considerable impact.

With all of these changes, the professional organizations of nursing took varied and sometimes uncoordinated action. A study to consider restructuring, reorganizing, and unifying the various organizations was initiated shortly after World War II. In 1952, the six major nursing organizations—ANA, NLNE, NOPHN, NACGN, the Association of Collegiate Schools of Nursing (ACSN), and the American Association of Industrial Nurses (AAIN)—finally came to a decision about organizational structure. Two major organizations emerged: the ANA, with only nurse members, and the renamed National League for Nursing (NLN), with nurse, nonnurse, and agency membership. The AAIN decided to continue, and the National Student

Nurses' Association was formed. Practical nurses had their own organization. (See Chapter 14 for details of the organizations.) Although there was an apparent realignment of responsibilities, the relationships between the ANA and NLN ebbed and flowed: sometimes they were in agreement, and sometimes they were not; sometimes they worked together, and at other times each appeared to make isolated unilateral pronouncements. Some nurses wanted one organization, but there seemed to be mutual organizational reluctance to go in that direction. Yet, each had some remarkable achievements: NLN in educational accreditation and ANA in its lobbying activities, its development of a model licensure law in the mid-1950s, and its increased action regarding nurses' economic security.

In 1965, ANA precipitated (or inflamed) an ongoing controversy. After years of increasingly firm statements on the place of nursing education in the mainstream of American education, ANA issued its first Position Paper on Education for Nursing. It stated, basically, that education for those who work in nursing should be in institutions of higher learning; that minimum education for professional nursing should be at least at the baccalaureate level; for technical nursing, at the associate degree level; and for assistants, in vocational education settings.

Although there had been increasing complaints by third-party payers about diploma education, and although diploma schools had declined as associate and baccalaureate degree programs increased, there was an outpouring of anger by diploma and practical nurses and those involved in their education. It was a battle that persisted and became another divisive force in nursing. But then, so was the beginning of the nurse practitioner movement. There were nurses who feared it or saw it as pseudomedicine, detracting from pure nursing professionalism. The issues remain unresolved to some extent.

Therefore, whether or not 1965 can be considered the gateway to a new era of nursing, it was the beginning of dramatic and inevitable changes in the education and practice of nursing and in the struggle for nursing autonomy—a revolution in nursing.

KEY POINTS

1. The work and ongoing interest of the "lady" volunteers who acted as nurses in the Civil War were influential in the establishment of the first training schools for nurses modeled (to some extent) on Nightingale principles.
2. Students in the early training schools worked long hours, did many menial nonnursing tasks, and gave almost all the nursing care in hospitals.

3. Twenty-five years after trained nursing had begun, nursing leaders in the United States were responsible for setting nursing standards, improving curricula, writing textbooks, starting two enduring nursing organizations and a nursing journal, inaugurating a teacher training program in a university, and initiating nursing licensure.

4. Studies about nursing that pointed out deficiencies in nursing education and practice were often ignored because of the students' economic benefit to the hospital, but they seem to have had a cumulative effect that eventually brought about change.

5. Because of the shortage of nurses that occurred during and after wars, reforms in both nursing education and practice were instituted.

6. AD nursing initiated in 1952 as an action research project produced a new kind of nurse and changed nursing education.

7. The first baccalaureate program in nursing was founded in 1909, but for decades a common pattern was a combination of two years of college and three years in a diploma school.

8. Before the Great Depression, most graduate nurses worked at private duty, but public health nursing, school nursing, industrial nursing, midwifery, and other specialties gradually emerged under the leadership of nursing pioneers.

9. Black nurses and men were often discriminated against in nursing but slowly gained status in the last half of the twentieth century.

REFERENCES

1. Selavan IC. Nurses in American history: The revolution. *Am J Nurs,* 75:592–594 (April 1975).

2. Kalisch P, Kalisch B. *The advance of American nursing,* 2nd ed. Boston: Little, Brown and Company, 1986, p. 79.

3. Kalisch P, Kalisch B. Untrained but undaunted: The women nurses of the blue and gray. *Nurs Forum,* 15(1):4–33 (1976); see p. 17.

4. Dolan JA, et al. *Nursing in society: A historical perspective,* 15th ed. Philadelphia: W.B. Saunders Company, 1983, pp. 173–174.

5. Carnegie ME. Black nurses at the front. *Am J Nurs,* 84:1250–1252 (October 1984).

6. Culpepper MM, Adams PG. Nursing in the Civil War. *Am J Nurs,* 88:981–984 (July 1988).

7. Bullough V, Bullough B. *The care of the sick; the emergence of modern nursing.* New York: Prodist, 1978, p. 114.

8. Dolan et al., op. cit., p. 202.

9. Kalisch and Kalisch (1986), op. cit., pp. 221–224.

10. Ibid., pp. 164–165.

11. Flaumenhaft E, Flaumenhaft C. American nursing's first text books. *Nurs Outlook,* 37:185–188 (July–August 1989).
12. Kalisch B, Kalisch P. Slaves, servants, or saints: An analysis of the system of nurse training in the United States, 1873–1948. *Nurs Forum,* 14(3):230–231 (1975); see p. 228.
13. Kalisch and Kalisch (1986). p. 171.
14. Ibid., pp. 315–318.
15. Ibid., p. 372.
16. Kelly L. *Dimensions of professional nursing,* 5th ed. New York: Macmillan Publishing Company, 1985, p. 71.
17. Bullough and Bullough, op. cit., p. 156.
18. Ingles T. The physician's view of the evolving nursing profession—1873–1913. *Nurs Forum,* 15(2):123–164 (1976); see p. 148.
19. Bullough B, Bullough V. Sex discrimination in health care. *Nurs Outlook,* 23:40–45 (January 1975); see p. 43.
20. Kelly L. *Dimensions of professional nursing,* 6th ed. Elmsford, NY: Pergamon Press, 1991, p. 67.
21. Nutting MA. Isabel Hampton Robb: Her work in organization and education. *Am J Nurse,* 10:19 (January 1910).
22. Poslusny S. Feminine friendship: Isabel Hampton Robb, Lavinia Lloyd Dock and Mary Adelaide Nutting. *Image,* 21:64–67 (Summer 1989).
23. Benson E. Nursing and the World's Columbian Exposition. *Nurs Outlook,* 34:88–90 (March–April 1986).
24. Christy TE. Portrait of a leader: Sophia F. Palmer. *Nurs Outlook,* 23:746–751 (December 1975); see pp. 746–747.
25. Flanagan L. *One strong voice: The story of the American Nurses' Association.* Kansas City, MO: American Nurses' Association, 1976, pp. 35–38.
26. Pryor EB. *Clara Barton, professional angel.* Philadelphia: University of Pennsylvania Press, 1987.
27. Kalisch and Kalisch (1986). op. cit., p. 292.
28. Christy TE. Portrait of a leader: Lillian D. Wald. *Nurs Outlook,* 18:50–54 (March 1970).
29. Ruffing-Rahal MA. Margaret Sanger: Nurse and feminist. *Nurs Outlook.* 34:246–249 (September–October 1986).
30. Christy TE. Portrait of a leader. Lavinia Lloyd Dock. *Nurs Outlook,* 17:72–75 (June 1969); see p. 74.
31. Ibid.
32. Pletsch PK. Mary Breckenridge: A pioneer who made her mark. *Am J Nurs,* 81:188–190 (February 1981).
33. Carnegie ME. *The path we tread: Blacks in nursing 1854–1984.* Philadelphia: J.B. Lippincott Company, 1986.
34. Kalisch and Kalisch (1986), op. cit., pp. 205–206.
35. Fitzpatrick ML. Nursing and the great depression. *Am J Nurs,* 75:2188–2190 (December 1975).
36. Gourney C. Military nursing: 211 years of commitment to the American soldier. *Imprint,* 34:36–45. (February–March 1987).

37. Kalisch and Kalisch (1986), op. cit., pp. 217–220.
38. Curtis D. Nurses and war: The way it was. *Am J Nurs,* 84:1253–1254 (October 1984).
39. Kalisch P, Kalisch B. Nurses under fire: The World War II experience of nurses on Bataan and Corregidor. *Nurs Res,* 25:409–429 (November–December 1976).
40. Kalisch B, Kalisch P. Nurses in American history: The Cadet Nurse Corps. *Am J Nurs,* 76:240–242 (February 1976).
41. Brown EL. *Nursing for the future.* New York: Russell Sage Foundation, 1948, p. 178.
42. Kelly (1991), op. cit., pp. 423–426.

PART II
NURSING IN THE HEALTH CARE SCENE

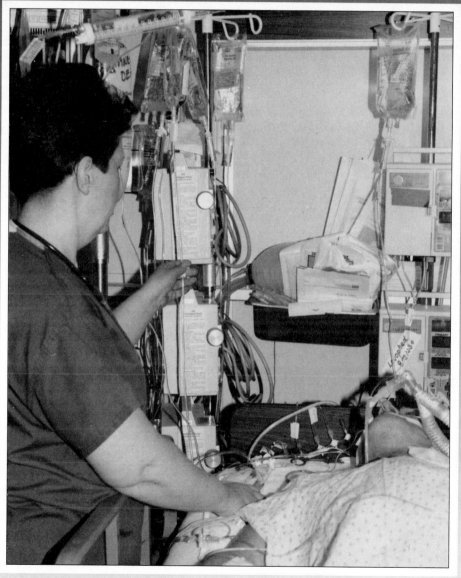

Complex medical care is being given in hospitals today.
(Courtesy of the Robert Wood Johnson Medical Center.)

C H A P T E R 3

THE HEALTH CARE SYSTEM

OBJECTIVES

After studying this chapter, you will be able to:

1. Explain how at least five social and economic factors affect health care.
2. Describe the impact of cost containment on health care.
3. Define self-care, primary care, secondary care, and tertiary care.
4. Describe the major settings in which health care is given.
5. Describe briefly the role of major personnel who are part of the health care team.
6. Identify three changes that are common to many health occupations.
7. Explain how at least five predictions for future health care are related to current trends.

Most people have no idea how complex health care is today, with its multiple settings and array of workers. Even those in the field often don't know much about what their colleagues do or how care is given in any place but their own. When a health care "crisis" hits the headlines periodically, health workers are, naturally, more interested in how this affects them personally than in the larger picture. Yet, no part of health care is untouched when problems become big enough to be called a crisis. To remain ignorant or indifferent about what is going on is a luxury no one in health care can afford.

This chapter provides an overview of American health care, the settings, the people, the issues, and how outside factors influence the system.

WHAT INFLUENCES HEALTH CARE?

As a part of society and as one of the health professions, nursing is affected by the changes, problems, and issues of society in general, as well as those that specifically influence health care. Some of the changes, such as an emphasis on the civil rights of minority groups and women, have been occurring for almost 100 years. Others, such as the changes in social attitudes and the growth of economic pressures, have been building up but were ignored until they created a crisis. Still others, such as new lifestyles and technological and scientific advances, appeared to emerge with a suddenness that has created what Toffler calls "future shock," the shattering stress and disorientation induced in individuals when they are subjected to too much change in too short a time.[1] Yet, even though it might be tempting simply to do your job and never mind the outside world, people (or professions) that do not pay attention to economic and social trends find themselves scrambling to catch up, rather than planning to move ahead—reacting, rather than acting. When the public accuses the professions of unresponsiveness to their needs, it is, in part, because those professions have not been acute enough to observe patterns of future development or have been too self-centered to see the necessity to become a part of them. Among the major factors to consider are changes in population, people's health, technology and scientific advances, education and employment, and social movements.

THE AMERICAN PEOPLE: A TIME OF CHANGE

Although the 1990 census is in the past, the correct U.S. population figure seems to be a matter of ongoing debate. Large cities such as New York maintain that many residents have gone uncounted, and everyone knows that there is no accurate count of the homeless, undocumented aliens, and even migrant workers. Nevertheless, the tentative figure for the total population is generally reported at about 250 million, over 9 percent greater than that stated in the 1980 census. There are some interesting differences that, while they may have been predicted, are quite dramatic and are expected to change the face of America into the next century.

The population will not be as white as before. Nearly one in four Americans has African, Asian, Hispanic, or native American ancestry; it was one in five in 1980. The rate of increase in the minority population has been nearly twice as fast as in the 1970s. The greatest surge is among Hispanics, who increased by 7.7 million people, or 56 percent, since 1980. Part of this increase is due to immigration (7 to 9 million over the decade), some to legalization of illegal immigrants, and some to a high birth rate. The wave of immigration from the Philippines, China, India, and southeast Asia and the generally high birth rate in these groups are additional factors that account for the prediction that in some states, like New Mexico and California, whites will be a minority by the year 2000. One report notes that by 2020, the number of U.S. residents who are Hispanic or nonwhite will have more than doubled to nearly 115 million, while the white population will not increase at all. Some call this the "browning" of America;[2] others see it as the dawn of the first universal nation.[3] But whatever this population change is called, a truly multiracial society is seen as being more difficult to govern. Racial and ethnic conflict, already a sad fact of life from the ghetto to schools to businesses, may increase, as may the rivalry and competitiveness among various minorities themselves. The concern of some is the tendency of new immigrant groups to stay culturally isolated, maintaining their language and mores without attempting to become part of "American" society. Traditionalists who accept the reality of a multiracial society deplore a multicultural society, arguing that strong nations need a universally accepted set of values. No doubt, the children of the old and new American societies will determine what those values are.

Other major changes that have been evolving and that affect nursing and health care are both geographic and social. The 1990 census data showed sharp rural losses, with big gains in Western and Southern metropolitan areas like Seattle, Los Angeles, and Orlando, Florida. As predicted by Naisbett in his 1982 best-seller,[4] the sunbelt continues its growth, in contrast to the decline in Northeastern and some Midwestern states. The census also reported that the family structure is different. Only 26 percent of the nation's 93.3 million households consist of the traditional family of a married couple and children under age 18, a drop from the 1970s and 1980s. There are 9.7 million single parents, mostly women. Single-parent households are three times more common among blacks than among whites, but black families have taken part in the overall trend toward family stability since the growth (not the number) of single families has slowed. Household size has continued to decline slightly, from 2.76 in 1980 to 2.63 in 1990.

The most dramatic change in age structure is the increase in the proportion of the elderly to more than 12 percent of the population, the highest in the nation's history. By the end of the century, there are likely to be 36 million Americans 65 years of age or older, about half of whom will be 76 or more. Those aged 85 or older are the fastest-growing segment of the population.

Over one-fifth of the elderly are poor or near-poor; women, blacks, and Hispanics have a higher poverty rate than men and whites. Only about 5 percent of the elderly live in institutions, but of those who do, a disproportionate number are unmarried or widowed women. However, the income level of the elderly varies greatly, and that, combined with the fact that they are better educated than ever, has enabled the elderly to influence legislation significantly, often through powerful lobbying organizations such as the American Association of Retired Persons (AARP). At the other end of the age spectrum is the declining number of persons between ages 18 and 24. The number of baby boomers (aged 25 to 44) has grown by over 25 percent. This group is seen as another potentially powerful political force, since it is the first such group to be mostly college educated; over half have attended college.

Unfortunately, there is another population that has an uncommon share of social and health problems. About one in seven Americans live below the poverty level. Child poverty is particularly sad, with one in five children under 18 and one in four under 3 being poor. One of every two black children and two of every five Hispanic children are poor. The fact that those who are already poor, undernourished, undereducated, and underemployed tend to have the most children increases the social consequences. Many of these families migrate to cities, where they become victims of drugs, AIDS, crime, prostitution, and other ills of the environment. Children of young, uneducated, unmarried mothers, little more than children themselves, may be born with crack addition, AIDS or, all too often, low birthweight, leading to mental and physical problems. Their future is bleak, for while ideas for helping the poor abound, a consensus is wanting, as is funding. (Funds for waging war and for bailing out the savings and loan industry seem to be found much more readily.

But at least the majority of the poor have homes of a sort. An estimated 600,000 to 1.2 million Americans are homeless. (Advocates of the homeless say that the figure is closer to 3 million.) Among these are youths who have come from chaotic or violent families, single males with alcohol or drug problems, and both men and women who are often mentally ill. Yet the fastest-growing segment are families, often single mothers and children, living in unsafe shelters and welfare hotels. Needless to say, the health problems of all the homeless are horrific, with tuberculosis (TB), accidents, drug-related conditions, violence, sexually transmitted diseases (STDs) including AIDS, and infections being common. Pregnancy occurs at twice the national average rate, and the babies are almost always born with serious health problems.[5] In many cities, and increasingly in suburban areas, soup kitchens are becoming common, and even those with homes come for food. People, especially children, are hungry, and this fact is beginning to reach Congress, with the hope that suitable action will follow.

There is little doubt that the poor not only lack adequate housing, nutrition, and jobs, but they also have a multitude of health problems for which they may not seek help until there is a serious need. A series of needs related to health has emerged because of their particular social, ethnic, and economic problems. The need is for readily available health services, such as neighborhood family health centers, health workers who understand the problems of the people and are able to communicate with them, understandable health teaching, and coordination of the multiple services required. Some of the more urgent health needs that have been cited are preventive, diagnostic, referral, and counseling services for pregnant women, infants, and preschool children. Equally vital are community mental health services to alleviate problems or redirect deviant behavior of individuals, families, or groups.

The Nation's Health

According to the U.S. Department of Health and Human Services (DHHS) report "Health U.S. 1990," the health status of the U.S. population as a whole is better than ever. However, the news is both good and bad. The good news is that life expectancy has reached a new height; infant mortality and the overall death rate have dropped. Two of the biggest killers of Americans, heart disease and stroke, have continued their decade-long decline, and cancer deaths, except those due to smoking-related lung cancer, are down. (Nevertheless, one startling statistic is that women's risk of developing breast cancer has risen from one in ten to one in nine).

The bad news is that the life expectancy of blacks born in 1990, although rising slightly, is still about six years less than the 75.5 years for whites. The difference seems to be due to the greater likelihood of blacks having heart attacks, cancer, and strokes, as well as an increase in auto accidents, TB and other infectious diseases, and particularly AIDS and homicide, which are the chief causes of death of black males. (In fact, the homicide rate in general increased to 9.8 slayings per 100,000 people in 1990 from 8.8 in 1989, with most concentrated in big cities. The accidental death rate did decrease. Another gap among races was in the overall death rate, with the lowest rates found among Asians in the United States in every age group and across nearly every cause of death. The death rates for whites and Hispanics were higher, with those of blacks and native Americans being almost twice as high, including the rates for children. The death rate for all races in the 25- to 34-year age group has risen, reflecting in part the AIDS epidemic. The greatest rise is in black males in this group (29 percent), with an even greater jump in the black 15- to 24-year group. However, human immunodeficiency virus (HIV) infection and AIDS is also rising for women.

There are other interesting statistics. Infant mortality (deaths of children under 1 year old) dropped by the largest amount in nearly a decade, from 9.7 deaths per 1000 in 1989 to 9.1 in 1990, a 6 percent decline, as opposed to a 2.5 decline throughout the 1980s. This is seen as very significant. Again, infant deaths are higher for blacks than for whites. The decline appears to be due to new drug therapy that helps prevent the death of premature infants and some increase in Medicaid spending for prenatal care. Still, many poor women and young girls still do not seek (or have access to) prenatal care, often resulting in premature births. As noted earlier, the birth of babies addicted to drugs and fatally infected with AIDS is becoming a growing problem. AIDS itself continues in epidemic proportions although new cases are expected to level off. Since it was first recognized in about 1981, it has killed more than 100,000 people. The Centers for Disease Control (CDC) estimates that perhaps 215,000 more will die by 1994. It is now the second leading cause of death of men 25 to 44 years of age and is probably among the top five killers of women of that age. Most of the deaths have occurred among men who have sex with other men; the next largest group are male and female intravenous drug users. Other diseases that are resurging are TB and syphilis, borne on a tide of AIDS, homelessness, and drug and alcohol abuse. According to the American Cancer Society, estimates of the highest incidence of cancer in 1991 show (in order) lung, colon/rectum, and prostate cancer leading in men and breast, colon/rectum, and lung cancer in women. These cause the most cancer deaths, but skin cancer, including melanoma, is the fastest-growing cancer. Mental illness also continues to be a problem, with one person in five affected, and according to the National Institute of Mental Health (NIMH), serious mental disorders are far more likely to strike before age 20 than experts previously believed. Teen health hazards such as suicide, accidents, and drug use may all be related to mental health problems. Another serious problem, births to teenagers, were reported as rising again in 1990 after some years of decline. There is some speculation as to whether the increase is due to decreasing availability of abortion providers or to publicity about parental consent laws. Since right-to-life groups frequently lobby against sex education as well as abortion, their successful efforts may also be a factor. One particularly controversial issue now is the availability of Norplant, a contraceptive consisting of thin capsules of a synthetic hormone implanted under the skin of a woman's upper arm that prevents contraception for five years but can be removed, and RU486, the so-called French abortion pill. These, of course, involve all women of childbearing age. (Further discussion of the related ethical/legal issues of abortion is found in Chapter 13.)

Affecting the health of all people are environmental hazards. Although few deny that pollutants of various kinds damage health, just what should be done when pollution control affects people's jobs or increases production costs has been a constant point of dispute among environmentalists, unions, industry, and government. In late 1985, the Environmental Protection Agency (EPA) listed 403 toxic chemicals manufactured, used, or stored in the United States that could pose an immediate threat to life and health. While those dealing in these toxic elements were urged to disclose the information and make changes to reduce excessive risks, compliance is voluntary. Health problems range from lung diseases to cancer to birth defects. Experts say that the highest risks to human health are outdoor and indoor air pollutants, worker exposure to chemicals in industry and agriculture, and pollutants in drinking water. Among these hazards are those to which nurses are exposed every day,[6,7] including chemicals, antineoplastic drugs, and communicable diseases. Some occupational diseases have been identified, and to varying degrees, safety standards have been set and are enforced by the Occupational Safety and Health Administration (OSHA), as well as the EPA. However, enforcement seems to vary according to the attitude of the federal government as administrations change. Under fire have been various OSHA actions, including OSHA rules on hepatitis B, AIDS, and other bloodborne diseases to which health care workers are exposed,[8] especially when the employer refuses to acknowledge responsibility. On the other hand, the fact that in 1991 OSHA was working on the issue of smoking in the workplace was generally approved by health care workers. Finally, many nurses are actively working to improve or eliminate environmental hazards in general. One example is the rapid depletion of the ozone layer that protects the earth from too much ultraviolet light. The Nurses' Environmental Watch provides nurses and others with information about such hazards.

Even though the impact of more sophisticated diagnostic tools, drugs, and surgery has been recognized, prevention is generally acknowledged to be a factor in improving health statistics. One-third of the deaths caused by heart disease, cancer, strokes, accidents, and pulmonary disease could have been prevented by modifying just three risk factors: smoking, hypertension, and alcohol abuse. There are data showing that a balanced diet and exercise also reduce cardiopulmonary disease. Therefore, it is not surprising that the country's official health objectives for 1990, as announced by DHHS, focused on health promotion and disease prevention.

The five broad national goals proposed in the DHHS document *Healthy People 2000: Health Promotion and Disease Prevention* are as follows:

- Reduce infant mortality to no more than 7 per 1000 live births.
- Increase life expectancy to at least 78 years.
- Reduce disability caused by chronic conditions to no more than 7 percent of all people.
- Increase the number of healthy years of life to at least 65.
- Decrease the disparity in life expectancy between white and minority populations to no more than 4 years.

Some of the most important specific objectives are as follows:

- Improve nutrition.
- Improve surveillance and data systems.
- Increase physical activity and fitness.
- Reduce tobacco use.
- Reduce alcohol and other drug problems.
- Encourage responsible sexual behavior.
- Reduce violent behavior.
- Maintain the vitality and independence of older people.
- Improve environmental health.
- Improve occupational safety and health.
- Prevent unintentional injuries.
- Improve maternal and infant health.
- Improve immunization for infectious diseases.
- Reduce HIV infection.
- Reduce the incidence of sexually transmitted diseases.
- Reduce high blood cholesterol and high blood pressure.
- Reduce the toll from cancer.
- Reduce other chronic disorders.
- Improve oral health.
- Prevent mental and behavioral disorders.
- Improve health education and preventive services.

This is a tall order, particularly when health-related organizations promptly began to suggest additions and changes. Nevertheless, it will be interesting to see how much can be accomplished in the 1990s, particularly since prevention activities have had their ups and downs. With the focus on health promotion and disease prevention, nurses should be especially involved, even taking a leadership position in working toward achievement of these goals.

Not resolved, but a serious issue for the people's health, is the problem of access to care; this is discussed later in this chapter and in Chapter 9.

Many of these social and health problems are international, with the addition of serious overpopulation, famine, and war in Third World countries.[9] While the World Health Organization (WHO) goal of health for all by the year 2000 (HFA/2000) does not seem possible, particularly when 40 million people are expected to be HIV-infected by then, there is hope that progress in child health is now a practical goal. One child in three is still malnourished, but successes have been achieved in saving lives through immunization and oral rehydration therapy. The World Bank and other agencies have pledged increased aid to poor children, for healthy people are seen as the key to development. American nurses, with increased interest and participation in international nursing, especially in the Third World, are often involved in these efforts.

Technological and Scientific Advances

The technological advances of the last quarter-century have been extraordinary. Some of the most significant advances affecting patient care can be categorized as follows:

1. Developments in diagnosis and patient care, such as automated clinical laboratory equipment; organ transplants; artificial human organs and parts; improved surgical techniques and equipment, such as microsurgery and laser beams; genetic engineering; and the use of the computer and new imaging techniques in diagnosis.
2. Hospital information management—mainly due to application of the computer for patient billing, accounting, and patient records. Methods are being developed to control the flow of information so that health care practitioners can have ready access to necessary data, and can have information transmitted quickly and accurately to all departments.
3. Developments affecting hospital supply and services, such as widespread adoption of plastic and other inexpensive disposable materials, and such equipment as specialized carts, conveyers, and pneumatic tubes.
4. Improvements in the management and structural design of health facilities aimed at more efficient utilization of personnel, equipment, and space. This involves improved concepts of management and construction of health facilities, based on advances in the organization of health care services.
5. Mass communication, making possible speedy transmission of health information and new knowledge, and exerting a powerful influence in molding public opinion. It can bring about positive results, such as providing information on communicable diseases and ways in which to get help; it can provide knowledge about other social and health problems, and even provide formal educational programs.

Although there is undeniable progress in health care directly attributable to technology, there is also great fear that the more machines do, the less human interaction there will be. Naisbitt commented on these points by noting that the enforced high technology in health care, especially in hospitals, has created an immediate counterpart that he calls "high-tech/high touch." Among examples of high-touch, he listed hospice care, birthing rooms, neighborhood clinics, and primary nursing.[10] He also noted that computers could allow for a more humanistic touch because of the ability to reach out and stay in touch with people and to share information. The information society has replaced the industrial society, he claims, with new jobs being created in the information and service sectors, not the manufacturing fields.[11] In a later follow-up, he noted that by 1990 women had already taken two-thirds of the new jobs created in the information era and would continue to do so into the millennium. Naisbett's predictions are discussed later in this chapter.

Computers have had a definite impact on organizational structures such as hospitals. Hospital information systems (HISs) are expected to promote efficiency, but have proved in some cases that they can be both disturbing and disruptive to those already employed. If they are not appropriately selected, introduced, and used, communication can be less effective than expected. The greatest impetus to the development of nursing information systems (NISs) came about when Medicare-Medicaid coverage required nurses to provide data needed for reimbursement and to document the care given both in hospitals and in community health agencies. Effective use of computer systems in health care organizations requires that nurses be critical of the systems they evaluate and use, which means that they must learn about computers and what they can do. They must also help clarify and standardize the nursing data base.

Over the last several years, a great deal has been written in the nursing literature about the use of computers in education and practice. The variety of uses continually increases, and more nurses are becoming computer experts.[12] An important point made is that nurses, like others, must find fast, effective ways to turn raw data into useful organized information. NISs can improve both the cost effectiveness and the quality of care, possibly even helping to alleviate the nursing shortage, as nurses can be helped to use their time in the most effective possible ways. Among the ways health care information systems (HCISs) can be applied are systems that assist in patient assessment and classification, care planning, charting and documenting care, quality assurance, discharge planning, staffing and scheduling and tracking acuity, cost, and quality data. Computer terminals at the patient's bedside, in the examining room, and even in the patient's home can ease data entry, improve accuracy, and eliminate duplication of information. If used properly, computers can also improve exchange of information between nurses and other health care professionals and staff.[13]

In addition, computer technology is increasingly being used in nursing education and research. Computer-assisted instruction (CAI) is used in such areas as drill and practice, simulations, and tutorials. Nursing informatics courses are being offered (or required) in many schools of nursing. Much nursing research also depends on competent use of computer technology, whether related to clinical data collection or to retrieval of information from libraries, as described in Chapter 14. The increase in the use of electronic media is demonstrated in the new Sigma Theta Tau Center for Nursing

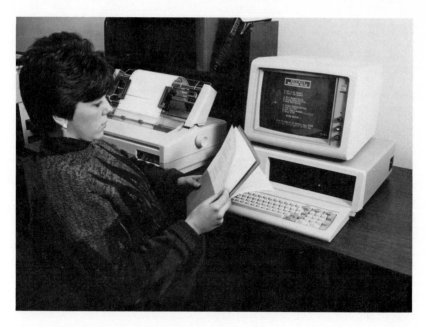

Computers are playing an important role in health care communications. (*Courtesy of the National Student Nurses' Association.*)

Scholarship International Library in Indianapolis, where just about all information will be in computerized form.

There is no question that the use of computers in health care institutions and agencies will escalate. Experts repeatedly identify computer technology as essential to improvement in health care. Particularly named are fully integrated information systems that link patient care with everything from accounting to materials management, computer-assisted clinical prescribing and monitoring of drug interactions, and computerized patient records, including bedside information systems. For nurses, this means learning to use the new technology for the benefit of the patient but continually maintaining the emphasis on individuality and human contact, which no machine can provide, as well as protecting the patient's privacy, that is, the question of security of information. In the last decade, computer experts have made headlines with their ability to invade the computers of banks, hospitals, industry, and even the government, in some cases changing or erasing data. While others had already used the computer to commit crimes (and were not always caught and punished), this new danger has reinforced earlier concerns about the confidentiality of computer-stored information. Would an employer, or simply a curious individual, be able to review another individual's credit record or hospital record? For that matter, would the record be accurate? Anyone who has had to deal with the unresponsive computers of businesses and the government knows the difficulty of catching and correcting errors; computer input still has a human component. All this has implications for nurses and their ethical responsibilities.

Education

Trends in education affect nursing in a number of ways: (1) the kind, number, and quality of students entering the nursing programs and the background they bring with them; (2) the development of educational technology, which frequently becomes a part of nursing education; and (3) the impact of social demands on education, which are eventually extended to education in the professions, including nursing. Usually it is not just one social or economic condition that brings about change in education, nor is there only one kind of change. For instance, overexpansion by most institutions of higher education when the baby boom was at its height created a large pool of unemployed college graduates in the early 1970s. Some of these, as well as college students with a worried eye to the future, looked for educational programs that seemed to promise immediate jobs with a future, among them nursing. Thus, what had once been a trickle of mature, second-degree students into nursing became a steady stream. As the baby boom group diminished, the overextended institutions of higher education and individual programs found it necessary to use marketing strategies of all kinds to attract enough students. They discovered the working adults in the community, who were a relatively untapped pool.

There were several definitive results. The diversity of age, background, education, and life experience in those seeking (or being sought for) advanced education has been an important factor in both social and political pressures for more flexibility in higher education. At the same time, providing such flexibility is one of the marketing strategies educational institutions are, after considerable resistance, relying on to attract the older prospective student. One focus is on liberalizing the ways in which individuals can receive academic credit for what they know, regardless of when, where, or how they acquired that knowledge. Credentials are viable currency in the struggle for upward mobility, and those in the health field are as eager as others in society to be a part of this movement. In general education, the concepts of independent study and credit by examination have been explored by an increasing number of colleges, and a variety of testing mechanisms are being used to grant credit, including teacher-made tests and standardized tests, which have wide acceptance. One example of the latter is the College Level Examination Program (CLEP), which includes tests of general education and numerous examinations in individuals courses for which a number of colleges and universities award credit.

Other examples are the so-called external degree programs. Some are marginally legitimate operations that have given the whole concept a bad name with meaningless mail-order degrees, but more and more respected, accredited educational institutions have established external degree programs using various modes: weekend, evening, summer, or other time periods for concentrated classes; outreach programs for isolated areas or even the workplace; self-study courses with examinations; and a process of combining educational credentials and examination results. A particularly successful example of the last is the Regents College Degrees, previously the New York Regents External Degree Program, which includes both associate and baccalaureate degrees in nursing. (See Chapter 5 for more detailed information on this and other open curriculum practices in nursing.)

It was predicted that an aid to these new educational or flexible patterns was the use of all types of audiovisual media, computers, programmed learning, and other new techniques that can enhance the teaching-learning process. Although these methods appear to be generally successful, they are expensive, and there is some argument as to whether the learning acquired is superior to that gained by more traditional methods. One great asset appears to be that learning can be individualized more easily through the use of these techniques and also that satisfactory learning can occur in places other than the classroom and in the teacher's presence.

Equally significant are other happenings in higher education. Cost, to students and institutions, is an ongoing controversial issue. As costs go up for institutions, governmental aid declines, and there are not as many tax benefits in charitable giving. Colleges and universities have a major problem in balancing costs, quality, and service to students. Two-year colleges, which have shown a decline in enrollment in recent years, are under particular pressure because of their very low tuitions. There are also criticisms that relatively few students continued their education in a four-year college and that the dropout rate is high. On the other hand, despite the cry for higher quality, there is less state interest (and sometimes simply a lack of funds) for improving the public community colleges. Thus, many junior colleges have found it necessary to raise tuition and to market themselves vigorously to attract more students. There now seems to be a trend toward enrollment of more traditional-age students, in part because of the relatively low costs and transferability of credits. The financial problems of some four-year colleges are also serious; many smaller colleges have been forced to close their doors, as have some nursing programs.

The cost of a college education is outpacing inflation. The nontraditional students, although welcomed by institutions of higher learning, have found costs particularly serious since they are often not eligible for funding, which is primarily reserved for full-time students. In testimony to Congress, the point was made that part-time students who must work often do not have the funds to pay high tuition. This may have had an impact in nursing; in

1989, some nurse traineeship funds were made available for the first time for part-time students, although certain restrictions were put on the grants. However, all students who need funding may have problems in the next few years, since federal funding has shifted from grants that do not have to be repaid to loans. Experts say that this will have a particular impact on the low-income group, since students from poor families are reluctant to go into debt for education. Consequently, many students take more than six years to complete a baccalaureate; over half of the black and Hispanic students drop out for good.

Another point of interest is information about the attitudes and characteristics of today's undergraduates.[14] The Chronicle of Higher Education publishes a survey of attitudes and characteristics of freshman every year. Although nursing still does not have enough appropriately prepared faculty in any of its educational programs (in fact, a shortage is looming), the economic pressures of the times affect these faculties, as well as others in higher education. They share common concerns: heavier teaching loads; salary reductions; attacks on tenure; attacks on collective bargaining; and criticisms of the quality of teaching. In addition, there seems to have been an increase in court decisions regarding sexual harassment, sexual discrimination (in salaries, promotion, and retirement benefits), faculty rights, and civil rights. How these trends, issues, and pressures affect nursing is specifically discussed in Chapters 5 and 13.

Finally the quality of students who enter nursing and what they are prepared for can also be traced back to what happens in general education. Concern about poor education was voiced in several major reports,[15] all of which made strong recommendations. Five years after the declaration that a "rising tide of mediocrity" had eroded the quality of American education, a new Secretary of Education stated that schools had improved, but not enough.[16] While this information might seem to be of only general interest, the reality is that such educational issues not only relate to the society in which we find ourselves, but for nurses, it has meaning, as do the college statistics, for the kinds of students who may or may not enter nursing as well as the kinds of patients they deal with.

The Consumer Revolution

The consumer revolution, said to have begun when Theodore Roosevelt signed the first Pure Food and Drug Act in 1906, has been an accelerating phenomenon since the 1950s. Although various interpretations are given to the term, it might be broadly defined as the concerted action of the public in response to a lack of satisfaction with the products and/or services of various groups. The groups comprising the "public" are, of course, different, but they often overlap: a woman unhappy about the cost and quality of auto repairs might be just as displeased by the services of her gynecologist, the cost of hospital care, or the use of dangerous food additives.

There have always been dissatisfied consumers, but the major difference now is that many are organized and have the power, through money, numbers, and influence, to force providers to be responsive to at least some of their demands. The methods vary but include lobbying for legislation, legal suits, boycotts, and media campaigns. There is an increasingly strong force moving in that direction, especially with the better-educated and more aggressive baby boomers and elderly consumers. Consumers, who first concentrated their efforts against the shoddy workmanship and indifferent services offered in material goods, have now turned to the quality, quantity, and cost of other services, particularly in health care. Fewer patient/clients are accepting without protest the "I know best" attitudes of health care providers. The self-help movement, in which people learn about health care and help each other ("stroke clubs" and Alcoholics Anonymous, for instance), has extended to self-examination—sometimes through classes sponsored by doctors, nurses, and health agencies. Interest in health promotion and illness prevention has also been demonstrated by the involvement of consumers in environmental concerns.

The dehumanization of patient care, which is contrary to all the stated beliefs of the professions involved, is repeatedly cited in studies of health care. Although complaints often are directed at the care of the poor, it is a universal health care deficiency. The concerted action of organized minority groups led to the development of the American Hospital Association's Patient Bill of Rights. It received widespread attention in 1973, followed by a rash of similar rights statements specifically directed to children, the mentally ill, the elderly, pregnant women, the dying, the handicapped, patients of various religions, and others. In some cases, presidential conferences and legislation followed. The whole area of the rights of people in health care settings, which focuses to a great extent on patients' rights, has major implications for nurses (see Chapter 13).

An excellent example of the rise of a health consumer group is the women's health movement, which emerged from women's disenchantment with their personal and institutional health relationships. It came into existence around 1970 and is now worldwide. Among the best known of its activities are the various feminist health centers and their know-your-body and self-help courses and books.

Other consumers are also concerned with the power issue and are insisting on such rights as participation in governing boards of hospitals and other community health institutions, accrediting boards, health planning groups, and licensing boards. Their successes are increasing, and Naisbitt predicted that this trend will continue.

Historically, nurses have been consumer advocates, both as individuals and through their organizations. This is a particularly good time to march together to improve or refocus health care, because both have similar concerns. For instance, the Conference of Consumer Organizations (COCO) has identified key issues that include the need for more preventive health care programs, primary health care centers, and alternatives to conventional health care delivery systems; better reimbursement for prevention; rectifying maldistribution of health personnel; and dealing with environmental hazards. Nurses are also addressing these issues. COCO has challenged nurses to work with them to gain input into such policy decisions that ultimately affect everyone.[17]

The Women's Movement

Nursing, from its American beginning, was primarily made up of women, and some nurses have always been involved in the women's movement to some degree. However, feminist women and nurses have historically had an uneasy alliance. A group of nurse activists describe this relationship as follows:

> Much of the energy in the women's movement has been directed toward opening up nontraditional fields of study and work for women. Nursing has been seen as one of the ultimate female ghettos from which women should be encouraged to escape. . . . Feminists have sometimes failed to look beyond the inaccurate sexist stereotypes of nurses and to acknowledge the multiple dimensions of professional nursing.[18]

Even today, there is a sense that many in the women's movement have been coopted into accepting men's values to define success and do not value traditional feminine values, such as caring.[19] Therefore, they look down on professions that consider caring an innate part of their practice. Obviously, nursing is one of these professions.

Women in all walks of life still face many formidable economic, social, and political barriers. But despite disagreements, the success of the women's movement attests to the fervor and commitment with which they have fought to improve women's status. It is no surprise that the women's movement has been considered one of the major phenomena of the mid-twentieth century. Over the years, there has been a proliferation of women's organizations concerned with women's rights. Among the most active groups is the National Organization for Women (NOW), founded in 1966 and made up of women and men who support "full equality for women in truly equal partnership with men" and ask for an end to discrimination and prejudice against women in every field of importance in American society.

The founding of NOW offered one of the most politically radical agendas of the twentieth century: men and women would share equally in public and private responsibilities—in paid work and in the rearing of children.

NOW's activities are directed toward legislative action to end discrimination, and it attempts to promote its views through demonstrations, research, litigation, and political pressure. Among actions taken are the development of a model rape law and endorsement of health education for women in self-help clinics. It is interesting that the first president of NOW, Wilma Scott Heide, was a nurse and feminist, demonstrating that nursing and feminism can find common ground.

Another prominent women's organization is the National Women's Political Caucus (NWPC). It was founded in 1971 as the first national political organization to promote women's entry into politics at leadership levels. The main thrust of the NWPC is to ensure that women's issues are given more attention by facilitating the election of women to political office.

In addition to the League of Women Voters and the American Association of University Women, there are other important women's organizations such as the Women's Research and Education Institute, the National Women's Educational Fund, over 600 women's business organizations, and hundreds of women's sections and networks of major organizations.

Although many of the issues that women have confronted over the past 25 years remain unresolved, the women's movement has been the major catalyst in raising awareness of women's issues and opening discussions on sex discrimination and women's rights. The impact of the movement can be observed in newspaper reports, which show that both legal and social changes are occurring, slowly but surely, in relation to women's roles. A sudden, overwhelming about-face by men (and women) in terms of what women are, and can be, is not expected; attitudes are too deeply embedded. There is also insurmountable evidence that children are socialized into stereotyped male and female roles by books, use of toys, and influence of parents, teachers, and others—a problem that feminists and others continue to address. According to NOW, "A feminist is a person who believes women (even as men) are primarily people; that human rights are indivisible by any category of sex, race, class or other designation irrelevant to our common humanity; a feminist is committed to creating the equality (not sameness) of the sexes legally, socially, educationally, psychologically, politically, religiously, economically in all the rights and responsibilities of life."

Certainly these negative attitudes are not merely American. Reports from the United Nations' Decade for Women Conference in 1985 show that discrimination and inequality are still widespread. In 1979, the United Nations General Assembly adopted "what is essentially an international bill of rights for women." However, the treaty, known as the United Nations Convention on Elimination of All Forms of Discrimination Against Women, has yet to gain worldwide recognition or acceptance. As of 1990, 101 countries had ratified the treaty, and few had made any significant efforts to eliminate discrimination against women. Notably, although the United States was part of the General Assembly consensus in adopting the convention, the U.S. Senate has yet to ratify it.

In the United States, resistance to the women's movement is epitomized by the death of the proposed Equal Rights Amendment (ERA) to the Constitution, 3 states short of the 38 needed for ratification. Ten years after it was passed by Congress, and despite an extension of the deadline for ratification from 1979 to 1982, Indiana in 1977 was the last state to ratify it. More than 450 national organizations endorsed the amendment, and polls showed that more than two-thirds of U.S. citizens supported it, but to no avail. The conservative opposition, including fundamentalist Christian churches, the so-called Moral Majority, the John Birch Society, the Mormon Church, and the American Farm Bureau, led a well-financed, smoothly organized, and politically astute campaign. Antiamendment forces assured state legislators that the Fourteenth Amendment offered sufficient protection to women and claimed that the ERA would cause the death of the family by removing a man's obligation to support his wife and children, would legalize homosexual marriages, would lead to unisex toilets, and most damaging, would lead to the drafting of women for combat duty. Advocates of the ERA were later criticized as lacking political finesse and alienating women who were potential supporters—blacks, pink-collar (office) workers, and housewives. Amendment supporters lay heavy blame on men, particularly in legislatures and business. After the defeat, the 50,000-member Eagle Forum, and its founder, Phyllis Schlafly, the woman considered the leader of the anti-ERA forces, laid plans to campaign against sex education, the nuclear freeze, and "undesirable" textbooks.

In the 1980s and early 1990s, feminists determined to concentrate women's new consciousness and resources in building legislative strength to eventually pass the ERA and to mount a campaign for reproductive freedom, democratization of families, more respect for work done in the home, and comparable pay for the work done outside it.

Some 25 years after Betty Friedan published *The Feminine Mystique* (called by the futurist Alvin Toffler "the book that pulled the trigger of history") changes can be clearly identified, even though some of the results have varied. In terms of the ERA, Congress voted down another ERA bill in 1983. The bill was defeated by six votes. Yet, both friends and foes of equal rights note that the campaign for the amendment, along with other social forces, made a definite impact on American life. For example, labor force participation has become the norm for most women. In 1989, women comprised 45 percent of the workforce, up from 38 percent in 1970. More women than ever before are combining responsibilities of raising children, keeping up a household, and working outside of the home. Seventy-five percent of working women work full-time. These female labor force participation rates seem to be increasing, and projections to the year 2000 call for continued increases and further convergences of male and female labor force patterns over the life cycle.

Although women's wages are still not commensurate with men's, they are improving in that regard. The ratio between what the average woman earns and what the average man earns has risen in recent years to 70 cents on the dollar, up from 62 cents in the late 1960s. In terms of education, young women aged 25 to 29 have just about closed the gap in educational attainment between men and women.

On the downside, many women and men report dissatisfaction with the toll that women's work outside the home takes on family and personal lives. In a 1989 survey, 48 percent of all women respondents said that they had to sacrifice too much for their gains, especially with regard to time spent with children and family. The labor force participation of women can be viewed as a further disadvantage when one considers the many single mothers who have no choice but to work outside of the home because they are facing severe financial hardships. These problems seem to be intensifying as the proportion of families maintained by women alone increases.

Finally, despite the narrowing of the wage gap between women and men, 59 percent of women work in low paying 'pink-collar' jobs because they are trained for nothing else, some because such jobs tend to be more compatible with childrearing. It is harder to explain why the higher women advance, the larger the wage gap between men and women. Corporate women at the vice-presidential level and above earn considerably less than their male peers.

A growing number of lawsuits and union negotiations have challenged the male-female pay ratio based on the *comparable worth* theory. This theory, going beyond equal pay for equal work, calls for equal pay for different jobs of comparable worth. The intent is to revalue *all* jobs on the basis of the skills and responsibility they require. Neither the Equal Pay Act nor the Civil Rights Act brought about reform at any level of the workforce. A landmark case resulted in the state of Washington being ordered in 1984 to pay female workers up to $1 billion in back wages and increases because of such pay inequity. However, shortly thereafter, the decision was reversed on appeal.

Generally, federal and state governments, as well as the courts, have not been supportive of the comparable worth concept. For example, in 1985, the U.S. Civil Rights Commission rejected it. That same year, a U.S. Court of Appeals ruling written by Judge Anthony M. Kennedy, who was later appointed to the Supreme Court, approved a state's relying on market rates in setting salaries even if it knowingly paid less to women as a result.

More recently, a federal judge in California ruled that California had not deliberately underpaid thousands of women in state jobs held predominantly by women, a serious blow to the country's largest lawsuit on this issue. Nonetheless, industry and business are becoming more interested in job evaluation studies, with presumably equal pay following. Also important are a series of Supreme Court rulings that ban employers from offering retirement plans that provide men and women with unequal benefits. As one justice wrote, "An individual woman may not be paid lower monthly benefits simply because women as a class live longer than men."

Certainly, individual women have made major breakthroughs on the political and scientific scenes.[20] However, despite the advances women have made over the past 30 years, the burdens of childrearing still fall disproportionately on the shoulders of women and in contrast to many Western European countries, the United States does not provide a childrearing allowance to help families with the costs of raising children. Moreover, the feminization of poverty is a very serious problem facing American society. In 1988, 53 percent of all poor families were maintained by a woman with no spouse present. This was one of the highest rates ever.

Therefore, the political and economic gains women have achieved cannot obscure (in fact, they even intensify) the need for a national consensus on family policy. Such a policy would include a guarantee that employed parents have the right to a leave after the birth or adoption of a child and are ensured of job security. In addition, child-care initiatives from the private and public sectors are important in easing the dual responsibilities of family and career that so many women face. For several years, Congress has wrestled with legislation for parental leave and child care without enacting any laws. However, the time seems ripe for laws in both of these areas as pressure from women's organizations and other groups intensifies. ANA has lobbied for passage of these laws, because of its predominantly female constituency and because of the importance of these laws for the health and welfare of the American people. In the meantime, some state legislatures and private companies have launched programs that assist families, and most often women, with regard to child care and parental leave. None of these initiatives would have evolved without the force and appeal of the women's movement.

In fact, the success of the movement is evidenced by John Naisbett, the author of *Megatrends 2000,* who referred to the 1990s as the "Decade of Women in Leadership."[21] He based his prediction on his belief that women were ready to break through the "glass ceiling," the invisible barrier that has kept them from the top, because their talents and abilities are being recognized and because they have already taken two-thirds of jobs in industries of the future. He also pointed out that the tendency to want to balance the top priorities of family and career along with other interests, once attributed to women, is becoming increasingly important in these times. He sees the emergence of a new leadership style, which focuses on quick responses to change and the ability to bring out the best in people, as symbolic of women's influence in the workplace. (These are certainly attributes that most nurses have mastered!) He describes a new type of work environment due to the growing numbers of women who work out of the home and the values they bring to their places of employment. In addition to citing the importance of the critical mass that women have reached in the professions, he predicts that benefits such as day care and family leave will increasingly be used as recruitment and retention strategies because of their importance to men and women alike, as women continue to increase their labor force participation. However, although women's issues are receiving increased attention, and changes are being made, there is still much to be done.[22]

The issue of women's rights is closely related to the problems, activities, and goals of women working in the health service industry. From 75 to 85 percent of all health service workers are women, and the largest health occupation, nursing, is almost totally female. These women-dominated occupations are also expanding most rapidly, but, as one writer indicated, "Health service is women's work but not women's power. . . The health service industry is run by a small minority. It is run primarily by physicians, who have traditionally held the power, but also by the increasingly powerful hospital administrators, insurance company directors, government regulators, medical school educators, and corporation managers. Most of these people are men."[23] Although the proportion of female physicians has increased, men continue to dominate the positions of authority within the medical system.

According to Brown, the reasons for so many women in health care is that, first, they are an inexpensive source of labor; second, they are available; and third, they are safe, that is, no threat to physicians who, in order to expand their power and income, "must be assured of subordinates who will stay subordinate."[24] The rise of nurses as autonomous practitioners certainly is a threat to that traditional power base.

Labor, Industry, and Economics

It is expected that the political pendulum that swung from liberal to conservative with the beginning of the Reagan administration will continue in that direction for some years before its inevitable return. There are a number of economic outcomes that are also expected to continue. One is more support for business and less for labor. As early as 1978, labor was losing members, primarily due to its inability to adjust to changing work patterns— a growth switch from industry to the white-collar, wholesale, and retail trades and service industries. Their loss of numbers meant a loss of political power, especially since they seemed to have less ability to influence their own members to vote a certain way. Legislators, therefore, have felt more free to vote for business interests and have done so. While union lobbying is still influential, the economic and political climate has emboldened employers in dealing with unions.[25]

What has also made it easier for management is the growing tendency of people to prefer to work part time, a trend that is predicted to increase.

Although this is particularly true of women, including nurses, who have young families or simply need to contribute to the family's income, there are also a surprising number of men who make this choice. Both women and men may be attending school, beginning their own businesses, testing a different field, working at a second job, or simply looking for more flexibility and independence. Some like the variety and the fact that they need not get involved in the politics and problems of the workplace. On the other hand, wages may be lower (not necessarily true for nurses), there is little opportunity for career advancement, and some temporary workers complain of being "dumped on" by regular employees. Industry has found these "contingency workers" economically advantageous. Employers do not usually pay for any benefits, which can be a considerable savings, and they can bring in these workers at busy times while maintaining a minimum workforce. Employing part-timers provides a way around union work rules and, at times, a way to confront striking unions. The negative side is that part-time or short-term workers may not have the same commitment to the company, and unless they return to the same place frequently, they need orientation and perhaps even training. Yet, it is quite possible that the availability of these workers and full-time replacements has made strikes a less popular union tool. In the 1970s, the average number of strikes per year was 289; in the late 1980s, it was 52.

Despite these problems, by the beginning of 1990 there was some optimism in the ranks of labor. For the first time in over a decade, younger, more sophisticated labor leaders had replaced nearly all the old guard. Also, both labor and industry were stressing the need for harmony. The year 1989 had seen union membership grow, although with a greater growth in the workforce, the percentage continued to diminish (16.4 percent as opposed to the previous low of 23 percent in 1977). There was considerable growth in governmental unions, but the service industries, accounting for most of the growth in the labor force, had only 6 percent union participation. All seemed to be good candidates for organization. Because women are a large part of the latter group (they are also considered easier to organize), the unions are beginning to tackle women's issues such as abortion, and the safety of women on the job. However, their interest has not extended to placing women in the top echelon of the labor federation's hierarchy.

All this has had several effects on health care. First, unions are busy trying to organize workers in health care, including the whole gamut of clerical, technical, and clinical workers and professionals, including nurses and physicians. The ANA has also stepped up its campaign to organize RNs, both because of the belief that ANA can serve nurses better and because these other unions could potentially influence the direction of nursing politically through their organized numbers of nurses. Both groups have had some success, in part because of the dissatisfaction of workers in health care.

This is also true in other fields. Management, criticized for its authoritarian approach, is trying new techniques to increase worker satisfaction. While far from widespread, there does seem to be growing interest in involving workers in decision making. Some labor experts say that these "reforms" (known by such names as *quality circles, job redesign, work humanization, employee participation, workplace democracy,* and *quality of work life*) are more cosmetic than real, since few workers participate in the companies' most important decisions, and that in a difficult situation most managers revert to an authoritarian stance. Others say that this new management style is necessary now that the nation is engaged in vigorous international competition. Whether there will be backsliding when economic times are better is the question. Nevertheless, one long-standing hit on the best-seller list in 1982, and still considered valid, was a book that delineated the management style of America's best-run and most successful corporations.[26] Emphasized were a bias for action; satisfying the consumer; fostering autonomy and entrepreneurship throughout the organization; showing respect for the individual; hands-on involvement (going to the workers); and clarity of company values. In later books, the authors added "flexibility" because of the chaotic times. Many of these qualities seem to tie in with worker satisfaction and commitment to the job, and are also seen in the studies of the successful magnet hospitals described in Chapter 8.

Future Trends

Preparing today for the future so that a profession, group, or individual will be in the forefront is often advised. Futurists have become popular writers and speakers, with their books often hitting the best-seller list. It has been noted that making predictions is a much more popular activity than evaluating their accuracy. Toffler's *Third Wave*[27] and *Powershift*[28] were popular publications and present some provocative ideas.

By 1990, a number of Toffler's predictions proved to be accurate. Naisbett, who feels that it is not possible to predict more than about 10 years in advance, recapped his predictions in a new book, *Megatrends 2000: Ten New Directions for the 1990's,* and noted that they were pretty much on schedule. His new trends related primarily to emerging international economic changes, but he also predicted a renaissance in the arts and a religious revival. As mentioned earlier, of particular interest to nurses is his designation of the 1990s as a decade of women in leadership. Another of his major trends focused on "the age of biology." While he praised the value of both current and emerging research in biotechnology, he also predicted that related ethical problems would increase. Finally, Naisbett celebrated the "triumph of the individual," stating that recognition of the individual was the thread connecting every trend in the book and that the new responsibility of society was to reward the initiative of the individual.[29]

Of the various reports about trends, especially commissioned for health care organizations, discussed later, several factors are mentioned repeatedly as having a major impact on health care: the more sophisticated activist consumers with their demand for quality; the changing demographics, especially the increased number of the aging; the cost of health care in competition with other social needs; and the changing involvement of government.

There are also those who say that in predicting the future, the only certainty is change. The futurists have said that no matter how strong trends seem, there is something called "unintended consequences," which occurs when people decide that they really don't like the direction of the trends and work to change them. As Naisbett says, "Today there is a new possibility: the individual can influence reality by identifying the direction in which society is headed. Knowledge is power. . . . even if you do not endorse the direction of a trend, you are empowered by your knowledge about it. You may choose to challenge the trends, but first you must know where they are headed.[30]

As you read the overview of the many elements of health care delivery that follow, it is useful to keep in mind all the changes that are putting pressure on the system and how they might affect nurses in this, their workplace, and beyond.

ISSUES IN HEALTH CARE

Before describing where and by whom health care is delivered, it is essential to understand some of the changes that have occurred in the last several decades—changes that relate directly to the public's concern about the cost and quality of health care. As often happens, the public's dissatisfaction with something becomes translated into legislation by those they elected. In this case, because the cost of health care was (and is) rising so rapidly, executive branch regulations, both on the national and state levels, also began to clamp down on the people (providers) and places delivering health care. (See Chapter 10 on how laws are made and how legislation affects health care.) The reason governmental impact is so great is that most health care facilities and many providers are funded, one way or another, by the government. Moreover, others who pay for health care (payers) such as health insurance companies, including the well-known Blue Cross and Blue Shield, tend to follow the patterns of payment set by the government.

Health care in the United States (frequently criticized as more likely to be "sick care") devours more than 11 percent of the gross national product (GNP), with a steady, sometimes massive increase in the last decades that exceeds that of any other advanced country. A variety of factors have been

blamed. Both Medicare and Medicaid and most health insurance plans traditionally have paid for the "full and reasonable" cost of care on a retrospective basis, that is, whatever the provider said it cost, within certain
limits. (Medicare/Medicaid law and its changes are described more fully in
Chapter 10.) With the high cost of new technology used for both diagnosis
and treatment and the consumer demand for the newest and the best, costs
soared. In 1983, because of fear that Medicare funds would run out, a new
form of payment was devised.[31] Under this prospective payment system
(PPS), disorders of the human body were divided into major diagnostic
categories with (currently) 477 subgroups called *diagnostic related groups
(DRGs)*. Now the payment for services that hospitals receive per discharge
patient is determined based on the patient's principal diagnosis and the
predetermined length of hospitalization considered suitable for that diagnosis. Certain other factors are considered (outliers), and some hospitals are
exempted. One problem for health care institutions, public health agencies,
and physicians is that reimbursement can be denied retroactively, after the
service has been given, and the amount of documentation needed is both
specific and voluminous. Another concern has been whether the relative
severity of the patient's illness is considered, especially in relation to the
nursing care needed.[32] "Acuity levels" are sometimes used to bill for nursing
services, as opposed to including nursing as a part of the room charge.) On
the other hand, if the patient is discharged more rapidly, hospitals may keep
the full amount of the designated reimbursement. This has resulted in accusations that patients are being discharged "sicker and quicker," with more
complex (and new), highly technological care required in the home or nursing
home. (Both of these services are also under tight fiscal constraints.)[33,34]
Hospital utilization was at first greatly reduced, and patients were considerably sicker since there were no grace periods of early admission for tests,
now to be done on an outpatient basis, and leisurely postacuity or postsurgical
recovery before discharge.

Since the Reagan administration encouraged competition and the introduction of cost-saving approaches, several changes resulted as some hospitals found themselves in a financial bind. One was aggressive marketing,
aimed particularly at self-paying patients and those with insurance. From
nothing in 1980, $1 *billion* a year was spent on marketing by 1990. Although
it is sometimes denied, administrators encouraged physicians to admit patients who were likely to be dischargeable early. Some hospitals, particularly
the for-profit chains, closed units that were costly and unlikely to be fully
reimbursed, such as burn units and trauma units. "Patient dumping," transferring certain patients to governmental hospitals, was another cost-saving
technique[35] although in 1989 a law was enacted penalizing hospitals that
dump. Hospitals looked for other ways to fill beds with paying patients,
such as those requiring long-term care. As described later, they formed
satellite clinics, emergicenters, surgicenters and home care services. They

used helicopters to bring in emergency patients from distant areas and advertised their services and their physicians in media campaigns. Some created profit-making components that included equipment rental, health promotion and teaching classes, and even hotels and contracts with noted fast-food companies. They merged with other hospitals or agencies to share services, sometimes even developing into national chains. In all these activities, they mimicked the more businesslike for-profit hospitals or hospital chains. These had long since used those tactics to increase profitability, even creating health-care malls, which include doctors' offices, a hospital, ambulatory care, laboratory, pharmacy, optometry, physical therapy and physical fitness services, as well as home care services, restaurants, gift shops, banking, and parking. While such "copy-cat economics" was criticized, nonprofit hospitals maintained that these approaches were needed for survival. In fact, in the 1980s, many small hospitals, especially in rural areas, simply went out of business, despite the needs of the population, and more closures are predicted for the 1990s.

Even with these limitations on reimbursements, health care costs continued to soar faster than the inflation rate. There were still too many empty beds and too much expensive technology used. To add to the costs, AIDS patients began to fill hospital beds and draw on complex home care services. According to an AHA report in 1990, the care for AIDS patients was $1.1 billion in 1989 and is expected to increase astronomically, more than half of it covered by Medicaid. (President Reagan's AIDS commission claimed that it might go up to $15 billion.) Only care for automobile accident victims and cardiac patients will be more costly, and it has been said that AIDS will be with us forever. Another major problem for private hospitals is the care of the uninsured, estimated by some at more than 37 million nationwide. These people are not unemployed but are the working poor, not covered by health insurance or federal programs and unable to afford private health insurance, or those with very limited insurance.[36] Then there are the homeless who come to emergency rooms, also without Medicaid, even though they may be eligible.

Hospitals have always given free care, and usually the cost was absorbed by increasing the bills of paying patients. Now this practice, too, is backfiring, since most of these patients are insured. Many health insurers have put into effect a system, somewhat like that of the government, in which a company employee, reviewing the patient's record and/or a predetermined list, approves or denies payment. In some cases, the approval must be received before treatment. Even so, as the cost of insurance premiums rises, employers, particularly large corporations, are resisting these increases and looking for ways to lower health care costs.[37] Small companies may simply drop this employee benefit. One approach, used especially by large corporations, has been "managed care." There are a number of versions, but the idea is for the large employer to come to an agreement with one or more hospitals, groups of physicians, or a health maintenance organization (HMO) in which a certain number of potential patients (the employees) are guaranteed at a set, discounted price. In some cases, employees choosing not to participate must pay a larger health insurance premium. Freedom of choice for such employees is declining because these preferred provider organizations (PPOs) are being used more and more often. In 1984, 85 percent of all employee coverage was by unmanaged fee-for-service plans allowing free choice; in 1988, only 28 percent had such choices. Some companies are also less likely to simply approve a bill or a procedure, since there is a known tendency for some physicians to perform unnecessary surgery; others reward employees who have healthy lifestyles or even pay back those who do not use their health benefits. In addition, employees are being required to pay for a greater part of their health insurance or a larger deductible.

A combination of all these factors has brought back interest in national health insurance, a concept that has not been popular since the Great Society years of the Johnson administration.[38] Except for South Africa, the United States is the only industrialized nation without a form of national health insurance. Nevertheless, the government expected to spend $156 billion on Medicare and Medicaid in 1991. While there seems to be a trend in those other countries to privatize a portion of their health care, and certainly there are problems, including high costs, several national polls of Americans showed that they were interested in a national health insurance system such as Canada's[39] although it also has gaps.[40] Actually, both the ANA and the NLN, as well as the American Public Health Association (APHA), have supported this concept for years, but the American Medical Association (AMA) and other powerful groups that influence health policy have opposed it. Only a few years ago, it was predicted that there would be no national health insurance in the foreseeable future. Whether such a system will indeed be put in place is not clear. However, given the burden of caring for the uninsured, there is a movement to provide some kind of program. Massachusetts and Hawaii were the first states to put one in place, requiring employers to provide insurance while providing some state support. Yet, financial problems plague many of these plans.[41] Meanwhile, just about everyone agrees that unnecessary use of health care should be curbed, and some of the power figures insist that the way to do that is to shift more of the financial burden to workers. There is some evidence that those who are insured make little effort to limit utilization or search for the best services for the least cost. Of course, such information is not always easy to come by, although consumer advocates are making some progress in having providers or the government present cost and quality information. Meanwhile, the issue of access to care, that is, who gets what when resources are limited, is becoming a serious ethical problem. (This is explored in more depth in Chapter 9.)

Perhaps because of this limited access for both uninsured and Medicaid patients, as well as for some others, there has been a surge of plans for various forms of health care coverage.[42,43] Some have been suggested by physicians, some by consumer groups, some by congressional committees, and some by nursing groups. They range from recommendations to expand Medicaid and Medicare, to employer-based financing approaches, to shared public-private financing. Nursing's National Health Proposal, developed primarily by the Tri Council for Nursing made up of the NLN, the ANA, the American Association of Colleges of Nursing (AACN), and the American Organization of Nurse Executives (AONE), was presented to the public in February 1991. Its major components were (1) a federally defined "standard package" of essential health care benefits, including primary care and prevention, available to all citizens and residents of the United States, and provided and financed by a mix of public and private sources; (2) improved consumer access by delivering primary care services in convenient settings such as schools, the workplace, the home, and others; (3) control of health care costs through managed care, incentives for consumers and providers, consumer freedom of choice concerning providers, settings, and delivery arrangements, reduced administrative costs via simplified bureaucratic controls and administrative procedures, and payment policies tied to the results of effectiveness and outcomes research; and (4) implementation of the plan though incremental steps, with priority status in allocation of resources given to pregnant women, infants, and children. Initial focus on these groups was seen as a cost-effective investment in the future health and prosperity of the nation.

The strategy was to involve consumers, who are often left out of such planning, and to position nurses as "cost-saving providers," who, as gatekeepers in a managed care system, would encourage more appropriate care.[44] Needless to say, there were criticisms of this plan, as well as of the others, based to a large extent on the questions of funding and cost. Even when there is no agreement about *which* plan is most feasible, almost no one believes that things can go on as they are. The federal government predicts that national health care expenditures will reach $1.5 *trillion* by the year 2000, 15 to 17 percent of the GNP. The task is formidable, especially for a country that prides itself on its autonomy, diversity, and pluralism, as shown in this chapter, in relation to health care delivery.

Another serious issue is quality of care. Accusations that quality is not commensurate with cost are heard from many sources. Beyond state licensing of hospitals and other health care facilities and agencies, which presumably represents some screening for quality, the Joint Commission on Accreditation of Healthcare Organizations (JCAHO), described later, puts its stamp of approval on institutions and agencies that meet specific criteria of quality. There is some cynicism as to whether this is simply a paper tiger, but the value of accreditation is certainly evident in some circumstances: federal funding of certain kinds may require accreditation. A number of consumer groups, some formal, some loosely organized, some interested in specific kinds of care, such as nursing homes, and some servicing a large group such as the AARP, which see high-quality health care as one of their concerns, are also active in evaluating health care and/or lobbying for improvements. In addition, the federal government has released the names of hospitals with high mortality rates, which some have said is unfair because certain hospitals have more at-risk patients. There are predictions that quality of care will be a major issue in the next decade and that the public expects health practitioners to take responsibility for ensuring high-quality care. Although both physicians and nurses have peer review systems in place, to one extent or another, the warning is that unless improvements are made, government oversight, such as the federally funded peer review organizations (PROs) that assess medical necessity, appropriateness, and quality of care provided to Medicare patients to determine if Medicare should pay the hospital, will increase.

Meanwhile, health care experts continue to present varying proposals to change what many call the disarray of the American health care system (although others maintain that it has never been otherwise). These include development of or increased use of alternative systems of delivering care, most of which are discussed in the following sections.

HEALTH CARE DELIVERY: AN EXPANDING MAZE

Health care is big business, sometimes said to be the second or third largest industry in the United States, with $1.7 billion spent on health care per day. There are now about 6500 hospitals, over 19,000 long-term care facilities, and almost 11,000 home health care agencies. Uncounted but growing are a wide variety of ambulatory care services, besides the physician's single and group practice that has been traditional. Among these are surgicenters and other "centers" for urgent care, mental health, alcohol/drug addiction, renal dialysis, women's health, childbearing, adult/geriatric day care, and wholistic health. HMOs and hospices, more concepts than places, are also on the rise, while free clinics and community health centers may come and go, depending on the economy and support. Add to this an estimated 8.7 million health-related employees, 37 of every 1000 Americans, and it is easy to see why people are confused and sometimes frightened about who and what to select for their health care needs. Even nurses, who can be found in every setting, are not always clear about the system and the choices available. Following is an overview of current health care delivery, its organization, and its workers. Specific details on how the nurse may function in these various settings are presented in Chapter 7.

Self-Care

Obviously, most people spend most of their lives in a relative state of health or at a level of self-care. The World Health Organization (WHO) defines health as a "state of complete physical, mental, and social well-being, and not merely the absence of disease or infirmity." Although it serves as a broad philosophical declaration, this definition is more an optimum goal than a reality. Also frequently quoted is Parson's definition: "a state of optimal capacity of an individual for effective performance of the roles and tasks for which he has been socialized."[45] On a practical level, the Public Health Services' National Center for Health Statistics defines health implicitly in its use of "disability days," when usual activities cannot be performed.

Self-care can be defined as "a process whereby a lay person can function effectively on his own behalf in health promotion and prevention and in disease detection and treatment at the level of the primary health resource

Definitions

Primary care: "(a) a person's first contact in any given episode of illness with the health care system that leads to a decision of what must be done to help resolve his problems: and (b) the responsibility for the continuum of care, i.e., maintenance of health, evaluation and management of symptoms, and appropriate referrals."[a]

Secondary care: the point at which consulting specialty and subspeciality services are provided in either an office (group practice) or community hospital inpatient setting.

Tertiary care: the point at which highly sophisticated diagnostic, treatment or rehabilitation services are provided, frequently in university medical centers or equivalent situations.

Acute care: "those services that treat the acute phase of illness or disability and has as its purpose the restoration of normal life processes and function."[a]

Long-term care: "those services designed to provide symptomatic treatment, maintenance, and rehabilitative services for patients of all age groups in a variety of health care settings."[a]

[a]U.S. Department of Health, Education, and Welfare, *Extending the Scope of Nursing Practice* (Washington, D.C.: The Department, 1971), pp. 3–11.

in the health care system."[46] It is not new, and ranges from simply resting when tired to a more careful judgment of selecting or omitting certain foods or activities, or a semiprimary-care activity of taking one or more medications self-prescribed or prescribed by a physician at some other point of care. Health care advice comes from family, friends, neighbors, and the media (often with a product to sell). People also seek information from a health professional acquaintance, but self-care often becomes a matter of trial and error. Increasingly, with the consumer mentality, people turn to others with similar conditions. The individual gets support and reinforcement as needed but can also detect at what point he or she needs professional help. There are even programs and courses teaching specific knowledge and skills that a lay person can learn and use. Included are such aspects as taking vital signs, use and abuse of medications, when to call a doctor, and methods of health risk appraisal.[47] The sale of do-it-yourself medical tests, stethoscopes, blood pressure devices, and other medical devices for home use has become a rapidly growing big business.

As noted earlier, health promotion and health education also play a large part in maintenance of health. Lifestyle has a major influence on most serious illnesses, and those who know what the risk factors are at least have the choice of making decisions leading to better health. Experts note that the role of parents as early models for children's health beliefs is undisputed and that early experiences structure people's personal beliefs and shape their attitudes. Because this learned behavior may be deep-seated, it is often resistant to reeducation. Thus, changing undesirable eating patterns, smoking and drinking, and other aspects of the lifestyle takes more than simple information. Other determinants influencing health attitudes and behavior are both cultural and socioeconomic. Evaluative research on health education health promotion, and self-care is being done and is expected to provide helpful information on overcoming some of these obstacles.

Various polls seem to indicate that business, industry, and the public in general believe that the health care system should give more emphasis to preventive rather than curative medicine. However, reimbursement for health education is still not common, in either the public or the private sector, despite the rhetoric. And there is evidence that interest in healthy living is primarily a middle-class and upper-class concern.

The role of government was noted earlier in this chapter, but the degree of governmental follow-through on these proposals fluctuates with the vagaries of political pressures. Thus, some of the objectives set forth in the 1980 health plan were underfunded or neglected because they were not popular with a particular administration. Yet, because of rising health costs, the *idea* of health promotion and education continues to receive overt support.

A philosophical point raised frequently is whether a government has the right to legislate individual choice. Attempts to mandate the use of seat belts and motorcycle helmets have not been completely successful. The more complex problems of smoking, drug use, and pollution control have not only personal but also economic ramifications. In the last several years, there has been more governmental intervention on this issue. According to various polls, most of the public approves.

Besides consumerism, another factor that encourages self-care is the cost of health care. It has been estimated that perhaps 85 percent of all health care could be self-provided and might be necessary to avoid flooding parts of the health care system. For instance, emergency rooms are frequently filled with patients who have minor conditions that could have been prevented or self-treated at home at an earlier stage.

One interesting approach to encouraging self-care is *holistic* or *wholistic* health care, which incorporates a number of precepts of the consumerist ethic. These include providing physical, psychological, and spiritual care, therapeutic approaches that involve the patient and encourage the patient's independence and capacity for self-healing, emphasis on self-care and education, consideration as an individual, and an environment that encompasses other activities besides health care. *Wholistic health care centers* were so named by their founder as a protest against the fragmentation of care.[48] These centers are actually described as primary care doctors' offices, generally located in a church, which offer pastoral counseling and health education as well as physical care.

Ambulatory Care: Physician's Offices

Ambulatory care is generally defined as care rendered to patients who come to physicians' offices, outpatient departments, and health centers of various kinds. Except for home care, most of these services currently involve patient contact with physicians in solo, partnership, or private practice. About 80 percent of patient visits are to specialists often referred by another physician. Although there is a growing acceptance of nurses practicing independently, most people must be educated to that concept.

Most private practitioners are paid by the patient or by some form of third-party insurance. Some contract for all or part of their practice with maintenance HMOs, PPOs, or an independent practice association (IPA). With the competition of freestanding emergency or walk-in centers, some are also extending their hours and increasing their walk-in services.

Ambulatory Care Alternatives to Institutions

Out of the social unrest of the 1960s and early 1970s emerged the *neighborhood health center (NHC)*, an ambulatory facility based on the concepts of full-time, salaried physician staffing, multidisciplinary team health practice, and community involvement in both policy making and facility operations. The NHC movement was stimulated by funding from the Office of Economic Opportunity (OEO) during the Johnson administration. Now more commonly called *community health centers (CHCs),* they serve some 6 million people at about 2000 primary care sites.[49] They may be freestanding, with a backup hospital for special services and hospital admissions, or legally part of a hospital or health department, functioning under that institution's governing board and license, but with a community advisory board.

CHCs are primarily found in medically underserved urban areas. Often they are at least partially staffed by the ethnic group served, so that communication is improved. A real effort is made to provide services when and where patients/clients need them in an atmosphere of care and understanding. Use of nontraditional workers such as family health workers and an emphasis on using a health care team have been characteristics of CHCs. Starting and maintaining CHCs is extremely expensive, and most patients can pay only through Medicare or Medicaid, if at all. Few are self-supporting. When external funds are not available, severe program and personnel cuts are often necessary. The future of CHCs remains uncertain, in part because of a sociological question: are they perpetuating a separate kind of care for the poor? Nevertheless, variations of CHCs are present in different parts of the country. *Rural health centers,* developed under federal financing or funded by communities or foundations, serve people, usually the poor, in medically underserved areas (MUAs). Since few physicians are available, care is often given by NPs and PAs linked to physicians at other sites.

The term *health maintenance organization (HMO)* may refer to a number of organizational entities, but essentially, an enrolled population of patients prepay for the use of all the HMO's services, including diagnosis and treatment with, if necessary, hospitalization.[50] A major emphasis is on prevention and health teaching, and nurse practitioners are involved in these as well as other aspects of primary care at HMOs. Research shows that the health outcomes for HMO subscribers are the same as or better than those in conventional settings; that consumer and provider satisfaction is generally good; and that the system is cost effective. Tremendous growth of HMOs is expected.

The 1980s brought increased complaints about the expense of health care, particularly in hospitals, and ushered in the *competitive model.* The idea is that consumer choice and market forces rather than regulation should be used to control health care costs.

As a result, alternative health care delivery modes, particularly in ambulatory care, developed and expanded. Among these are the *surgicenters,* originally independent proprietary facilities. Some are specialized, such as plastic surgery centers, but in general, the centers can perform any surgery that does not require prolonged anesthesia. Because of their low overhead, surgicenters can charge as little as one-third of hospital costs for the same procedure. Patients like being able to return to home, or even work, the same day. Surgicenters were seen to be the most cost-saving innovation in health care. However, because the unregulated fees soon soared, the government is now stepping in, with DRG-type payment pending. Tentatively, 2509 ambulatory patient groups (APGs) are being suggested, with payment accordingly for all types of ambulatory care.

Private, for-profit, freestanding emergency centers (FECs), also called *emergicenters* or *urgicenters,* first appeared in 1976. Designed to treat episodic, nonurgent health problems, they are among the fastest-growing forms of U.S. health care. The term *freestanding* may refer either to an independent, physician-owned emergicenter or to one that is hospital sponsored or affiliated. Typically, the emergicenters are located in shopping centers or commercial and industrial areas, have a high patient turnover, a short (15- to 20-minute) waiting period, and a cost that may be 30 to 40 percent lower than that of hospital emergency rooms.

Although some women are again turning to home births attended by midwives, a more popular and growing alternative to hospital births is the *childbearing center,* also called *birth center* or *childbirthing center.* These centers appeared in 1973, when the alienated and questioning middle class became disenchanted with hospital maternity care. The demonstration nurse-midwifery model was the Maternity Center of New York. Now out-of-hospital centers are operating in an increasing number of states. About one-third are operated by or utilize nurse-midwives; others are sponsored by physicians and/or lay midwives. There are freestanding centers or variations of them in hospitals. Both allow for more humane care in a high-quality, homelike setting with the father and other children present—all costing considerably less than regular hospital care.[51]

Renal dialysis centers were spurred into massive growth by their inclusion in the 1972 Medicare amendment. Once, the treatment of those with chronic kidney disease by using expensive artificial kidneys was a sensitive matter of deciding who shall live. When Congress decided that all patients should have that opportunity and funded it, the cost rose to unexpected millions of dollars. Many centers are freestanding, mostly physician owned or developed by proprietary organizations, but they also exist in hospitals. A whole new group of specialists at all levels has developed. The desired alternative now is less expensive home dialysis.

Mental health centers or *community mental health centers* are intended to provide a wide range of mental health services to a particular geographic catchment area. They may be sponsored by state mental health departments, psychiatric hospitals or departments of hospitals, or the federal government. They are staffed by teams of mental health personnel, such as psychiatrists, clinical psychologists, psychiatric nurses, social workers, marriage and family counselors, and community workers. They may consist of single physical entities or networks but are usually for short-term care, including crisis intervention. These centers were originally intended, in part, to prevent the warehousing of mental patients and assist their reintroduction into the community. Unfortunately, deinstitutionalization moved faster than the available community services. Even today there are discharged mental patients living on the streets or in terrible single-room occupancy hotels (SROs). While there are good halfway houses, day-care centers, and semisupervised living services, the services have not caught up with the demand.

Free clinics, often functioning in informal settings and sites, provide health care services to transient youths, minority groups, and students. They are usually staffed by volunteers. Their peak was reached in the early 1970s with the "flower child" generation; many of those that survived became more formally organized. Some now serve the homeless.

Women's clinics are usually owned and operated by women concerned about women's health problems and dissatisfied with the quality of care for women and the attitudes of many male health care providers. Most emerged out of the women's movement, along with the consumer and self-care movements. Services may include routine gynecological and maternity care and family planning, as well as some general health care. Emphasis is on self-help, mutual support, and noninstitutional personal care. Both nurse-midwives and lay midwives are used, as are supportive physicians, although many staff members are lay people. In a number of cities and towns, the clinics have been harassed by conservative groups and medical societies, and have had to become involved in lengthy and expensive legal suits.

Family-planning clinics, of which the clinics of Planned Parenthood are best known, provide birth control services and information. *Abortion clinics* increased with the legalization of abortion, but are now decreasing due to more restrictive antiabortion actions and laws. They are sponsored by community and other groups, as well as proprietary organizations.

Nurse-managed centers (NMCs) were initiated about a decade ago when faculty in schools of nursing offered nursing services to the community and at the same time provided model teaching centers for their students. NPs in private practice may also practice in such centers, whether or not they are university affiliated. Often the centers serve inner-city communities and, more rarely, middle-class clients. Patterns of practice for NMCs vary but usually include health maintenance and health promotion services, such as risk factor screening, health education, and counseling for a variety of populations including the elderly, children, employees, and pregnant women.[52]

Community nursing organizations (CNOs) came into existence in 1987 under the Omnibus Reconciliation Bill (P.L. 100-203) when Congress approved their establishment under the Medicare program. A CNO is a model of care similar to nurse-managed centers, in that nurses are the mainstay of care and coordination. However, a CNO also provides services in addition to nursing that Medicare beneficiaries often require. Under the CNO model, community nursing and ambulatory care include part-time or intermittent nursing care furnished by or under the supervision of a registered professional nurse; physical, occupational, or speech therapy; social support services; part-time or intermittent services of a home health aide; medical supplies and equipment; and certain medical services. The CNO model allows patients to receive comprehensive community care, with the advantages of improved quality and cost containment over the more fragmented existing arrangements.

The 1987 law called for the establishment of at least four demonstration sites to provide payment on a prepaid, capitated basis for community nursing and ambulatory care rendered to Medicare Part B beneficiaries. The legislation was the culmination of several years of lobbying, led by the ANA, to secure financial recognition for the services of RNs under Medicare.

However, despite their advantages, by 1991 the CNOs had yet to be implemented because of the federal government's delays in devising the capitated payment rates. Basically, CNOs presented the challenges of obtaining sufficient numbers of enrollees and establishing capitation rates that would ensure CNO viability, yet be acceptable to the federal government.

Whether under Medicare or the auspices of other programs, CNOs serve as a prototype for comprehensive noninstitutional care in which nurses can play a key role in both development and administration. Once the demonstration sites are established, the merits of such care will undoubtedly become even more evident.

Another humanistically oriented as well as cost-saving type of care is the *hospice*. The hospice movement was pioneered in Great Britain. The first widely recognized hospice in the United States was Hospice, Inc., established in 1971 in New Haven, Connecticut. Modeled after St. Christopher's in London, it concentrated on improving the quality of patients' last days or months of life so that they could "live until they die."[53]

The Hospice Association of America estimates that there are between 1700 and 1900 hospices in the United States; about 800 hospitals have hospice services. Medicare classifies hospices into four types: hospital based; home health agency based; skilled nursing facility based; and independent. The first three are part of a larger institution; the independents, of which there are very few, are corporate entities. Hospices may offer inpatient care, home care, or a mix of the two. But whatever the setting, in reality it is a concept, an attitude, a belief that involves support of the family as well as the dying patient. Two-thirds of the patients die at home, surrounded by their families and free of technological, life-prolonging devices. Symptom control is a vital first step, and pain-relieving medications are not withheld.

The hospice functions on a 24-hour, 7-day-a-week basis; backup medical, nursing, and counseling services are always available. The typical hospice team consists of a physician and some combination of nurses; medical social workers; psychiatrists; nutritionists; pharmacists; speech, physical, and occupational therapists; and clergy or pastoral counselors. Most hospices serve cancer patients primarily, but many also care for patients with progressive neurological diseases and, now, AIDS. Except for the latter two groups, the majority of hospice patients are elderly. Any patient whose physician certifies that he or she has a life expectancy of less than six months is eligible for hospice care. Studies show that hospice care is less expensive than traditional care, and slowly reimbursement is being offered. Most major private insurance companies and some HMOs reimburse at least partially; however, since hospice care can be an "add-on" benefit, very few patients receive full reimbursement. In 1986, hospice care became a permanent Medicare benefit and an optional Medicaid benefit, but at least 80 percent of the care is supposed to be provided in the home. One problem is that only about 400 hospices have become Medicare certified because of fiscal constraints and inability to meet all the criteria.

Other facilities that are increasing in number are those for rehabilitation of drug abusers. Most common are the *methadone maintenance programs* (substituting methadone for heroin, along with certain rehabilitative measures), which have had varying success. *Drug-free programs* include self-help and therapeutic resident programs, halfway houses, counseling centers, and hot lines.

Adult day-care centers are agencies that provide health, social, psychiatric, and nutritional services to infirm but ambulatory individuals who are able to be transported between the home and the center. Psychogeriatric day-care centers were first opened in 1947. Funding now comes from a variety of uncoordinated sources, and therefore some communities have set priorities as to who can use the services. Yet, day care has been shown to be superior to nursing homes for eligible individuals because of lesser cost, improved health and functional outcomes, and an enhanced quality of life. Unresolved issues are related to their use for young adults with debilitating diseases, the feasibility of rural centers, and the need for regulation and licensing.

Government Facilities

In the federal government, at least 25 agencies have some involvement in delivering health services. Those with the largest expenditures in direct federal hospital and medical services are the Veterans Administration, which operates the largest centrally directed hospital and clinic system in the United States, the Department of Defense (members of the military and dependents), the Indian Health Service (IHS), and the Health Resources and Services Administration (HRSA) of DHHS, which operates one Public Health Service (PHS) hospital and provides care for federal prisoners and Coast Guard personnel. Other DHHS agencies provide indirect funding or contracts for a variety of clinics and the National Health Service Corps.

State and local governments also have multiple functions and multiple services in health care delivery, directly through grants and funding to finance their own programs, and indirectly as third-party payers. Although most states have some version of a state health agency (SHA) or department of public health, health services are often provided through other state agencies, a situation that has created territorial battles, duplication, and gaps.

In providing direct services, some states operate mental, tuberculosis, or other hospitals and alcohol and drug abuse programs, provide noninstitutional mental health services, fund public health nursing programs and laboratories, and provide services for maternal and child health, family planning, crippled children, immunization, tuberculosis, chronic respiratory disease control, and venereal disease control. All are considered traditional public health services, in addition to environmental health activities.

On a local level, services offered by a health department depend a great deal on the size, needs, and demands of the constituency. Some large municipalities operate hospitals that provide for the indigent or working poor who are not covered by Medicaid or private insurance. Some health departments run school health services and screening programs. Some duplicate services offered by the state.

Although there is a great deal of criticism of most local health services in relation to high cost, waste, corruption, and poor quality, attempts to terminate any of them, particularly hospitals in medically underserved areas, become political conflicts, with representatives of the poor complaining that no other services are available and that the loss of local jobs will create other hardships. With all the politically sensitive issues involved, most health care experts are pessimistic about reorganization or major improvement of the health systems at any governmental level.

Home Health Care

Home health care is probably more of a nurse-oriented health service than any other, originating with Florence Nightingale's "health nurses" and the pioneer efforts of such American nurses as Lillian Wald. (Today the term *public health nurse* or *community health nurse* is used.) Nevertheless, what Wald worked for in the late nineteenth century—comprehensive services for the patient and family that extend beyond simple care of the sick—is even more pertinent today.

Home care includes a broad spectrum of services from home birthings to hospice care. Medical services are primarily provided by the individual's private or clinic physician, although in some instances agencies will employ or contract for a physician's services. In addition, there are homemaker-home health aide services, required in addition to (or sometimes following) nursing and therapy and consisting of providing personal grooming needs, helping with the practice of self-help skills, and general housekeeping services. Among the other home health services that may be available are medical supplies and equipment (expendable and durable), nutrition, oc-

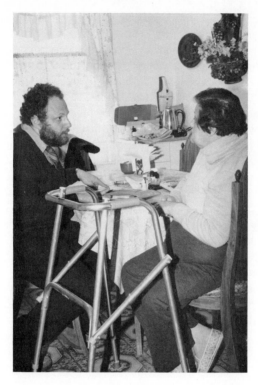

A social worker visits a disabled client in her home. (*Courtesy of the Visiting Nurse Service of New York.*)

cupational therapy, physical therapy, speech pathology services, and social work. Other services, which may be provided through coordinated efforts of the agency and the community, include audiological services, dental services, home-delivered meals (Meals on Wheels), housekeeping services, information and referral services, laboratory services, ophthalmological services, patient transportation and escort services, podiatry services, prescription drugs, prosthetic/orthotic services, respiratory therapy services, and x-ray services.

Agencies that provide home care (almost 11,000) have various organizational bases. As noted earlier, some cities, counties, and states provide home health care, but the general trend there is emphasis on services related to case finding, health teaching, and well-baby care, much of which is now clinic based. Visiting nurse associations (VNAs) of various names, which are nonprofit voluntary agencies, have been the classic providers of home care and provide services to 43 percent of all Medicare-eligible patients. Depending on the location and resources, the spectrum of services varies greatly but includes personal health services and patient/family teaching.

They also operate adult day-care centers, wellness clinics, hospices, and Meals on Wheels programs. VNAs ensure quality care by being overseen by professional advisory committees composed of local physicians and nurses. They are governed by voluntary boards of directors. Community volunteers assist the VNAs by serving on the board of directors, raising funds for indigent care, visiting patients in their homes, assisting at wellness clinics, delivering meals to patients, running errands for patients, doing VNA office work, and providing tender, loving care to patients.

The mission of VNAs is to provide quality care to all people, regardless of their ability to pay. Because for-profit agencies dump patients who are no longer reimbursable, which the VNAs then pick up, such as terminal AIDS patients and long-term stroke patients, many VNAs find themselves functioning under tight financial constraints. Nevertheless, VNAs are noted for their high quality of care. They were among the first home health agencies to seek accreditation. Accreditation is offered by both the NLN and JCAHO.

Other home care providers are hospital-based home health services, the "hospital without walls" concept. A prototype program was established at Montefiore Hospital in New York City in the late 1940s. Since then, a large number of hospitals have initiated such programs, but the number of services may be limited. In some cases, most services, including nursing, are con-tracted for, using established voluntary or proprietary agencies already in operation. At times, the program is little more than a coordination of services for continuity of care, which is nevertheless a vast improvement over what is still common—discharge with no follow-up except for a clinic or physician appointment. In part because of the prospective reimbursement system and the consequent pressure to discharge patients as soon as possible, more hospitals have become interested in setting up home care programs as a means of increasing income.

Most aggressive in providing services are the large number of proprietary agencies that are springing up throughout the country. Some offer compre-hensive services; others concentrate their efforts on training and deploying home workers and home health aides. In these agencies, operated for profit, marketing is brisk and sophisticated. Although there have been complaints of poor-quality care, the readily available services on a 24-hour-a-day, 7-day-a-week basis have proved to be highly competitive (VNAs are now also providing this round-the-clock service in many places).

One reason for the increase in interest is the financial support of Medi-care/Medicaid. On the other hand, as in the HMOs, the complex restric-tiveness of the regulations, particularly in relation to reimbursable services, leads to quality problems and severe financial burdens for the homebound patient and sometimes the agency.[54] Determining the need for home care is not a simple matter, and varies in terms of both the patient and the envi-ronment; in addition, retroactive cost adjustment according to new Medicare rules has sometimes caused severe losses. Some of the VNAs and other agencies that have survived best now plan on a more businesslike basis, and new organizational patterns have emerged. One includes the development of a holding company or major corporation with both a nonprofit (traditional VNA) and a for-profit subsidiary, and others as necessary, somewhat similar to the new hospital models. The for-profit corporation may provide a variety of profitable services, such as home-health aides, chore services for the frail elderly, presurgery counseling before hospital admission, and vocational rehabilitation. The after-tax profits from this corporation are then donated to the nonprofit corporation to provide the free services that have sometimes kept VNAs on the point of bankruptcy.

Both voluntary and official (governmental) agencies have been affected by the financial squeeze, and although total restructuring is not always possible, approaches have been used that were never even considered previously. Some have successfully marketed health teaching-health promotion services to industry and the public. Another developed a new market and gained increased economy by developing "neighborhood nurse" offices.[55] Other variations are block nursing[56] and nurses working out of the home. Computers have become essential for keeping records and statistics and for case management. Seen as the key by many is marketing of services based on the needs of the consumer.[57]

Comprehensive home health care is being hailed as less expensive than institutional care and as a more effective, humane approach, especially for the elderly and chronically ill, groups expected to expand the home care market to $16 billion by 1995. Whether it is indeed cheaper may depend on what supportive services are needed, an issue that is now the focus of serious study.

Emergency Medical Services (EMS)

Ambulance services, originally a profit venture of funeral directors, are a vital link in transporting accident victims or those suffering acute overwhelming illnesses (such as myocardial infarctions) to a medical facility. In most cases, providing for such services, either directly or through contracts, has now become the responsibility of a community, a responsibility that is not consistently assumed. The unnecessary deaths due to delayed and/or inept care have received considerable attention, which was probably responsible for some important federal legislation.

With continued federal and state funding and regulation, the previous diverse ambulance and rescue services of volunteers, firemen, police, and commercial companies are being coordinated with regional systems. Several hundred are now in place. Criteria include training of appropriate personnel; education of the public; appropriate communication systems, transportation vehicles, and facilities; adequate record keeping; and some participation by the public in policymaking.

Under these laws, a variety of emergency medical technicians (EMTs) have been trained and staff many ambulance services, including mobile intensive-care units, which have very sophisticated equipment.

Hospitals

Hospitals are generally classified according to size (number of beds, exclusive of bassinets for newborns); type (general, mental, tuberculosis, or other specialty, such as maternity, orthopedic, eye and ear, rehabilitation, chronic disease, alcoholism, or narcotic addiction); ownership (public or private, including the for-profit, investor-owned proprietary hospital or not-for-profit voluntary hospital, which may be owned by religious, fraternity, or community groups); and length of stay (short-term, with an average stay less than 30 days, or long-term, 30 days or more). Hospitals vary from fewer than 25 to more than 2000 beds. The most common type of hospital has been the voluntary, general, short-term hospital. Between 1980 and 1990, almost 500 hospitals, mostly small, closed. Causes cited by the American Hospital Association (AHA) included financial cutbacks in federal funding, pressure by insurance companies and business to reduce health expenditures, and changing health care practices (such as those described earlier). If not closed, the small hospitals are likely to become part of a multi-institutional system, a major trend in health care delivery. These systems may comprise two or more hospitals owned, leased, sponsored, or contract-managed by a central organization. They can be for profit or nonprofit. Advantages can include improved access to capital markets, shared purchasing, technology, economics of scale, and use of technical and management staff.[58] In 1990, there were over 300 multihospital systems, representing over 2500 hospitals.

The primary purpose of hospitals is to provide patient services. However, many also assume a major responsibility for education and research. The term *teaching hospital* is applied to those hospitals with accredited medical residency programs in which medical students and/or residents and specialty fellows (house staff) are taught. It does not include those that provide educational programs or experiences for other health professionals or allied health workers.

Administrative organization of services varies greatly according to administrative philosophy and types of services. Figure 3–1 shows a common organizational pattern of a general hospital, which illustrates both the lines of authority and the kinds of services available. However, not all of these services or units exist in all hospitals. Size is a factor, but another is the fact that hospitals that are part of a chain sometimes purchase certain services, like food and laundry. The nursing service has the largest number of personnel in the hospital, in part because of round-the-clock, 7-days-a-week staffing. Other departments, such as radiology and clinical laboratories, may maintain some services on evenings and weekends and may be on call at

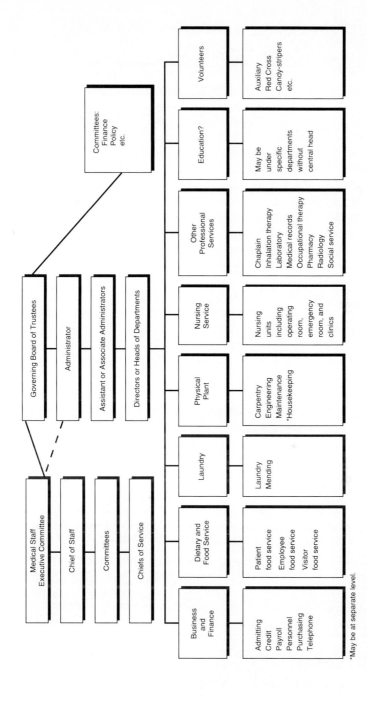

Figure 3-1 One pattern of hospital organization.

*May be at separate level.

night. There is a trend toward having other clinical services available at least on weekends.

The physical layout of a hospital varies from one-story to high-rise, and may include large or small general or specialized patient units, special intensive care units, operating rooms, recovery rooms, an emergency department, offices (sometimes including doctors' private offices), space for diagnostic and treatment facilities, storage rooms, kitchens and dining rooms, maintenance equipment workrooms, meeting rooms, classrooms, a chapel, waiting rooms, and gift and snack shops. To expand, build, or remodel extensively, hospitals need a certificate of need (CON) from the state. The approval of the planning agency is based on a set of planning criteria and community need.[59]

Hospitals are licensed by the state and presumably are not permitted to function unless they maintain the minimum standards prescribed by the licensing authority. ("Presumably" because the process of closing a hospital due to inadequate facilities and/or staff is long, difficult, and not always successful.) However, to be eligible for many federal grants, such as Medicare, and to be affiliated with educational programs, including medical residency programs, accreditation is necessary. Accreditation by the Joint Commission on Accreditation of Health Care (JCAHO) is voluntary and is intended to indicate excellence in patient care. Specific standards, usually more rigorous than those of the state, are set to measure hospital efficiency,

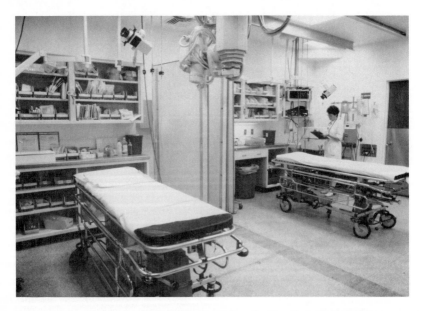

Trauma Suite. (*Courtesy of Presbyterian University Hospital, Pittsburgh.*)

professional performance, and facilities, and must be met in all facets of health care services (including nursing). Visits are made by an inspection team (that may or may not have a multidisciplinary makeup) that reviews various records and minutes of meetings, interviews key people, and generally scrutinizes the hospital. Reports are made that include criticisms and recommendations for action. Accreditation may be postponed, withheld, revoked, granted, or renewed on the basis of the inspection and review of the hospital's report and self-evaluation. Nurses are now usually included on the inspection team, and there is nursing input into the standards for nursing service. Another external quality check is the federal PRO program. An internal *utilization review committee* is expected to monitor the quality of care (and cost) of federally insured patients, using chart reviews. Nurses are often employed in these positions.

Voluntary hospitals are usually organized under a constitution and by-laws that invest the board of trustees with the responsibility for patient care. This governing board is generally made up of individuals representing various professional and business groups interested in the community. Although unsalaried and volunteer (except for proprietary hospitals, in which members are often stockholders), board members are usually extremely influential citizens and are often self-perpetuating on the board. This type of membership originated because at one time administrators of hospitals did not have a business background, and because of the still-present need to raise money to support hospitals. (Most trustees still see recovery of operating costs as their most crucial hospital problem.) Some consumer groups have complained that most members are businessmen, bankers, brokers, lawyers, and accountants, with almost nonexistent representation of women, consumers in general, and labor. Physicians also complain of lack of medical representation, although they work closely with the board and are subordinate to it only in certain matters. Because of these pressures, boards are gradually acquiring broader representation.

It is also possible that there will be some lessening of trustee power as hospitals adopt the corporate model, integrating the board of trustees and the administration of the hospital, with the board having full-time and salaried presidents and vice-presidents. The growth of mergers, consortia, and holding companies that are creating new business-oriented hospital systems may also change the role of trustees.

Public hospitals usually do not have boards of trustees. Hospital administrators are directly responsible to their administrative supervisors in the governmental hierarchy, which may be a state board of health, a commissioner, a department such as the Veterans Administration, or a public corporation with appointed officials. All are ultimately responsible to the public.

Although *administrator* is still the generic term for the managerial head of a hospital, in recent years this title has included a variety of designations such as *president* and *chief executive officer,* usually called *CEO.* The hospital administrator, the direct agent of a governing board, implements its policies, advises on new policies, and is responsible for the day-to-day operations of the hospital. Department heads or supervisors are next in the line of authority; these individuals are also gradually becoming specialists by education and experience in their area of responsibility. Nurses, in charge of the largest department, are either department heads or assistant/associate administrators.

The medical staff organization is made up of selected physicians and dentists who are granted the privilege of using the hospital's facilities for their patients. They, in turn, evaluate the credentials of other physicians who wish to join the staff and recommend appointment to the hospital's governing board, which legally makes the appointments. In some institutions, nurse-midwives, NPs, and other health professionals, such as podiatrists, have been given these admitting privileges with certain restrictions, usually as adjuncts.

Long-Term Care Facilities

Long-term care services for chronic diseases and conditions are one of the fastest-growing areas of health care. In part this is due to the success of medical science in saving those who once might have died, and in part to the fact that the nuclear family has no place for those who, years ago, were simply cared for at home with no public help. While the use of ambulatory care facilities and a return to home are being recommended, such care requires a considerable number of social and health-related backup services. These are not easy to organize or coordinate and are even less easy to be reimbursed for. Therefore, institutional care for long-term patients, while considerably more expensive and often lessening the individual's quality of life, still appears to be necessary for part of the population.

There are two major categories of long-term care institutions: long-stay hospitals (for example, psychiatric, rehabilitation, chronic disease, and tuberculosis hospitals) and nursing homes. There are approximately 600 long-stay hospitals, mostly psychiatric and mostly government owned. Over 19,000, mostly small nursing homes, about 75 percent of which are proprietary, account for 70 percent of the institutionalized population. This does not refer to residential facilities that may provide some degree of nursing services over and above room, board, and personal care or "custodial" services. Although over half are still independently owned and operated, this trend is decreasing as chains buy more and more of them.

Nursing homes can be classified according to the level of care offered and whether they are certified for the Medicare and/or Medicaid programs. According to these regulations, a skilled nursing facility (SNF) which provides inpatient skilled nursing and restorative and rehabilitative services must provide 24-hour nursing services, have transfer agreements with a hospital, and fulfill other specific requirements. An intermediate care facility (ICF) provides inpatient health-related care and services to individuals not requiring SNF care. Nursing homes may be certified for either or both levels; about 25 percent are not certified at all. If certified, PROs monitor them; some are also JCAHO accredited.

The organizational structure of a nursing home is often much like that of a hospital, but there are fewer diagnostic and therapeutic departments, depending on the major purpose of the institution. Usually both short-term and long-term care are offered. The nursing home may or may not be associated with a particular hospital. Some extended-care facilities have expansive services providing a continuum of care from skilled nursing to home care. For those who can afford it, there are complexes in which older people can live in their own apartments for life; health care services, including skilled nursing, are made available when needed. Sometimes a nursing home and even a hospital are on site.

Most of the 1 million employees who care for nursing home residents are unskilled and untrained aides. Almost no direct hands-on care is given by licensed nurses, although at least one RN must be employed by every licensed nursing home. That one RN may also be the director of nursing and probably has no degree. Neither do most nursing home administrators. Medical care is also minimal, with few physicians employed by nursing homes. Although it represents a minority of the elderly, the nursing home population is very old, with 85 percent over 75 years and more than 10 percent over 90. Patients usually have three to four chronic illnesses; half have psychiatric diagnoses. However, a major predictor of nursing home admission is inability to manage activities of daily living (ADL).[60] The majority of residents are poor, white, unmarried women, whose sole significant source of income is a survivor (not retiree) Social Security check. The lack of Hispanics and blacks is seen as due to inequity in services, not cultural preferences. In almost all cases, residents in a nursing home lack financial resources and/or family members to care for them outside. Over half of the patients stay less than six months, but after three years, discharge is usually to a terminal hospital stay or "discharged dead." Except in the best nursing homes, there is minimal social activity.

The cost of nursing home care is quite high on a long-term basis, and often the patient and spouse must "spend down" their assets until the patient is eligible for Medicaid. Not long ago, this practice could have reduced the spouse to poverty, but recent legislation allows the spouse to keep both assets and a monthly income at a more reasonable (but still not generous) level. Some elderly people are still often upset that their hard-earned savings, which they have hoped to leave to their children, are almost wiped out when nursing home care is necessary. Whether or not another law like the Catastrophic Coverage Act (enacted in 1988 and repealed in 1989, because some elderly people objected to the surcharge all would need to pay) would again cover long-term care is problematic. It is difficult to get agreement on what people need and what the government and taxpayers are willing to pay.

Nursing homes are considered good business opportunities for investors, many of whom believe that more elderly people will have good investments in years to come and can pay the ever-increasing rates. And these are the kinds of clients they seek—not the Medicaid patients, with relatively low reimbursement and more governmental oversight. There are now some insurance plans (rather expensive) that cover nursing home care, but Medicare covers very little. This situation may change, since a number of SNFs now care for patients who require complex care and technology that was once seen only in hospitals. Giving intravenous (IV) fluids is common, as are tube feedings. Some extended-care facilities have set up geriatric-intensive-care units (GICUs) for ventilator-dependent patients. Caring for these patients usually requires coordination with the hospital, where the nursing home staff may receive appropriate training. For such GICUs, the staff mix is different, with more nurses and often a geriatric nurse practitioner (GNP). The variation in care needed by LTC patients will also probably affect the prospective payment systems used by some states, such as the resource utilization groups (RUGs) plan based on a classification according to patient needs.

Aside from the cost, another issue is the quality of nursing homes. In 1989, the Health Care Financing Administration (HCFA) released a 75-volume report on the 15,000 nursing homes that then participated in Medicare and Medicaid programs. This, like earlier investigations, revealed many serious discrepancies in both the environment and care. Regulations for the 1987 OBRA nursing home reform law were then finally put into effect, but they drew fire from almost everyone: nursing homes said they were too tough and expensive, health groups that they were too weak.[61] One key element was the requirement for 24-hour "licensed nurse" coverage, with an RN on duty on the day shift. Coupled with a generous waiver clause, it was possible that nursing home patients could be entirely without an RN. One happier note was that physicians could designate an NP (or PA) to make some of the required visits to nursing home residents, and that nurses' aides must be given a minimum of 75 hours of training. Nurses' aides give up to 85 percent of the care and are often given little or no training. Among other improvements were requirements for a full-time social worker in facilities with more than 120 beds; rehabilitation and dental services; no admissions of mentally ill patients except those with Alzheimer's or related dementia; and residents' guarantee of freedom from abuse, excessive medication, and punitive physical or chemical restraints. Other rights were also spelled out.

There will probably still be complaints about the quality of life, if not always the quality of physical care, in nursing homes. In some areas, voluntary ombudsmen regularly make checks to prevent or detect abuses. There are also a few adopt-a-grandparent or similar programs that give the residents caring social contacts outside the home. It has been noted that the factors generally listed by residents as important to quality of care—an adequate, competent, caring staff, a homelike environment, properly prepared and varied food, activities, and medical care—were rated most highly. No doubt, if these were present in most nursing homes, people would not be as reluctant, even frightened, to be admitted to them.[62]

Experts disagree on the future of nursing homes. Nursing homes serve socially isolated women, a group that is increasing, but no one seems to want to expand the nursing home system because of concerns about cost and quality of care. Yet if all home care and support services were reimbursed, the latent demand might cause a financial catastrophe, since almost all of that care is now given without reimbursement by family and friends. As the older population increases, so does the need for a reasonable plan for their long-term care needs.

THE CAREGIVERS: A GROWING NUMBER

A hundred years ago, trained caregivers consisted of physicians, dentists, some pharmacists, and nurses. Now there are more than 250 acknowledged health occupations, with more being developed every day. In 1990, the number of health-related employees was over 8.7 million, 37 of every 1000 Americans. This figure includes certain supportive services. Health care facilities, like other places of business, employ secretaries, clerks, accountants, receptionists, messengers, and others to carry on business operations. In addition, institutions need laundry workers, dietary workers, cooks, plumbers, electricians, carpenters, maids, porters, and similar kinds of employees to function in the hotel-keeping aspect of their services. Not included in any category are faith healers, root doctors, or certain untrained healers who rely on herbs, meditation, or other semi–self-care techniques of healing. Nor does it include independent practitioners or others who are self-employed.

The overwhelming growth of personnel is in direct health services. Many of the health occupations and suboccupations have emerged because of increased specialization in health care, others on the peculiar assumption that several less-prepared workers can substitute for one scarcer professional. Some of these workers can be employed in almost any health setting—hospitals, nursing homes, clinics, doctors' offices, occupational health, and school health. Some work primarily in one setting. Most of these workers are not licensed; many are trained in on-the-job programs, and even more are trained in a variety of programs with no consistent standards. Others have standardized programs approved by the AMA and/or other health organizations. This entire group, categorized as *allied health manpower (AHM)* by the federal government, includes almost any health worker engaged in activities that support, complement, or supplement the professional functions of physicians, dentists, and registered nurses.

Services rendered by AHM range across the entire spectrum of service delivery and include every aspect of patient care, as well as services provided as part of community health promotion and protection. AHM range from personnel with complex functions and the highest educational degrees, who have always had a great deal of autonomy, to those who function in relatively simple assisting roles and must be supervised, sometimes by others categorized as AHM. Because of this diversity, as well as changes in health care, there are also many changes occurring within occupations/professions so identified. Since such a large percentage of health care personnel are AHM, it is ironic that there are so little fundamental data. This is blamed on the elasticity of supply and the constant evaluation of the roles and responsibilities of certain occupations.

At one time, most AHM were educated in almost apprentice-like programs in hospitals. Many AHM programs are now offered in a junior college setting, with the hospital remaining as a clinical practice site. Credentialing of health care providers and their educational programs is under a variety of auspices: the state, a single professional organization, or a coalition of professional organizations, such as the Committee on Allied Health Education and Accreditation (CAHEA), a collaborative effort of national health organizations and medical specialty organizations with the American Medical Association (AMA). Practitioners who are not licensed may become certified or registered on a voluntary basis by the occupation's national organization or a parent medical group. The inconsistency of these various processes is the focus of some of the complaints about health care credentialing. In 1990, AHA listed the following as health personnel licensed in every state: nursing home administrators, chiropractors, dentists, dental hygienists, practical nurses, professional nurses, optometrists, pharmacists, physical therapists, physicians (MD and DO), podiatrists, psychologists, and veterinarians, but many others are licensed in *some* state. This does not necessarily mean that licensure is required, only that it is available (see Chapter 11).

The largest categories of health workers, in order, are nursing (all types, including aides), physicians, dentists and their allied services, clinical laboratory workers, pharmacists, and radiological technicians. As feminists are the first to point out, *manpower* is a misnomer; from 75 to 85 percent are women. However, they are, or have been, in the lower-paid and less powerful positions. Except for the independent practitioners who are primarily self-employed, the mass of health workers are employed in institutions and agencies, with the greatest number concentrated in hospitals.

It would be unrealistic to attempt to describe all the professional and technical workers with whom nurses work or interact. However, an introduction to the most prevalent health occupations should provide a better understanding of the complex relationships in health care. Appendix 2 puts these in a format that allows comparison of numbers, education, credentials, and issues.

The organization of this section is primarily alphabetical, although two closely related groups may be described in logical succession. Good brief descriptions of almost every health occupation can be found in *200 Ways to Put Your Talent to Work in the Health Field* (New York: National Health Council, Inc., 1990). One is published periodically. The education of RNs and practical nurses is described in Chapter 5 and the practice of nursing in Chapter 7.

Administration

Health services administrators manage organizations, agencies, institutions, programs, and services within the health care delivery system. They may work in any setting but are probably more visible in hospitals, academic medical centers, nursing homes, neighborhood health centers, and community health agencies.

Other positions in the operation of health facilities and plants are the usual business positions, finance, data processing, personnel, public relations, and admissions, with all types of jobs and educational levels.

Chiropractic

Chiropractic is described by the American Chiropractic Association (ACA) as "a branch of the healing arts which is concerned with human health and disease processes. Doctors of chiropractic are physicians who consider man as an integrated being, but give special attention to spinal mechanics and neurological, muscular, and vascular relationships." Chiropractors use standard diagnostic measures, but treatment methods, determined by law, do not include prescription drugs and surgery. Essentially, treatment includes "the chiropractic adjustment, necessary dietary advice and nutritional supplementation, necessary physiotherapeutic measures, and necessary professional counsel." Most chiropractors are in private practice. All 50 states, the District of Columbia, and Puerto Rico recognize chiropractic as a health profession and authorize these services for workmen's compensation. They are also reimbursable by Medicare and Medicaid.

Clinical Laboratory Sciences

There are a number of technicians or technologists working in the clinical laboratories in such specialties as immunohematology, hematology, clinical chemistry, serology, microbiology, and histology. The physician in charge is a pathologist, although technologists may have specific responsibilities for technicians. *Medical technologists* are prepared for all phases of clinical laboratory work. *Certified laboratory assistants,* who perform routine laboratory tests, and *histological technicians,* who prepare body tissues for microscopic examination by pathologists, are usually prepared in one-year hospital programs. All these programs may be CAHEA accredited.

Dentistry

Dentists treat oral diseases and disorders. They may fill cavities, extract teeth, and provide dentures for patients. About 13 percent of dentists specialize. These specialties usually require two or more additional years of training and a specialty board examination. Nine out of ten dentists are in private practice; the others practice in institutions, the armed forces, and health agencies, teach, or do research. Most are located in large cities. An increasing number of minorities and women are entering the field.

Dental hygienists, almost all women, provide dental services under a dentist's supervision. They examine and clean teeth, give fluoride treatments, take x-rays, and educate patients about proper care of teeth and gums. In many states, hygienists' responsibilities have been expanded to include duties traditionally performed by dentists, such as giving local anesthetics.

Dental assistants maintain supplies, keep dental records, schedule appointments, prepare patients for examinations, process x-rays, and assist the dentist at chairside, but their functions are also expanding.

Dental technicians or *denturists* make and repair dentures, crowns, bridges, and other appliances, usually according to dentists' prescriptions. They are lobbying to work directly with patients and have become licensed in some states.

Dietetics and Nutrition

Nutritionist is a general occupational title for health professionals concerned with food science and human nutrition. They include dietitians, home economists, and food technologists.

Dietitians may have a general dietary background or preparation in medical dietetics. Medical or therapeutic dietitians are responsible for selection of appropriate foods for special diets, patient counseling, and sometimes management of the dietary service. More and more are becoming licensed and are seeking third-party reimbursement.

Clinical dietitians work with patients not only in the hospital, but in clinics, neighborhood health centers, or in the patient's own home.

Dietetic technicians graduate from one of two kinds of ADA-approved technical programs with an associate degree. A program with food service management emphasis allows the individual to serve as a technical assistant to a food service director and, with experience, to become a director. The program with nutritional care emphasis enables the individual to become a technical assistant to the clinical dietitian.

Most *dietetic assistants* serve as *food service supervisors* in hospitals, schools of nursing, schools, and nursing homes. However, a number of food service supervisors currently functioning in that position lack such preparation.

Health Educators

Community health educators help identify the health learning needs of the community, particularly in terms of prevention of disease and injury. They may then plan, organize, and implement appropriate programs, for example, screening devices, health fairs, classes, and self-help groups. Some health educators are employed by the state as consultants, others by insurance companies, voluntary health organizations such as the American Heart Association, the school system (school health educators), and, occasionally, industry.

A number of hospitals are employing *patient educators* or health educators to develop and direct programs of both patient education and community health education. Frequently, these people are nurses with or without training in health education and administration. In a few states, health educators are registered and/or certified.

Medical Records

Medical record administrators are responsible for preparation, collation, and organization of patient records, maintaining an efficient filing system, and making records available to those concerned with the patient's subsequent care. They may also classify and compile data for review committees and researchers.

Medical record technicians assist the physician and the administrator in preparing reports and transcribing histories and physicals. They also work closely with others using patient records.

Medical record transcriptionists have specialized courses in terminology, in addition to typing and filing.

Medicine

Doctors of medicine and osteopathy practice prevention, diagnosis, and treatment of disease and injury. *Doctor of medicine degrees (MDs),* awarded in more than 100 allopathic medical schools, are considered the first professional degree. Some physicians may later decide to acquire advanced degrees (master's or doctorates) in an advanced science or public health.

The formalized program of education after the MD degree is titled *graduate medical education* and consists primarily of the residency, which involves preparation for specialties, a period of two to five years. On completion of the specified years of residency, the physician may take certification exams in the specialty and is board certified. If exams are not taken (or failed), he or she is board eligible. In some cases, continuing medical education is required for recertification. Most American physicians choose specialties as their field of practice. In medical centers, a *fellow* is a post-residency physician who enters even more advanced, highly specialized, or research-oriented programs, although presumably still involved in teaching and patient care. Graduate medical education is under the direction of medical school faculty recognized as specialists or subspecialists.

Physicians practice in every setting where medical care is provided, as well as in medical or public health education, public health practice, and research. About 50 percent are now employees (not in private practice). Some positions, such as that of medical director, are primarily administrative and are beginning to be recognized as such.

The number of women in medical schools has increased, but the percentage of minorities has been dropping, in part due to lack of financial support.

Doctors of osteopathy (DO) are qualified to be licensed as physicians and to practice all branches of medicine and surgery. DOs graduate from colleges of osteopathic medicine (now 15), accredited by the Bureau of Professional Education of the American Osteopathic Association (AOA).

After graduation, almost all DOs serve a 12-month rotating internship, with primary emphasis on medicine, obstetrics/gynecology, and surgery, conducted in an approved osteopathic hospital. Those wishing to specialize must serve an additional three to five years of residency. Continuing education is required by the AOA for all DOs in practice.

Osteopathic physicians are considered separate but equal in American medicine; they are licensed in all states and have the same rights and obligations as allopathic (MD) physicians. The "something extra" they claim is emphasis on biological mechanisms by which the musculoskeletal system interacts with all body organs and systems in both health and disease. They prescribe drugs, use routine diagnostic measures, perform surgery, and selectively utilize accepted scientific modalities of care. DOs comprise about

4 percent of all physicians; most are general practitioners who provide primary care, usually in towns and cities with populations less than 50,000.

Medical assistants (MAs) are usually employed in physicians' offices, where they perform a variety of administrative and clinical tasks to help the doctor; however, some work in hospitals and clinics. They perform tasks required by the doctor and are supervised by the doctor. The medical assistant, among other things, answers the telephone; greets patients and other callers; makes appointments; handles correspondence and filing; arranges for diagnostic tests, hospital admissions, and surgery; handles patients' accounts and other billings; processes insurance claims, including Medicare claims; maintains patient records; prepares patients for examinations or treatment; takes patients' temperature, height, and weight; sterilizes instruments; assists the physician in examining or treating patients; and, if trained, performs laboratory procedures. Most are trained in one- or two-year programs.

Physician Assistants (PAs)

In 1965, Dr. Eugene A. Stead, Jr., of Duke University inaugurated a program for *physician's assistants (PAs),* later called *physician's associates,* designed to assist physicians in their practice, either to enable them to expand that practice, or to give them time to pursue continuing education, or to have more time for themselves and their families. The generally accepted name now is *physician assistant.*

PA programs are found primarily in schools of allied health, four-year colleges, and allopathic medical schools, with a few each in community colleges, teaching hospitals, and federal facilities. All these accredited programs have medical facilities and clinical medical teaching affiliations of some kind. The clinical rotations or preceptorships introduce the student to potential areas of expertise, including family medicine, internal medicine, surgery, pediatrics, psychiatry, obstetrics/gynecology, and emergency medicine. This is intended to prepare the PA to:

1. Elicit a comprehensive health history.
2. Perform a comprehensive physical examination.
3. Order and interpret simple diagnostic laboratory tests.
4. Develop diagnoses and management plans.
5. Provide basic treatment for individuals with common illnesses.
6. Provide clinical care for individuals with commonly encountered emergency needs.
7. Develop treatment plans and explain them to patients. They may recommend medications and drug therapies and, in more than one-half of the states, have the authority to write prescriptions.

In addition to specific technical procedures that PAs perform, which vary with the practice setting, they carry out a variety of minor surgical procedures. They also may provide pre- and postoperative care. Surgeon assistants (graduates of specialized training programs) and PAs with surgical training often act as first or second assistants in major surgery. By law, all activities must be done under the supervision of a physician.

In recent years, PA residency programs ranging from 9 to 12 months have been developed that provide further classroom and clinical education in various specialties. Some offer certificates and a few offer a master's degree. PA education is not seen as part of a career ladder leading to MD licensure, although some PAs may go to medical school later, just as they may turn to schools of public health or nursing in a career change. Lack of career choices without shifting to another discipline is a PA complaint.

Most PA graduates take the certification exam given by the National Commission on Certification of Physician Assistants (NCCPA), which requires that educational programs be accredited by CAHEA. Although not all PAs are certified, most states (and employers) require certification in order to practice. The statutory provisions for utilization of PAs vary from state to state, but because PAs cannot practice without the supervision of a physician, licensure is almost unheard of. This may change; the Federation of State Medical Board's model Medical Practice Act includes PAs.

Most PAs are employed in one of three specialty areas: family medicine; surgery, including subspecialties; and internal medicine. Surgery is increasingly favored. Although about 35 percent work with physicians in private or group offices and another 30 percent in a variety of clinics, the trend is toward employment by hospitals. One reason is that medical residents' hours are being limited and PAs are being hired to fill in the gap for patient care, especially in the emergency room and in assisting the doctor in the operating room (OR). There are still a large percentage practicing in rural areas or small towns (mostly men), but hospital employment in larger cities and suburbs is becoming more common, especially for women. Some say that demand is a major factor; others point out that PAs must go where there is a doctor to supervise them, and doctors prefer urban and suburban areas over rural ones. In reality, though, those in rural clinics are "supervised" from a distance. Salaries of PAs have increased in the last few years differing with the specialty, setting, and geographic location. Women consistently earn less than men, even when they have the same education and experience. (Sometimes PAs earn more than NPs in the same setting.) Medicare and Medicaid policies governing coverage for PA services in hospitals and other institutions encourage their employment. PAs are also caring for underserved populations in rural areas, inner-city neighborhoods, substance abuse clinics, prison systems, and long-term care facilities. They are also actively involved in the treatment of HIV-infected persons at all levels, from ordering tests to counseling patients. A new, related career is anesthesiologist assistant, with two programs recently accredited by CAHEA.

There are still many unresolved issues related to PA practice, particularly in relation to role and functions. The AHA has published a statement on PAs in hospitals, which, overall, indicates that the medical staff and administration should formulate guidelines under which the PA can operate, with the request for the PA to be permitted to practice in the hospital being handled by the medical staff credentials committee. Emphasis is on medical supervision; however, current reality has shown that PAs go unsupervised in busy urban hospitals where they handle many emergency and other ambulatory patients. This has created a problem for nurses, for the authority of the PA vis-à-vis the nurse is frequently not clear. Although the nurses' associations, some state boards, some courts, and attorneys general have indicated that nurses do not take orders from PAs, in other states the rulings are the reverse. Because the PA usually functions according to a protocol specified by the employer-physician, an operational agreement may be reached similar to the basis on which a nurse carries out standing orders or some verbal orders from the physician. Nevertheless, there is frequently interdisciplinary conflict when roles are not clarified.

Emergency Medical Care

Emergency medical technicians-ambulance (EMT-As) respond to medical emergencies and provide immediate care to the critically ill or injured. They may administer cardiac resuscitation, treat shock, provide initial care to poison or burn victims, and transport patients to a health facility. They act under MD and nurse voice direction when necessary. Those who are certified may apply to a CAHEA-accredited program for EMT paramedic training of 600 to 1000 hours plus an internship. *EMT paramedics* are competent in assessing an emergency situation and managing the care, initiating appropriate treatment. They are employed by community fire and police departments, by private ambulance services, and in hospital emergency departments. Salaries are generally under $20,000.

Nursing Support Personnel

Nursing assistants, nurse's aides, orderlies, and attendants functioning under the direction of nurses are all part of the group of ancillary workers prepared to assist in nursing care, performing many simple nursing tasks, as well as other helping activities besides nursing. Usually training occurs on the job and is geared to the needs of the particular employing institution, but there has been some increase in public school programs within vocational high school tracks or as outside public education services. The program may vary in length from six to eight weeks or more and costs little or nothing. Commercial programs usually cost the student an unreasonable amount, make unrealistic promises of jobs, and frequently give no clinical experience; therefore these "graduates" are seldom employed. Sometimes students who drop out of certain practical nurse programs after six weeks receive a certificate as aides. In-service education during employment is relatively common. The difference in training, patient care assignment, and ability may be enormous on both an individual and an institutional basis. These workers are not licensed or certified as a rule, although there is a move to do so. Programs have been developed for LTC aides leading to certification.

Community health aides of various kinds are found in ambulatory care settings, especially in disadvantaged areas. Community residents are sometimes recruited and trained as health aides. Many are women not previously trained as vocational nurses or hospital aides. There is usually a limited period of instruction with ongoing supervision and on-the-job instruction. Certain technical skills are learned, such as auditory and visual screening, but the primary purpose is to identify health problems or deficiencies, such as lack of immunization, poor oral hygiene, dermatological problems, and child development problems, and to assist and encourage families to seek and continue necessary medical, nursing, and other services. Community health aides may also go into the community to do case finding rather than wait for the client to appear in the formal health facility.

As more attention is focused on keeping people at home rather than in institutions, the services of *homemaker/home health aides* have become reimbursable by Medicaid, Medicare, or other governmental funding sources under certain circumstances. The aide is assigned to the home of a family or individual when home life is disrupted by illness, disability, or other problems, or if the family unit is in danger of breakdown because of stress. Specific tasks include parenting, performing or helping with household tasks, providing personal care such as bed baths or helping with prescribed exercises, and providing emotional support. Educational programs are usually developed by the employing agency in a 60-hour (or less) course. Most aides are women who already have housekeeping skills; even so, there is some question as to how effectively they can be prepared in the limited time suggested. In 1989, New Jersey was the first state to certify this group, requiring certain criteria. As others follow, educational requirements will probably be raised.

There is an increasing tendency for proprietary agencies to offer homemaker/home health care services and to contract these workers out to voluntary agencies. Although there is evidence that a well-trained, conscientious home/health aide can be extremely helpful to a sick person or disrupted family, there are also some serious problems in the selection of workers, the quality of training, and supervision. There are also some reimbursement problems when the homemaking part of the aide's function is reimbursable

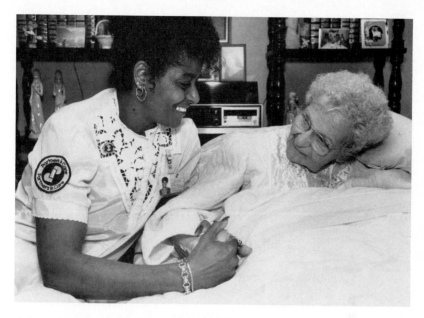

A home health aide is often a key factor in enabling an elderly person to stay at home (*Courtesy of the Visiting Nurse Service of New York.*)

and the health part is not, or vice versa. However, the homemaker/home health aide is usually one person doing whichever aspect of the job is needed and is reimbursed in a particular situation. Most often, a combination of the services is needed by the client. Ongoing assessment by health professionals is intended to evaluate the need of the family/client for specific services.

The lack of reimbursement often prevents the use of homemaker/home health aides, for this can cost hundreds of dollars a month. Still, it is a less costly health service than institutional care.

Surgical technicians or *surgical technologists* function in the operating room and sometimes the delivery room. Under the direction of the operating room supervisor, an RN, they perform required tasks, such as setting up for surgery, preparing instruments and other equipment before surgery, "scrubbing in" for surgery (assisting the surgeons by handing instruments, sutures, and so on), and otherwise assisting in the operating room.

The psychiatric/mental health technician is found in psychiatric and general hospitals, community mental health centers, and the home, working with the mentally disturbed, disabled, or retarded under the direction of a physician and/or nurse. In hospitals, he or she is concerned with the patient's daily life as it affects his or her physical, mental, and emotional well-being, including eating, sleeping, recreation, development of work skills, adjustments, and individual and social relations. In the community, the focus is on social relationships and adjustments. In the hospital, psychiatric technicians are expected to give some routine and emergency physical nursing care, but their close contact with patients makes observation and reporting of the patient's behavior particularly important. In some institutions they function almost independently in group therapy and counseling, seeking consultation as necessary. They may be skilled in nursing, communication techniques, counseling, training techniques, and group therapy.

Ward (unit) clerks or *ward (unit) secretaries* are usually trained on the job in an inservice program to assist in the clerical duties involved in the administration of a nursing unit. Ward clerks order supplies, keep certain records, answer telephones, take messages, attend to the massive amount of routine paperwork and, in some cases, copy doctors' orders.

Unit managers take even broader responsibilities in the management of a patient unit (usually in a larger institution) and may report directly to the hospital administration instead of the nursing service administration. Unit clerks often function under the direction of unit managers. In some institutions, unit management is an early step in an administrative career, and managers have full administrative responsibilities.

Pharmacy

Pharmacists are specialists in the science of drugs and require a thorough knowledge of chemistry and physiology. They may dispense prescription and nonprescription drugs, compound special preparations or dosage forms, serve as consultants, and advise physicians on the selection and effects of drugs.

With the increase of prepackaged drugs and the use of pharmacy assistants, pharmacists in hospitals and clinics are becoming interested in a more patient-oriented approach to their practice. They may be involved in patient rounds, patient teaching, and consultation with nurses and physicians. Pharmacists working in (or owning) drugstores have also been encouraged to increase their client education efforts in terms of explaining medications.

Besides the traditional responsibilities of pharmacists, the doctor of pharmacy (Pharm D) or clinical pharmacist provides consultation with the physician, maintains patient drug histories and reviews the total drug regimen of patients, monitors patient charts in ECFs and recommends drug therapy, makes patient rounds, and provides individualized dosage regimens. In some states, such as California, clinical pharmacists may also prescribe (as do NPs and PAs), with certain limitations.

Podiatry

Podiatrists, doctors of podiatric medicine (DPM) (once called *chiropodists*), are professionally trained foot care specialists who diagnose, treat, and try to prevent diseases, injuries, and deformities of the feet. Treatment may include surgery, medication, physical therapy, setting fractures, and preparing orthoses (supporting devices that mechanically rearrange the weight-bearing structures of the foot). Podiatrists may note symptoms of diseases manifested in the feet and legs and refer the patient to a physician. Most podiatrists are in private practice; others practice in institutions, agencies, the military, education, and research.

Podiatric assistants aid podiatrists in office management and patient care.

Mental Health Practitioners

Besides the physician (the psychiatrist), clinical psychologists, psychotherapists, nurses, social workers, and a variety of semiprofessionals trained in mental health participate in individual and group therapy. Psychologists may also give and interpret various personality and behavioral tests, as might a *psychometrician,* who is skilled in the testing and measuring of mental and psychological ability, efficiency, potentials, and functions.

Public Health

Industrial hygienists deal with the effects of noise, dust, vapor, radiation, and other hazards common to industry on workers' health. They are usually employed by industry, laboratories, insurance companies, or government to detect and correct these hazards.

Sanitarians, sometimes called *environmentalists,* apply technical knowledge to solve problems of sanitation in a community. They develop and implement methods to control those factors in the environment that affect health and safety, such as rodent control, sanitary conditions in schools, hotels, restaurants, and areas of food production and sales. Most work in government under the direction of a health officer or administrator.

Biostatisticians apply mathematics and statistics to research problems related to health. *Epidemiologists* study the factors that influence the occurrence and course of human health problems, including not only acute and chronic diseases but also accidents, addictions, and suicides.

Radiology

Radiologists are physicians who deal with all forms of radiant energy, from x-rays to radioactive isotopes; they interpret radiographic studies and prescribe therapy for diseases, particularly malignancies. A number of technicians work under the direction of a radiologist in radiology departments. They operate equipment, prepare patients, and keep records. These include the *radiologic technologist,* sometimes called *x-ray technician* or *radiology technician; radiation therapy technician* or *technologist;* and *nuclear medicine technologist.*

Rehabilitation Services

Occupational therapy is concerned with the use of purposeful activity in the promotion and maintenance of health, prevention of disability, and evaluation of behavior. Persons with physical or psychosocial dysfunction are treated using procedures based on social, self-care, educational, and vocational principles. One important responsibility is helping patients with activities of daily living. Adaptive tools such as aids for eating or dressing may also be provided.

Occupational therapists (OTs), the professional workers, and *occupational therapy assistants and aides* are usually employed in hospitals. However, OTs may also work in private practice or for nursing homes or community agencies.

Physical therapy (PT) is concerned with the restoration of function and the prevention of disability following disease, injury, or loss of a body part. The goal is to improve circulation, strengthen muscles, encourage return of motion, and train or retrain the patient with the use of prosthetics, crutches,

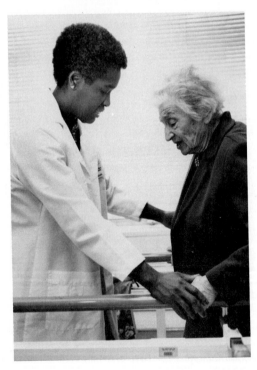

A physical therapist encourages a patient to walk again. (*Courtesy of the Jewish Home and Hospital for Aged, New York; photo by Phyllis Belkin.*)

walkers, exercise, heat, cold, electricity, ultrasound, and massage. Most *physical therapists (PTs)* and *PT aides* work in hospitals, but PTs may also work in private practice or for other agencies. The physical therapist designs the patient's program of treatment, based on the physician's stated prescription of objectives. He or she may participate in giving the therapy and/or evaluate the patient's needs and capacities and provide psychological support. The aides work directly under the PT's supervision, with limited participation in the therapeutic program.

Prosthetists make artificial limb substitutes. *Orthotists* make and fit braces. Both work with physicians and other therapists, and have direct patient contact to promote total rehabilitation services. *Orthotic/prosthetic technicians* make and repair devices but usually have no patient contact.

Rehabilitation counselors help people with physical, mental, or social disabilities begin or return to a satisfying life, including an appropriate job. They may counsel about job opportunities and training, assist in job placement, and help the person adjust to a new work situation. Others assisting in patient rehabilitation include *art therapists, dance therapists,* and *music therapists* who work primarily with the emotionally disturbed, mentally retarded, or physically handicapped. *Recreational therapists* or *therapeutic recreationists* may plan and supervise recreation programs that include athletics, arts and crafts, parties, gardening, or camping.

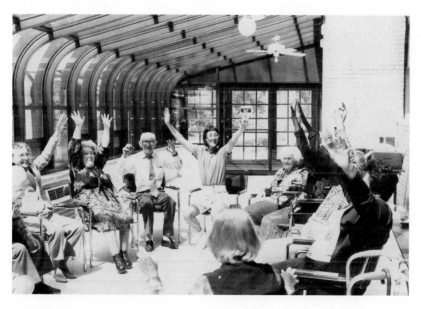

A recreational therapist helps patients in a nursing home exercise. (*Courtesy of the Jewish Home and Hospital for Aged, New York; photo by Ranete Koster.*)

Respiratory Therapy

Respiratory therapy personnel perform procedures essential in maintaining life in seriously ill patients with respiratory problems and assist in the treatment of heart and lung ailments. Under medical supervision, the *respiratory therapy technician* administers various types of gas, aerosol, and breathing treatments; assists with long-term continuous artificial ventilation; cleans, sterilizes, and maintains equipment; and keeps patients' records. The *respiratory therapist* may be engaged in similar tasks, but exercises more judgment and accepts greater responsibility in performing therapeutic procedures. Respiratory therapy personnel usually work in hospitals and clinics.

Social Work

The *social worker* attempts to help individuals and their families resolve their social problems, using community and governmental resources as necessary. Social workers are employed by community and governmental agencies as well as hospitals, clinics, and nursing homes. If the social worker's focus is on patients and families, he or she may be called a *medical* or *psychiatric social worker*.

Social workers also have assistants and aides, who sometimes carry a client load in certain agencies. There may be only on-the-job training available for these workers, but in order to move up, they must acquire additional education.

Speech Pathology and Audiology

Speech therapists and *audiologists* are specialists in communication disorders. Speech pathologists or therapists diagnose and treat speech and language disorders that may stem from a variety of causes. Speech therapists are particularly valuable in assisting patients whose speech has been affected by a cerebrovascular accident or patients with laryngectomies. Audiologists often work with children, and may detect and assist with the hearing disorder of a child who has been mistakenly labeled retarded.

Vision Care

Ophthalmologists are physicians who treat diseases of the eye and perform surgery, but they may also examine eyes and prescribe corrective glasses and exercises. *Opticians* grind lenses, make eyeglasses, and fit and adjust them. *Optometrists,* doctors of optometry (OD), are educated and clinically trained to examine, diagnose, and treat conditions of the vision system, but they refer clients with eye diseases and other health problems to physicians. After a variety of diagnostic tests, they may prescribe corrective lenses, contact lenses, and special optical aids, as well as corrective eye exercises, to provide maximum vision. Some may specialize in such areas as prescribing and fitting contact lenses. The majority of optometrists are in private office practice; but they are increasingly found in institutional settings. All of these professionals are aided by technicians and assistants.

Other Health Workers

There are a number of other health workers not described in this chapter, such as those in science and engineering: anatomists, biologists, biomedical engineers (who design patient care equipment such as dialysis machines, pacemakers, and heart-lung machines), biomedical technicians (who maintain and repair the equipment), and technicians dealing with instrumentation. There are also diagnostic medical sonographers, electrocardiograph (EKG/ECG) technicians, electroencephalographic (EEG) technologists and technicians; clinical perfusionists, who operate equipment to support or replace temporarily a patient's circulatory or respiratory functions; specialists in dealing with the visually handicapped; biological photographers; medical illustrators; patient advocates; acupuncturists; health science librarians; and computer specialists, to name just a few. In addition, volunteers provide many useful services.

All of these specialties are part of what the federal government calls *health manpower* and for which federal funds are often distributed for educational programs. The fact that this list is not complete and is expanding may help to explain why the public often becomes angered by the fragmentation of services. It is clear that if the public is to receive the services it requires, expects, and deserves, direction must be given through the health care delivery maze.

ISSUES IN HEALTH MANPOWER

Many of the most serious issues in health manpower—numbers, distribution, proliferation, and especially quality of care—have been focused on credentialing. This complex process is discussed in Chapter 11. However, the problem of health manpower planning has even greater priority. Why, over and over, are there shortages and then oversupplies of health care workers? Is it because administrators encourage the training of quickly prepared assistants without thinking ahead to their future place in health care? Does the government artificially expand the growth of certain categories by providing funds for education and reimbursement of services? The answer to both questions is probably yes, but for many reasons, predicting demand and supply is not easy. The data used are often inexact and out of date. When the need for a certain kind of worker is met, there are still many students in the educational pipeline. Lobbying for continued funding, perhaps unnecessary, is powerful because those who have started programs don't want to lose them. The need may shift because of unexpected social or economic changes. Because of costs, administrators now look for a multipurpose worker. For the least-educated, lowest-paid workers this may mean increased union activity or even unemployment, because there is little job mobility. For the highly educated, it is a shaky start to a career that may need to go in a totally different direction. For all those employed, oversupply also affects salaries and job security. The climate of competition has added to the pressures, with practitioners in and across various health occupations struggling with their colleagues for a piece of the health care action. Theoretically, legally clear distinctions of each profession would be helpful; practically, this has proved to be impossible.

It is true that in the 1960s improved salaries were a major budget item, and the need to move from what were often below-poverty wages to living wages was largely responsible for the jump. Since that catch-up period, the masses of workers have gained a new aggressiveness that affects not only monetary considerations but also power issues. Some are not necessarily in the best interests of the consumer. Nevertheless, one of the trends that has been widely predicted is aggressive action by unions to organize every type of health worker—professional, technical, aide, clerical, maintenance, and housekeeping. The likelihood that this will be successful is now in doubt because of the tight economic constraints of health care institutions and their preference for multipurpose workers.

Now, with some current shortages and major shortages expected for RNs, LPNs, PTs, OTs, medical lab personnel, clinical perfusionists, speech pathologists, respiratory therapists, nurse anesthetists, nurses' aides, computer specialists, and according to AHA, 14 other health care occupations close behind, hospitals particularly are demanding action. (It is interesting that the nonclinical computer specialists are one of those most in demand.) There is concern that patients everywhere will suffer if the needs are not met. Yet, as discussed earlier, the shortage of young people available to enter these fields and the strong possibility that those interested may not have an adequate education does not make for a good prognosis.

The nursing shortage will be discussed in Chapter 7, but solutions proposed by AHA and AMA present a picture of their involvement (not to be seen as always bad). In 1989, the AHA co-sponsored a pilot project with the Illinois Hospital Association to test a new employee group, an all-purpose worker to make beds, empty trash, serve meals, and take over other nonclinical chores to help nurses. The idea was to cross-train staff to handle anything from transport to housekeeping. (How the unions reacted was not reported.) It was expected that other hospitals would replicate this plan. Meanwhile, some hospitals produced other kinds of assistants called *general medical technicians* or *unit helpers* to do all the nonnursing tasks nurses are forced to do. The idea has merit, but will it create one more set of low-paying jobs that go nowhere?

Less beneficent is the AMA's brainchild, the registered medical technologist (RCT), a bedside caregiver who would execute physicians' orders at the bedside with special emphasis on technical skills.[63] The nursing protests were strong and united.[64] Many state and local medical associations dissociated themselves from the plan, as did individual physicians, health care advocates, and some influential lay people. Finally, in 1990, the AMA abandoned its plan to develop RCTs. The lost energy, time, and money that could have been spent on supporting nursing in its plans to alleviate the shortage are appalling, yet the AMA's action is not atypical.

On the other side of the shortage issue is oversupply, still being predicted for physicians, dentists, and some administrators; given the uncertainties of the health care future, others could be included. The reactions of those concerned follow a pattern: denial or prediction of a later shortage, as in medicine; a tendency to warn off potential students; disillusionment with the field; an attempt to hold on to their own territory and resist others' encroachment, coupled with an attempt to encroach on others; efforts to expand their services to meet previously unnoted or unattractive needs (such as serving the elderly); or making some aspect of their services attractive to consumers (such as cosmetic dentistry). Because real health care needs may begin to be met, there are good aspects to the situation; however, the dissension and the cost to the public are not desirable.

The issue of maldistribution is also not easily resolved. Maldistribution of professionals toward attractive urban and suburban places and away from isolated, poor, or ghetto areas is a major problem. In some cases, nurses, PAs, physician-nurse, or physician-PA and/or nurse teams are giving care that is as good as or better than that provided by solo practitioners, but the service gap still exists. Even federal intervention, such as requiring service in medically underserved areas (about 30 percent of the United States) in return for supporting the practitioners' education, has had only short-term results; practitioners leave after their required service. It may be, however, that the oversupply of physicians and others will make these less attractive settings suddenly look better.

Health manpower education is a major issue. How many? What kind? Prepared where? Financed by whom? The education for all levels of health service practitioners is under scrutiny. Why is this education so costly? Could institutions develop more economical teaching-learning methods? Are minority groups being actively recruited? Are the types of workers in proper proportion? Should the government continue to subsidize the education of high-earning professionals? How much should any health profession be subsidized, and for whom—the programs or students? Are the practitioners appropriately prepared to give safe and effective care? The trend toward increased educational criteria seems to permeate each occupational group, but almost all face the questions asked by the cost-conscious: Will it cost the consumer more? Will it keep out the poor?

Another concern is the workability of the health care team. It is naive to expect that bringing together a highly diverse group of people and calling them a team will cause them to behave like a team. One obvious gap is their lack of communication and practice together, either as students or as full practitioners. Sports teams practice together intensively for long periods of time, both to develop a team spirit and to mesh their individual skills to produce an effective unit. Not only do health care teams not have (or take) time to practice together, but often there are serious territorial disputes as areas of responsibility overlap more and more. As for patients, who should be members of the team, unless they are assertive, their only participation is as recipients of care.

Exhibit 3-1

What's Next for Health Care: Predictions for the New Century

- Technology, particularly computers, will have a major impact. Future improvements in technology will lead to faster-acting, safer anesthetics; sutureless surgery; improved cancer therapies; new genetic screening and engineering; microsurgical techniques that will allow correction of fetal abnormalities in the uterus; and alternative, less invasive means of delivering drug therapy.
- Technological advances will create additional ethical problems in terms of access to care and right-to-live and right-to-die issues. The government may step in and define life and death.
- All patients can expect access to a *minimum* level of care, although a multitiered system will probably be even more evident. There may be some kind of national health insurance in the century's last decade, but at any rate, the federal government will mandate minimum health coverage for employees of small businesses.
- Interest in self-care and personal responsibility for wellness will grow.
- Financial concerns will shape the health care agenda. There will be covert rationing of care as health policymakers limit funds for medical technology. Limits may be based on nonmedical factors such as age and ability to pay.
- More health professionals, including nurses, will provide reimbursable services on an entrepreneurial basis.

It has been said that society can no longer afford to use the physician as gatekeeper to control the flow of patients into and out of the health care system. Physician services should be saved to assist patients who need that level and kind of services. In other words, there must be others, like NPs, who are reimbursable by third-party payers and who have the same types of privileges held by physicians. Then the consumer will have a choice without being financially penalized. But who has power or should have power to make these decisions? The consumer? But who advises the consumer? All too often, the power figures in health care, such as the AHA, AMA, and IOM, make policy, even if indirectly, by their input into legislation or major influential groups.

Another major issue is quality of care. This inevitably involves health care personnel. Related to this issue is not only practice but education. Health care personnel, experts say, must develop some special skills to deal

---

- The cost of care will increase and patients will be expected to pay more of it. Insurance premiums will be based in part on lifestyle. Institutions and providers will continue to seek ways to cut costs and find other revenue. They will do more extensive marketing.

- Alternative systems will provide more competition to hospitals.

- Patients will rely more on self-diagnosis and treatment, using artificial intelligence and computers to keep in touch with their physicians. They will be admitted to hospitals less frequently and stay for shorter periods. They will challenge their doctors more, seeking second opinions.

- AIDS testing will be required for immigrants and for marriage license and insurance policy applicants.

- There will be a growing demand for geriatric and mental health services.

- Senior citizens will have more clout in determining health care policy and more options for care. However, the age for Medicare eligibility will be raised, and a means test may be used (the well-to-do may get less coverage).

- More sophisticated consumers will demand quality care, and if the providers are not accountable, the government will set regulations and/or the courts will set standards.

- There will be increasing concern about the effects of the environment on health.

- Home care will grow dramatically. Hospitals will become giant intensive care units.

with the future, for instance, the new "age wave,"[65] and educators should take note.

If there are any good answers to these questions and issues, they have not been found or accepted. Consumers' restlessness with professional indecision and evasion of their concerns and complaints is reaching a critical stage.

In the 1980s, the "crisis in health care" was the subject of concern, complaint, and predictions. Several impressive surveys were done then[66-68] and later[69] to advise health care executives about trends and to suggest strategies for coping with or even taking advantage of them. Several did suggest that the only certainty was uncertainty and ongoing change. However, there was a remarkable amount of agreement on the major predictions. These are seen in Exhibit 3–1.

What would be the impact on nursing if any of the predictions become reality? Or, perhaps a better question would be, given the trends and predictions discussed, how can nurses help move the health care system toward a more equitable, high-quality service to the public?

KEY POINTS

1. Being aware of population patterns, as well as social and economic trends, helps in anticipating the kinds of patients who will enter the health care system and how to give the best care.
2. Social trends like the women's movement and changes in the economy affect not only health care delivery but also the economic security of the workers.
3. The prospective payment method of reimbursement has changed the way patients are admitted to and discharged from hospitals, resulting in shorter stays and a greater likelihood of their going home sicker.
4. Competition and cost containment in the health care system have resulted in marketing of services, a trend toward conglomerates, and the growth of investor-owned health care corporations and nonprofit chains.
5. Health care services are now being provided in many places besides traditional doctors' offices and institutional agency settings. There is increased emphasis on more cost-effective delivery modes such as HMOs, surgicenters, and emergicenters.
6. The large numbers of caregivers and the overlapping of their activities add to the public's confusion about the selection and cost of services.
7. Health manpower needs are seldom predicted accurately, with a resulting cycle of shortage and oversupply.

8. Many of the common issues that concern health care providers are related to competition—the desire of some to expand their scope of practice and others to hold on to their territory. Therefore many of those striving for a better place in the system are looking to educational and other credentialing.

9. Predictions about the directions for health care focus on economic issues, public demand, and the conflicting pull of health promotion ideals, on the one hand, and the complex, expensive treatments made possible by technology on the other.

REFERENCES

1. Toffler A. *Future shock*. New York: Random House, 1970, p. 2.
2. Beyond the melting pot. *Time* (April 9, 1990), pp. 28–31; see p. 29.
3. Barringer F. Census shows profound changes in social makeup of the nation. *New York Times* (March 11, 1991), pp. A1, B8); see p. A1.
4. Naisbitt J. *Megatrends*. New York: Warner Books, 1982.
5. Rafferty M. Standing up for America's homeless. *Am J Nurs*, 89:1614–1617 (December 1989).
6. Jacobson E. New hospital hazards: How to protect yourself, Part 1. *Am J Nurs*, 90:36–41 (February 1990).
7. Jacobson E. Hospital hazards: How to protect yourself, Part 2. *Am J Nurs*, 90:48–53 (April 1990).
8. New OSHA rules under fire from all angles. *Am J Nurs*, 91:18, 22 (January 1991).
9. Kelly LY. *Dimensions of professional nursing*, 6th ed. Elmsford, NY: Pergamon Press, 1991, pp. 94–97.
10. Naisbitt, op cit., pp. 40–42.
11. Ibid., pp. 19–21.
12. Entire issue. *Nurs and Health Care*, 9:477–521 (November–December 1988).
13. Andreoli K, Musser L. Computers in health care: The state of the art. *Nurs Outlook*, 33:16–21 (January–February 1985).
14. Kelly, op. cit., pp. 111–112.
15. A nation at risk: The imperative for educational reform. *Chron Higher Ed*, 26:11–16 (May 4, 1983).
16. Wilson R. Bennett notes improvement of schools in past 5 years but paints bleak portrait of U.S. education in report. *Chron Higher Ed*, 31:A29–42 (May 4, 1988).
17. Meyer L. Untangling communication lines to connect consumer and provider. *Nurs and Health Care*, 6:367–368 (September 1985).
18. Vance C, et al. An uneasy alliance: Nursing and the women's movement. *Nurs Outlook*, 33:281–285 (November–December 1985).

19. Gordon S. *Prisoners of men's dreams.* Boston: Little, Brown and Company, 1991.
20. Kelly, op. cit., p. 116.
21. Naisbett J, Aburdene P. *Megatrends 2000: Ten new directions for the 1990's.* New York: William Morrow and Company, 1990, pp. 216–240.
22. Women: The road ahead. *Time* special issue (Fall, 1990).
23. Brown C. Women workers in the health service industry. *Int J Health Serv,* 5(4):173–174 (1975).
24. Ibid.
25. Kelly, op. cit., p. 118.
26. Peters T, Waterman R Jr. *In search of excellence.* New York: Harper and Row, 1982.
27. Toffler A. *The third wave.* New York: William Morrow and Company, 1980.
28. Toffler A. *Powershift: Knowledge, wealth, and violence at the edge of the 21st century.* New York: Bantam Books, 1990.
29. Naisbett and Aburdene, op. cit.
30. Ibid., p. 309.
31. Shaffer F. DRGs: History and overview. *Nurs and Health Care,* 4:388–396 (September 1983).
32. Joel L. Reshaping nursing practice. *Am J Nurs,* 87:793–795 (June 1987).
33. Kent V, Hanley B. Home health care. *Nurs and Health Care,* 11:234–240 (May 1990).
34. Rantz M. Inadequate reimbursement for long-term care; The impact since hospital DRGs. *Nurs and Health Care,* 11:470–472 (November 1990).
35. Brider P. Too poor to pay: The scandal of patient dumping. *Am J Nurs,* 87:1447–1450 (November 1987).
36. Weis D. Who are the working poor? *Am J Nurs,* 87:1451–1453 (November 1987).
37. Califano J. Guiding the forces of the healthcare revolution. *Nurs and Health Care,* 8:401–404 (September 1987).
38. Harrington C. A national health care program: Has its time come? *Nurs Outlook,* 36:214–216, 255 (September–October 1988).
39. Poll shows desire for change in U.S. health system. *The Nation's Health,* 19:1, 9 (March 1989).
40. Ward D. National health insurance: Where do nurses fit in? *Nurs Outlook,* 38:206–207 (September–October 1990).
41. Braunstein J. National health care: Necessary but not sufficient. *Nurs Outlook,* 39:54–55 (March–April 1991).
42. Harrington C. Policy options for a national health care plan. *Nurs Outlook,* 38:223–228 (September–October 1990).
43. Johnson P. A national health insurance program: A nursing perspective. *Nurs and Health Care,* 11:416–418, 427–429 (October 1990).
44. *Public Policy Bulletin.* New York: National League for Nursing, March 1991.

45. Parsons T. Definition of health and illness in the light of American values and social structure. In: Jaco EG, ed. *Patients, physicians, and illness*. Glencoe, IL: Free Press, 1958, p. 176.

46. Levin L. Self-care: Towards fundamental changes in national strategies. *Int J Health Ed*, 24(4):219–228 (1981).

47. Goeppinger J. Self-health care through risk appraisal and reduction: Implications for community health nursing. In: Stanhope M, Lancaster J, ed. *Community health nursing*. St. Louis: C.V. Mosby Company, 1984, pp. 316–329.

48. Gordon JS. Holistic health centers. In: Hastings A, et al, eds. *Health for the whole person*. Boulder: Westview Press, 1980, pp. 467–482.

49. Roemer M. Resistance to innovation: The case of the community health center. *Am J Public Health*, 78:1234–1239 (September 1988).

50. Drew J. Health maintenance organizations: History, evolution, and survival. *Nurs and Health Care*, 11:144–149 (March 1990).

51. Lubic R. Childbirthing centers: Delivering more for less. *Am J Nurs*, 83:1053–1056 (July 1983).

52. Lang N. Nurse-managed centers—Will they thrive? *Am J Nurs*, 83:1290–1296 (September 1983).

53. Corr C, Corr D, eds. *Hospice Care*. New York: Springer Publishing Company, 1983.

54. Lowe-Phelps K. Dismantling the Medicare home health benefit. *Am J Nurs*, 88:1364–1367 (October 1988).

55. Grimes EE. Developing neighborhood nurse offices. *Nurs and Health Care*, 3:138–141 (March 1983).

56. Jamieson MK. Block nursing: Practicing autonomous professional nursing in the community. *Nurs and Health Care*, 11:250–253 (May 1990).

57. Griffith E. Home care in crisis: Turning it around. *Nurs Outlook*, 36:272–274 (November–December 1988).

58. Freund C, Mitchell J. Multi-institutional systems: The new arrangement. *Nurs Economics*, 3:24–32 (January–February 1985).

59. Simpson J. State certificate-of-need programs: The current status. *Am J Pub Health*, 10:1225–1229 (October 1985).

60. Richardson H. Long-term care. In Kovner AR, ed. *Health care delivery in the United States*, 4th ed. New York: Springer Publishing Company, 1990, pp. 175–208.

61. Harrington C. Nursing home reform: Addressing critical staffing issues. *Nurs Outlook*, 35:208–209 (September–October 1987).

62. Kayser-Jones J. The environment of life in long-term care institutions. *Nurs and Health Care*, 10:125–130 (March 1989).

63. Chavigny K. RCTs—A resource for nurses at the bedside? *Imprint*, 35:19–25 (November 1988).

64. Maraldo P, Binder L. Nursing's response to the RCT proposal. *Imprint*, 35:19–25 (November 1988).

65. Dychtwald K. *Age wave: The challenge and opportunities of an aging America*. Los Angeles: Jeremy P. Tarcher, Inc., 1989.

66. *Health care in the 1990s: Trends and strategies*. Chicago: Arthur Anderson and ACHE, 1984.

67. *The future of healthcare: Changes and choices*. Chicago: Arthur Anderson and ACHE, 1987.
68. Amara R, et al. *Looking ahead at America's health*. Washington, DC: McGraw-Hill Book Company, 1988.
69. *Managing care and costs: Strategic choices and issues*. Minneapolis: Health One Corporation, 1991.

C H A P T E R 4

NURSING IN THEORY AND PRACTICE

OBJECTIVES

After studying this chapter, you will be able to:

1. Give a definition of nursing that is based on your beliefs about nursing.
2. Give examples of how nursing meets or doesn't meet the criteria for characteristics of a profession.
3. List nursing functions common to all nurses.
4. Briefly describe the nursing process and nursing diagnosis.
5. Name five major nursing theorists.
6. Describe how today's image of nursing differs from the reality and how it might be accurate.

THE NEW-OLD QUESTION: WHAT IS NURSING?

If asked what a nurse does, probably most people entering nursing would, like the general public, say, "Take care of the sick." That is a common dictionary definition, a common media image, and a large part of reality. That nurses do health teaching and want to keep people well is also part of the reality. So is the fact that they hold nursing positions in education, administration, research, and publication in many settings that aren't too different in basic responsibilities from similar jobs in other fields. And more are becoming entrepreneurs. Yet the historical orientation of nursing has been one of mother surrogate, of tending and watching over a dependent ward, of a helping person.[1] Although the caring, helping part of the role is basic to nursing, it is confusing to some that nurses can also be powerful, assertive professionals cutting out a piece of the health care pie for *nursing*, controlled by *nurses*.

Some nurses still tend to cherish a traditional image even as they move into new roles, and may then live uncomfortably with a blurred self-image. Others, as they enter this changing field, have more contemporary ideas about what nursing is, without discarding the caring concept, which is seen as the heart of nursing. Thus, there are many interpretations of nursing. Why not? There are many facets to nursing, and perhaps it isn't logical or accurate to settle on one point of view. All nurses must eventually determine their own philosophies of nursing, whether or not these are formalized. The public and others outside nursing will probably continue to adopt an image that is nurtured by contact, hearsay, or education about the profession. The first may be the most powerful influence. This chapter presents an overview of the components of nursing, the theory, the image, and the reality.

PROFESSIONS AND PROFESSIONALISM

Almost everyone talks about the *nursing profession* in the sense of an organized group of persons, all of whom are engaged in nursing. Yet, an ongoing debate centers on whether or not nursing as a whole is an occupation, rather than a profession, in the same sense that medicine, theology, and law have been called professions since the Middle Ages.

Professions have been historically linked with universities or other specialized institutions of learning, implying a high level of scholarly learning and study, including research. The specific criteria for a profession vary, but there is fairly general agreement that professionalism centers on specialized expertise, autonomy, and service. Bixler and Bixler's characteristics of a profession, modeled after Flexner's classic criteria,[2] are widely accepted.

1. A profession utilizes in its practice a well-defined and well-organized body of knowledge which is on the intellectual level of higher learning.

2. A profession constantly enlarges the body of knowledge it uses and improves its techniques of education and service by the use of the scientific method.
3. A profession entrusts the education of its practitioners to institutions of higher education.
4. A profession applies its body of knowledge in practical services that are vital to human and social welfare.
5. A profession functions autonomously in the formulation of professional policy and in the control of professional activity thereby.
6. A profession attracts individuals of intellectual and personal qualities who exalt service above personal gain and who recognize their chosen occupation as a life work.
7. A profession strives to compensate its practitioners by providing freedom of action, opportunity for continuous professional growth and economic security.[3]

Other models and criteria of professionalism have been developed, frequently by sociologists and usually using criteria similar to the classic ones. It has also been popular to use the term *semiprofession,* with the implication that there are steps that a group must go through to become professional. One interesting model shows the independent professional at the top of a "crown" of what might be stages of professionalism. Encroaching on this elite area are groups that have some of the desired attributes. At the bottom are the unskilled or semiskilled. The further away from the top, the more dependent that group is on a bureaucracy. Significantly, the lines are broken, showing the mobility of each group from level to level.[4] This approach is in agreement with what many sociologists are saying, which is that professionalism is not a matter of either/or but rather a continuum, with some criteria being much more important than others.

Which criteria are most important? Looking at them objectively, it is clear that nursing does not totally fulfill all of them. It has been pointed out that nursing's theory base is still developing, that the public does not always see the nurse as a professional, that not all nurses are educated in institutions of higher learning, that not all nurses consider nursing a lifetime career, and that in many practice settings, nursing does not control its own policies and activities.[5] The last, a lack of autonomy, is considered the most serious weakness. Sociologists have long contended that an occupation has not become a profession unless the members of that occupation are the ones who make the final decisions in the field of activity in which they are engaged. For instance, Goode identifies two "core characteristics of a profession: a prolonged specialized training in a body of abstract knowledge, and a collectivity or service orientation." However he focuses on characteristics that relate to autonomy:

- The profession determines its own standards of education.
- Professional practice is often legally recognized by some form of licensure.
- Licensing and admission boards are manned by members of the profession.
- Most legislation concerned with the profession is shaped by that profession.[6]

Friedson argues that the only "truly important and uniform criteria for distinguishing professions from other occupations is the fact of autonomy—a position of legitimate control over work."[7] Noted sociologist, Robert Merton, made a similar statement earlier.[8]

The importance of autonomy is also seen in the legal interpretation of nursing. Whereas nurse practice acts have traditionally used the term *profession of nursing* when defining nursing, the courts often have not considered nursing a profession. In a review of various cases across the country, Murphy concluded that the courts regarded nursing as an occupation that possesses a body of knowledge not known to lay persons, yet not held exclusively, since this knowledge is also possessed by physicians who have superior nursing knowledge. Often they were confused as to the independence of nurses from physicians, although one supreme court did differentiate NP practice as separate from that of a physician even when performing medical acts.[9] This has legal ramifications, as discussed in Chapter 12, but it also identifies nursing to the public in a particular way. Since the law is changing constantly, new opinions will emerge. In the end, whether or not such legal opinions will influence how nursing is perceived may well depend on whether the autonomy of nurses is strengthened.

That there has been some progress in changing the legal interpretation of nursing is related to the fact that there has also been progress in achieving autonomy. Perhaps more crucial is nurses' recognition of how autonomy or its absence affects not only the profession but how they practice. (See Chapter 8.) This mental turnaround is related to the fact that more nurses are seeking advanced education and planning nursing careers as opposed to simply taking nursing jobs. There is also more professional involvement, research, and theory development. Nurses are also becoming more aggressive about getting recognition for what they *have* accomplished. Both nurses and others are convinced that the fact that nursing is predominantly female is also a factor in why nurses have had difficulty achieving high professional status. However, with changes in society, including the effect of the women's movement, that have had at least some impact on the stereotyping of women, as well as the progress of nurses themselves, this is seen as a time to move the profession forward.[10] If nursing is not considered a profession in the strictest sense of the word, it is well on the way to becoming so. One author commented thoughtfully, "On the continuum of professionalization, qualitatively nursing and many individual nurses excel far beyond contemporary recognized professions in many areas. Quantitatively, the road ahead is very long."[11] Whether or not (or when) it will become a full profession depends on whether its practitioners choose this demanding status and continue to make progress.

It should be pointed out, however, that the term *profession* is essentially a social concept and has no meaning apart from society. Society decides that for its needs to be met in a certain respect, a body undertaking to meet these particular needs will be given special consideration. The contract is that the individuals of that favored group continually use their best efforts to meet those obligations, constantly reexamining and scrutinizing their functions for appropriateness and always maintaining competence. When they fail to honor these obligations and/or slip into demanding status, authority, and privileges that have no connection with carrying out their professional work satisfactorily, society may reconsider.

Violation of this code eventually brings retribution from society, as seen today in the tightening of laws regulating professional practice and reimbursement. Certain behaviors, such as unprofessional conduct, may be specifically punished by removal of the practitioner's legal right to practice— licensure (see Chapter 11).

On the other hand, despite the prestige of professionalism, many concepts that were traditionally held are fading. For instance, collective bargaining, unionism, and strikes, once seen as unprofessional, have been gradually accepted as legitimate activities by professionals who are employed. Obviously, the very fact that more professionals, even physicians, are employed, and thus lack a degree of autonomy, is a factor. In addition, there is an increasing tendency to use the term *professional* in another context to describe someone who has recognized competence in a particular field or occupation, such as a hairdresser, or someone who participates in an activity for pay as opposed to an amateur—a musician, artist, or baseball player.

Looking at it in the pure sense, however, the idea of professionalism has been called the most important and powerful in the belief system of nursing. But this ideology does not seem to provide all nurses with universal beliefs and ideals about the profession. Nurses themselves do not hold a common concept of professionalism. Six thousand nurses responding to a survey all felt that they were professional, but their concept varied from the majority view of professionalism as an "amalgam of competence, high ethical standards, medical knowledge, and compassion" to individual qualities such as sense of humor, well groomed, cheerful, courteous, capable, and confident.[12]

In a scholarly but personalized treatise on her beliefs about nursing, Margretta Styles introduces new and challenging thoughts about professionalism. One provocative point is that professionalism is not, as perceived, rooted in a two-party arrangement between the professional and the client.

Because today professions are practiced predominantly in some type of institutional setting, there are other factors to consider, such as multiple client systems. Faculty members, for instance, may have as clients students, the university, the health care agency, and the patient, to all of whom they owe some accountability.[13] (What if their demands conflict?)

Styles' key point is that nurses should not set their sights on an external ideal—professionalism—and on externally applied qualifications, but rather should compete with themselves to be the best they can in accomplishing goals set by themselves—"self-actualized professionals forming an actualized profession." She calls this *professionhood.*

Professionalism, Styles maintains, emphasizes the *composite character of the profession* and "allows us to lose ourselves in the crowd . . . it even encourages a nonproductive or counterproductive range of responses from passivism, escapism, and blamism. On the other hand, professionhood [focusing on the characteristics of the individual] . . . forces us to pay attention to our own image as the dominant figure in the mirror of nursing. It recognizes that the professionalism of nursing will be achieved only through the professionhood of its members."[14]

Therefore, we return to the basic ingredient of professionalism—the individual nurse. Regardless of which term is preferred, professionalism is more than a theoretical notion; it is a way of life that demands commitment. (There are also those who say that once nurses never doubted that they were professionals, but have now allowed themselves to be intimidated by accepting other American professions as a standard.)[15]

Definitions of Nursing

Causing almost as much disagreement as the question of whether nursing is a profession is "How do you define nursing?" Definitions of nursing vary according to the philosophy of an individual or group. How people see the roles and functions of nursing is based on what they think nursing is. Exhibit 4-1[16–19] gives an overview of some of the best-known definitions. Most nurses would probably accept any of these in principle, although they might argue that some are more ideal than real. In the ANA position paper of 1965, the terms *care, cure,* and *coordination* were used as part of a definition of *professional practice,* and this phrase has been used numerous times, with individual interpretation of the components.

As nurses expanded their functions into the new nurse practitioner role, *cure* acquired a different meaning for some nurses as management of the patient's care, which includes aspects of what has been medical diagnosis and treatment. Some nurses, like Rogers, feel that such medical (not nursing) diagnosis and treatment diminishes the role of the nurse as a nurse. (The same opponents also usually reject the term *nurse practitioner* or *NP.*)

However, Ford, a pioneer of the NP movement, immediately responding, called this "semantic roulette" and added, "I'm not so concerned about the words. I'm convinced that nursing can take on that level of accountability of professional practice that involves the consumer in decision-making in his care and also demands sophisticated clinical judgment to determine levels of illness and wellness and design a plan of management."[20]

Coordination has a particular importance in the case manager role, which has received increasing attention, since the case manager's major responsibility is to meet the needs of a patient's continuum of care. Coordinating the many diverse aspects of patient care is an important facet.[21]

Care is also translated in a number of ways, sometimes as a physical activity, such as in giving care, but it is considered by nursing experts as much more. The concept has been given considerable attention in the last several years, with research exploring the meaning and entire curricula based on related theory. Watson, who has written extensively on caring (some see her concepts as a new theory), says: "Caring is a normal ideal that guides and directs human actions, not just as a means but a human end in and of itself that is of intrinsic value to human civilization . . . human caring values and actions contribute to the health and healing of individuals."[22] Caring is also seen as invisible or hidden, and therefore often undervalued. Says Roberts, "It is necessary that we 'uncover' more of the characteristics of this caring practice, so that it can be recognized, rewarded, and taught to students of nursing."[23] In a much praised book that presents an analysis of expert nursing, based on vivid examples of excellence in actual nursing practice, Benner remarks on "the nature of the power associated with the caring provided by the nurses" in the study and concludes: "One thing is clear: Almost no intervention will work if the nurse-patient relationship is not based on mutual respect and genuine caring."[24]

One concern that has been voiced about emphasizing caring as a major part of nursing is that people will revert to the old notion that nursing does not require intelligence—just love. Therefore, while the NCNIP nursing image campaign of 1990 emphasized caring, posters also carried the tag line, "If caring were enough, anyone could be a nurse." The other side of the coin is presented by a distinguished historian, who contends that nursing's problem is being "ordered to care" in a society that refuses to value caring.[25]

Although, over the years, nursing has been defined in specific situations according to the functions of nurses or the clinical fields in which they practice, or the specific job titles they may hold, there is a thread running throughout the definitions that indicates that the focus of nursing is the health of whole human beings in interaction with their environment—a holistic, humanistic focus. The ANA 1973 *Standards of Practice* states:

Nursing practice is a direct service, goal-directed, and adaptable to the needs of the individual, family, and community during health and illness. Professional practitioners of nursing bear primary responsibility and accountability for the nursing care clients/patients receive.

An extremely significant step in the definition of nursing occurred in 1980 when ANA published *Nursing: A Social Policy Statement*. It was intended to "assist nurses in conceptualizing their practice; to provide direction to educators, administrators, and researchers within nursing; and to inform other health professionals, legislators, funding bodies, and the public about nursing's contribution to health care."[26] Based on the "diagnosis and treatment of human responses" concept, it detailed what this encompassed. It

---

Exhibit 4-1

Definitions of Nursing by Nurses

"(to have) charge of the personal health of somebody . . . and what nursing has to do . . . is to put the patient in the best condition for nature to act upon him." *(Florence Nightingale, 1859.)*

Nursing in its broadest sense may be defined as an art and science which involves the whole patient—body, mind, and spirit; promotes his spiritual, mental and physical health by teaching and by example; stresses health education and health preservation as well as ministration to the sick; involves the care of the patient's environment—social and spiritual as well as physical; and gives health services to the family and the community as well as to the individual.[16] *(Sister M. Olivia Gowan, 1944.)*

The unique function of the nurse is to assist the individual, sick or well, in the performance of those activities contributing to health or its recovery (or to peaceful death) that he would perform unaided if he had the necessary strength, will, or knowledge. And to do this in such a way as to help him gain independence as rapidly as possible. This aspect of her work, this part of her function, she initiates and controls; of this she is master. In addition she helps the patient to carry out the therapeutic plan as initiated by the physician. She also, as a member of a medical team,

was also noted that all nurses are responsible for including preventive nursing in their practice, that nurses provide care across the life span and in a variety of settings, and that they are ethically and legally accountable for actions taken in practice or delegated.

A separate section was on specialization, called a mark of the advancement of the nursing profession. It stated:

Specialization in nursing practice assists in clarifying, revising, and strengthening existing practice. It also permits new applications of knowledge and refined nursing practice to flow from the specialist to

helps other members, as they in turn help her, to plan and carry out the total program whether it be for the improvement of health or the recovery from illness or support in death.[17] *(Virginia Henderson, 1961.)*

The essential components of professional nursing are care, cure, and coordination. *(ANA Position Paper, 1965.)*

Nursing's first line of defense is promotion of health and prevention of illness. Care of the sick is resorted to when our first line of defense fails.[18] *(Martha Rogers, 1966.)*

Nursing is the diagnosis and treatment of human responses to actual or potential health problems. *(New York State Nurse Practice Act, 1972.)*

The first level nurse is responsible for planning, providing, and evaluating

nursing care in all settings for the promotion of health, prevention of illness, care of the sick and rehabilitation; and functions as a member of the health team. *(International Council of Nursing, 1973.)*

Nursing is an essential service to all of mankind. That service can be succinctly described in terms of its focus, goal, jurisdiction, and outcomes as that of assessing and enhancing the general health status, health assets, and health potentials of all human beings.[19] *(Rozella Schlotfeldt, 1978.)*

The "Practice of Nursing" means assisting individuals or groups to maintain or attain optimal health, implementing a strategy of care to accomplish defined goals, and evaluating responses to care and treatment. *(Model Practice Act, National Council of State Boards of Nursing, 1988.)*

the generalist in nursing practice and graduate to basic education, thus ensuring progress in the general practice in nursing.[27]

Despite its somewhat obscure language at certain points, which made it less than totally understandable to some nurses, much less nonnurses, the *Social Policy Statement* was another major step in defining contemporary nursing.

NURSING FUNCTIONS

Nursing functions can be described in broad or specific terms. For instance, classically, the common elements have included maintaining or restoring normal life function; observing and reporting signs of actual or potential change in a patient's status; assessing his or her physical and emotional state and immediate environment; formulating and carrying out a plan of nursing care based on a medical regimen, including administration of medications and treatments and interpretation of treatment and rehabilitative regimens; counseling families in relation to other health-related services; and teaching. Some of these are referred to in the *Social Policy Statement*.

Of course, some nurses (and administrators) still see the nurse more as a manager of nursing care than as a face-to-face clinical practitioner—in other words, responsible for nursing care, supervising and coordinating the work of others, but not personally giving care. While in recent years there has been a return to a clinical emphasis, now, during a major nursing shortage and rising salaries, the issue has emerged again. This notion that nurses are too expensive to give bedside care assumes that today's very sick patients don't need the most expert nursing care—clearly a fallacy.

In defining functions that should be common to all nurses, Schlotfeldt identifies the following:

1. Interviewing to obtain accurate health histories.
2. Examining, with use of all senses and technological aids, to ascertain the health status of persons served.
3. Evaluating to draw valid inferences concerning individuals' health assets and potentials.
4. Referring to physicians and dentists those persons whose health status indicates the need for differential diagnoses and the institution of therapies.
5. Referring to other helping professionals those persons who need assistance with problems that fall within the province of clergymen, social workers, homemakers, lawyers, and others.

6. Caring for persons during periods of their dependence to include:
   a. compensating for deficits of those unable to maintain normal functions and to execute their prescribed therapies;
   b. sustaining and supporting persons while reinforcing the natural, developmental, and reparative processes available to human beings in their quest for wholeness, function, comfort, and self-fulfillment;
   c. teaching and guiding persons in their pursuit of optimal wellness;
   d. motivating persons toward active, knowledgeable involvement in seeking health and in executing their needed therapies.
7. Collaborating with other health professionals and with persons served in planning and executing programs of health care and diagnostic and treatment services.
8. Evaluating in concert with consumers, other providers, and policy-makers the efficacy of the health care system and planning for its continuous improvement.[28]

The degree of expertise with which nurses carry out these functions depends on their level of knowledge and skills, but the profession has the responsibility of setting standards for its practitioners. In its 1991 *Standards of Clinical Nursing Practice,* the ANA incorporated standards of care and standards of professional performance.

THE NURSING PROCESS AND NURSING DIAGNOSIS

Yura and Walsh state that the term *nursing process* was not prevalent in the nursing literature until the mid-1960s, with limited mention in the 1950s.[29] Orlando was one of the earliest authors to use the term, but it was slow to be adopted. In the next few years, models of the activities in which nurses engaged were developed, and in 1967, a faculty group at the Catholic University of America specifically identified the phases of the nursing process as assessing, planning, implementing, and evaluating. The nursing process is described as "an orderly, systematic manner of determining the client's problems, making plans to solve them, initiating the plan or assigning others to implement it, and evaluating the extent to which the plan was effective in resolving the problems identified."[30]

At this point, there is considerable information in the nursing literature about the use of the nursing process, and many schools of nursing use it as a framework for teaching. However, there are those who feel that other approaches are more suitable to today's complex care.[31]

Nursing diagnosis is seen as part of the nursing process:

> Provision of nursing care is a problem-solving process. The nurse first gathers data about her patient, then identifies the problem. An approach to the problem is selected and carried out. Finally, the results of this approach, in terms of consequences for the patient, are evaluated. By using this process the nurse can individualize her care and be accountable for providing a scientifically based service. Nursing diagnosis is the title given to the stage of identifying the problem.[32]

A diagnostic taxonomy (a set of classifications that are ordered and arranged on the basis of a single principle or set of principles) has been in the development stage for several years. Its development is currently under the direction of the North American Nursing Diagnosis Association (NANDA) and may serve as a major communication tool among nurses. It could also help the public understand what nurses do; just as physicians can pinpoint what they do in relation to treating diseases, nurses can point out nursing diagnosis as the patient problems they try to resolve. However, interesting developments have occurred in recent years, with some argument about the usefulness and appropriateness of nursing diagnosis either as a concept or in practical application in the specialty field.[33-35] Need for validation is another concern.[36] Nevertheless there are those who say that the ability to make a *nursing* diagnosis and to prescribe *nursing* actions is basic to the development of nursing science, and there are many sophisticated studies about its various dimensions.[37]

MAJOR NURSING THEORIES

As nursing has developed in professionalism, nursing scholars have developed theories of nursing based on research, and the science of nursing is coming of age. A scientific body of knowledge unique to nursing is important to provide a basis for clear differentiation between medicine and nursing, on the one hand, and nursing and nurturing, on the other. Research and theory building unique to a discipline are elements required for that discipline to be recognized by a profession.

Although Florence Nightingale identified a body of knowledge specific to the nursing of her time and used this as the basis for instruction in the Nightingale schools, it was not until the 1950s and 1960s that there was a proliferation of nursing concepts and theories. Nursing scholars argued that without research and theory building, nursing would be unable to carve out a role for itself in the future health care system, and would thus allow itself to be defined, instructed, and controlled by other disciplines.

Theory building in nursing takes several forms and has several purposes. Mid-level theory, for example, focuses on the improvement of direct patient/client care through research on patient/client care modalities, such as effective methods of decubitus care or patient education. Findings of this type of research are essential to the development of specialized knowledge in nursing.

Grand theory is not built on research findings as much as it is built on ideologies and concepts. Grand theory takes a world view that attempts to explain and define nursing and analyze the interrelationships between patient, nurse, illness, health, and support mechanisms. Nursing theorists are those who are involved with developing theories or models of nursing. Nursing theorists may explain all or some of the interrelationships listed above.

Exhibit 4-2 summarizes the contributions of selected nursing theorists who have greatly influenced the current practice of nursing. The emphasis of nursing on the holistic approach to patient/client care is evident as a consistent element since the time of Florence Nightingale. For further details, see the Bibliography.

NURSING IMAGE: TRUE OR FALSE

Considering how much responsibility nurses have in health care, their constant presence in every place that care is given, and their numbers, you might expect that people would have a reasonably accurate idea about what nurses do. Yet they don't. One reason may be the extreme diversity of nurses' responsibilities. There simply isn't just one kind of nurse, but almost no one in the general public is in contact with nurses in every field. Therefore, people's image of the nurse is formed in many ways and from many sources: personal acquaintance, contact during their own or someone else's illness, or the media—books, magazines, newspapers, radio, and television.

In the last few years, the nursing profession has been disturbed about the inaccurate picture of nursing in the media to the point where various nursing groups have made image making a priority. The Kalisches have presented an excellent overview of how nurses have been portrayed over the years in all the media, especially television. (See the partial list in the Bibliography.) The nurse, almost always a woman, is everything from angel to devil, sexpot to sexless, stupid to brilliant, tender to terrible—much like characters representing any other field. Although sometimes these nurses do seem to function as autonomous practitioners, more frequently they are physicians' handmaidens, technology tenders, and pillow plumpers. The story lines about personal relationships, problems, and successes are what is important; the rest is background. What is surprising is why anyone should really expect any other priority. Other disciplines are probably treated just as well or

Exhibit 4-2

An Interpretation of Nursing Theories

Theorist	Concept	Patients/Clients	Nursing	Health/Illness	Support
Florence Nightingale	Adaptation; environmental theory	Individuals who are unable to manipulate the environment to promote health.	A profession for women. Modification of the environment to provide the best possible conditions. Using nature's laws governing health in the service of humanity.	Disability related to environmental factors.	Changing the environment to allow the body to repair itself.
Virginia Henderson	Developmental theory; interpersonal relationships	Individuals who would care for themselves if possible. Biological beings with inseparable mind and body.	Assists patients with 14 essential functions toward independence. Doing for patients what they cannot do for themselves.	Wholeness of mind and body, completeness; health is the ability to function independently in relation to 14 components.	Complement the patient to supply what is needed.

Sister Callista Roy	Adaptation; general systems theory	Biopsychosocial beings interacting with a dynamic environment.	Supports the individual's adaptation to stimuli.	A state or a process of being and becoming an integrated and whole person through adaptation.	Emphasis on maximizing coping mechanisms to free energy for promoting adaptation.
Dorothea Orem	Self-care nursing theory (*self-care*: a consciously chosen behavior)	An integrated whole interacting with the environment; performs self-care to maintain health and well-being.	A human service assisting patients in overcoming deficits in self-care action for health-related reasons.	Maintenance and promotion of structural integrity, functioning, and development.	Ranges from wholly compensatory to educative-supportive nursing interventions.
Betty Neuman	Systems theory; stress/adaptation	An open system interacting with the environment.	Interventions that depend upon the patient's/client's interaction with stressors.	Internal and external harmony and balance viewed as a continuum of health.	Readaptation, maintenance, stability.

Exhibit 4-2 (Continued)

An Interpretation of Nursing Theories

Theorist	Concept	Patients/Clients	Nursing	Health/Illness	Support
Myra Levine	Basic sciences; holism	Persons with illness or disease that requires adaptation to environmental factors. Actively participate in care.	Application of principles of conservation to promote adjustment of client by supportive and therapeutic interventions.	Response of the individual to the environment. Maintenance and promotion of client's unity and integrity.	Supportive and therapeutic interventions to promote patient's adjustment.
Martha Rogers	Science of Unitary Beings; open systems continually interacting with the environment	More than the sum of their parts; wholeness is reflected in pattern and organization	Learned profession based on application of a science and an art; a continuous, mutual, simultaneous interaction.	Interchange and repatterning between the individual and the environment to prevent illness and promote health.	Emphasis on health promotion and illness prevention.

Josephine Patterson and Loretta Zderad	Nursology: inter-subjectivity of nurse and client.	Persons with needs in the process of becoming in an environment of time and space.	Responsive transactional relationship founded on the nurse's awareness of self and others aimed at the development of human potential	Well-being, rather than freedom from disease. Becoming more, as possible in particular life situations.	Interact with client to assist in reaching full potential as a human.
Margaret Newman	Movement, consciousness, time and space, expanded consciousness	Increasingly complex person evolving in the environment.	Mutual nurse-client relationship to recognize and augment the person-environment interaction in order to enhance expanding consciousness.	A fusion of disease-nondisease that explicates the basic pattern of person-environment interaction.	Evolving together with the client to reach expanding consciousness.
Jean Watson	Human care	Persons possessing three spheres: mind, body, and soul; Continually striving to actualize the higher self.	Human science and caring activity modified by professional, personal, aesthetic, scientific, and ethical transactions.	The feeling of being at one with what is. A unity of mind, body, and soul.	Human-to-human caring relationship that allows for detection, empathy, and response to the patient's condition.

badly in fiction and are just as unhappy about it. At times doctors, nurses, and others in the health field are pleased with their images in shows where real issues are tackled (not always realistically). That does not mean that the nurses are shown as what we'd like nurses to be.

Books about nursing, from simplistic preteenage novels to those such as *One Flew Over the Cuckoo's Nest,* are also seen to impress the public.[38] The Kalisches have also done an interesting analysis of movies and novels about nursing.[39,40] Both media seemed to follow similar patterns. In six time periods from 1854 to the late 1980s, nurse stereotypes ranged through the stages of angel of mercy, girl Friday, heroine, mother, sex object, and, finally, careerist, which is seen as the ideal image for this decade. Needless to say, this was not necessarily consistent in each time period. In fact, Dorothy Canfield Fisher, who ranked with the most noted authors of the time and was published from 1907 to 1953, "wrote with clarity and compassion about nursing and its contribution to the well-being of individuals and society."[41] A former public health nurse administrator, Mary Sewall Gardner, wrote realistic novels about public health nurses in the 1940s (as well as textbooks).

Yet, perhaps because television is so pervasive in almost everyone's life today, attracting all age groups, there is some fear that, of all the media, this one is most likely to influence the public concerning the image of nurses. Nursing was concerned enough that in the late 1980s it took massive action against a TV show called *Nightingales,* which portrayed nurses as promiscuous birdbrains and tinsel handmaidens.[42,43] Nursing organizations and individuals offered to provide script consultation and other help, and were turned down. The surge of nursing protests led commercial sponsors to back out, and eventually the show was canceled. (Lone's lucid "op-ed" commentary in the *New York Times,* widely reported, was seen as particularly useful in affecting public opinion.) At the same time, another series, *China Beach,* was praised as a realistic and sensitive portrayal of nurses in the Vietnam War. Its star later did commercials to promote nursing as a career. Ironically, however, this program, too, was eventually canceled, and the protests of nurses could not revive it.

Does the public believe that such fiction is reality? Probably not. Even children are beginning to regard some aspects of television cynically. More serious might be the nonfiction or news programs and articles that show what is new in medicine and health care, and where nurses are shadowy background figures or have limited exposure, to show what they do to help patients recover. In addition, when nurses become involved in criminal cases related to patients, the news coverage can be unfair or slanted toward the sensational.[44]

Magazines publishing feature stories have often taken a "pity the poor nurse" point of view, although more recently the emphasis has been on new nursing roles. In fact, in nonfiction of all kinds, the portrayals of nurses have become more positive and up-to-date (while not totally eliminating the "poor nurse" aspect). No breakthrough seems to have come from greeting card manufacturers, who often portray nurses as devastating cartoons in get-well cards.[45] Some have complained that the protesters had no sense of humor.

The power of the media and the numerous shows that continue to portray nurses in a negative and unrealistic manner led to the organizing of a group called Nurses of America (NOA) and their publication, *Media Watch*. NOA was sponsored by the Tri-Council organizations (see Chapter 27). It was funded by a grant from the Pew Charitable Trusts and administered by the NLN. NOA described itself as "a national, multi-media effort designed to inform the public about the role contemporary nursing plays in the delivery of high quality, cost-effective health care services. . . . NOA's media efforts are designed to demonstrate the real drama of nursing; the vital work that nurses do every day."

NOA worked with a variety of media, ranging from newspapers and magazines to TV and community forums. A large component of their activities included monitoring the media for health-related issues and the portrayal of nurses and nursing practice.[46] Although its funding ceased in 1991, the nurses involved hope for continued support from the Tri-Council.

Does all this have any effect on how the public sees the nurse? Hard data are not easy to come by. Questions have been raised as to how much a prestige rating is influenced by personal contact and how much by reputation or image. Overall, the public seems to have a positive view of nurses, more so than of many other professions, but the cumulative effect of the various media may still influence the public, without people knowing just where they got their wrong ideas about nursing. One survey showed that "the image of the nurse continues to turn on feminine and nurturant qualities,"[47] which is not completely wrong, while another showed that university professors held a more positive image of nurses than that typically portrayed in the media.[48] Since the nursing shortage, still another factor affecting nursing's image, may have been the advertising about nursing under the aegis of the Advertising Council and NCNIP. The purpose was to portray nursing as a "discipline that offers excitement, clinical substance, and authority and responsibility, all tied up in the richness of interpersonal closeness with patients."[49] This seems to have had a positive impact on nursing enrollments.

Another encouraging factor is the result of a nationwide survey of the public's attitudes toward health care and nurses done for the Pew Charitable Trusts in May 1990. Although people reacted negatively about many aspects of health care, its institutions and providers, nurses were the most widely respected and supported. They were seen as caring, competent practitioners who are underutilized and should be given more responsibility. People also thought that nurses could reduce the cost of health care if they were better used.

In addition to the image of nursing in the media and the public's viewpoint, another concern of nurses is how physicians perceive them and their profession. It is clear that the perceptions of some physicians are as confused as they were 100 years ago. However, now, as then, there are physicians and leaders in organized medicine who see and applaud the changes in nursing toward full professionalism; others find this trend either threatening, incongruent with what they think a nurse's role should be, or not as desirable as the situation in the "good old days."[50] But there is good news. In a survey of hospital CEOs, nursing was named as the most significant factor in providing quality care,[51] and the AHA noted that good nursing care was what most attracted physicians to a particular hospital. Another survey reported that nurses showing personal concern for patients in the emergency room was the most important factor in patients recommending those emergency room services (a big source of admissions).

What about the impact of the "real" nurse on the *perception* of the nurse? Emerging research indicates that direct contact with a group, like nurses, may be the most influential factor in image making. Such contact may actually not provide a more objective view. Personal acquaintance almost always introduces the factors of liking or disliking, with little relation to, or knowledge of, professional performance. For others, emotionalism involved in contacts during illness is inevitable, because neither patient nor family and friends can be objective at such times. People do have expectations about what they want from a nurse, most often competence and caring. If their expectations aren't met, a bad image may replace a good one. For instance, whether a nurse is pleasant or unpleasant, patient or hurried, gentle or rough are factors. If buzzers aren't answered promptly or a patient is left in pain or discomfort, an image of uncaring nurses is formed and often communicated to others. (Note the surveys mentioned above.) It does not help that some caregivers today are difficult to identify and that the "nurse" may not be an RN. Moreover, unimportant as it may seem, *how* a nurse looks makes an important first impression. Findings from a 1985 survey indicated that both patients and professionals prefer the white uniform and see it as a powerful symbol in the health field.[52] (Of course, this may not be seen as important in some of the specialty areas, where color or a different type of garb is more appropriate.) The point is to make an impression that communicates professionalism. Kalisch and Kalisch wrote about the changes in nursing uniforms over time, and they were quick to note that "clothing is a form of nonverbal communication that stimulates judgmental or behavioral responses in others. Our clothing makes it possible for a stranger to categorize us—at least tentatively—and set the stage for further interactions. . . . For better or worse, clothing communicates. Now, as before, it is important that nurses dress for success.[53] Other points that are made about how nurses can improve their image are these: they should be more visible and active in community activities and organizations; converse more easily on a broad range of subjects, rather than be focused on nursing alone; and learn how to handle the media.[54]

What creating a positive image of nursing comes down to, then, is, more than anything else, the individual, as aptly expressed by one nursing leader:

> Let us recognize that the major change agent, as we so glibly use the term, is the individual who carries the title nurse and provides nursing care to the individual who requires it. The power to change the image lies in that practitioner. It is true that the media can help, but only a limited amount. The media will cling to the conservative, traditional view of nurses and women until what we want, professional clinical nursing practice, becomes the usual practice.[55]

THE REALITY: FACTS, FIGURES, GUESSES

The information we have about the *real* nurse can also cause confusion. Demographic data, such as numbers, age, marital status, and employment, are usually acquired by taking a sample and then projecting to the total number. By the time that these and other facts are published, they may be somewhat outdated. However, by comparing them with earlier data, a trend or a change can be detected. Exhibit 4-3 shows some of the latest information available on nurses. Some of the interesting trends in the employed population over the last 10 years are a slow increase in the number of men, fewer nonwhite nurses, and more married nurses with children at home. A dramatic drop in the number of nurses with a diploma as the highest degree reflects educational trends, as does the older average age. Hospitals have consistently employed the largest number of nurses, with the percentages not varying much in this time period; private duty has decreased the most dramatically. Even though the percentage of NPs and clinical specialists has remained quite small in the last several years, this category was not even listed before the 1977 surveys.

A Nursing Profile

The most current, general, comprehensive demographic data about nurses come from the Division of Nursing of DHHS. The most recent (as of 1991) is the 1988 National Sample Survey of Registered Nurses, summarized in Exhibit 4-3. It is also the source of other important data.[56]

Certain past studies of nurses are useful in identifying the background of nurses in the workforce. One of the most comprehensive studies of nurses was the longitudinal NLN Nursing Career Pattern Study, begun in 1962. It was designed to obtain definitive biographical characteristics of nursing

Exhibit 4-3

Who Are the Nurses?

	1988	1980
Total RN population	2.0 million	1.7 million
Employed in nursing[1]	80.0%	76.6%
	(about 26% part time)	(about 32% part time)
Sex		
Female	96.6%	96.1%
Male	3.3%	3.0%
Ethnic-racial background		
White/ non-Hispanic	91.7%	90.4%
Black	3.6%	4.3%
Asian/Islander	2.3%	2.4%
Hispanic	1.3%	1.4%
American Indian/ Alaskan Native	.4%	0.28%
Age		
Under 25	3.9%	9.6%
25–34	29.8%	36.2%
35–44	29.5%	23.3%
45–54	19.1%	17.2%
55–64	12.3%	15.7%
65 or over	5.0%	4.5%
Marital status		
Married	70.6%	70.6%
Divorced, separated, widowed	15.4%	13.8%
Never married	13.0%	14.8%
Places of employment		
Hospital	67.9%	65.6%

students, their occupational goals, and the reasons for their choice of nursing as a career. Later, the Department of Health, Education and Welfare (DHEW) supported extension of the study to include students who entered associate degree, diploma, and baccalaureate RN programs in 1965 and 1967. The 6893 students who graduated from the 259 basic nursing programs in the 1962 group became part of the cohort that was surveyed 1, 5, 10, and 15 years after graduation. Although declining over that period, from 96 percent the first year, the response rate for the 15-year segment was still at 70

	1988	1980
Nursing home	6.6%	8.0%
Community health	6.8%	6.6%
Physician's office/		
ambulatory care	7.7%	5.7%[2]
Nursing education	1.8%	3.7%
Student health service	2.9%	3.5%
Occupational health	1.3%	2.3%
Private duty nursing	1.2%	1.6%
Other	3.6%	1.7%
Type of position		
Staff nurse	66.9%	65.0%
Heads nurse and supervisor	10.9%	13.1%
Administration (service and		
education)	6.6%	4.8%
Instructor	3.8%	4.7%
Clinical specialist/clinician	2.9%	2.1%
Nurse practitioner/midwife	1.5%	1.3%
Nurse anesthetist	1.0%	1.1%
Other	6.6%	6.8%
Higher educational preparation		
Doctorate	0.3%	0.2%
Master's	6.2%	5.1%
Baccalaureate in nursing	25.1%	20.7%
Other baccalaureate	2.3%	2.6%
Diploma	40.4%	50.7%
Associate degree	25.2%	20.1%

Source: DHHS Division of Nursing, National Sample Survey of Registered Nurses, 1988.

[1]Data refer to *employed* nurses. Some figures do not total 100% because of no response and rounding of figures.

[2]Refers to physician's office only.

percent. The study was completed in 1981 and was one of the most comprehensive studies of nursing ever done.[57]

The final phase of the study showed some trends in career patterns that are of interest even today.[58] Six out of 10 of the nurses reported working for 10 or more years, with 27 percent having worked the entire time. For instance, those who had continued their education were more likely to be in the nurse labor force at the end of the 15-year interval, but they were also slightly more likely to be working in nonnursing positions.

Knopf noted several disturbing findings. Three out of 10 stated that they would not choose nursing again as a career. Whether that was due to dissatisfaction, the availability of other career opportunities today, or some other reason was not determined.

More recently, another comprehensive study on nursing is the NLN's newly licensed nurse survey.[59] It provides details on the employment, mobility, and demographic characteristics of all newly licensed nurses in the country on a regional basis. In 1990, each nurse who was newly licensed after taking the July 1989 licensure exam, received a questionnaire covering demographic, employment, educational, and geographic characteristics. Over 28,000 nurses responded, for a response rate of 64 percent.

The study's findings reinforced the previous perceptions of demand also reported in a similar NLN survey published in 1989.[60] Specifically, new RNs were overwhelmingly eager to work in hospitals for their first job, and only a few were seeking nonnurse employment. Hence, new RNs were committed to nursing and lacked the oft-cited tendency to want to change professions. The study's findings provide impressive evidence that the demand for new RNs was still very strong. Their major satisfaction was that they were able to work in their desired specialty. They were most unhappy about poor working conditions, for instance, forced overtime. In distant second place was inadequate salaries.

As in previous years, the overwhelming number of new graduates, although generally older than previously, are still white women. Although the second-degree students may account for some of the older group, the AD programs also attract older students. For instance, over 41 percent of AD graduates held licenses as licensed practical/vocational nurses (LPN/LVNs). The majority of AD graduates are married and have children living at home; the BSN graduates are mostly single. This may also account for the fact that most AD nurses tended to choose a nursing program close by, whereas baccalaureate students were more mobile. Most RNs stayed in the same locale after graduation, with blacks and Hispanics being most likely to stay.

Another group of nurses that warrants discussion is nurses professionally involved in public policy. As nurses have become more visible participants in the political arena, many have come to hold positions in regulatory agencies, state legislatures, and congressional offices. A recent study of 33 of these nurses revealed that they were not similar to employed nurses in general. They were typically older, had more formal education, and were more likely to be unmarried and without children. Additional differences were noted between nurses working in state and congressional offices.[61]

Minority Groups in Nursing

Studies on the general population of nursing students and graduates are inevitably influenced by the fact that the majority of nurses are both women

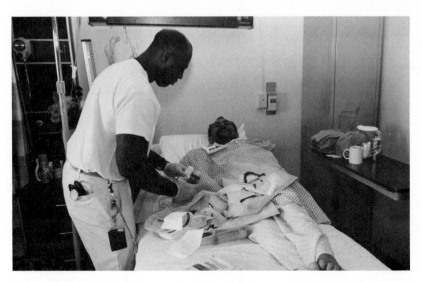

An increasing number of men and ethnic minorities are entering nursing. (*Courtesy of the New York State Nurses' Association; photo by Ricky Flores.*)

and white. There is increasing interest in both the ethnic minority groups in nursing, such as blacks, native Americans, and Hispanics, and the male minority. One question is why minorities do or don't enter nursing and why they often do not complete nursing education programs. Reasons given to explain why many of the racial and ethnic minorities, who are often also considered socioeconomically deprived, do not enter nursing include lack of role models, lack of understanding of what nursing is, lack of proper counseling, and inability to qualify because of poor academic records.

Nursing recruitment for all ethnic minorities has gradually increased, stimulated by federal grants available since 1965 and, perhaps, by the presence of more role models. Even so, the *proportion* of ethnic minorities has *not* increased. Cost is a serious concern to black and Hispanic students and loss of funding may again cause a downturn, although the Advertising Council campaign, in cooperation with the National Commission on Nursing Implementation Project (NCNIP), has made a special effort to recruit them. (See Appendix 1.) Carnegie points out that a number of blacks hold doctorates, serve in high offices in nursing organizations, and hold very prestigious positions in academia and health care institutions.[62] A very positive factor in the increase of doctoral minority nurses has been the ANA Minority Fellowship Program that began in 1974. It provided stipends and other forms of support to ethnic-minority students seeking doctoral education.

Minority nurses at all educational levels continue to exhibit higher employment patterns, with about 89 percent employed in nursing. Those employed in nursing are younger than those not employed; most are married, but over 20 percent have never married. Other demographic data available are similar to those of the general nursing population.

Men have been neglected as potential sources of nurse power, although male nurses have existed almost as long as female nurses in the United States. By 1910, about 7 percent of all student and graduate nurses were men, but in succeeding years the percentage declined, until by 1940 it had dropped to 2 percent. Most men were graduates of hospital schools connected with mental institutions; not many schools (for men) were affiliated with general hospitals, and few coeducational ones existed (see Chapter 2). By 1960, male nurses (not including students) comprised 0.91 percent of the nursing workforce. The current 3.3 percent level reflects a significant increase in the number of male nurses and a gradual increase in their proportion of the total employed RN population over the past 30 years.[63]

Men suffered the same discrimination in nursing that women encountered in male-dominated fields, although this was not always the fault of nursing. For instance, male nurses were kept in the enlisted ranks in the regular armed services until 1966, when, with the continuous pressure of the ANA, commissions were finally available to them in the Regular Nurse Corps.

Some surveys and studies show that overall, female nurses recognize that male nurses are accepted by both patients and physicians and believe that they can make a valuable contribution to nursing. Discrimination has been highlighted primarily in assignment of private duty nurses and in the care of women in obstetrics and gynecology.[64] Some men have gone to court, with varied results. (See Chapter 13.) One serious concern is that men comprised 18 percent of the disciplinary cases reported by state boards, most relating to substance abuse.[65]

It seems that men are influenced to enter nursing through previous contacts or work in the health field. Their families seldom encourage them but usually do not object. Men report that although friends are generally supportive, they get negative reactions from other classmates and strangers, who sometimes show a tendency to view them as homosexuals. These attitudes have created some role strain for the men, as have women in authority. Indeed, one nursing leader described how the fact that nursing is composed of mainly white women "poses both a social and an ethical problem for the profession." He contended that

women, when they are in power, are just as reluctant to share power with men as men have been accused of doing in their relationships with women.[66]

He added:

The recruitment of men into the profession is not a panacea. Men candidates range from exceptional competence to borderline ability.

They bring with them all the positive and negative variables that are indigenous to all humans.[67]

When looking at the issues regarding the role of minorities in nursing, it is important to remember that cultural differences stem from myriad components in all our backgrounds—gender, religion, ethnicity, and even geographic locale. Separating the causes and effects of any one component is probably impossible. Studies that try to do so are flawed by small sample sizes and inconsistent findings..

Personality and Attitude

About 30 years ago, nurses were often the subjects of personality studies,[68] but interest in them has faded. It is questionable if the results would still be valid even though the nurses studied are still in practice, simply because rapidly changing social factors have probably influenced changes in their attitude and behavior.

The tendency now is for nursing journals to publish surveys. These are often popular with readers because nurses like to know what other nurses think about an issue. Over a period of time, if the same issue is addressed, such as baccalaureate education, differences in attitude can also be detected. However, interesting though they may be, results should be taken with the proverbial grain of salt. First, all survey questions are subject to varied interpretation, and some are slanted to get a certain type of answer. Most of all, unlike a scientific sample, only those who are interested and happen to find that particular survey answer, leaving hundreds of thousands of nurses whose opinion is not known.

One kind of research on nurses that has been done continually explores their attitudes about nursing in general, work situations, and reactions toward certain kinds of patients. The finding of the NLN study previously cited, indicating that individuals entered nursing because they wanted to help others, has been consistent over the years. Therefore, because it is evident that a number of students left nursing before completing the program, or did not work in nursing after graduation, and because nurses have also been accused of some indifference to quality care, the basic question arises: why? A number of writers have cited "disillusionment with nursing" as a major reason why nurses leave jobs or nursing itself. Yet, further investigation seems to show that the disillusionment, for graduates as for students, is related more to the practice setting than to the practice. This is discussed more fully in Chapter 7. Whether the study is almost 20 years old or one of the many new studies (see Appendix 1), nurses still appear to find their greatest satisfaction in caring for patients. In nursing, as in any profession, there are some who are primarily interested in nursing as a job or as a way to earn money—the so-called utilizer, migrant, or appliance nurse (one who works only long enough to buy a new home appliance). However, the majority of nurses still apparently have some of the same motivations with which they entered nursing. This is reinforced in a 1991 survey showing that a desire to help people was the primary reason most nurses entered the field; providing high quality care ranked first in importance in their practice.[69]

A word should be said about nurses' attitudes toward certain types of patients. There has been some evidence that nurses do not view all types of patients equally favorably; for example, they tend to be more negative toward the elderly, alcoholic, criminal, mentally ill, or those with certain kinds of conditions. A number of studies, usually small, have been done on these topics. The purpose is primarily to determine what these attitudes are and why, how they affect patient care, and how to encourage or change particular attitudes. One such study reported on nurses' descriptions of unpopular behavior, and on their emotional and behavioral responses to certain vignettes. The researchers found that the majority of nurses' reports of their reactions were classic fight-or-flight responses.[70] Several researchers have explored nurses' attitudes and concerns regarding AIDS. A number of nurses described their thoughts, fears, and satisfactions in caring for AIDS patients.[71] Another study found that many nurses were fearful of contracting AIDS and did not have confidence in their ability to meet the intense physical and psychological needs of AIDS patients.[72] Nurses' attitudes toward homosexuality, drug abusers, ethnic minorities, "unattractive" people, and terminally ill patients complicate the picture even more.[73]

Finally, it is necessary for nurses to acknowledge the importance of our attitudes toward each other, especially when such attitudes affect clinical care, the advancement of the profession, and an individual nurse's practice. We need to question if we govern our professional interrelationships with the same guidelines that regulate our performance in patient care.[74] Other areas to consider are attitudes toward nurses who are impaired,[75] handicapped, or of different ethnic or national origin, and even nurses of different educational backgrounds.

How do nurses feel about doctors? One survey indicated that over half of the respondents were dissatisfied with their professional relationships, citing a subordinate rather than a collegial relationship. Over half also said that it was better with younger doctors but not necessarily with female doctors. Most felt that there were channels for resolving conflicts and for reporting incompetent doctors. The respondents were primarily young hospital staff nurses about evenly divided in relation to their basic education.[76]

Obviously, there is no one profile of today's nurse, particularly in these dynamic times. However, the information obtained from the various studies and reports tells us a great deal about the practitioners of nursing. This can help both nurses and others understand the profession better.

WHAT IS NURSING?

It can easily be seen that there may not be a single definition of nursing. Perhaps there never will be, since nursing is a multifaceted profession. This is one problem legislators have had in writing a nurse practice act, which is, after all, the legal definition of nursing. (These definitions, along with other aspects of licensure, are discussed in Chapter 11.) Nevertheless, at some point, every nurse has to decide what nursing is to him or her and how to interpret it to others. Here are some nurses' observations.[77]

> The essential nature of nursing is love. It is the love of knowledge about health, disease, and treatment. It is the love of people and of life and growth.

> When I nurse another human being, I feel that I am the closest person in the world to them. I do what a loved one would do if only he or she had the skill, intuition, and stamina to do so.

> Nursing lets me savor the essence of caring.

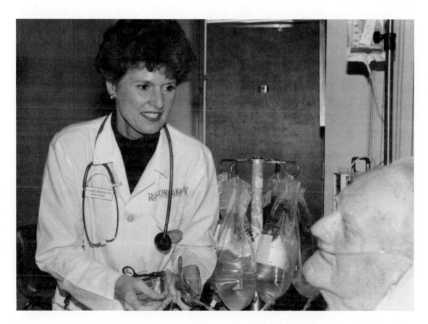

The nurse is a professional person who is technically competent, intellectually able, and caring. (*Courtesy of the Robert Wood Johnson Medical Center.*)

A nurse directly helps people to understand their disease or health status and to adapt to and prepare for changes during life. A nurse is key in helping people to reach higher levels of functioning.

Nursing means helping people out when it really matters.

This chapter, its references, and its bibliography may provide a basis for working out your own definition, but the final determination is yours.

KEY POINTS

1. The basic criteria of professionalism include the concepts of autonomy, altruism, a defined body of knowledge, research, career commitment, social value, and ethics.
2. Nursing is defined in many ways, but the concept of caring for the individual as a whole is generally consistent.
3. Basic nursing functions include interviewing, examining, evaluating, referring, collaborating, and caring for persons during their periods of dependence.
4. The nursing process and nursing diagnosis are a way of organizing data for nursing care.
5. The emphasis of nursing on the holistic approach is evident in the work of the nursing theorists, beginning with Florence Nightingale.
6. The image of nursing in the media is often distorted, but the public may also form a more lasting image, whether positive or negative, through direct contact.
7. Nurses must take some responsibility for creating a true, positive image of nursing.
8. Changes in the growing RN population include an older average age for working nurses and a higher level of education.
9. Since nursing is a large profession made up of a diverse population, information about the background and attitudes of subgroups, as well as of the majority, helps nurses understand one another better.

REFERENCES

1. Schulman S. Basic functional roles in nursing: Mother surrogate and healer. In: Jaco EG, ed. *Patients, physicians and illness: Behavioral sciences and medicine.* Glencoe, IL: Free Press, 1963, p. 532.

2. Flexner A. *Is social work a profession? Proceedings of the National Conference of Charities and Correction*. New York: New York School of Philanthropy, 1915, pp. 576–581.
3. Bixler GK, Bixler RW. The professional status of nursing. *Am J Nurs*, 45:730–735 (September 1945).
4. Buick-Constable B. The professionalism spectre. *Int Nurs Rev*, 16(2):133–144 (1969).
5. Beletz E. Professionalism—A license is not enough. In Chaska N, ed. *The nursing profession: Turning points*. St. Louis: C.V. Mosby Company, 1990, pp. 16–23.
6. Goode W. Encroachment, charlatanism and the emerging professions: Psychology, medicine and sociology. *Am Soc Rev*, 25:902–914 (December 1960).
7. Friedson E. *Profession of medicine: A study of the sociology of applied knowledge*. New York: Dodd, Mead and Company, 1970, p. 82.
8. Merton R. Issues in the growth of a profession. Summary proceedings, American Nurses' Association Convention, 1958 (New York: American Nurses' Association), 1958, p. 298.
9. Murphy E. The professional status of nursing: A view from the courts. *Nurs Outlook*, 35:12–15 (January 1987).
10. Rosenfield P. Nursing and professionalism: On the road to recovery. *Nurs and Health Care*, 7:485–488 (November 1986).
11. Beletz, op. cit., p. 21.
12. Gulack R. I'm a professional. *RN*, 16:29–35 (September 1983).
13. Styles M. *On nursing: Toward a new endowment*. St. Louis: C.V. Mosby Company, 1982, pp. 19–20.
14. Ibid., p. 8.
15. Parsons M. The profession in a class by itself. *Nurs Outlook*, 6:270–275 (November–December 1986).
16. Gowan MO. *Proceedings of the workshop on administration of college programs in nursing, June 21–24, 1944*. Washington, DC: Catholic University of America Press, 1946.
17. Henderson V. *ICN basic principles of nursing care*. London: International Council of Nurses, 1961. Expanded in Henderson V. *The nature of nursing*. New York: Macmillan Publishing Company, 1967.
18. Rogers M. Doctoral education in nursing. *Nurs. Forum*, 5:77 (January, 1966).
19. Schlotfeldt R. The professional doctorate: Rationale and characteristics. *Nurs Outlook*, 26:303 (May 1978).
20. The nurse practitioner question. *Am J Nurs*, 74:2188 (December 1974).
21. Grau L. Case management and the nurse. *Ger Nurs*, 5:372–375 (November–December 1984).
22. Watson J. The moral failure of the patriarchy. *Nurs Outlook*, 38:62–66 (March–April 1990).
23. Roberts J. Uncovering hidden caring. *Nurs Outlook*, 38:67–69 (March–April 1990).
24. Benner P. *From novice to expert*. Menlo Park, CA: Addison-Wesley Publishing Company, 1984, p. 209.

25. Reverby S. *Ordered to care: The dilemma of American nursing.* New York: Basic Books, 1987.
26. *Nursing: A social policy statement.* Kansas City, MO: American Nurses' Association, 1980, p. 30.
27. Ibid., p. 22.
28. Schlotfeldt, op. cit.
29. Yura H, Walsh M. *The nursing process,* 2nd ed. New York: Appleton-Century Crofts, 1973.
30. Yura H, Walsh M. *The nursing process: Assessing, planning, implementing, evaluating.* Norwalk, CT: Appleton-Century-Crofts, 1988, p. 1.
31. McHugh M. Has nursing outgrown the nursing process? *Nurs 87,* 17:50–51 (August 1987).
32. Roy C. A diagnostic classification system for nursing. *Nurs Outlook,* 23:91 (February 1985).
33. Entire issue. *Topics C1 Nurs* (January, 1984).
34. Hagey E, McDonough P. The problem of professional labeling. *Nurs Outlook,* 32:151–157 (May–June 1984).
35. Bruckhorst B, et al. Who's using nursing diagnosis? *Am J Nurs,* 89:267–268 (February 1989).
36. Derdiarian A. A valid profession needs valid diagnoses. *Nurs and Health Care,* 9:137–140 (March 1988).
37. O'Hearn C. Nursing diagnosis: A phenomenological structural description and multidimensional taxonomy or typological redefinition. In Chaska N. ed. *The nursing profession: Turning points.* St. Louis: C.V. Mosby Company, 1990.
38. Eichenberger J, Parker JE. The making of an image. *AAOHN J,* 35:113–115 (March 1987).
39. Kalisch PA, Kalisch BJ *The changing image of the nurse.* Palo Alto, CA: Addison-Wesley Publishing Company, 1987.
40. Kalisch PA, Kalisch BJ. The image of the nurse in motion pictures. *Am J Nurs* 82:605–611 (April 1982).
41. Benson ER. An early 20th century view of nursing. *Nurs Outlook,* 38:275 (December 1990).
42. Lone P. TV's Nightingales—or birdbrains? *New York Times* (Apr. 7, 1989), p. A31.
43. Mallison MB. NBC's tinsel handmaidens. *Am J Nurs,* 89:453 (April 1989).
44. Kalisch B. When nurses are accused of murder. *Nurs Life,* 2:44–47 (September–October 1982).
45. Hott J. "To see ourselves as others see us." *Imprint,* 31:45–48 (February–March 1984).
46. What Nurses of America is all about. *Media Watch,* 1:1–2 (Winter 1990).
47. Kaler SR, et al. Stereotypes of professional roles. *Image,* 21:85–89 (Summer 1989).

48. Lippman DT, Ponton KS. Nursing's image on the university campus. *Nurs Outlook*, 37:24–27 (January 1989).
49. Joel L. NCNIP/Advertising Council campaign challenges resistant stereotypes. *Am J Nurs*, 22:13 (February 1990).
50. Stein LI, et al. The doctor-nurse game revisited. *Nurs Outlook*, 38:264–268 (November–December 1990).
51. Nursing tops CEO's quality list. *Am J Nurs*, 89:468 (April 1989).
52. Levine D. Getting extra mileage from your uniform. *Am J Nurs*, 87:1310–1311 (October 1987).
53. Kalisch BJ, Kalisch PA. Dressing for success. *Am J Nurs*, 85:887–893 (August 1985).
54. Kalisch BJ, Kalisch PA. Good news, bad news, or no news: Improving radio and TV coverage of nursing issues. *Nurs and Health Care*, 6:255–260 (May 1985).
55. Aydelotte MK. Book review, The changing image of the nurse, by Kalisch PA, Kalisch BJ. *Image*, 4:214 (Winter 1987).
56. Moses EB. *The registered nurse population*. Bethesda, MD: U.S. Department of Health and Human Services, 1990.
57. Knopf L. *From student to RN*. Bethesda, MD: Department of Health, Education, and Welfare, 1972.
58. Knopf L. Registered nurses fifteen years after graduation: Findings from the nurse career-pattern study. *Nurs and Health Care*, 4:72–76 (February 1983).
59. Rosenfeld P. *Licensed to care: An executive report on the new nurse*. New York: National League for Nursing, 1991.
60. Rosenfeld P. *Profiles of the newly licensed nurse*. New York: National League for Nursing, 1989.
61. Barry CT. Profiles of nurses professionally involved in public policy. *Nurs Economics*, 8:174–176 (May 1990).
62. Carnegie ME. Blacks in nursing: An update. *The Am Nurse*, 22:6 (February 1990).
63. Halloran EJ. Men in nursing. In McCloskey J, Grace H, eds. *Current issues in nursing*. St. Louis: C.V. Mosby Company, 1990, p. 547.
64. Ibid., pp. 552–553.
65. Lewis JD, et al. Men in nursing: Some troubling data. *Am J Nurs*, 90:30 (August 1990).
66. Christman L. Men in nursing. *Imprint*, 35:75 (September 1988).
67. Ibid.
68. Kelly LY. *Dimensions of professional nursing*, 5th ed. New York: Macmillan Publishing Company, 1985, pp. 229–232.
69. Yeast C. Nurses: who are we and what motivates us? *Am Nurse* Supplement 23:14 (October 1991).
70. Podrasky DL, Sexton DL. Nurses' reactions to difficult patients. *Image*, 20:16–21 (Spring 1988).
71. Bennett JA. Nurses talk about the challenge of AIDS. *Am J Nurs*, 87:1148–1155 (September 1987).

72. Scherer YK, et al. AIDS: What are nurses' concerns? *Clin Nurs Specialist* 3(1):48–50 (1989).

73. Baer ED, Lowery BJ. Patient and situational factors that affect nursing students' like or dislike of caring for patients. *Nurs Res,* 36:298–302 (September–October 1987).

74. Sharkey L. Nurses in the closet: Is nursing open and receptive to gay and lesbian nurses? *Imprint,* 37:38–39 (September 1987).

75. Cannon BL, Brown JS. Nurses' attitudes toward impaired colleagues. *Image,* 20:96–101 (Summer 1988).

76. The doctor-nurse game. *Nurs 91,* 21:60–64 (June 1991).

77. How do I sell nursing? Listen to this. *Am Nurse,* 20:14–15 (October 1988).

PART III
NURSING EDUCATION AND PRACTICE

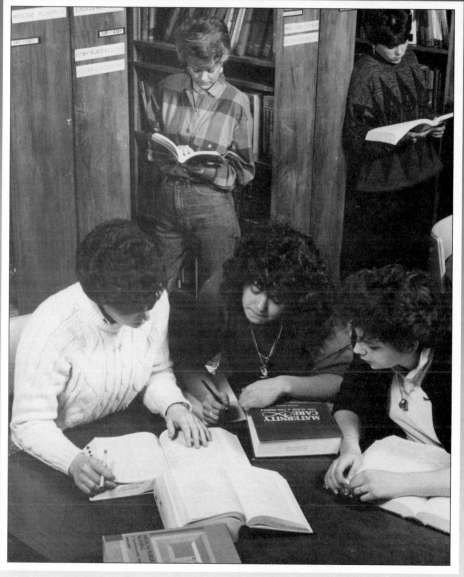

Students in nursing schools today spend considerable time in studying.
(Courtesy of the National Student Nurses' Association.)

CHAPTER 5

EDUCATION AND RESEARCH IN NURSING

OBJECTIVES

After studying this chapter, you will be able to:

1. Identify four ways in which nursing education programs are alike.
2. Compare the major types of education programs leading to RN licensure.
3. Explain briefly the various alternatives for RNs seeking a baccalaureate.
4. Discuss the controversies surrounding continuing education.
5. Present the key points in landmark actions related to entry into practice.
6. Give the pros and cons of a two-tier educational system for nursing.
7. Define nursing research.
8. Identify the problems in putting nursing research into practice.
9. Describe briefly two trends or issues in nursing education and how they may affect future education.

Unlike most professions, nursing has a variety of programs for entry into the profession (also called *basic, preservice,* or *generic education*). This situation confuses the public, some nurses, and employers. The three major educational routes that lead to RN licensure are the diploma programs operated by hospitals, the baccalaureate degree programs offered by four-year colleges and universities, and the associate degree programs usually offered by junior (or community) colleges. A master's degree program for beginning practitioners, once available at only a few colleges, is becoming more popular as schools try to attract students with other degrees. There are still only a few professional doctorate programs that also admit students with baccalaureate or higher degrees in fields other than nursing.

Although at one time diploma schools educated the largest number of nurses (more than 72 percent of the total number of schools in 1964 were diploma schools), the movement of nursing programs into institutions of higher learning has been consistent. Between 1964 and 1990, associate degree (AD) programs expanded from 130 to 829; BSN programs grew from 187 to 489. At the same time, diploma programs decreased from 833 to 139. Admission rates vary. Such unpredictable factors as a sudden shortage of nurses or a decreased amount of federal aid to schools often change the picture.

This chapter gives an overview of the various educational programs in nursing, continuing education, the open curriculum, research, and related issues and trends. Appendix 3 presents a comparison of programs, including what each type of graduate is prepared to do after completion.

PROGRAM COMMONALITIES

There are certain similarities that all basic nursing programs share, in part because all are affected by the same societal changes.

1. Nursing education is becoming more expensive, and financial support is less available for schools and students. Both state and federal governments have been tightening the financial reins on programs. Tuition seldom covers the cost of education, but, even so, it has been rising consistently. Students are finding it more and more difficult to receive scholarships, loans, and grants, particularly with the great cutback in federal funds. Also, because of both costs and social trends, fewer students live in dormitories, and those who do, pay for room and board.
2. The student population is more heterogeneous. Few, if any, schools refuse admission or matriculation to married students with or without families. It is not unusual to have a grandparent in a class as more mature individuals look for a new or better career. The tight job market in many fields brings to nursing individuals with degrees and sometimes careers in related or unrelated fields. All programs are including more men and other minority groups, by a small but definite percentage. In all cases, the diploma programs admit the lowest percentage of these groups.

3. Educational programs are generally more flexible. Trends in this direction, plus the admission of a very mixed student body, including aides, LPNs, and RNs seeking advanced education, have required a second look at proficiency and equivalency testing, self-paced learning, new techniques in teaching, and the external degree program.

4. State approval is required and national accreditation is available for all basic programs. Every school of professional nursing, in all three categories as well as practical nurse programs, must meet the standards of the legally constituted body in each state authorized to regulate nursing education and practice within that state. These agencies are usually called *state boards of nursing* or some similar title. Without the approval of these boards, a school cannot operate, because the graduates would not be eligible to take the licensing examination. In addition, many schools of nursing seek accreditation by the NLN. Accreditation by the League is a voluntary matter, not required by law. Increasing numbers of schools seek it, however, because it represents nationally determined standards of excellence, and nonaccreditation may affect the school's eligibility for outside funding or retard the graduates' entrance into BSN or graduate programs. Today, most schools are accredited. Nevertheless, accreditation is often criticized (see Chapter 11).

5. Faculty and clinical facilities are scarce resources. Faculty with the recommended doctoral degree for baccalaureate and graduate programs and the master's degree for other programs are increasing in number, but the total need has not been met. Clinical facilities are at a premium. Most schools, including diploma programs, use a variety of facilities. In large cities, several schools may be using one specialty hospital or clinical area (particularly obstetrics and pediatrics) for student experience. In rural areas, distance, small hospitals, and fewer patients are problems. Community health resources are very limited. Schools are also searching for new types of clinical experiences with various ethnic groups and in new settings such as hospices.

6. There is a slow but perceptible trend toward involving students in curriculum development, policymaking, and program evaluation. Social trends and the maturity of students, with their demands to have a part in shaping the educational program, are making some inroads on faculty and administrative control of schools.

7. All nursing students have learning experiences in clinical settings. Somewhere a myth arose that only practical nurse and diploma students gave "real" patient care in their educational programs, that AD students barely saw patients, and that baccalaureate students prepared only for teaching and administration. In fact, the time spent in the clinical area differs among programs within a particular credential as much as it does among various types of programs. In all good programs, students care for selected patients in order to gain certain skills and knowledge.

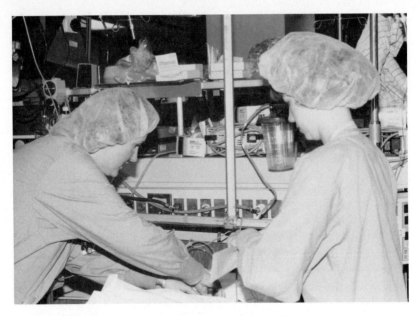

All nursing programs give students experience in clinical practice. (*Courtesy of the Robert Wood Johnson Medical Center.*)

8. It is generally agreed that the standards by which nursing education programs are judged should all include the same basic criteria related to the administration of the institution; facilities and resources; quality of faculty; student selection; retention and evaluation; and appropriateness and quality of the program.

PROGRAMS FOR PRACTICAL NURSES

Professional nurses work closely with practical nurses (PNs) in many practice settings. Both PN education and licensure are different from those of RNs, but because of changes in health care, an increasing number of PNs have been entering RN programs at either a beginning or an advanced level.

PNs (called *vocational nurses* in Texas and California) fall into four general groups: (1) those whose only teacher has been experience and who are not licensed to practice (this type of PN is disappearing); (2) those with experience but no formal education who have taken state-approved courses to qualify them to take state board examinations and become licensed; (3) those who have been licensed through a grandfather clause; and (4) those who have graduated from approved schools of practical nursing and, by passing state board examinations, have become licensed in the state or states in which they practice. There are also a few who were enrolled in RN programs and were permitted by their state law to take the PN examination after a certain number of courses. The large majority of LPNs/LVNs are licensed by examination (NCLEX-PN). Although LPNs in the third category can be legally employed, employers with a choice usually prefer graduates from an approved school who have been licensed by examination. (A grandfather clause is a legal device that allows persons who can show evidence that they have been practicing in a field to attain or maintain licensure even though the requirements have been changed and made more stringent.)

Formal PN education actually came later than that of the trained nurse. Although many women who nursed family and friends in the last 100 years were probably considered a type of PN, the first formal training programs were started by the Brooklyn, New York, YMCA in 1893. The three-month course taught home care of chronic invalids, the elderly, and children. Included were cooking, care of the house, dietetics, simple science, and simple nursing procedures. The program's success inspired similar courses in other states, but the first school was not organized until 1897. By 1947, there were only 36 schools, and only a few states had any kind of legislation regulating PN practice. After World War II, the nursing shortage and considerable amounts of federal vocational education funds set the stage for extraordinary expansion. Most of the early postwar programs, of about one year's duration, were in public schools, with practical experiences supervised by graduate nurses in cooperating hospitals. Generally no tuition was charged, although exploitive trade schools often charged much and gave little. By the 1950s there was more pressure for regulation, with states gradually requiring licensure.

Today the 1154 LPN programs are distributed throughout the nation, although most are in the South and fewest in the West. LPN education takes place primarily in vocational/technical schools and community colleges, with fewer programs offered in secondary schools and hospitals, and is commonly one year in length. Most programs are publicly funded. Interestingly, tuition at community colleges is about the same per year for LPN and ADN programs. In 1984, "concern for job safety" due to the layoffs that followed DRGs prompted the National Federation of Licensed Practical Nurses (NFLPN) House of Delegates to endorse two levels of nursing (RN and LPN) and the expansion of the PN curriculum to at least 18 months. An implementation date of 10 years was set, but no real action followed. (In 1986, North Dakota was the first state to change its licensure requirements for LPN to the AD level; other states are planning to take similar action.)

Not all LPNs or LPN faculty agreed with this decision. However, some programs began planning to phase into an AD level. Already existing are PN programs that are the first year of a two-year AD program. A student may exit at the end of the year, become licensed and work, or become licensed and not work and continue into the second year, becoming eligible for the RN licensure examination (NCLEX-RN). Some RN programs, particularly for the AD, give partial or total credit for the PN program (often only if the PN has also passed the licensing examination). Actually, over 41 percent of recent ADN graduates already held LPN licenses. A concerted effort has also been made to upgrade nurses' aides, home health aides, and other paraprofessional health care workers to LPN status through career ladders (discussed later).

Legitimate PN programs must be approved by the appropriate state nursing authority and may also be accredited, usually by the NLN. Upon graduation, the student is eligible to take the licensing examination (NCLEX-PN) to become an LPN or LVN. The licensing law is now mandatory in all states.

PN programs emphasize technical skills and direct patient care, but a (usually) simple background of the physical and social sciences is often integrated into the program. Clinical experience is provided in one or more hospitals and other agencies. The number of skills that are taught increases each year, probably because of employers' demands. The NLN has published statements on LPN entry-level competencies; the key points are found in Appendix 3.

LPNs work primarily in hospitals, extended care facilities, doctors' offices, private homes, and other health facilities, including to some extent community health agencies. They care for patients of all ages, but mostly adults. According to a survey done by the National Council of State Boards, entry-level PNs are primarily involved in basic nursing activities, including personal hygiene, measuring vital signs, giving medications, and carrying out such treatments as enemas, catheterizations, applications of heat and cold, and providing aspects of emotional support. They are least likely to be involved in activities that require technological skills.[1] Legally, LPNs are supposed to be supervised by an RN, physician, or dentist. Unfortunately, such supervision is often remote or absent.

The decline of LPN programs from a peak of 1319 in 1982 appears to have reached its limit for the time being. With the current nursing shortage and the dramatic increase in RN salaries, employers seem to feel that the LPN carrying out technical tasks will free the more expensive RN to perform those vital tasks that only a professional nurse can do. On the other hand, LPNs, who are often forced to do more complex nursing tasks than they were trained for, and who are frequently in charge of a unit (when, legally, they shouldn't be), will probably also demand better salaries. They are highly unionized and a target for more unionization. Furthermore, the federal government predicts an increased need for LPNs because of the growing elderly population; LPNs are a significant part of the nursing labor force in long-term care. Currently, it is estimated that there are about 608,000 LPNs, and the population is growing. It is, and will be, a diverse population in terms of age and racial background. A larger percentage of black, Hispanic, and native American students enter LPN programs as opposed to RN programs; more men also enter LPN programs. There is some conjecture that LPN education is seen by many as a quick, inexpensive, and useful first step on a nursing career ladder, so this diversity will also affect the RN population in the future.

DIPLOMA PROGRAMS

The diploma or hospital school of nursing was the first type of nursing school in this country. Before the opening of the first hospital schools in the late 1800s, there was no formal preparation for nursing. But after Florence Nightingale established the first school of nursing at St. Thomas's Hospital, England, in 1860, the idea spread quickly to the United States.

Hospitals, of course, welcomed the idea of training schools because, in the early years, such schools represented an almost free supply of nurse power. With some outstanding exceptions, the education offered was largely of the apprenticeship type; there was some theory and formal classroom work, but for the most part students learned by doing, providing the majority of the nursing care for the hospitals' patients in the process.

Gradually these conditions improved, faculty were better educated, and students had more classroom teaching. Yet, even as late as the 1950s, many classes were taught by doctors, and the focus was on giving care in the hospital, with the how sometimes more important than the why. When sciences were taught by a nearby college, courses were designed especially for nurses, often at a lower level than for other students. The student was typically a white, single, 18-year-old female who had to live in the dormitory. Breaking rules about curfew, smoking, drinking, and especially marrying meant dismissal, no matter how excellent the student.

This is no longer true. Today, in order to meet standards set in each state for operation of a nursing school and to prepare students to pass the licensing examinations, diploma schools must offer their students a truly educational program, not just an apprenticeship. Hospitals conducting such schools employ a full-time nurse faculty, offer students a balanced mixture of coursework (in nursing and related subjects in the physical and social sciences) and supervised practice, and look to their graduate nursing staff, not their students, to provide the nursing service needed by patients. The educational program has been generally three years in length, although most diploma schools have now adopted a shortened program. Upon satisfactory completion of the program, the student is awarded a diploma by the school.

This diploma, it should be understood, is not an academic degree. Because most hospitals operating schools of nursing are not chartered to grant degrees, *no* academic (college) credit is usually given for courses taught by the school's faculty. (Exceptions are some external degree programs and some nonnursing baccalaureate programs that offer "blanket credit" to RNs. The latter type of degree may be a problem when seeking graduate education.) For this and economic and educational reasons, large numbers of diploma schools enter into cooperative relations with colleges or universities for educational courses and/or services. It is not uncommon for diploma students to take regular physical and social science courses and, occasionally, liberal arts courses at a college. If these courses are part of the general offerings of the college, college credit is granted. Credit is usually transferable if the nursing student decides to transfer to a college or continue in advanced education. If the course is tailored to nursing only, it is often not transferable to an advanced nursing program but is sometimes counted as an elective.

The primary clinical facility is the hospital, although the school may contract with other hospitals or agencies for additional educational experiences. Advocates of diploma education usually say that early and substantial experiences with patients seem to foster a strong identification with nursing, particularly hospital nursing, and thus graduates are expected to adjust to the employee role without difficulty.

Hospital schools usually provide other necessary educational resources, facilities, and services to students and faculty, such as libraries, classrooms, audiovisual materials, and practice laboratories. When it was taken for granted that students would be housed, good schools had dormitory and recreational space, as well as educational facilities, in a separate building. Such housing must now be paid for and may also be used by others educated in or involved with the hospital.

The perceptible shift away from diploma school preparation for nursing can be explained (in an oversimplified way) by three factors: (1) some hospitals are terminating their schools, either because of the expense involved in maintaining a quality program and the objections of third-party payers, such as insurance companies and the government, to having the cost of nursing education absorbed in the patient's bill or because of difficulty in meeting professional standards, particularly in employing qualified faculty; (2) increasing numbers of high school graduates are seeking some kind of collegiate education; and (3) the nursing profession is becoming more and more committed to the belief that preparation for nursing, as for all other professions, should take place in institutions of higher education.

These social and educational trends will probably continue, but it is expected that diploma programs will be on the scene for some time and that quality programs will continue to prepare quality graduates. In fact, diploma schools have reported a dramatic increase in admissions in the last several years. Indeed, the vast majority of current diploma programs are NLN accredited, and many of the schools that dissolved or were "phased into" AD or baccalaureate programs were also accredited. The 1970 National

Commission study recommended that strong, vital schools be encouraged to seek regional accreditation and degree-granting status, but only a few have done so. Another recommendation, that other hospital schools move to effect interinstitutional arrangements with collegiate institutions, has been acted upon more readily.

Although hospitals are less likely to operate schools, they continue as the clinical laboratories for nursing education programs. In the communities where new AD or baccalaureate programs are opening, there is often planning for new programs to evolve as diploma programs close—a phasing-in process. This cooperation enables prospective candidates for the diploma program to be directed to the new program, qualified diploma faculty to be employed by the college, and arrangements made to use space in the hospital previously occupied by the diploma school. Cooperative planning provides for continuity in the output of nurses to meet the needs of the community.

ASSOCIATE DEGREE PROGRAMS

A relative newcomer to the scene of nursing education is the associate degree (AD) program that is usually offered by a junior or community college, is two years in length, and prepares graduates for the RN licensing examination. This type of program, offered in a college setting but not leading to a baccalaureate degree, was not even envisioned by nursing educators of the late nineteenth and early twentieth centuries.

The AD program is the first nursing education program to be developed under a systematic plan and with carefully controlled experimentation. In 1951 Mildred Montag published her doctoral dissertation describing a nursing technician able to perform nursing functions that are seen as considerably more prescribed and narrower in scope than those of the professional nurse and broader than those of the PN. This nurse was intended to be a bedside nurse who was not burdened with administrative responsibilities. Montag listed the functions as (1) assisting in the planning of nursing care for patients, (2) giving general nursing care with supervision, and (3) assisting in the evaluation of the nursing care given.[2] Previous experiences with the Cadet Nurse Corps supported the concept of providing a shortened nursing program. The emerging community college was seen as a suitable setting for this education since it would place nursing education in the mainstream of education, and the burden of cost would be on the public in general rather than on the patients, as was the case with diploma programs. An AD would be awarded at the end of the two years. As originally conceived, the program was considered to be terminal and not a first step toward the baccalaureate.

A five-year project to test this idea was started in 1952, with seven junior colleges and a diploma school participating. The results of the project showed that AD nursing graduates could carry on the intended nursing functions, that the program could be suitably set up in community colleges, with the use of clinical facilities in the community without charge or student service, and that the program attracted students. The success of the experiment plus the rapid growth of community colleges combined to give impetus to these new programs.

Over the years there have been changes in philosophy as to what the graduate of these programs is prepared to do. Many AD deans do not see the program as terminal or technical, perceiving a difference in amount rather than kind of professional education. The entire concept of the AD nursing program as terminal has changed over the last 25 years. Obviously, no educational program should be terminal in the sense that graduates cannot continue their education toward another degree. Trends have developed toward enhancing articulation opportunities for AD RNs into baccalaureate nursing programs. However, the AD nurse need not continue formal education to hold a valuable place in the health care system.

The practice of the AD graduate has often been called technical as differentiated from professional. Montag viewed nursing functions on a continuum, placing technical training in the middle of the continuum:[3] (See Exhibit 5-1.) The boundaries of the continuum are not totally fixed, and some overlap. Many nurse educators at all levels agree that there is a common core of knowledge drawn upon by all RN education.

The controversial ANA position paper on nursing education defined technical nursing practice in the following way:

> Technical nursing practice is carrying out nursing measures as well as medically delegated techniques with a high degree of skill, using principles from an ever-expanding body of science. It is understanding the physics of machines as well as the physiologic reactions of patients. It is using all treatment modalities with knowledge and precision.
>
> Technical nursing practice is evaluating patients' immediate physical and emotional reactions to therapy and taking measures to alleviate distress. It is knowing when to act and when to seek more expert guidance.
>
> Technical nursing practice involves working with professional nurse practitioners and others in planning the day-to-day care of patients. It is supervising other workers in the technical aspects of care.
>
> Technical nursing practice is unlimited in depth but limited in scope. Its complexity and extent are tremendous. It must be rendered under the direction of professional nurse practitioners, by persons who are selected with care and educated within the system of higher education; only thus can the safety of patients be assured. Education for this practice requires attention to scientific laws and principles with em-

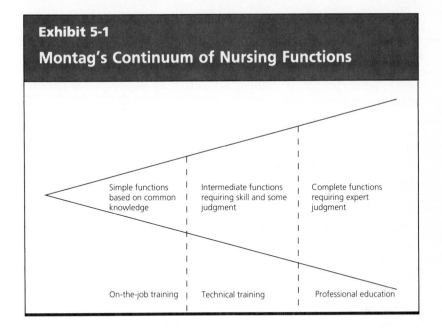

Exhibit 5-1

Montag's Continuum of Nursing Functions

Simple functions based on common knowledge

Intermediate functions requiring skill and some judgment

Complete functions requiring expert judgment

On-the-job training   Technical training   Professional education

phasis on skill. It is education which is technically oriented and scientifically founded, but not primarily concerned with evolving theory.

Whether the term *technical* will continue to be used is not clear. The concept of a technical worker, honored in other fields, has not been fully accepted in nursing, possibly because it is considered a step down from the *professional* label that has been attached to all nurses through licensing definitions and common usage over the years. Montag, noting the difficulty of choosing an appropriate term for the new type of proposed nurse, said, "It is also probable that the term 'nursing technician' will not satisfy forever, but it is proposed as one which indicates more accurately the person who has semi-professional preparation and whose functions are predominantly technical."[4]

The use of the term *technical* was rejected by the NLN Council of Associate Degree Programs in a 1976 action and the term *associate degree nurse (AD nurse)* was suggested. This term is frequently used now, although *associate nurse* is also used, especially in terms of licensing.

More important than the name are the role and functions of the AD nurse. Because of nursing shortages, as well as lack of understanding of the abilities and preparation of technical nurses, a tendency to use the diploma nurse of previous years as a standard, and general traditionalized concepts of nursing roles, employers have often not assigned AD nurses in the manner that best utilized their preparation. Like nurses throughout the centuries, AD nurses have been placed quickly as team leaders and charge nurses, positions in which they were not intended to function.

The NLN has published a new role and competencies statement for AD nurses, which provides guidelines for identifying their expected level of practice at graduation and six months later. The document is very comprehensive. The introduction notes that AD education is still based on Montag's "middle range" of nursing functions and states: "the goal of associate degree nursing programs continues to be preparation of registered nurses to provide direct client care. Although associate degree nursing students receive preparation to provide care for clients across the life span, the majority of the graduates are employed in settings where the focus of care is on adult clients."[5]

Like other RNs, AD nurses are accountable for their own practice and are expected to function ethically and legally. In addition, the NLN Council has made a point of saying that although these nurses work within the policies of an employing institution, they would also work within the organizational framework to initiate change in policies or nursing protocols.

Over the years, as Montag predicted, the AD curricula have varied and changed.[6] For instance, when college policies permit, there is a tendency to put a heavier emphasis and more time on the nursing subjects and clinical experiences, sometimes through the addition of summer sessions or clinical preceptorships. Some programs are also adding team leadership and managerial principles because their graduates are put in positions requiring these skills. Today, most AD programs are between 18 and 24 months in length, but some require that all science and general education courses be completed before the nursing program is begun, which may lengthen the AD program to over 2 years.[7]

Although there has been some complaint that AD nurses are not proficient in certain technical skills and require too much orientation to the responsibilities of a staff nurse, many AD educators believe that the need for additional clinical experiences is not suggested more frequently than for graduates of other programs. It is generally unrealistic for new graduates or their employers to expect newcomers to function as seasoned practitioners. Almost everyone agrees that AD graduates have a good grasp of basic nursing theory, have inquiring minds, and are self-directed in finding out what they don't know. It is also generally agreed that a good orientation program is the key to satisfactory adjustment to the work setting by new graduates from any type of RN program. One realistic concern is that the majority of AD programs do not appear to teach their students how to carry out complex technological procedures that both staff nurses and nurse executives consider an essential part of nursing practice, even for a new graduate.[8] Yet it is expected that a similar situation exists in other kinds of nursing programs.

AD programs are the fastest-growing segment of nursing education for a variety of reasons. Clearly, the availability of AD programs in a community; the low cost of about $1000 a year (most programs are publicly funded); the fact that this is usually the shortest way to RN licensure; the increasing possibilities of educational career ladders; and the reality that most employers do not differentiate much, if at all, in salaries for RNs with different kinds of education are all important factors. AD programs are distributed throughout the United States, with most in the West and fewest in the North Atlantic region; however, they make up the majority of nursing programs in *all* regions. The makeup of AD students (and graduates) is distinctly different from that of the other programs. In relation to minority enrollment, there are a larger number of Hispanics and native Americans in two-year institutions as opposed to Asian-Americans and blacks, who gravitate to baccalaureate programs. Percentages vary in different regions of the country. AD students are also more likely to be older, married with children, and working part-time. There is some indication that they are more likely to continue working in nursing than graduates in other programs. An interesting point is that, like diploma programs, AD programs have been attracting second-career students, perhaps, in part, because of the brevity of the program. The long-term implications of all these factors for nursing in general are discussed later.

BACCALAUREATE NURSING PROGRAMS

The first baccalaureate program in nursing was established in 1909 under the control of the University of Minnesota, through the efforts of Dr. Richard Olding Beard. Since then, these programs have become an increasingly important part of nursing education and have grown steadily in numbers.

The baccalaureate graduate obtains both a college education with a bachelor's degree and preparation for licensure and practice as a registered professional nurse. The most notable differences between baccalaureate education and the other basic nursing programs are related to liberal education, development of intellectual skills, and the addition of public health practice and teaching and management concepts, although some of the other programs do include a limited amount of such content. Baccalaureate nurses have the opportunity to become liberally educated; almost all programs allow free electives in the humanities and the sciences, as well as nursing courses. Nursing students are able to participate in the college/university cultural and social activities throughout their whole program and develop relationships with professors and students in other disciplines. Nursing majors meet the same admission requirements and are held to the same academic standards as all other students. The nursing program is an integral part of the college or university as a whole and is usually four years in length.

The baccalaureate degree program includes courses in general education and the liberal arts, the sciences germane to and related to nursing, and nursing. In some programs, the student is not admitted to the nursing major (nursing courses) until the conclusion of the first two years of college study. In other programs, nursing content is integrated throughout the four years.

As in the other nursing programs, the baccalaureate program has both theoretical content and clinical experience. The baccalaureate student who takes courses in the physical and social sciences will have greater depth and breadth, because students majoring in nursing take the college courses in the sciences and humanities with students majoring in biology or English literature.

Although technical skills are essential to nursing, learning activities that assist students to develop skills in recognizing and solving problems, applying general principles to particular situations, and establishing a basis for making sound clinical judgments are also emphasized. This enables the nurse to function more easily when a familiar situation takes an unexpected turn or when it is necessary to deal with an unfamiliar situation.

Like other nurse educators, those in baccalaureate programs constantly review (and often revise) their nursing curriculum, but they have given relatively little attention to the liberal arts component, even though this part of the program is supposed to be important in making the baccalaureate nurse an educated person as well as a clinical practitioner. However, in 1986, an interdisciplinary "Panel for Essentials of College and University Education for Professional Nursing" reported the recommendations of its two-year study to the AACN, its sponsor. The report had two components: one related to nursing knowledge and the other to liberal education.[9] What long-term action will come from this report remains to be seen. Since its release, most schools have been so involved in reversing the big drop in enrollment that there has not been as much discussion of the report as might be expected.

Most BSN graduates select hospitals as their first place of employment but then often turn to public health nursing. Those hospitals that have primary nursing, which gives nurses individual responsibility for a group of patients, seem most likely to attract and retain baccalaureate nurses. Graduates with long-term plans for teaching, administration, or clinical specialization continue into graduate study.

A baccalaureate degree in nursing offers many career opportunities, a fact that is widely acknowledged. Equally important is the fact that in the last 10 years, when nursing has been under particular scrutiny, the many reports and studies looking at the nursing shortage agree that what is needed to meet the nursing needs in today's complex health care is more baccalaureate nurses. However, this program, considered by the ANA as minimum preparation for professional nursing, is usually more expensive for students than other basic programs. This is a serious problem, as funding cuts lessen student aid.

A major phenomenon in baccalaureate nursing is the increase in the number of RNs entering these programs. In part, this is due to the trends and reports mentioned, the need for new knowledge given the increased complexity of care, and the fact that nurses are more eager to advance in their careers and want the greater options available with a nursing baccalaureate. Since employers are aware of this and look for ways to keep their nurses, more and more offer tuition reimbursement as a fringe benefit. When this is added to the new flexibility offered RNs by baccalaureate educators, nurses find it less difficult to go to school, work, and maintain family responsibilities (although it's never easy).[10] About 140 programs are designed especially for returning RNs. Other BRN or BS-RN tracks exist within regular baccalaureate programs, with the nurses mainstreamed into the basic curriculum. In most nursing programs, RNs receive some credit and/or advanced standing for their previous education through challenge examinations. Frequently, courses and clinical experiences are individualized to meet RNs' needs and goals. The degree is the same for basic and RN students. In 1989, 38 percent of the nursing baccalaureates were conferred on RNs. Other options will be described later. It is unfortunate that some RNs, because of circumstances, desire, or lack of counseling, choose nonnursing majors, which generally precludes their acceptance into a graduate program in nursing.

Another noticeable trend, which began in the 1980s, is the increase of students with baccalaureate or advanced degrees in fields other than nursing. These students, of course, receive a second baccalaureate. Depending on how many of their previous courses satisfy the BSN requirements, their program may consist primarily of upper-division major nursing courses. A few baccalaureate programs have been especially designed for the baccalaureate graduate. Actually, such programs may not take much more time than an AD program. Often these second-careerists do not realize, or are not told, that they will need a nursing baccalaureate for career advancement, regardless of their nonnursing degrees. More of them are looking at the generic masters as an option or at an accelerated master's program in which they acquire a nursing baccalaureate on the way to a nursing master's degree. These programs are described next.

OTHER PROGRAMS LEADING TO RN LICENSURE

A number of years ago, several nursing education programs, such as those at Yale and Western Reserve University, admitted only baccalaureate graduates and granted a master's degree in nursing as the basic educational credential. Today there is renewed interest in such programs. Some prepare for a generalist role, others for a specialty as clinical specialist or nurse practitioner. Depending on the school's philosophy and state law, the student may take the licensing examination before completion of the master's.[11] There are also *articulation* programs in which a student may get a license after completion of an AD or baccalaureate and then continue directly to the master's degree.

The first program for a professional doctorate (ND) for college graduates was established at Case-Western Reserve in 1979. It was designed for "liberally educated men and women who are gifted intellectually, willing to invest themselves in a rigorous, demanding, rewarding program of study, and committed to a sustained professional career."[12] As described, the program should be located only in universities with health science centers preparing several types of health professionals. Because such universities also offer advanced graduate education, ND students are prepared in an academic climate of scholarship and research. Faculty are prepared at the highest level of scholarship, with some engaged in teaching and research and others, jointly appointed, master's-prepared clinicians engaged in clinical practice, teaching, and some aspect of research. The curriculum prepares the ND graduates to become proficient in the delivery of primary, episodic, and long-term nursing care, and to evaluate their own practices and those of their assistants, since they are accountable for the outcomes of all nursing practice. Graduates of this program would continue graduate study in a specialization and/or a functional area such as teaching or administration. As is true of medical students whose professional degree is a doctorate, they may also obtain a master's or Ph.D. concurrently with the first doctorate.[13] This innovative approach, seen as a major step toward the emergence of nursing as a full-fledged profession, has now been adopted by several other universities, but many questions are still raised as to the functions, role, and job market for the graduates and the best organizational structure for the program.[14]

GRADUATE EDUCATION

An important ANA statement describes graduate education as

the preparation of highly competent individuals who can function in diverse roles, such as clinical nurse generalists or specialists, researchers, theoreticians, teachers, administrators, consultants, public policy makers, system managers, and colleagues on multidisciplinary teams . . . prepared through master's, doctoral, and postdoctoral programs in nursing that subscribe to clearly defined standards of scholarship.[15]

It is interesting to note that programs in *nursing* are specified, signaling that master's and doctoral degrees in other fields, without a nursing component, are not encouraged. Nevertheless, this is broader than an earlier document that endorsed only *clinical* graduate education.[16] The trends in graduate nursing education over the years, from simply being programs for graduate nurses, through the nurse scientist, to nursing doctorates, are interesting to explore.[17]

Graduate programs in nursing vary in admission requirements, organization of curriculum, length of program, and costs.[18] Admission usually requires RN licensure, graduation from an approved (or accredited) baccalaureate program with an upper-division major in nursing, a satisfactory grade point average, achievement on selected tests, and sometimes nursing experience. Some programs admit a few nurses without BSNs and assist them in making up deficiencies. Part-time study is available in many, perhaps most, programs, but often certain courses must be taken in sequence, and at least some full-time study may be required. Reduced federal support and fewer traineeships have stimulated faculty to develop more part-time study options. Since 1970, when about 75 percent of students went to school full-time, there has been a total reversal of numbers. Not all graduate programs offer all possible majors. The degrees granted are usually the MS (master of science with a nursing major); MSN (master of science in nursing); MNSc (master's in nursing science); MN (master's in nursing); MA (master of arts with a nursing major); and MPH (master of public health with a nursing major). The differences are sometimes obscure.

Most NLN-accredited master's programs offer a study of a clinical area, such as adult medical-surgical nursing, (with the most graduates), maternal-child nursing, community health nursing, or psychiatric nursing with advanced experience, based on a theoretical framework developed by that faculty and including relevant advanced courses in the natural and social sciences. The depth of clinical study varies in relation to whether the nurse plans to become a clinical specialist or NP or wishes to concentrate on a functional area such as teaching, administration, or consultation, for which other appropriate courses will also be offered. Increasingly, a practicum (planned, guided learning experiences in a setting that allow a student to practice in the role) is being recommended for the functional as well as the clinical areas. The length of the practicum varies from program to program, from one day a week for a semester to almost a year's full-time residency. In general, master's education in nursing includes concentrated study of a specific area of nursing, introduction to research methods, and independent study of a nursing problem, using research techniques. The latter is called a *master's thesis, project,* or *study.*

Although some nurses obtain graduate degrees outside the field of nursing, advanced positions in nursing, especially in nursing education, usually require a nursing degree, preferably with advanced clinical content and experience. In 1990, there were some 231 nursing master's programs in the United States, most with clinical majors. An NLN pamphlet, "Master's Education in Nursing, Route to Opportunities in Contemporary Nursing," updated frequently, presents an overview of all accredited nursing master's programs, including curricula, clinical and functional majors, admission requirements, availability of part-time study, length of program, approximate cost, and availability of housing.

Although many nurses are still enrolled in nonnursing doctoral programs, the pendulum may have swung toward doctoral degrees in nursing in the last few years. They have shown remarkable growth: 2 in 1946, 27 in 1983, and 50 in 1990. There have also been many changes during that time.[19,20] Among other things, the "appropriate" doctoral degree for nurses has been a matter of debate. Some nursing leaders favor granting a PhD in nursing with a minor in a relevant discipline. Others have felt that although the nursing PhD is an ultimate goal, nursing science is not sufficiently developed to make this practical immediately. Instead they suggest either a PhD in some other discipline with a minor in nursing or a strictly professional degree such as the DNS (Doctor of Nursing Science).[21] It is believed that a nurse with an academic degree (PhD) could help to generate knowledge, and the nurse with a professional degree such as the Doctor of Education or Doctor of Science in Nursing (EdD, DNSc) would apply this new knowledge. There are a variety of nursing doctorates offered today, as opinions vary. Several schools offer both the PhD and the DNS and have identified the differences.

PhDs and EdDs, not necessarily in nursing, are still the degrees most commonly held by nurses. As more doctoral programs evolve, the debate becomes more heated. Schools starting doctoral programs must consider what best suits their educational philosophy and the qualifications and interests of their faculty members. Yet, many schools choose a PhD program because it is still considered the most prestigious degree in academia.[22] Sometimes the university denies nursing this option because of the notion that nursing science is not advanced enough; therefore the school chooses a DNS or DNSc instead. Is this important? Some think it is.[23] Graduates of both are expected to become researchers, teachers, and administrators. (Most contemporary doctoral students are preparing primarily for education and research, not advanced clinical practice.) In actuality, the differences blur. Even nurses with a PhD employed in beginning positions in a nursing school may be teaching undergraduate students and may have little interest or time for research.[24] In fact, a doctorate of any kind has been called a "union card" for admission to a teaching position in higher education. Whether or not the person does research of any kind depends on personal inclination or professional pressure (the publish-or-perish syndrome). Some select post-doctoral fellowships to get adequate research training and experience.[25]

One consistent concern is quality in doctoral programs, particularly as they proliferate, perhaps in schools that do not have an adequate number of faculty properly prepared to guide the education and research of doctoral students. Monitoring of doctoral programs is usually a university preroga-tive, but it is not clear how well this is done. One thing that *is* made clear in all major reports is the continuing need for doctorally prepared nurses.

NURSING RESEARCH

With the growth of graduate education, nursing research has grown tre-mendously over the years, and it is important to have at least a basic understanding of where it is and where it's going. A more detailed discussion of nursing research is found in many sources and is useful as background.[26] It is also interesting to look at how nursing research evolved in the United States, beginning perhaps with Adelaide Nutting in 1906.[27]

Schlotfeldt's definition of the term *research* is classic: all systematic inquiry designed for the purpose of advancing knowledge.[28] Notter makes a useful comparison between problem solving related to patient care (some-times also described as the *nursing process*) and scientific inquiries.[29] Both go through such steps as (1) identifying a problem, (2) analyzing its various aspects, (3) collecting facts or data, (4) determining action on the basis of analysis of the data, and (5) evaluating the result. These steps may be relatively simple or very complex; they may involve laboratory equipment, human experimentation, or neither. Research may be designated as *basic,* the establishment of new knowledge or theory that is not immediately ap-plicable, or *applied,* the attempt to solve a practical problem. Either way, the same steps are taken.

One definition of *nursing* research is "research that arises from the practice of nursing for the purpose of solving patient care problems."[30] A noted nurse researcher describes nursing research as a "systematic inquiry into the prob-lems encountered in nursing practice and into the modalities of patient care, such as support and comfort, prevention of trauma, promotion of recovery, health education, health appraisal, and coordination of health care."[31] She emphasizes as key words *patient* and *effect,* calling them the critical nucleus of nursing research. This type of research is also defined as clinical nursing research. However, it has been pointed out that *clinical* can have different meanings for different people: involving a place such as a hospital or clinic; pertaining to some form of disease or symptom; or the testing of an action considered a nursing action. Newman maintains that if the criterion "relevance to practice" is applied, then all nursing research is clinical research, but "the distinguishing factor between basic and clinical research is the purpose of the research: whether it is knowledge for the sake of knowledge or knowledge for a specific purpose."[32] Johnson and others see nursing research in a more abstract vein, leading to development of "theories of nursing intervention which will yield predictable responses in patients when implemented in nursing care."[33]

There are a number of other variations on the definition of nursing research and how it might be classified, and probably the arguments will persist. One of the most thoughtful nurse researchers (and one with a sense of humor) suggests that perhaps the best answer to "What is nursing research?" is "A good question."[34]

Why nursing research? As one multidisciplinary group said: "Through research, nurses can test, refine, and advance the knowledge base on which improved education and practice must rest."[35] Practice disciplines have always needed to develop their own bodies of verified knowledge and to evaluate that knowledge in practice, both for survival as a profession and for the well-being of their clients. This has been said repeatedly by nursing leaders and scholars in the last few decades. However, the lack of understanding about nursing research common to most nurses presents some problems.

Over the years, a major issue has been the utilization of nursing research. After all, no matter how critical the findings of research studies may seem, if they are not tested in practice over a period of time, in a variety of settings, the results might still be questioned. If they are not used at all, practice may change, but it will not change as a result of research. The first step is communication, especially from researcher to practitioner. In the last few years, means of reporting research have increased considerably, with many more publications and conferences sponsored by organizations, universities, the government and others. Nevertheless, putting research into practice has made slow progress. Most nurses giving direct patient care do not read research journals or have contact with nurse researchers. Obstacles most frequently reported by them in relation to using research findings are reading and understanding the report, relevance of findings for practical situations, inability to find research findings, suggestions too costly or time-consuming to implement, resistance to change in the workplace, and lack of worthwhile rewards for using nursing research.

Probably in the majority of practice sites, this outlook is still prevalent. Most nurses in practice today, including nurse administrators, were not educated at a time when research was considered a part of nursing's responsibility and certainly were not trained to carry out any type of research. Moreover, since most hospitals are not affiliated with university programs, where most of the research has been done, and since even in programs of higher education most nurse faculty members do not do substantive research, it is small wonder that research has not been a part of nursing practice.

Some clear trends are now emerging that may turn this situation around. First, some researchers are beginning to realize that they have a responsibility for translating the research into terms and concepts understandable to the clinician and presenting their research results in places other than research conferences. They must make a distinct effort to reach out to nurses who are known as innovators and early adopters.[36]

Second, more practitioners are being oriented to nursing research in their educational programs.[37] And, perhaps most important, nursing research is being done in clinical sites, with nurse researchers and staff working together.[38] Having organized research programs in a significant number of hospitals will take time, but the advances that have been made in less than 10 years are impressive, especially given the interest of farsighted nurse executives.[39]

One dramatic acknowledgment of this is that in 1986, a National Center for Nursing Research (NCNR) was established at the National Institutes of Health (NIH). Congress not only overrode a presidential veto (and NIH objections), but key senators on both sides of the aisle spoke to the value of nursing research and the need for a visible national center. The Secretary of DHHS announced the establishment of the NCNR "for the purpose of conducting a program of grants and awards supporting nursing research and research training related to patient care, the promotion of health, the prevention of disease, and the mitigation of the effects of acute and chronic illnesses and disabilities. In support of studies on nursing interventions, procedures, delivery methods and ethics of patient care, the NCNR programs are expected to complement other biomedical research programs that are primarily concerned with the causes and treatment of disease."[40]

The NCNR supports research, research training, and career development in health promotion and disease prevention, acute and chronic illness, and nursing systems, which include such areas as innovative approaches to delivery of quality nursing services, strategies to improve patient outcome, interventions to ensure availability of resources, and bioethics research, a special initiative. A number of research training awards exist for beginning and advanced nurse researchers through individual and institutional predoctoral, postdoctoral, and senior fellowships. Among the research priorities targeted for the next several years are AIDS and HIV-positive patients, families, and partners; low-birth-weight infants and their mothers; long-term care; symptom management; information systems; health promotion; and technology dependency across the life span. As President Bush did recommend an increase in funding following the report, nursing research may begin to be integrated into the scientific community, something that has been lacking for a long time.[41]

EDUCATIONAL MOBILITY AND OPEN CURRICULUM PRACTICES

One of the key developments in nursing education is the open curriculum, which began in the 1970s. The NLN defines this as a system "which incorporates an educational approach designed to accommodate the learning needs and career goals of students by providing flexible opportunities for entry into and exit from the educational program, and by capitalizing on their previous relevant education and experiences."[42] The concept emerged only gradually as nurse educators who were aware of social and economic trends and sympathetic to the goals of those struggling for upward mobility began to plan and implement programs. Soon nursing was responding to the mandate for more flexibility. Innovative faculties have designed new methods for measurement of knowledge and competency or have developed entirely new programs.

There are a variety of approaches for providing flexibility in nursing education. The ladder approach, which provides direct articulation between programs, is used to move from nursing assistant to practical nurse to AD or diploma nurse to baccalaureate nurse, with any combination in between. For some, this means the ability to begin at a basic level and move one step at a time to the highest achievable level. For others, it means aiming at a particular level but being able to exit at distinct points, become licensed, and earn a living if necessary. (This exit opportunity is less common now.) An increasing number of baccalaureate programs are also being developed that enroll only RNs into the upper division, accepting past nursing education as the lower division to be built on.

There are nurses, especially nurse educators, who object to the ladder concept. They believe that each program in nursing has its own basis, content, and goals, that one cannot be based on another, and that the ladder tends to belittle the role of workers at each level, implying the necessity to move up. One solution seems to be using standardized and teacher-made tests to measure the individual's knowledge, according to clearly stated competency goals. There are a number of standardized tests available in both the liberal arts and nursing, but there is still some question as to how to test for clinical competency. Methods used include the use of videotapes, simulated experiences, practicums, and minicourses in the clinical setting. Also being used are the performance assessment centers of the Regent's College Degree program, as well as their paper-and-pencil exams.[43]

Other ways of giving students more opportunities are to offer courses more frequently, during evening hours, weekends, and in summer, to allow part-time study, and to have class sessions off the main campus in areas convenient to students living in communities not easily accessible to the main campus.[44] In addition, junior and senior colleges are cooperating to assist students who want baccalaureates.[45]

Another approach is to allow students to proceed through a course at their own pace through testing, self-study, and the use of media and computers. A number of schools are experimenting with self-pacing and self-learning, and reports indicate that students find it stimulating and satisfying, although sometimes stressful.[46]

Another version of the open curriculum concept is the external degree, sometimes called a "university without walls." This is independent study validated by testing, an approach long used in other countries (as early as 1836). In the United States the *Regents College Degree,* formerly called the *New York State Regents External Degree,* is a respected and successful example. Regents College (RC), The University of the State of New York (USNY), shares many goals and activities with conventional campus-based programs. However, it differs significantly in the ways students learn and the methods used to recognize and credential that learning. Rather than providing classroom instruction, RC provides the focus for learning through its degree requirements and related study materials. It provides a comprehensive system of objective assessment of college-level knowledge and skills, using transfer credits from regionally accredited colleges, recognized proficiency examinations, nursing performance examinations, and other specialized evaluation procedures. Sometimes referred to as "a national examining university," RC grants credits whenever college-level knowledge is validated through the use of faculty-approved, objective, academic assessment methods.

RC offers the only national total assessment nursing programs, and thus it is unique. Since 1972, RC has developed associate and baccalaureate programs in nursing through grants and federal funds. Both degrees are NLN accredited. ADN graduates, who are primarily LPNs, are eligible for licensure in 48 states; since 1975 the pass rate on licensure examinations has averaged 94 percent, with scores typically higher than the New York State and national averages.

As of 1990, over 3000 nurses from throughout the United States and several countries abroad had earned the Regents College BSN degree. Nearly 80 percent were RNs from diploma or AD programs, with an average of 10 years experience in nursing. Many BSN students had baccalaureate, master's, or doctoral degrees in other fields. The passing rate on the licensure exam, for those who need it, is 100 percent. Approximately three-fourths of the graduates stated intentions of continuing with graduate school.[47]

The performance examinations are administered by some 250 nurse faculty members, all of whom have completed the extensive training developed and administered by RC. Approximately 2100 nursing performance examinations are administered on weekends throughout the year at the national network of Regional Performance Assessment Centers created and established by RC. The written nursing examinations are administered by The American College Testing Program (ACT PEP tests) at some 160 locations throughout the country and at embassies and military bases throughout the world. Further information may be obtained by writing to Regents College Degrees, Nursing Office, Cultural Education Center, Albany, New York 12230.

Although some educators oppose the external degree on philosophical grounds and others fear the competition in the tight market for students, studies conducted relative to the program are providing data of significance to other states contemplating external degree programs that include nursing. Cooperative ventures with various colleges, service institutions, and service systems (such as the Air Force Nurse Corps) are part of the extensive Regents outreach.[48] Other external degree programs have also been developed, including one under the California State University Consortium.

If, as expected, the trend toward accepting baccalaureate education as the entry point in nursing education continues, the necessity for upward mobility becomes even more essential. However, RN students must beware of diploma mills. With nontraditional students comprising a major portion of the nursing education market, there should be plenty of options for RNs and others to continue formal education that is of good quality.[49]

CONTINUING EDUCATION

Professional practitioners of any kind must continue to learn because they are accountable to the public for minimum safe practice. This is impossible to maintain if pertinent aspects of the tremendous flow of new knowledge are not used. For nurses, specifically, continuing education (CE) is needed primarily to keep them abreast of changes in nursing roles and functions, acquire new knowledge and skills (and/or renew that which has been lost), and modify attitudes and understanding. To achieve these goals, various approaches to CE can be used, such as formal academic studies that might lead to a degree; short-term courses or programs given by institutions of higher learning that do not necessarily provide academic credit; and independent or informal study through opportunities made available by professional organizations and employing agencies.

Stressing the need for flexibility in order to meet both practice needs and career goals, the ANA stated:

> Continuing education in nursing consists of planned, organized learning experiences designed to augment the knowledge, skills, and attitudes of registered nurses for the enhancement of nursing practice,

education, administration, and research, to the end of improving health care to the public.[50]

In the 1970s, a number of states enacted legislation requiring evidence of CE for relicensure of nurses (and of certain other professional and occupational groups). Under the stimulus of this legislative mandate, formalized programs increased. They are given under the auspices of educational institutions, professional organizations, and commercial for-profit groups. Generally they must be self-supporting.[51] Most now have some sort of recognition or accreditation so that their programs will be acknowledged by licensing boards as legitimate sources of continuing education. Most programs use the Continuing Education Unit (CEU), nationally accepted for unit measurement of all kinds of CE programs. (Ten contract hours equal one unit.)

Both the ANA and NLN and their constituent organizations have developed a voluntary system of CE for nurses. The ICN has also urged its members to take the lead in initiating, promoting, or further developing a national system of CE in nursing.

Now, for a variety of reasons (often related to cost), there has been somewhat of a backlash against mandatory CE, and several states have rescinded the requirement of CE for relicensure.[52]

Still, more nurses seem to be attending formal programs. How much CE improves practice is still an arguable question, for measurement of direct results is seldom practical. However, it has been shown that the motivation of the learner and the opportunity to apply what is learned are key factors.

Although in-service programs are not always accepted for formal CE requirements, most employers make such programs available (or mandatory) for improvement of nursing practice. Because all CE programs can be quite costly, there is increased interest in providing educationally sound programs directed toward meeting specific practice goals and building in an evaluation mechanism.[53] In some cases, evidence of CE is a job requirement or a necessity for promotion. In other cases (fire prevention and infection control), formal CE is required by the Joint Commission for the Accreditation of Health Care Organizations.

Opportunities and funds to attend programs are often part of some collective bargaining agreements. However, nurses, if they consider themselves professionals, should be prepared to pay for their own CE.

Is CE readily available to most nurses? Despite some justifiable complaints that formal programs are not always available in certain geographic areas, there are many ways for nurses to continue their professional development. Examples of self-directed learning activities include self-guided, focused reading, independent learning projects, individual scientific research, informal investigation of a specific nursing problem, correspondence courses, self-contained learning packages using various media, directed reading, computer-assisted instruction, programmed instruction, study tours, and group work projects. Some nursing journals have developed self-learning programs that include evaluation, for a minimal fee. There are also other innovative ways in which nurses are offered learning opportunities, such as through mobile vans, television, telephone systems, satellites, and other forms of telecommunication, as well as increased regional programs by nursing organizations.

The opportunities for CE in nursing are considerably greater than they were some years ago. What kind of CE a nurse chooses will remain, to a large extent, an individual decision. However, the need to be currently competent is both a legal and an ethical requirement for any professional.

TRENDS AND ISSUES

The 100-Year Debate

Of all the issues that create heated debate within nursing (and outside), the one that causes the strongest reactions is also the oldest. The question of how nurses should be educated to enter the nursing field, often abbreviated as "entry into practice," has been going on for almost 100 years.[54] With the first training programs, hospital based and controlled, there were early concerns about the need to move away from the apprenticeship model. These programs had never been totally like the Nightingale model. Nightingale, for instance, advocated a better-prepared, career-oriented nurse, as well as a bedside nurse. The first baccalaureate program in 1909 added liberal arts and a degree to the nurses' education, but not much, if any, change in the nursing part of the curriculum. Nevertheless, there were now two kinds of programs. With the initiation of the AD program, there were three that produced masses of nurses; a generic master's was already in existence.

What's wrong with having choices? The postgraduation confusion. With several distinctly different ways of educating nurses, which presumably produce different outcomes, all graduates still take the same licensing examination and have the same title, RN. Then they may hold the same kinds of jobs with the same expectations, the same responsibilities, and often the same salary. If so, what justification is there for three major educational programs, not to mention the generic masters and doctorate?

In the late 1950s and early 1960s, both ANA and NLN made a variety of statements that focused primarily on the baccalaureate as the necessary educational degree for professional nursing. Since an important function of ANA is that of setting standards and policies for nursing education, it was the ANA that made the definitive statement in 1965. A strong recommendation, by the Committee on Education resulted in the ANA position that nursing education should take place within the general educational system. Reaction to the "position paper" was decidedly mixed. (This is actually correctly titled "Educational Preparation for Nurse Practitioners and Assistants to Nurses—A Position Paper.") Although the concept underlying the paper had been enunciated by leaders in nursing since the profession's inception, reiterated through the years, and accepted as a goal by the 1960 House of Delegates, many nurses misunderstood the paper's intent and considered it a threat. Probably the greatest area of misinterpretation lay in the separation of nursing education and practice into professional, technical, and assisting components. Minimum preparation for professional nursing practice was designated at the baccalaureate level, technical nursing practice at the AD level, and education for assistants in health service occupations was to be given in short, intensive preservice programs in vocational education settings rather than in on-the-job training. An obvious omission in the position paper was the place of diploma and PN education. A large number of hospital-based diploma graduates, students, faculty, and hospital administrators were angered by this. A major source of resentment was that the term *professional nurse* was to be reserved for the baccalaureate graduate.

Even in this period of confusion, it was recognized that the largest system of nursing education at the time, the hospital school, could not be overlooked or eliminated by the writing of a position paper. Later, both the ANA and the NLN prepared statements that advocated careful community planning for phasing diploma programs into institutions of higher learning. It was also pointed out that as PN programs improved and increased their course content, their length would be close to that of the AD program. Nevertheless, the storm raged for 20 years, although repeated attempts were made to clarify the content and intent of the position paper. ANA probably suffered a membership loss due to the alienation of many diploma nurses. As expected, social and economic trends gradually brought about many of the changes suggested by the position paper, and the definitions of *professional nurse* and *technical nurse* were widely used in the literature (although there was no major indication that employers were assigning nurses according to technical or professional responsibilities).

In 1976, the New York State Nurses' Association's voting body overwhelmingly approved introduction of a "1985 Proposal" in the 1977 legislative session. Although variations of the proposal evolved over the next few years, the basic purpose of the legislation was to establish licensure for two kinds of nursing. The professional nurse would require a baccalaureate degree, and the other, whose title changed with various objections, would require an AD. The target date for full implementation was 1985; currently licensed nurses would be covered by the traditional grandfather clause, which would allow them to retain their current title and status (RN). The bill did not pass but was consistently reintroduced during each legislative session.

Immediately, the 1985 Proposal became both a term symbolizing baccalaureate education as the entry level into *professional* nursing and a rallying point for nurses who opposed this change. There was, and is, considerable opposition from some diploma and AD nurses and faculty, some hospital administrators, and some physicians. Nursing organizations were formed whose major focus was opposition to such proposals. Nevertheless, an increasing number of state nurses' organizations, primarily made up of diploma nurses, voted in convention to work toward the goal of baccalaureate education for professional nursing.

The NLN has played an interesting role in the entry into practice debate. In 1979, it supported all pathways (baccalaureate, associate, diploma, and practical nursing). Given the structure of the NLN and its historic position as the accrediting body for each level of nursing education, this statement is understandable. In 1982, however, the board of directors endorsed the baccalaureate degree as the criterion for professional practice. This position was affirmed when the voting body met in June 1983. (See the convention reports published in *Nursing Outlook* in the odd years during that period.)

Later reaffirmations by the board that called for two separate licensing exams infuriated the AD programs and community college presidents, who threatened to pull out of NLN agency membership.[55] There was a demand for clarification and objections that this action downgraded AD nurses for the sake of elevating BSN nurses.[56] (From all this agitation came a number of organizations whose purpose was basically to support AD nursing and to protect AD nurses and programs from ANA and NLN actions they saw as detrimental.) The LPNs were not happy either. What resulted was a compromise statement that seemed reasonably acceptable. An interesting nonaction occurred at the next convention, where the issue was tabled and other issues related to a major reorganization were given priority. At the same time, where once ANA conventions were consumed with entry into practice debates, gradually the question in education became: how do we facilitate transition? (See the reports of ANA conventions in *Nursing Outlook,* and the *American Journal of Nursing* in the even years.) The 1980 Social Policy Statement,[57] which clearly stated that baccalaureate education was the basis of professional nursing practice, was accepted, and the Cabinet on Nursing Education continued to work toward this goal. In the next biennium, ANA provided grants to several SNAs to implement their plans to establish the baccalaureate as the minimum educational qualification for professional nursing and set its timetable for implementation in all states before the end of the century. A number of reports by interdisciplinary commissions and groups also supported baccalaureate education for nurses.[58] The final report of the interdisciplinary National Commission for Nursing saw pursuit of the baccalaureate as an "achievable goal." A three-year project funded by the W. K. Kellogg Foundation in late 1984 to carry out selected Commission recommendations included the objective, "to outline the common body of knowledge and skills essential for basic nursing practice, the curriculum content that supports it, and a credentialing process that reinforces it." (These reports and others relating to nursing education are summarized in Appendix 1.) In later meetings, the House of Delegates became involved in trying to agree on how the two types of nurses could be accommodated as members. Eventually, this was more or less resolved by changes in the bylaws (see Chapter 14).

Entry into practice and its inevitable corollary, changes in nurse licensure, continue to be major issues in nursing. Most organizations at the state and national levels have taken a stand supporting the 1985 Proposal, or its concept of baccalaureate education as the appropriate education for the professional nurse. After that, there is still disagreement as to whether the "other" nurse would be the technical nurse, with separate licensing, and whether the PN would remain the same. Some think that AD education should be required for the practical nurse, leaving only two levels of nursing for the time being. Because this means a major change in nurse licensure, which is always a political as well as a legal issue, only a few (small) states have taken that big step. As discussed in Chapter 11, the North Dakota Board of Nursing changed its administrative rules, stating that after January 1987 the appropriate educational program for those wishing to take the RN licensure exam is the baccalaureate, and that for the PN, it is the AD. While there was a legal attempt by several hospitals to prevent this ruling from going into effect, the North Dakota attorney general ruled that this decision was within the purview of the board.[59] Also in 1986, the Maine legislature stated its intent that there be two levels of nursing (AD and baccalaureate) by 1995 or as soon as possible thereafter. In 1985, a number of other state nurses' associations thought that legislation for entry-level changes was possible within a few years. This did not occur, perhaps because a more immediate concern was the nursing shortage. Opponents also seized on the shortage to maintain that this was not the time to make such changes because all types of nursing education programs were needed. Even when some of the study reports recognized the need for baccalaureate nurses, the approach suggested was often like that of the AHA—encouragement of educational mobility. As discussed earlier, this refers to articulation of diploma and AD programs with those programs awarding baccalaureate or higher degrees, as well as more high-quality external degree programs and flexible campus-based instructional programs for nurses who want baccalaureate education.

In the long debate about the nature of education for practice,[60] it is not surprising that there are those who think that the system should stay as it is, others who opt for changing the baccalaureate nurse's title and license to indicate advanced preparation, and a few who are anticipating the time when a professional nurse doctorate, like the MD and DDS of physicians and dentists, will be the entry level to the profession.[61]

Yet, if we follow the trail of the entry-into-practice issue, we see a little backtracking and a lot of sidetracking, but overall, a firm path toward higher education—a historical inevitability. Step by step, nurses, the public, legislators, and even reluctant physicians and administrators have moved toward that goal. The path has been, and may continue to be, rough.

Among the obstacles is titling, with its personal and political sensitivities, especially during a transitional period. There simply is no agreement about who should be called (and licensed as) what among nurses (or anyone). Another obstacle is cost. Will costs limit access to baccalaureate education, with a resulting shortage there and an oversupply of technical nurses? Even more serious is the need for clear delineation of the differences between (or among) the various practitioners. A number of nursing groups have worked on this, and some of the outcomes are included in Appendix 3. Unfortunately, too often these studies are not coordinated, and the terms and phrases used are not consistent. Then there is the care. Some people object to separate licensure because, they say, there is no evidence that the variously educated RNs are any different in how they pass the licensure exams and practice; in fact, some insist, maybe the baccalaureate is not as good as the others. This is and has been an ongoing argument for years.

Surprisingly, the scanty research that has been done doesn't help much, since the studies are small, with different objectives, criteria, and population samples. Even nationally recorded state board results are indefinite, showing more differences among programs of the same type than among all. Finally, there is the problem of the inevitable confusion during the years of transition when nurses with a certain legal title will hold a mixture of degrees and diplomas and other qualifications among them. Even nurses' cherished easy mobility from state to state will be in jeopardy as each state changes the law at its own pace and with its own peculiarities. Only close cooperation of nursing organizations and state boards will prevent unhappy consequences.

Some natural fears of nonbaccalaureate nurses are to be expected: that they will lose status and job opportunities despite the grandfather clause and those who desire baccalaureate education will find it too expensive, unavailable, or rigidly repetitive. As to the first, there is already some pro-baccalaureate selectiveness; as to the second, there is slow but definite progress. These issues will not be quickly resolved, but inevitable societal and professional changes, such as the decrease in diploma schools and the expectations of professional practice,[62] (nursing is the only health profession for which entry is less than a baccalaureate), will be major factors in the final outcome.

In the meantime, there has been a quiet revolution, one that may end the recurrence of the entry-into-practice issue. It is the steady move toward advanced education that both RNs and LPNs are making. While many RNs are not convinced that baccalaureate education necessarily equates with professionalism,[63] others feel differently, and back to school they go.[64]

The New Crisis

The supply of health care workers, including nurses, is always difficult to predict, even when social and economic factors are considered. What might or might not have been predicted was the combination of a serious nursing shortage in the late 1980s (after a short period of alarm that nurses were in oversupply and might not be able to get or retain jobs) and the dramatic drop in nursing program admissions. Some initially blamed this on the reports that, with the inception of prospective payment (see Chapter 3), hospitals were closing units and laying off nurses, so nursing could no longer be seen as an occupation where you could always get a job. However, there were more significant factors relating to social trends, reported in Chapter 3. These include a decrease in the number of high school graduates who were traditionally college bound or at least ready for some occupational training; multiple career options open to women who would once have chosen nursing; young people's interest in more lucrative careers; a poor image of nursing (hard work, little status, poor salary, limited opportunities for advancement, not a profession); and less financial support for nursing education. Whatever the reason, admissions to nursing programs dipped dramatically, beginning in 1983. In 1986, the NLN reported as much as a 30 percent drop in enrollments in all basic RN programs but particularly in baccalaureate programs, and this continued until 1989. Then enrollment of first-time nursing students rose by almost 9 percent, the largest increase occurring in ADN programs. Considering the decline for the previous five years, admissions were still not up to what they had been and new students were not replacing each year's graduating class (graduation numbers were also still declining).

Another change during this shortage period was that more students were going to school part time, which, of course, delayed graduation and sometimes made attrition more likely. Although more RNs were returning to school to get their baccalaureates, as discussed earlier, the emphasis on new students occurred both because an increase would show that people saw nursing as a good career choice and, certainly, because the nurse workforce would be enlarged.

One major outcome of the drop in admissions was participation of schools in the gigantic marketing effort of NCNIP (see Appendix 1), and various nursing and other health care organizations and groups, aimed at attracting prospective students to nursing and generally enhancing the image of nursing. However, individual schools also used many new techniques to recruit students to their own particular programs. Among these were establishing relationships with liberal arts programs or schools to funnel students directly into nursing education more easily; "adopting" a high school or even middle school, or "mentoring" specific students in these schools to orient them to nursing careers; and working with unions to encourage and assist LPNs or aides to move on to RN education. One well-funded program united the forces of over 100 hospitals, long-term care facilities, and nursing programs into consortia to provide educational advancement opportunities for aides and PNs, with the expectation that since they had already chosen nursing, they would, as RNs, stay on the job. Included were accelerated training, loan/service payback programs, support services, remedial help, and counseling.[65] In addition, schools used both radio and TV spots, mail campaigns, and booths at shopping malls and health clubs. There were also much discussion and lobbying for more student financial aid from the state and national governments, since there was considerable evidence that this was needed. (Among others, NSNA has reported for years that most nursing students require financial aid.) Launching a new Cadet Nurse Corps, which had increased nursing enrollment so much during World War II, was also suggested.[66] Some hospitals provided scholarships or made arrangements with potential students to pay back funding by promising to work in that institution for a specific period of time. One diploma school even recruited students in Ireland and other foreign countries, granting them full scholarships in return for a promise to work in the hospital for three years after graduation.

As is true of colleges in general, special attention was (and is) given to recruiting the nontraditional pool of potential applicants such as second careerists and older men and women.[67] College graduates were also seen as likely to be attracted to accelerated BSN or generic master's programs.[68] Minorities and men, still not a large percentage of the nursing population, were also targeted for recruitment. According to the NLN, of all graduating students, about 8 percent are black, 3 percent Hispanic, 2 percent Asian, and 5 percent native American. The largest percentage of black students (about 11 percent) are in BSN programs. Most men (7 percent) choose AD education, with slightly fewer in diploma programs and only 2 percent in baccalaureate programs. About 6 percent of all graduates are men. Attrition is a serious problem for many minority students, both for academic and financial reasons and also because they may require considerable support, for which schools are not always prepared or seem unable to provide.[69] More than minority students may need help, however, since there is some evidence of lowering of general admission standards.[70] One interesting outcome, as described earlier, is the speed with which some rather rigid programs have managed to adjust to the need for flexibility in curriculum, class scheduling, and meeting the needs of nontraditional students as well as returning RNs.

Whether the number of generic students entering and, more important, graduating from nursing schools will continue to grow is unknown. But just how this new mix of future nurses will affect the profession is already a big point of speculation.

Does Nursing Education Prepare Competent Practitioners?

There are other issues that seem to recur in nursing education. From the time that the last diploma program gave up the apprenticeship to nursing education, there have been accusations that the new graduates of modern nursing programs are not competent. Further investigation usually shows the new graduates are not as technically skillful or as able to assume responsibilities for a large group of patients as the nurses with whom they are compared—the diploma graduates of yesterday. Nevertheless, the criticisms are understandable. For the director of nursing with fiscal constraints, a lengthy orientation and in-service program is a strain on the budget; for the staff nurse and supervisor, someone who requires extra help or supervision on a usually short-staffed unit is an impediment.

Although graduates from all three types of programs are the targets of employer disapproval, the diploma graduate, whose program is focused on the hospital and who frequently stays at the hospital, may find adjustment a little easier. AD graduates who have been PNs and have had experience in caring for many patients are also somewhat immune from criticisms about slow adjustment. However, because most graduates today do not have these backgrounds, how justified are the criticisms? How differently do the graduates of the RN programs perform?

The nursing literature is full of articles on content and methods; nurse educators are certainly concerned about preparing the best possible practitioner. Everyone agrees that new graduates should be competent to give both physical and psychological/emotional care. Just how much of this is best taught in a clinical setting is a point of controversy. How much of what kind of clinical experience prepares nurses best? It has been suggested that additional emphasis be given to the physical care needed because of patients' pathophysiological problems. There is also some indication that students need practice in basic technical skills, which some schools deal with by encouraging additional self-study in labs. In others, a concentrated period of time in one or two clinical areas at the end of the program eases students into the work situation. It also allows them to integrate their clinical knowledge and skills over a continuum of time and to learn to organize the care of larger groups of patients, setting appropriate priorities. Certain programs also have cooperative arrangements with clinical facilities to allow students a paid work-study period in the summer or specific academic terms in which they work full time while being supervised in practice. Field placements, or clinical electives, are other options. There are mixed feelings about whether working as an aide or ward clerk is helpful because of the limited legal scope of practice and the possibility that students are subtly forced into assuming more responsibility than is legal.

Giving the added clinical experience in one mode or another seems to please both students and future employers. There are a number of variations of these methods. A *preceptorship* is usually a one-to-one experience for the student, with a staff nurse preceptor guiding the learning in the clinical facility. The carefully selected preceptor, who is often a clinical faculty appointment (without pay), has an orientation and sometimes classes on clinical teaching strategies.[71] Preceptorships seem to enhance the student's learning, if properly done, but they require careful preparation and monitoring.[72]

An *externship*, also involving preceptors, gives students full-time work experience in a real-world environment, often in the summers, for which they are paid. Since the latter involves no academic faculty if it is not part of the curriculum, both the facility and the student must be careful to adhere to the legal limitations of what the student can do. An *internship* generally occurs after the student has graduated and eases the new graduate into the work setting by providing a variety of supervised experiences. Usually the new nurse is paid less during this time, and if the internship is not carefully planned to meet both the employee's and the employer's needs, it can become nonproductive. Preceptors are often a part of this practice as well.[73]

There is also the question as to whether the various kinds of programs actually prepare different kinds of practitioners. Nurse educators say they do, but often the statements of philosophy and objectives or the various "official" competency statements have obvious areas of overlap. Moreover, some believe that there is a lack of clarity in how heads of AD and baccalaureate programs see their type of program as different from the other. Specifically, most programs do not seem to adhere to the differences spelled out in the literature. For instance, some AD program directors think their graduates have as broad a judgment base as the baccalaureate nurse, and many prepare these nurses for administrative functions without the necessary educational base. On the other hand, this is probably a matter of catching up with reality, because many employers given AD nurses responsibilities for which they are not prepared. But should the teacher then educate the employer instead of reeducating the student?

If success in state boards is considered to be a criterion for competency, the results are no more definitive; differences within each type of program are greater than those among the programs. As to differences in practice among diploma, AD, and BSN nurses, this has been difficult to determine because most studies have been done by graduate students. Not only are the numbers and the studies seldom replicated, but what is being measured is usually different from study to study.[74] Some researchers have concluded that, if properly defined, the leadership/management role could be a viable area of differentiation.[75]

Although the specific competencies of ADN and BSN nurses are discussed more in Appendix 3, one interesting project has differentiated the two, with the cooperation of both nursing education and nursing service. The general approach is categorization in terms of direct care, communication, and management competencies. The BSN competencies include and build on those of the ADN, with BSN nurses also assuming leadership and giving more advanced care in complex situations.[76] The very fact that nursing care is becoming increasingly complex and that AD nurses will considerably outnumber baccalaureate nurses if current trends continue has concerned many nursing leaders, who wonder whether very sick patients can be properly cared for.

Is faculty preparation and expertise part of the problem? There are still teachers without graduate education. Moreover, because of the kind of graduate education available at a particular time, there are nursing faculty who have learned curriculum and teaching skills but who shy away from actual patient care because they feel inadequate. There are also clinicians with graduate degrees who have difficulty communicating their know-how or who are forced to teach in a specialty area for which they were not educated. In some areas, joint appointments of faculty and clinicians enables each to contribute to the goals of the other, but this practice is largely limited to medical centers and university programs. One trend, particularly in college and university programs is the encouragement, sometimes the requirement, that clinical faculty maintain their clinical competence by regular practice beyond their clinical teaching. There are many versions of what is generally called *faculty practice*. (See the Bibliography for an overview of articles on faculty practice.) In some cases of faculty practice, faculty members simply give a few lectures, serve on committees, or make themselves generally helpful to a clinical facility in terms of their own expertise. In others, individual faculty may practice for set periods of time (a day, a week, in the summer, during holiday breaks) in staff nurse, clinical specialist, or NP roles, either being permitted to keep the money earned or required to give it to the school toward their salaries. A number of faculty have started a faculty group practice, delivering holistic care in the community to the poor, the homeless, the elderly, children, or even college students, faculty, and staff. Some are free, and some are fee-for-service, but almost all are non-profit. Some are part of an established health care facility, some are independent. It may be an interdisciplinary group that also has other nurses and paid employees. Students usually have part of their clinical experience there.[77] Clearly, such practices are not only good experience for the students but enable them to see their teachers as clinical role models. For the teachers, who may find this practice, although often stressful,[78] stimulating and rewarding, there is one drawback: they must usually still carry a full teaching load and often find themselves pressed for time to do the necessary research and writing required for promotion. Faculty practice is not considered a scholarly activity by university promotion and tenure committees. However, the assumption is that a teacher who practices clinically on an ongoing basis prepares more competent students.

Other Issues

There are a number of ongoing issues in nursing education, such as those related to continuing education. What kind of continuing education do nurses need? Who decides? Who is best qualified to provide it? Who should pay? Should it be mandatory for relicensure? Who is responsible for ensuring that it is available to all nurses? Will it improve practice?

Other issues relate to recruitment and retention of minority students who may or may not fall into the "disadvantaged" category, such as the handicapped; legal aspects of admission and student and faculty rights (Chapter 13); what kind and how much preparation is needed for specific clinical areas, such as operating room nursing, public health nursing, and occupational health nursing; the kind of education for RNs entering baccalaureate programs (basically the same as for the generic student? advanced? specialized?); and intradisciplinary education (should PN and various types of RN students learn together?). Interdisciplinary education with other health team members has also been a point of discussion for some time, with relatively little action taken.[79] There is also continued concern about the quality and cost of nursing education. (Reduced resources are forcing some baccalaureate programs to turn away qualified students.)

WHAT DOES THE FUTURE HOLD?

Taking into account what we see happening to nursing education now, and tying in external trends, some predictions about nursing education in the 1990s can be hazarded. These are:

- Nursing education will continue moving toward preparing two types of nurses both educationally and legally.
- Federal funding for all kinds of nursing education will be tighter. More students will choose part-time education and will look for scholarships and loans. Cost-effective teaching methods will be demanded.
- More RNs will seek advanced education, and more educational programs will provide the flexibility to accommodate their needs.

- There will be a closer relationship between school and clinical site, with qualified staff providing more clinical teaching and more faculty involved in clinical practice of some kind.
- Continuing education will be seen as increasingly important to maintain competence, and individual nurses will be expected to get what they need and pay for it.
- The generalist nurse will continue to be needed and educated, but specialization at a technical level will be necessary through continuing education or in-service education. Graduate-level specialization will have a steady but slow growth.
- Nursing research will make continued but not dramatic progress.
- More men and women will find nursing an attractive career choice, but because of program length and cost, the impetus will be toward non-baccalaureate generic education.

KEY POINTS

1. Nursing education programs share certain similarities: regulation, changes in student mix, need for clinical facilities, and educational trends.
2. Nursing education programs also differ in many ways, particularly in the expected competencies of their graduates.
3. RNs seeking baccalaureate education have more choices than they did 15 years ago, including self-learning activities and external degrees.
4. Continuing education is an ethical and professional responsibility whether or not it is legally required.
5. Entry into practice issues center on whether baccalaureate education should be required for the professional nurse and AD education for a technical or associate nurse, and how and when this should be accomplished.
6. The resolution of the entry-into-practice issues will have a great impact on both nursing education programs and all graduates.
7. Beginning with the ANA's position paper on education in 1965, the actions of the various nursing organizations have tended to support baccalaureate education for professional nursing.
8. Nursing research is a systematic inquiry into questions and problems arising from the practice of nursing.
9. Problems of translating the findings of nursing research into action are related to the lack of knowledge about nursing research held by many practicing nurses.
10. Issues in nursing education include perceived problems in student and faculty competence, desirable content in curriculum, costs, and how and by whom programs should be evaluated.

REFERENCES

1. Ference H. What LPNs do. *Am J Nurs,* 84:799 (June 1984).
2. Montag M. *The education of nursing technicians.* New York: G.P. Putnam's Sons, 1951, p. 70.
3. Ibid., p. 6.
4. Ibid., p. 13.
5. *Educational outcomes of associate degree nursing programs: Roles and competencies.* New York: National League for Nursing, 1990.
6. Brown E. The economics of change: Associate degree education today and tomorrow. *Nurs and Health Care,* 8:147–150 (March 1987).
7. Wajdawicz E. The Americanization of Florence: A look at associate degree nurses. *Nurs and Health Care,* 7:96–99 (February 1986).
8. Neighbors M, et al. Nursing skills necessary for competencies in the high-tech health care system. *Nurs and Health Care,* 12:92–97 (February 1991).
9. Kelly LY. *Dimensions of professional nursing,* 6th ed. Elmsford, NY: Pergamon Press, 1991, pp. 266–267.
10. Rich J. In pursuit of a BSN. *Nurs 90,* 9:118, 120 (February 1990).
11. Slavinsky AT, Diers D. Nursing education for college graduates. *Nurs Outlook,* 39:292–297 (May 1982).
12. Schlotfeldt R. The professional doctorate: Rationale and characteristics. *Nurs Outlook,* 26:309 (May 1978).
13. Fitzpatrick J, et al. An experiment in nursing revisited. *Nurs Outlook,* 35:29–33 (January–February 1987).
14. Forni P. Models for doctoral programs; First professional degree or terminal degree? *Nurs and Health Care,* 10:429–434 (October 1989).
15. American Nurses' Association. *Statement on graduate education in nursing.* Kansas City, MO: The Association, 1978.
16. American Nurses' Association. *Statement on graduate education in nursing.* New York: The Association, 1969.
17. Kelly, op. cit., pp. 268–272.
18. Forni P. Nursing's diverse master's programs: The state of the art. *Nurs and Health Care,* 8:70–75 (February 1987).
19. Marriner-Tomey A. Historical development of doctoral programs from the Middle Ages to nursing education today. *Nurs and Health Care,* 11:133–137 (March 1990).
20. Gortner SR. Historical development of doctoral programs: Shaping our expectations. *J Prof Nurs,* 7:45–53 (January–February 1991).
21. Andreoli K. Specialization and graduate curricula: Finding the fit. *Nurs and Health Care,* 8:68 (February 1987).
22. Fields W. The PhD.: The ultimate nursing doctorate. *Nurs Outlook,* 36:188–189 (July–August 1988).
23. Meleis A. Doctoral education in nursing: Its present and its future. *J Prof Nurs,* 6:436–446 (November–December 1988).
24. Taira F, Reed S. Is that doctorate necessary? *Nurs Outlook,* 31:12–15 (January–February 1983).

25. Lev E, et al. The postdoctoral fellowship experience. *Image,* 22:116–120 (Spring 1990).
26. Kelly, op. cit., pp. 278–289.
27. Reilly DE. Research in nursing education: Yesterday—today—tomorrow. *Nurs and Health Care,* 11:138–143 (March 1990).
28. Schlotfeldt R. Research in nursing and research training for nurses: Retrospect and prospect. *Nurs Res,* 24:177 (May–June 1975).
29. Notter L. *Essentials of nursing research,* 2nd ed. New York: Springer Publishing Company, 1978, pp. 20–23.
30. Larson E. Nursing research outside academia: A panel presentation. *Image,* 13:75 (October 1981).
31. Gortner S. Research for a practice profession. *Nurs Res,* 24:193–196 (May–June 1975).
32. Newman M. What differentiates clinical research? *Image,* 14:88 (October 1982).
33. Johnson D. Development of theory: A requisite for nursing as a primary health profession. *Nurs Res,* 23:373 (September–October 1974).
34. Downs F, Fleming J, eds. *Issues in nursing research.* New York: Appleton-Century-Crofts, 1979, p. 75.
35. National Commission on Nursing. *Summary report and recommendations.* Chicago: The Commission, 1983, p. 11.
36. King D, et al. Disseminating the results of nursing research. *Nurs Outlook,* 29:164–169 (March 1981).
37. Sneed N. Curiosity and the yen to discover. *Nurs Outlook,* 38:36–39 (January–February 1990).
38. Beckstrand J, McBride AB. How to form a research interest group. *Nurs Outlook,* 38:168–171 (July–August 1990).
39. Betz CL, et al. Nursing research productivity in clinical settings. *Nurs Outlook,* 38:180–183 (July–August 1990).
40. Merritt D. The National Center for Nursing Research. *Image,* 18:84–85 (Fall 1986).
41. Jacox A. The coming of age of nursing research. *Nurs Outlook,* 34:276–281 (November–December 1986).
42. Lenburg C, Johnson W. Career mobility through nursing education. *Nurs Outlook,* 22:266 (April 1974).
43. Lenburg CB, Mitchell CA. Assessment of outcomes: The design and use of real and simulation nursing performance examinations. *Nurs and Health Care,* 12:68–74 (February 1991).
44. Almost the entire issue of *Nursing Outlook* (September–October 1984) is devoted to descriptions of alternative educational patterns for RNs.
45. Davids SL, Laeger E. Developing a BSN program across two institutions: Arizona State University West Campus/Glendale Community College—the adjuvant model. *Nurs and Health Care,* 11:84–88 (February 1990).
46. Brubaker B. A faculty learns to make self-pacing work. *Nurs and Health Care,* 11:74–77 (February 1990).
47. Lenburg C. Do external degree programs really work? *Nurs Outlook,* 38:234–238 (September–October 1990).

48. Lenburg C. Preparation for professionalism through Regents External Degrees. *Nurs and Health Care*, 5:319–325 (June 1984).

49. Mitchell CA. One view of the future: Nontraditional education as the norm. *Nurs and Health Care*, 9:187–190 (April 1988).

50. American Nurses' Association. *Self-directed continuing education in nursing*. Kansas City, MO: The Association, 1978.

51. Newbern V. The future of nursing continuing education. *Nurs Outlook*, 37:182–184 (July–August 1989).

52. Woodruff D. Continuing education: How do we make it work? *Nurs 87*, 17:83 (September 1987).

53. Kristjanson L, Scanlon J. Assessment of continuing nursing education needs: A literature review. *J Cont Ed in Nurs*, 20:118–123 (May–June 1989).

54. Christy T. Entry into practice: A recurring issue in nursing history. *Am J Nurs*, 80:485–488 (March 1980).

55. Two-year colleges prepare for battle over nursing programs. *Chr Higher Ed*. (April 23, 1986), p. 2.

56. Waters V. Restricting the RN license to BSN graduates could cloud nursing's future. *Nurs and Health Care*, 7:142–146 (March 1986).

57. American Nurses' Association. *Nursing: A social policy statement*. Kansas City, MO: The Association, 1980.

58. Kelly, op. cit., pp. 71–85.

59. Wakefield-Fisher M, et al. A first for the nation: North Dakota and entry into nursing practice. *Nurs and Health Care*, 7:135–141 (March 1986).

60. Warner S, et al. An analysis of entry into practice arguments. *Image*, 20:212–216 (Winter 1988).

61. Schlotfeldt (1978), op. cit.

62. Butts P, et al. Tracking down the right degree for the job. *Nurs and Health Care*, 7:91–95 (February 1986).

63. Schoen D. A study of nurses' attitudes toward the BSN requirement. *Nurs and Health Care*, 3:382–387 (September 1982).

64. Smullen B. Second-step education for RNs: The quiet revolution. *Nurs and Health Care*, 3:369–373 (September 1982).

65. Dixon A. Project LINC (Ladders in Nursing Careers): An innovative model of educational mobility. *Nurs and Health Care*, 10:398–402 (September 1989).

66. Kalisch P. Why not launch a new Cadet Nurse Corps? *Am J Nurs*, 88:316–317 (March 1988).

67. Whitley M, Malen A. Market research and nursing's dwindling applicant pool. *Nurs Economics* 5:130–135 (May–June 1987).

68. Salvinsky A, et al. College graduates: The hidden nursing population. *Nurs and Health Care*, 4:373–378 (September 1983).

69. Tucker-Allen S. Losses incurred through minority student nurse attrition. *Nurs and Health Care*, 10:395–397 (September 1989).

70. Rosenfeld P. Nursing education in crisis—A look at recruitment and retention. *Nurs and Health Care*, 8:283–286 (May 1989).

71. Fire N, et al. The Presbyterian Hospital Program. *Nurs Outlook,* 32:209–211 (July–August 1984).
72. Goldenberg D. Preceptorship: A one-to-one relationship with a triple "P" rating (preceptor, preceptee, patient). *Nurs Forum,* 23(1):10–15 (1987–1988).
73. Davis L, Barham P. Get the most from your preceptorship program. *Nurs Outlook,* 37:167–178 (July–August 1989).
74. Rose MA. ADN vs. BSN: The search for differentiation. *Nurs Outlook,* 36:275–279 (November–December 1988).
75. Schank MJ, Stollenwerk R. The leadership/management role: A differentiating factor for ADN/BSN programs. *J Nurs Ed,* 27:253–257 (June 1988).
76. Primm P. Entry into practice: Competency statements for BSNs and ADNs. *Nurs Outlook,* 34:135–137 (May–June 1986).
77. Rosswurm MA. Characteristics of 23 faculty group nurse practices. *Nurs and Health Care,* 2:327–330 (June 1981).
78. Steele RL. Attitudes about faculty practice, perceptions of role, and role strain. *J Nurs Ed,* 30:15–21 (January 1991).
79. Barnum BJ. At New York University, the Division of Nursing develop a model for nursing and medical school collaboration. *Nurs and Health Care,* 11:89–90 (February 1990).

CHAPTER 6

EMPLOYMENT GUIDELINES

OBJECTIVES

After studying this chapter, you will be able to:

1. Prepare for a job interview.
2. Put together a professional résumé.
3. Write an application letter.
4. Identify sources of information about jobs.
5. Terminate employment in an appropriate manner.
6. Assess your talents and interests in planning for your career.

Graduation at last! And now what? For most nurses, "what" means it's now time to get a job. For some, the job is predetermined—commitment to the armed services, the Veterans Administration, or another agency that funded their education. Others may have decided early on exactly the kind of nursing they prefer and the place they want to do it. If all goes well and there are no problems, such as an oversupply of nurses for that specialty or geographic area, at least one major decision is made. But for all graduates, choosing that crucial first job and preparing for it are big considerations.

There are many employment opportunities for nurses today, although the place of employment preferred may not offer the exact hours, specialty, opportunities, or assistance a new graduate may want. Pockets of unemployment most often result from budgeting factors and a tightening of the economy. Nurses may be *needed,* sometimes seriously, but some employers still tend to retain less qualified workers on lower salaries and to eliminate patient care services. Another problem is maldistribution, with not enough nurses opting to work in ghettos or poor rural areas, although the need there is serious. On the other hand, small communities may be flooded by nursing graduates of a community college who wish to stay in that area.

Even with these social and economic factors, new nursing opportunities are constantly emerging (these are described in some detail in Chapter 7). How, then, can you decide what is the best job for you? How do you maximize the chances of getting it?

BASIC CONSIDERATIONS

Personal and Occupational Assessment

It's a good idea to start thinking about career choices while you are still in your educational program. Since most schools have rotations through the various clinical specialty areas, this gives you a chance to compare as you learn. Generally, there is also access to someone who can advise you about the pros and cons of certain types of nursing—or at least there's a more experienced nurse, often a faculty member, to talk to.

More important than anything else, though, is to take a considered look at yourself—your own qualities and what you want out of life. There are a variety of approaches to this sort of self-assessment that are interesting to explore in depth,[1] but there are generally certain commonalities. Some questions you might ask are:

What are my personality characteristics? Do I like to do things with people or by myself? Am I patient? Do I like to do things quickly? Am I good at details, or do I like to take the broad view? Do I like a structured and quiet environment or one that is constantly changing? Am I relatively confident in what I undertake or do I look for support? Am I easily bored? Do I like to tackle problem situations or avoid them? Do I have a sense of humor? Am I emotional? Am I a risk taker? Do I care about the way I look? Do I care what others think of me?

What are my values? Do I believe in the right to life or the right to die? Do I think everyone should have access to health care? Do I have some religious orientation? Do I think that too many people today are too rigid or too loose in their beliefs and behavior? Can I accept and work with those who have very different values? How do I feel about my responsibility to myself, my employer, my patient, the doctors, my profession, and society? Do I believe strongly that my way is the right way? Am I intolerant of others' beliefs?

What are my interests? In the broad field of nursing? In certain specialties? In the health field? In my private and social life? In the community? Do I like to travel?

What are my needs? Am I ambitious? Do I like to boss? Is money important to me? Status? Do I need intellectual stimulation? Is academic success important? What about academic credentials? Am I willing to relocate? Does a city, suburb, or rural area fit my desired lifestyle? Is success in my field important? Am I willing to sacrifice personal and family time for success? Do I think that my first responsibility is to my family at this point? Do my spouse and I plan to have dual careers? Is part-time work an option? Do I want plenty of time for family, friends, and leisure activities? Do I see nursing as a career or a way to earn a living as long as that is necessary? Do I really like nursing? If not, why not, and what can I do about it?

What kinds of abilities do I have? In manual skills? In communication? In intellectual/cognitive skills? In analyzing? In coordinating? In organizing? In supervising? In dealing with people? Do I have a great deal of energy and stamina? Are there certain times, situations, or climate conditions in which I have less? Am I good at comforting people? Am I able to give some of myself to others?

It's good to prioritize some of these lists, since life and a job are usually a compromise. What's most important? What would make you miserable? It might also be very helpful to share this list with others. Is this the way you are seen by them? Have you missed something? If some of your friends and peers are involved in their own decision making, get together with them and/or a trusted teacher or mentor to brainstorm about the possibilities in the field now or later in order to match your own profile most accurately with nursing opportunities. When compromises are necessary, you can decide ahead of time which ones are tenable or even perfectly acceptable at that point.

Since there will probably be economic constraints in the health care system for a long time, one way to look at the job market is in terms of future growth. For instance, you may choose a community hospital for a first job in order to hone your new skills, but have you considered an investor-owned hospital or, later, a long-term care facility, home care, or an ambulatory-care outreach center? All are part of a trend in health care. You should examine those job prospects as carefully as any other. They may have components that do not fit in with your own self-assessment. But don't close doors because of preconceived notions.

Licensure

Regardless of the results of your self-study, a basic and essential step in your professional nursing career is becoming licensed, since you cannot practice in any state without an RN. Information about how to apply to take the state board examination leading to licensure is found in Chapter 11. The procedure for becoming licensed, either initially or later, may take from four to six months. State boards of nursing in most states permit nurses to practice temporarily while their application for licensure is being processed. You can usually be employed as a *graduate nurse* until you pass the licensure exam. In some places, you can continue in that status, if you fail, until you take the next scheduled examination. More frequently now, this is not done, and you are dismissed or must work as some type of nursing assistant.

What if you decide not to work right away—for example, to stay home with your family or to take a long vacation? It's probably wise to study for and take the exam anyway. Unused knowledge has a way of disappearing from the mind, and it might be much more difficult to pass the exam later, without some ongoing learning and practice. Should you take a nursing board review course? It depends on the confidence you have in your nursing knowledge and test-taking ability. The *good* courses can be very helpful, and may provide backup materials as well as lectures. However, be careful to select a reputable company. Remember that these are profit-making operations, expensive to you, and always attracting some borderline operators. Another way of preparing is to study with a group of peers, perhaps using board review workbooks or texts designed for that purpose.[2]

PROFESSIONAL BIOGRAPHIES AND RÉSUMÉS

Now that you have done your self-assessment and thought about career alternatives, it's time to write your résumé. No matter how you obtain a position in nursing, you will probably be asked to submit a résumé or summary of your qualifications for the job. This might include a personal history, education and experience, character and performance references, professional credentials such as the license registration number, and a transcript of your education records.

Some universities and other educational programs still maintain a file with updated information about your career provided by you, as well as references that you have solicited. This has the advantage of eliminating the need to ask for repeated references from teachers who may scarcely re-member you or to write again and again to a variety of places for records. However, this service is gradually fading away and that may not be bad. As you and your career develop, a reference from your first teacher or your first staff position says little other than how you were evaluated at that time. Newer references may be far more useful. Your academic record or simply evidence of your graduation may still be requested, and your school always provides that information. But today a well-prepared résumé is considered more appropriate.

A résumé is a relatively short professional or business biography. In academia, a curriculum vitae (CV), which is somewhat lengthier and con-tains different and more detailed information, is the appropriate form of professional biography.[3] Résumés are usually shorter than CVs.

The résumé should be businesslike, typed neatly on one side of good-

---

Exhibit 6-1

Résumé

LESLIE B. SMITH

120 Pine Street   Home Phone (413) 456-7890
North Ridge, MA 01302   Message Phone (413) 482-6132

PROFESSIONAL
OBJECTIVE: Staff nursing in a community hospital.

EXPERIENCE:
1989–1991   University Hospital Los Angeles

                        Unit clerk on medical-surgical units, evening shift.
                        Assisted charge nurse in (list activities); trained new
                        clerks; developed end-of-shift report between clerks.

1988   Williams General Hospital, Williams, Maine
(Summer)
                        Nurse's aide on medical-surgical units. Responsible
                        for care of thirty patients under direction of RNs
                        including (list major activities).

quality plain white, off-white, or light gray paper measuring 8½ by 11 inches, with a good margin all around. No more than two pages are usually recommended. A word processor is useful in writing résumés because it allows you to tailor the résumé to a particular job opportunity without making a total revision. However, make sure that the word processor prepares a good-looking résumé.

There are various ways to write a résumé.[4] Remember that it is a marketing tool and should show you to advantage. Therefore, while you must never be dishonest,[5] the way you present your talents and credentials, especially after you have had additional work experience, may make the difference between whether you are even interviewed or ignored, especially in a competitive situation. While format is a matter of taste, a sample résumé is shown in Exhibit 6-1.

Some suggestions may be helpful. The professional objective is not a

---

EDUCATION:

| 1991–1993 | Blank Community College |
| | Associate in Science, May 1993 |

HONORS:

1991–1993	Dean's List
1992–1993	Member, Wings, college honor society
1991–1993	Honor Scholarship
1992	Outstanding Student Leader Award, Blank Community College

PROFESSIONAL ACTIVITIES:

1991–1993	Member, National Student Nurses' Association
1992–1993	Chair, Program Committee, NSNA
March 1993	Presented paper "When Students Teach Patients." Blank Hospital
1985	Chair, Program Committee at College
1992	Attended ANA Convention
April 1992	Debate: "Be It Resolved: Everyone Has a Right to Health Care." NSNA convention, Denver

COMMUNITY ACTIVITIES:

1985–1992	Volunteer for public television telethon
1984–1993	Volunteer for March of Dimes
1985–1988	Candy-striper at Blank Hospital, Blank Town

must, especially if you are not sure exactly what you want to do. If you choose to write a résumé , it should match the job for which you are applying, and thus may need to be changed accordingly. For instance, someone with a master's degree in perinatal nursing may be interested in either a teaching or a clinical specialist position. Both the objective and the emphasis in the résumé must focus on the position for which the person is applying. Needless to say, if you are applying for your first or second staff nurse position in a hospital, the decision on what to write is less complex.

All relevant work experiences should be included, with the most recent listed first. The usual format is to list the agency and date, followed by a brief description of the duties performed, using "action" verbs—*developed, initiated, supervised*. Some experts suggest that if you have not had impressive positions, you should attempt to bury this fact in statements that focus on your personal qualities, such as "Leadership—Demonstrated my ability to lead others as night nurse on a pediatric unit at X hospital, such and such address." No one really knows whether this is more effective, but again, style is a matter of personal choice.

The education section should also begin with the most recent academic credential, and should include the major and such additions as research projects, special awards, academic honors, extracurricular activities, and offices held. There is no need to go as far back as high school. Information on other honors, professional memberships and activities, and community activities might also be given in separate sections. Don't put down a heading such as "honors" and then write "none." Just omit such categories.

Under federal law, you cannot be required to include personal data such as your age, marital status, place of birth, religion, sex, race, color, national origin, or handicap. If you choose to do so, decide whether this makes you a more desirable candidate. For instance, a second language or extensive travel might be a plus in certain situations. When you are licensed as an RN, or if you later become certified in a specialty, that can be listed as well. It is usually best not to list specific references on your résumé, since this omission allows you to select the most appropriate reference for a particular position. It is not necessary to say "References on request"; you would hardly refuse to give them. If your school does maintain a file, you can state this, giving the correct address. When you do give the references, include the full names, titles, and business addresses of three persons who are qualified to evaluate your professional ability, scholarship, character, and personality. Most suitable are teachers and former employers. Ask permission to use their names as references in advance. Choose carefully.[6] If the individual, no matter how prestigious, really doesn't know you, your talents, and your abilities, and the reference is noncommittal, it can do more harm than good. When you contact a reference, however, it is acceptable, even good sense, to offer to send a résumé to refresh that person's memory. For instance, almost everyone forgets the dates they knew you, as you are not likely to be the only student or employee they know. If the individual is reluctant, don't push; the result can be a reference that says nothing much, and the potential employer may read it as negative. You should also keep in mind that employers frequently telephone the reference, either because they want a quick answer or because they want to ask questions that are not on a reference form or to explore some aspect of the written reference (particularly if it was noncommittal). Therefore, if your reference is inclined to be abrupt, unpleasant, or irritated on the phone, choose another. As a rule, don't ask for a "To whom it may concern" letter and have it recopied. Most sophisticated employers see that as an uninterested response.

Suppose that you didn't get along with your last employer and, even though you left with appropriate notice, you fear a poor reference. Sometimes someone else who was your positional superior, or another person such as a clinical specialist who knows your work, can be substituted. (A peer's opinion may be discounted.) However, administrators often know each other, and your potential employer may know that you did not name the person who would be the usual reference and may check with him or her by phone. That could result in a really negative reference. Therefore, as lists of references are often not requested until after the interview, you could simply say then that you did not have a positive relationship. Be careful not to speak negatively of the former employer; try to be objective or neutral. Though references can be important, the impression you make in an interview can be much more important in the long run.

LOOKING OVER THE JOB MARKET

It's sensible to assess the potential for a particular job both before and after applying for and/or being offered a nursing position. Chapter 7 should be helpful as an overview of the opportunities available in terms of both specialties and professional development (career ladder, internships), but reading the literature, talking to practitioners in the field, and, if possible, getting exposure to the actual practice during your educational program will help answer some specific questions.

Today, even if an employer is actively recruiting for nurses, an application, a formal letter of interest, and often a résumé are necessary before a position is actually offered. Although there are those who feel that going through the entire process is worthwhile for the experience alone, unless you have at least some interest, it is unfair to take an employer's time to review an application and go through an interview for nothing. Therefore, after self-assessment, do at least a potential job assessment in advance. The first logical consideration is a place with which you have already had experience.

Hospitals or other agencies affiliated with schools of nursing may offer new graduates staff positions. That has several advantages for the employer and usually for the student as well. Nurses who are familiar with the personnel, procedures, and physical facilities may require a shorter orientation period, which saves time and money. And, of course, to an extent, the former student is already known. There are also benefits for new graduates. During these first months after graduation, you can gain valuable experience in familiar surroundings. There are opportunities to develop leadership and teaching skills and to practice clinical skills under less pressure because the people, places, and routines will not be totally unknown. The potential trauma of relocating and readjusting your personal life is not combined with the tension of being both a new, untried graduate and a new employee. And it may be a wonderful place to work.

However, if the experiences offered do not help you to develop, if the environment is one that eventually makes you resistant, resentful, indifferent, unhappy, or disinterested, the tone may be set for a lifetime of nursing jobs, not a professional career. Of course, that can also happen in other places, but if you're alert, you can often get a pretty good notion of how it would be to work at the agencies in which you have had student or work experience. This evaluation can be a little more difficult if you don't know a place at all, but the opinion of someone you respect, word-of-mouth information, the institution's newsletter and brochures, and even the way someone replies to your inquiry provides indirect as well as direct information.

On a more concrete level, you can give some thought to what you are willing to accept in terms of salary, shifts, benefits, and travel time. (Don't underestimate the value of the fringe benefits, which may not be taxable). Balancing these with other advantages and disadvantages as determined by your self-assessment is important. And realistically, if the job market is tight, your choices may be fewer than they would be in times of nursing shortage.

All of these factors must be considered seriously. You'll never have another first job in nursing, a job that could set the tone of your professional future. At best, you'll have wasted time. It's much better to act carefully and make sure that your choice is the best possible one for moving you toward your goal, whatever it may be.[7]

SOURCES OF INFORMATION ABOUT POSITIONS

Three principal sources of information are available to nurses who are looking for a position: (1) personal contacts and inquiries; (2) advertisements and recruiters; and (3) commercial placement agencies.

Personal Contacts and Inquiries

The nursing service director or someone on the nursing staff of a student-affiliated agency, instructors, other nurses, friends, neighbors, and family members may suggest available positions in health agencies or make other job suggestions. Hospitals not affiliated with schools of nursing sometimes ask the heads of nursing schools to refer graduates to them for possible placement on their staff. Often, letters or announcements of such positions are posted on the school bulletin board or are available in a file. Your own inquiries are likely to be equally productive in turning up the right position.

Never underestimate the value of personal contacts. People seldom suggest a position unless they know something about it. That gives you the opportunity to ask questions early on, and the information can help you decide as well as prepare you better for the interview. Moreover, if your contact knows the employer and is willing (better yet, pleased) to recommend you, your chances of getting the position are immediately improved. (This kind of networking, discussed more fully in Chapter 8, will be useful throughout your career.) One business executive has said, "Eighty percent of all jobs are filled through a grapevine . . . a system of referrals that never see the light of day." When equally qualified people compete for the same position, the network recommendation could make the crucial difference. Asking for job-seeking help is neither pushy nor presumptuous, but you should be prepared to discuss your interests intelligently. A résumé will help, too. Most people like to be asked for advice and want to be helpful, but they have to be asked. On the other hand, you need to use some common sense in deciding how much and how often you ask for help from whom.

Advertisements

Local newspapers and official organs of district and state nurses' associations often carry advertisements of positions for professional nurses. National nursing magazines list positions in all categories of employment, usually classified into the various geographic areas of the country. National medical, public health, and hospital magazines also carry advertisements for nurses, but they usually are for head nurse positions or higher, or for special personnel such as nurse anesthetists or nurse consultants.

All publications carry classified advertisements for information only, and, of course, as a source of revenue. Rarely, if ever, does the publisher assume responsibility for the information in the advertisement beyond its conformity to such legal requirements as may apply. If you accept an advertised position that does not turn out to be what was expected, you cannot hold the publication responsible. Read the advertisement very carefully. Is the hospital or health agency well known and of good reputation? Is the information clear and inclusive? Does it sound effusive and overstress the advantages and delights of joining the staff? What can be read between the lines? How much more information is needed before deciding whether the job is suitable? Some of these questions can be resolved through correspondence or telephone contact or your network.

At some time, you may want to place an advertisement in the "Positions Wanted" column of a professional publication. In that case, obtain a copy of the magazine and read the directions for submitting a classified advertisement. The editor will arrange the information to conform to the publication's style but will not change the material sent unless asked to. Therefore, all the information needed to attract a prospective employer within the limits of professional ethics should be included clearly and concisely.

Career directories published periodically by some nursing journals or other commercial sources are free to job seekers. They have relatively extensive advertisements with much more detailed information than appears in the usual ad. The other advantage is instant comparison and geographic separation, with preprinted, prepaid postcards that can be sent to the health agency of interest. (Most are geared to hospital recruitment). Directories are frequently available in the exhibit section of student and other nursing conventions. Some carry reprints of articles on careers, licensure, job seeking, and other pertinent information. Some journals also do periodic surveys on job salaries and fringe benefits that can be useful when considering various geographic areas.

Recruiters for hospitals and other agencies are usually present at representative booths in the exhibit areas of conventions; some have suites where they have an open house. Recruiters, who may or may not be nurses, also visit nursing schools or arrange for space in a hotel for preliminary interviews. Notices are placed in newspapers or sent to schools. There are advantages to the personalized recruiter approach because your questions can be answered directly, and you can get "a feel" for the employer's attitude, especially if nurses accompany the recruiter. However, remember the recruiters are selected for their recruiting ability.

Commercial Placement Agencies

There are commercial placement agencies in some places that maintain a list of nurses who are looking for part-time work or who are job hunting. As might be expected, some are reliable and some are not. They can be checked out with the Better Business Bureau and your network. Almost always a fee must be paid to the registry, sometimes based on a percentage of the nurse's earnings. At another level of job seeking—executive positions—well-known agencies of good reputation (headhunters) are used by both employers and potential employees to match the best possible person to a suitable position.[8]

Under ordinary circumstances, however, the so-called temporary nurse service is another option (see Chapter 7). These services function quite differently from agencies or registries, since they themselves employ the nurses and then, according to requests and a nurse's choices, send her or him to an institution or other agency for a specific period of time. Nurses are usually placed in short-term situations in hospitals, but some services advertise home care. The single most important factor that seems to attract nurses to temporary nurse services is control over working conditions, including the time, place, type of assignment, and so on. New graduates may find this type of employment attractive as a temporary measure, since the nonavailability of fringe benefits may not be important to them. There is also an opportunity to try out different types of nursing, but for the new nurse, the lack of individual support and supervision is a disadvantage.

PROFESSIONAL CORRESPONDENCE

New nursing graduates today have a wider variety of personal and educational backgrounds than they did a few years ago. Many have held responsible positions in other fields, and even more have worked part or full time before or during their educational programs. Therefore, the suggested procedures for application and resignation presented are just that. They review generally accepted ways to handle certain inevitable professional matters in a sophisticated and businesslike way, and may serve as a refresher for those already familiar with these or other equally acceptable ways of relating and communicating in professional business relationships. For the younger less experienced nurse, this material provides a convenient reference and guide.

The first contact with a prospective employer is usually made by letter, followed by a personal interview, telephone conversation, and, occasionally, telegrams, mailgrams, or, perhaps, a fax. Every business letter makes an impression on its reader, an impression that may be favorable, unfavorable, or indifferent. To achieve the best effect, the stationery on which it is written should be in good taste; the message accurate and complete, yet concise; the tone appropriate; and the form, grammar, and spelling correct.

Stationery and Format

Business letters should be neatly and legibly typed or handwritten in black or blue ink on unlined white stationery. Single sheets no smaller than 7 by 9 inches or larger than $8\frac{1}{2}$ by 11 inches are more suitable than folded sheets. Personal stationery is acceptable if it is of the right size and color (white, light gray, or off-white) and used with unlined envelopes. Notebook paper should never be used for business correspondence; neither should someone else's personal stationery or the stationery of a hospital, hotel, or place of business. Good-quality typing paper is always in good taste if a suitable envelope is used with it.

If you type the letter, which is often considered most desirable, use a fresh black typewriter ribbon and avoid erasures or carelessness in the general appearance of the letter. Use of a word processor is becoming more common. There is mixed feedback on its acceptance in formal correspondence, in part because of the variability in appearance. If it looks good, it's worth considering; it can certainly save a lot of time.

An attractive handwritten letter may have certain advantages over a typed one. For example, it can show your ability to prepare neat and legible records and reports, and can indicate precision and careful attention to details. A nicely handprinted letter may also make a good impression, perhaps because so few individuals have the patience and skill to do it. However, usually, a typed letter is recommended. Regardless of what you do, keep a copy for future reference.

Books on English composition and secretary's handbooks include correct forms for writing business letters. Two or more variations may be given; the choice is yours. The block form is employed most widely in business correspondence, and therefore is selected for one illustration here (Exhibit 6-2). The left-hand words or margins are aligned throughout the letter, with extra space between paragraphs. Commas are used sparingly in this form, and a colon is used following the salutation. No abbreviations are used. If personal stationery on which the name and address are engraved or printed is used, this information should be omitted from the heading of the letter and only the date is given. Another acceptable format is shown in Exhibit 6-3.

In doing business correspondence, it is always advisable to address a person exactly as the name appears on her or his own letters. The full title and position should be used, no matter how long they may be. It is better to place the lengthy name of a position on the line below the addressee's name, and break up a long address, in the interest of a neat appearance, remembering to indent continuation lines as follows:

Selma T. Henderson, RN MS

Director, School of Nursing and Inservice Education Program for
    Nurses

The Reddington J. Mason Memorial Hospital School of Nursing

1763 Avenue of the Nineteenth Century

Smithtown, OH 00000

Exhibit 6-2

Cover Letter

Date of letter
Applicant's address
Applicant's phone number

Employer's name and title   (Use complete title and address)
Employer's address

Salutation:

Opening paragraph: State why you are writing. Name the position or type of work for which you are applying. Mention how you learned of the opening.

Middle paragraph: Explain your interest in working for this employer and the specific reason for desiring this type of work. Describe relevant work experience, pointing out any other job skills or abilities that relate to the position for which you are applying. If appropriate, state your academic preparation and how it relates to the job description. Be brief but specific; your résumé contains details. Refer the reader to your enclosed résumé.

Closing paragraph: Have an appropriate closing to pave the way for an interview and indicate dates and times of availability. A telephone number is useful. If you cannot be reached during the day, give a number for messages.

Sincerely,

Signature
Name typed

Enc. (probably your résumé)

It is always best to address your correspondent by name. This may be more difficult at a distance. If you are within reasonable telephoning distance, call and get the correct name and title from the person's secretary or other staff. However, if the name of the person to whom you are writing to inquire about a position is not known, the letter may be addressed to the director or supervisor of the appropriate division, for example, "Director of the Department of Nursing." The salutation could then be "Dear Director." Using "Dear Sir" or "Dear Madam" may be incorrect, since you don't know whether the recipient is male or female. The inside address and the envelope address should be identical. People are sensitive about their names and titles; be accurate.

There is no agreement as to whether it is only correct to give a title before the name in an address in the heading and on the envelope—not in the form of initials after the name—for example, "Dr. Constance E. Wright" rather than "Constance E. Wright, EdD." Both forms seem to be used. In a signature, however, it is preferable to place the degree initials after the name of the signer of the letter. Never use both the title and the initials in an address; "Dr. Constance E. Wright, EdD" is incorrect.

It is quite suitable, and even desirable, for a (licensed) nurse to use "RN" after his or her name, particularly in professional correspondence. Many nurses with doctorates place after their names RN PhD, or EdD RN to clarify that they are nurses as well as holders of a doctorate. They should be addressed as "Dear Dr. Whatever:"

A professional or businesswoman usually does not use her husband's name at all in connection with her work. However, she may use the title "Mrs." to identify herself as a person who is, or has been, married if she desires. "Mrs." goes in parentheses before her typed name. Many women prefer "Ms.," but this is not included in the signature.

Content and Tone

The information included in a business letter should be presented with great care, giving all pertinent data but avoiding unnecessary details. It is often helpful to outline, draft, and edit a business letter, just as you would a term paper. This requires you to think it through from beginning to end in order to ensure completeness and accuracy. It is also helpful to tailor it to fit a well-spaced single page, if possible, or two at the most.

Your writing style is your own, and how you word your message may be part of what you are judged on. The tone of a business letter has considerable influence on the impression it makes and the attention it receives. It is probably better to lean toward formality rather than informality. Friendliness without undue familiarity, cordiality without overenthusiasm, sincerity, frankness, and obvious respect for the person to whom the letter is addressed set the most appropriate tone for correspondence about a position in nursing. Although there are those who suggest very unusual dramatic, or "different" formats, the reality is that they may backfire.

If you feel that you need more information before seriously considering a position (for instance, whether tuition reimbursement is a benefit or a particular specialty area has an opening), you can indicate your interest in a letter, simply asking for the information, or ask directly within the same application letter. The kind of response you get in terms of courtesy, promptness, and general tone will tell you a lot about the prospective employer.

If you decide not to apply for the position after all, or not to follow through with an interview, it is courteous to inform the person with whom you have corresponded. Specific reasons need be given (briefly) only if such a decision is made after first accepting the position. This is not only courteous but advisable, because you may wish to join that staff at another time or may have other contacts with the nurse executive.

Applications

Applications are not just routine red tape. Whether or not a résumé is requested or submitted, the formal application, which is developed to give the employing agency the information it wants, can be critical in determining who is finally hired. Even if the information repeats information offered in the résumé, it should be entered. It is usually acceptable to attach the résumé or a separate sheet if there is not adequate space to give complete information. It's a good idea to read the application first so that the information is put in the correct place. Neatness is essential. Erasures, misspellings, and wrinkled forms leave a poor impression. Abbreviations, except for state names and dates, should not be used as a rule.

If the form must be completed away from home, think ahead and bring anticipated data—Social Security and registration numbers, places, dates, and names. Although occupational counselors say that it is not necessary to give all the information requested (such as arrests, health, or race, some of which are illegal to request), it is probably not wise to leave big gaps in your work history without explanation. (See Chapter 13 regarding federal legislation on employment rights.)

PERSONAL INTERVIEW

An interview may be the deciding factor in getting a job. Anyone who has an appointment for a personal interview should be prepared for it physically, mentally, emotionally, and psychologically. The degree of preparation will depend on the purpose of the interview and what has preceded it. Assuming that you have written to a prospective employer about a position and an interview has been arranged, preparation might include the following:

Physical Preparation. Be rested, alert, and in good health. Dress suitably for the job, but wear something in which you feel at ease. It is important to be well groomed and as attractive as possible. First appearances are important, and given a choice, no one selects a sloppy or overdressed person in preference to someone who is neat and appropriately dressed. Have enough money with you to meet all anticipated expenses. If you are to be reimbursed by the employing agency, keep an itemized record of expenses for submission later. Arrive at your destination well ahead of time, but do not go to your prospective employer's office earlier than five minutes before the designated time.

Mental Preparation. Review all information and previous communications about the position. Showing that you know about the hospital or agency is desirable and impressive. Make certain that you know the exact name or names of the persons you expect to meet and can pronounce them properly. (You can always ask the secretary.) Decide what additional information you want to obtain during the interview. Consider how you will phrase your leading questions. Carry a small notebook or card on which you have listed the names of references and other data that you may need during the interview. If you bring an application form with you, place it in a fresh envelope, which you leave unsealed. Have it ready to hand to the interviewer when she or he asks for it; otherwise, offer it at an appropriate time.

Emotional and Psychological Preparation: If you have any worries or fears in connection with the interview, try to overcome them by thinking calmly and objectively about what is likely to take place. (Role-playing an interview with a colleague who may have been through the experience can be helpful.) Be ready to adjust to whatever situation may develop during the interview. For example, you may expect to have an extended conversation with the director of nurses and find when you arrive that a personnel officer who is not a nurse will interview you. She or he may interview you in a very few minutes and in what seems to be an impersonal way. Or you may have visualized the job setting as quite different.

Accept things as you find them, reserving the privilege of making a decision after consideration of the total job situation. If a stimulating challenge is inherent in the position, you will sense it during the interview, or you may have reason to believe that it will develop. However, you can't demand a challenge, and if one is "created" for you spontaneously by the interviewer, regard the promise with some reservations; an employment situation rarely adjusts to the new employee.

During the Interview

Usually the interviewer will take the initiative in starting the conference and closing it. You should follow that lead courteously and attentively. Shake hands. Be prepared to give a brief overview of your experiences and interests, if asked. At some point, you will be asked if you have any questions, and you should be prepared to ask for additional information if you would like to have it. Should the interviewer appear to be about to close the conference without giving you this opportunity, say, "May I ask a question, please?" It is perfectly acceptable to ask, before the interview is over, about salary, fringe benefits, and other conditions of employment if a contract or explanatory paper has not been given to you. In fact, it would be foolish to appear indifferent. A contract is desirable (see Chapter 13), but if that is not the accepted procedure, it is important to understand what is involved in the job. The job description should be accessible in writing, and it is best that you have a copy.

Most interviewers agree that an outgoing candidate who volunteers appropriate information is likeable. On the other hand, many use the technique of selective silence, which is anxiety provoking to most people, to see what the interviewee will say or do. A good interviewer will try to make you comfortable, in part to relax you into self-revelation; most do not favor aggressive methods. Good eye contact is fine, but don't stare. Be sensitive to the interviewer's being disinterested in a certain response; maybe it's too lengthy. Don't interrupt. Don't smoke. Don't mumble.

Some questions that are likely to be asked in an average one-hour interview are:[9,10]

- What position interests you most? (Be specific.)
- Why do you want to work here? (Know something positive.)
- What are your strengths and weaknesses? (Play up your strengths, and, although you should be honest, play down your weaknesses. Give examples, perhaps of what people say about you.)
- What would you do if . . . ? (Show your decision-making and judgmental skills.)
- What can you do for us? (Tell about your special qualities and experience.)
- Tell me about yourself. (Keep it short; don't give more information than necessary to reassure the interviewer that you are suitable for the job physically, mentally, and in terms of preparation. Stress your reliability.)
- What did you like most and least in school or on your last job? (Be honest, but don't list a series of gripes.)

- How would you describe your ideal job? (Take the opportunity to do so, but let the interviewer know that you know that nothing's perfect.)
- Where do you think you'll be five years from now? (Emphasize goals that show your interest in growing professionally.)
- Do you have any questions? (Be prepared.)

In a survey of directors of nursing service in various settings, the characteristics valued most highly in rating a nursing job applicant were punctuality, completion of the application prior to the interview, neatness and completeness of the application, well-groomed personal appearance, and questions asked. As other qualities that might be more important were bypassed, this list may show how important the external aspects of an interview can be.[11]

When the interview is over, thank the interviewer, shake hands, and leave promptly. You may or may not have been offered the position. If it was offered to you, it's usually well to delay your decision for at least a day or two until you have had time to think the matter over carefully from every practical point of view. Perhaps you'll want more information, in which case you may write a letter, send a fax, a telegram or mailgram, or make a phone call to your prospective employer. It's always courteous and sometimes acts as a reminder to send a thank-you letter.

Telephones and Telegrams

Sometimes during the procedure of acquiring a position, you may have occasion to discuss some aspect of it over the telephone with the prospective employer. If you make the call, be brief, courteous, and to the point, with notes handy, if needed. It may be helpful to make notations on the conversation. It's sensible to listen carefully and not interrupt. If you receive a call and are unprepared for it, be courteous but cautious and, perhaps, ask for time to think over the proposal—or whatever may have been the purpose of the call.

Agreements about a position made over the phone should be confirmed promptly in writing. If it's your place to do so, you might say, while speaking with the person, "I'll send you a confirming letter tomorrow." If it's the responsibility of the other person to confirm an agreement but she or he doesn't mention it, ask, "May I have a letter of confirmation, please?"

After any interview or conversation, make notes about what happened for future use and reference. If any business arrangements are made by fax, mailgram, or telegram, file this information with other related correspondence.

For positions sought through a registry or employment agency, the same courteous, thorough, and businesslike procedures used when dealing directly with a prospective employer are appropriate. A brief thank-you note for help received shows consideration of the agency's efforts in your behalf.

Evaluation

What if you didn't get the job you wanted? There may simply have been someone better suited or better qualified. Still, it is helpful to review the experience in order to refine your interview skills. Were you prepared? Did you present yourself as someone sensitive to the employer's goals? Did you make known your personal strengths and objectives? Did you look your best? Sometimes discussing what happened with another person also gives you a different perspective. And there's no reason why you can't reapply another time.[12]

CHANGING POSITIONS

There seems to be an unwritten rule that nurses should remain in any permanent position they accept for at least a year. Certainly, this is not too long—except in the most unusual circumstances—for you to adjust to the employment situation and find a place on the staff in which to use your ability and talents to their fullest. Furthermore, persons who change jobs too frequently may find that some employers are reluctant to hire them. However, should it be desirable or necessary to change positions, a number of points might be observed. Consider your employer and coworkers as well as yourself, and leave under friendly and constructive circumstances.

Depending on the reasons for leaving and how eager you are to make a change, some writers suggest that before you definitely accept a new position, the present employer should be informed about your desire to leave and why. It may be that, depending on the employer's concept of your value to the institution, a new, more desirable position might be offered. However, it is important to give reasonable notice of your intention to resign. If there is a contract, the length of the notice will probably be stipulated. Two weeks to a month is the usual period, depending principally on the position held and the anticipated difficulty in hiring a replacement. Don't tell everyone else before you tell your immediate superior, privately and courteously.

Try to finish any major projects you have started; arrange in good order the equipment and materials your successor will inherit; and prepare memos and helpful guides to assist the nurse who will assume your duties. Check out employment policies about benefits, including accrued vacation or sick leave.

A letter of resignation should state simply and briefly, but in a professional manner, your intention of leaving, the date on which the resignation will

Exhibit 6-3

Sample Letter of Resignation

240 North Street
San Diego, CA 00000
Date

Ms. Carol Winter, RN, MSN
Vice President of Nursing
West Central Hospital
20 California Avenue
San Diego, CA 00000

Dear Ms. Green:

I will be relocating to Phoenix, Arizona, in May and have accepted a position there at General Hospital as head nurse of the pediatric unit. Therefore, I wish to resign effective April 18, 1993.

Being at Central Hospital has been a very satisfying personal and professional experience. The atmosphere is one in which a nurse can grow, and I appreciate the support given by the staff of 4B and the head nurse, Melanie Jones. She has especially helped me to develop my managerial skills and encouraged me to take advantage of the hospital's tuition reimbursement. I expect to finish my degree in Phoenix. I am proud to have been a part of a group of practitioners and administrators who are committed to caring, competent patient care.

If there is anything I can do to help in the transition, I will be happy to do so.

Sincerely,

(Signature)
Alan Collins, RN

cc: Melanie Jones
Head Nurse 4B

become effective, and the reasons for making the change. A sincere comment or two about the satisfactions experienced in the position and regrets at leaving will close the letter graciously. There should be no hint of animosity or resentment, because this will serve no constructive purpose and may boomerang.[13] (See Exhibit 6-3.)

Don't burn your bridges. You may want to come back to that place at another time. At the least, you may need a reference, and if you appear vindictive or childish, the employer is unlikely to give you an enthusiastic reference, even if you did your job satisfactorily. In these days of litigation, nothing may be written specifically, but employers are adept at reading between the lines of a bland reference. The administrative network (via a personal phone call) may paint you as an undesirable employee, and you'll never know.

Terminal interviews are considered good administrative practice, and are sometimes used for a final performance evaluation and/or a means to determine the reasons for resignation. There is some question of how open employees are about discussing their resignation (unless the reason is illness, necessary relocation, and so on), perhaps because of fear of reprisal in references or even a simple desire to avoid unpleasantness. This is a decision you must make in each situation.

What if you're fired? The most common reasons for being fired are poor job performance, chronic tardiness, excessive absenteeism, substance abuse, or inappropriate behavior.[14] Usually you are given a warning about any of these problems, and if you haven't done anything about correcting your problem (assuming that the charge is justified), you had better take a good look at yourself. Those kinds of uncorrected problems may make your future prospects look dim.

Whether or not you're caught by surprise when you're told, try to maintain your composure. If you can't pull your thoughts together, request another interview to ask questions and find out about the termination procedure. If you are at fault, make a clean, fast break. If you are not at fault, try to clarify the situation to avoid negative references. You may choose to contest the action and file a grievance, particularly if you are part of a union. This process is described in Chapter 13. However, weigh whether it's worth it. You may need to clear your name, but it might be unpleasant or impossible to stay in that setting and work productively. If the dismissal is a layoff for economic reasons, it is a good idea to have a letter to this effect, both in terms of professional security and in order to get unemployment benefits, if necessary.

When leaving a job is not your choice, it sometimes helps to talk with a supportive person, to ventilate and analyze what happened. Choose someone you can trust but who can help you see things as objectively as possible. Then it's time to get back to career planning. Perhaps you should look at the possibility of further education or training in a different kind of nursing.[15]

If not, be sensible about conserving your economic resources until you find another job. Try to select the next job, keeping in mind what made you unhappy in the last one and, of course, correcting those problems that got you fired. You need not volunteer to your prospective employer that you were fired, but if asked, don't lie. Just say that you were asked to leave and why. Don't criticize your previous employer and try to be as positive as possible about your last job. Your honesty and determination to do well could be a plus.

It's doubtful that you will stay in the same institution throughout your career. This is a very mobile society, and there are many job opportunities for nurses throughout the country (and world). Without closing the doors to unexpected opportunities, beginning early to think in terms of a career will make nursing more satisfying and interesting in the long run.[16]

KEY POINTS

1. Assessing yourself in terms of abilities, interests, characteristics, and values is a good idea before starting a job hunt.
2. A professional résumé and appropriate letters of application are factors in being selected for a job.
3. Some of the best sources of information about the job market are advertisements, personal contacts, job fairs, and recruiters.
4. In interviewing for a job, it is important to be prepared physically and psychologically and to know, or get, as much information as possible about the position and environment.
5. Consideration of its effect on future employment is an important factor in how a job should be terminated.

REFERENCES

1. Esche CA. SHARE your way to success: An approach for finding your first job. *Imprint,* 32:19–22 (December–January 1986).
2. Henley J, Anema M. Blueprint for success on the NCLEX-RN. *Imprint,* 37:165–167 (April–May 1990).
3. Gay J, Edgil A. Is your curriculum vitae or résumé working for you? *Imprint,* 32:8–17 (December–January 1986).
4. Nowak J, Grindel C. *Career planning in nursing.* Philadelphia: J.B. Lippincott Company, 1984, pp. 127–195.
5. Kelly L. The Pinocchio principle. *Nurs Outlook,* 32:307 (November–December 1984).
6. Nowak and Grindel, op. cit., pp. 145–146.

7. Huey F. Your first job: Great news or giant nightmare? *Am J Nurs*, 88:452–457 (April 1988).

8. Filoromo T. Changing jobs? A look at employment agencies and executive search firms. *Nurs Economics*, 1:202–205 (November–December 1983).

9. Bruce S. A blueprint for better job interviews. *Nurs 87*, 17:64B–64F (June 1987).

10. Weis D. 10 questions recruiters will ask and how you should respond. *Nurs Life*, 7:22–23 (May–June 1987).

11. Brydon P, Myli A. After the interview, who gets the job? *Am J Nurs*, 84:736–738 (June 1984).

12. Hanger T. How to market yourself. *Am J Nurs Guide*, 18–23 (1984).

13. Williams A, Pellicciotta B. Resigning with style. *Nurs Economics*, 3:173–176 (May–June 1985).

14. Marriner A. Surviving being fired. *Nurs 86*, 16:16N, 16P (January 1986).

15. Davis J. Getting hired after getting fired. *Am J Nurs*, 84:514 (April 1984).

16. Filoromo T. Career pathing (or, finding a job). *Imprint*, 31:1347 (December 1985–January 1986).

CHAPTER 7

THE PRACTICE OF NURSING

OBJECTIVES

After studying this chapter, you will be able to:

1. Identify at least two problems related to nursing supply and demand.
2. List the basic competencies most employers expect the new graduate to have.
3. Identify job opportunities available in the first years after graduation.
4. Recognize the types of positions that require advanced study.

A TIME OF UNLIMITED OPPORTUNITIES

One of the most exciting aspects of nursing is the variety of career opportunities available. Nurses, as generalists or specialists, work in almost every place where health care is given, and new types of positions or modes of practice seem to arise yearly. In part, this is in response to external social and scientific changes—for instance, shifts in the makeup of the population, new demands for health care, discovery of new treatments for disease conditions, recognition of health hazards, and health legislation. In part, these roles for nurses have emerged because nurses saw a gap in health care and stepped in (NP, nurse epidemiologist) or simply formalized a role that they had always filled (nurse thanatologist).

Usually further education is required to practice competently in specialized areas, which are expected to grow.[1] Sometimes this is part of on-the-job training, but frequently it requires formal or other continuing education. Practice in areas of clinical specialization will vary to some extent according to the site of practice and the level and degree of specialization. For instance, in a small community hospital, a nurse may work comfortably on a maternity unit, giving care to both mothers and babies; in a tertiary care setting, perinatal nurse specialists, psychiatric nurse specialists, and nurses specializing in the care of high-risk mothers may work together; in a neighborhood health center, the nurse-midwife may assume complete care of a normal mother and work with both the pediatric NP and hospital nurses.

In addition, nurses hold many positions not directly related to patient care as consultants, administrators, teachers, editors, writers, patient-care educators, executive directors of professional organizations or state boards, lobbyists, health planners, utilization review coordinators, nurse epidemiologists, sex educators, and even anatomic artists, airline attendants, and legislators.

There are few careers that can offer the diversity of nursing. Almost always, a switch to a different kind of practice or a different setting means building on your basic nursing and experience, learning some new theory, and getting some new practice. This is a good way to be stimulated and remotivated. Even if you stay in the same job, there are opportunities to try new techniques or broaden your responsibilities. The frequent crises in health care delivery present unlimited opportunities for nurses to show what they can do. With all these choices, it is difficult to find any one way to present areas of practice. In this chapter, the approach used is first to describe positions and the responsibilities and conditions of employment for each of the types of positions that graduates can hold at graduation or shortly afterward. (You may wish to refer to Chapter 3, to review the settings in which health care is given, and Chapter 4, Exhibit 4-3, to see where nurses work.) Then an overview of other nursing opportunities is given. Exhibit 7-1 describes some of the major positions that require advanced education and experience, such as the clinical specialties.[2] Further information is available from the specialty nursing organizations, educational programs, and career articles published in various nursing journals, some of which are listed in the Bibliography, as well as in Chapter 15 of L.Y. Kelly, *Dimensions of professional nursing,* 6th edition (Elmsford, NY: Pergamon Press, 1991).

In discussing conditions of employment, specific salaries are usually not

Exhibit 7-1
Positions in Nursing Requiring Advanced Preparation

Position	Qualifications[a]	Places	Responsibilities	Salary, benefits, and conditions of work[b]
Nurse anesthetist	Graduation from an approved nurse anesthetist program; certification; baccalaureate degrees and master's preparation for anesthetist are increasing.	Operating and delivery rooms in hospitals, surgicenters, emergency rooms, some doctors' offices if surgery done.	Preoperative visits/teaching of patient and sometimes family. Administration of anesthesia, oxygen, and other appropriate drugs under direction of anesthesiologist.	Salary among highest in nursing. Usually not under nursing service. On day shift or into early evening. Could be on call frequently. Very high malpractice insurance needed.
Student health service (school or college nurse)	Usually baccalaureate (same as for teachers); may require special courses as designated by state or other governmental regulations; may be a school NP with a master's degree or certificate.	Any type of school, public or private, kindergarten through high school. Also colleges, universities.	Vary with requirements of board of education; may be first-aid-type care with some health teaching; routine screening for visual and hearing problems; record keeping. For NPs, same as NP responsibilities.	Depends on types of schools— salary/benefits (health plans, retirement). Could be same as for teachers; salary often lower without master's degree. Same holidays and vacations as teachers. Usually work only days except in higher education.

| Nursing education (faculty) | Depends on educational program. Baccalaureate for LPN to doctorate for universities (usually). Nursing degree (BSN and/or MSN) preferred, sometimes required. Usually require experience, sometimes specialization. | Trade schools, hospitals, junior colleges, colleges, universities. | Develop and carry out curriculum; prepare for and teach courses in classroom, laboratory, and clinical settings; recruit, select, promote, counsel, and evaluate students; develop special projects; work on committees to meet needs of program and/or students; may be expected to do research, write, and be involved in nursing and community activities, especially in colleges and universities; may be expected to hold joint positions in the clinical setting, especially in higher education; also involved in campus activities. | In higher education, salaries vary according to rank (instructor or associate to professor); education (doctoral/nondoctoral) and whether a 10-months or one-year contract is given. Range, $25,000 (lecturer)–$60,000+ (professor). Deans to $100,000+. Other schools usually offer lower salaries. Hours flexible; may have evening classes; may do much work at home. May work during academic year only. May become tenured if criteria are met (beginning of associate professor rank). |

Exhibit 7-1 (Continued)

Positions in Nursing Requiring Advanced Preparation

Position	Qualifications[a]	Places	Responsibilities	Salary, benefits, and conditions of work[b]
Nursing education (*Continued*)			Administrative head is responsible for recruiting and selecting faculty; has overall responsibility for program, budget, general well-being of school. Works with faculty on curriculum, student affairs.	
Staff development (in-service education)	From simply good clinical experience to a master's, the latter especially for a director.	Hospitals, nursing homes, public health/community health.	Sees to orientation and ongoing education of nursing staff as related to job. May require similar preparation as above for teaching classes.	May have salary and benefits somewhat in range of middle management if director; teachers usually have less. Most programs given during the day, but may also include evenings and nights for other shifts.

Nurse executive/nurse administrator (director of nursing; vice president for nursing; assistant administrator)	Preferred: baccalaureate in nursing with master's or doctorate in nursing administration. Other degrees in administration, business also acceptable. In smaller settings, baccalaureate and experience. For nursing home, varies from job experience and RN only to master's degree.	Any place that nursing services are given. Most employed in hospitals, nursing homes, public health/community health agencies (PH/CH). Some corporate positions with responsibilities for nursing in several settings.	Varies with size of operation. May include direct or indirect activities. Planning, organizing, controlling, evaluating nursing services; includes personnel management, labor relations, budget, working with other administrators and public. May be limited to nursing department or include other departments. Should be part of top management.	Negotiable salary and benefits; $25,000–$100,000 +. Flexible hours (may be long). Executive benefit plans and usual benefits. Lowest salaries/benefits usually in nursing homes.

Exhibit 7-1 (Continued)

Positions in Nursing Requiring Advanced Preparation

Position	Qualifications[a]	Places	Responsibilities	Salary, benefits, and conditions of work[b]
Middle management. Supervisor, clinical coordinator (various titles)	Nursing baccalaureate and master's preferred with clinical and/or administrative focus; experience. Still some acceptance of baccalaureate or no degree (especially in nursing homes) with good clinical and/or head nurse track record.	Usually hospitals, PH/CH. In nursing homes, may be the only nurse at night.	Participate in nursing policymaking and problem solving; supervising and evaluating delivery of nursing care; collaborating with other departments; coordinating staff activities, possibly scheduling staff; recruiting, selecting, evaluating personnel; sometimes facilitating research, coordinating student learning experiences.	Salary: should be higher than that of staff nurse but isn't always if nurses are unionized. May have same benefits as staff nurses plus meeting expenses, retirement benefits, major medical plan, more vacation than staff.

Clinical nurse specialist (CNS): psychiatric/mental health; medical-surgical; community health; perinatal; oncology; geriatric; pediatric; obstetric subspecialties	Master's degree in nursing specialty; certification desirable. Sometimes specialty experience and certification accepted without graduate education.	Usually hospitals, especially medical centers; increasing number are PH/CH; some ambulatory care; private practice; rarely, nursing home.	Direct care of selected patients in specialty; consultation with nurses and other health professionals; identification of populations at risk; sometimes research; may include middle management functions.	Salary: usually middle manager level. Hours may be flexible. Benefits depend on setting. If position includes management, may be structured into eight-hour shifts; hours may be long. Sometimes called at home. If self-employed, must arrange own benefits.
Nurse practitioner (NP); obstetric/gynecologic; midwife; psychiatric-mental health; pediatric; family; subspecialties	Specialized training, usually with certificate or diploma; master's preferred. Certification desirable; experience in field.	Primarily ambulatory care settings; some physicians' offices; private practice; PH/CH; rarely nursing home.	Assess health status of families and clients through history taking, physical examination; define health problems; provide treatment of chronic conditions, sometimes under medical supervision; teach patients and families; collaborate with other nurses and health professionals; refer as necessary.	May be negotiable; salary and benefits generally about same as for CN. Hours may be flexible, depending on setting.

Exhibit 7-1 (Continued)

Positions in Nursing Requiring Advanced Preparation

Position	Qualifications[a]	Places	Responsibilities	Salary, benefits, and conditions of work[b]
Nurse practitioner (*Continued*)			(Midwife does perinatal care and sometimes delivery of maternity patient.)	
Nurse researcher	Usually a doctorate; sometimes advanced research training and experience.	Any health care setting; universities; NIH; private research groups.	Develop and carry out research. Assist others in applying research findings. Train nurses in research.	Negotiable, except for governmental positions. Hours flexible.

[a]All require current licensure and generally, experience in nursing.

[b]Common fringe benefits at these levels are holidays, vacations, health insurance (with or without major medical), tuition reimbursement, meeting expenses, life insurance, disability plan. The package of benefits may vary more from place to place than among positions. Factors are location, size, and private, public, or nonprofit ownership.

given or are presented as a range or average because they are changing rapidly in the unstable economic climate and because they vary geographically (highest in the West, lowest in the North Central and Southern states, but rising in the Sunbelt) and according to whether they are urban, rural, or suburban. There is agreement that nursing salaries have been climbing, in part due to the nursing shortage. They may level off or continue to rise. Listings of current salaries are reported periodically in many nursing journals, in federal statistics, in the current ANA *Facts About Nursing,* and in ANA reports.

NURSING SUPPLY AND DEMAND

Throughout the history of nursing, there have been repeated shortages. Other than in times of war, most often a shortage was caused by the fact that nurses were underpaid, overworked, and lacked status. In that general sense, until recently, things had not changed significantly. One major problem of apparent oversupply occurred during the Great Depression years, when families could not afford private duty nurses and hospital nursing was done primarily by students. Another, more recent one, had a short life: the prospective payment system described in Chapter 3 panicked hospitals, and as they closed units and sometimes laid off nurses, there was talk of a nurse oversupply. This panic lasted for about a year, because it was soon clear that, under the new system, even more nurses were needed to care for the very ill patients. Therefore in 1986, as one nursing journal surveyed nurses about their fears of layoffs and found that almost half of those whose jobs were in jeopardy were considering leaving the field,[3] another reported, "RN Shortage Suddenly Surfaces in Many States."[4] What seemed to start with a shortage of specialty nurses, particularly in ICUs, soon included every type of nurse, particularly in hospitals. Even at that early stage, it was agreed that, after leveling off, hospital admissions were rebounding, patient acuity was increasing, alternative health care facilities that required nurses were expanding, and new nonnursing opportunities were opening up for nurses. Moreover, at this time more nurses were choosing to work part-time and nursing enrollments were sagging. When these factors showed no signs of changing, the situation suddenly became a crisis. How do you define a crisis in what has always been a recurring nursing shortage? Probably not only when nurses and hospitals see a problem, but when it becomes headline news in *The New York Times, Time* magazine and *The Wall Street Journal.*

At any rate, this shortage did not vanish, and it seemed to be a shortage without an immediate end, as demand continued to rise and the number of nurses did not. (It wasn't that nurses weren't working, as 80 percent were, but that there were a great number of options for nurses.) Private and governmental commissions and study groups were formed, as finding a solution became a major effort of nursing, health care administration, and public and private agencies (see Appendix 1).

Although the nursing shortage involved almost every facet of health care, it appeared to be most acute in hospitals and long-term care facilities. In hospitals, the specialty areas especially reported shortages. Among other problems was the high turnover rate of about 20 percent (more in some regions and particular hospitals), which was costly both in terms of the time and money required to recruit and orient new nurses and in interrupted nursing care and lowered staff morale. It seemed to be a vicious cycle: as discontented nurses left, those remaining worked harder and longer, grew discouraged, and left for another position. That new position was often in a supplemental staffing agency that gave nurses a choice of when, where, and how often they wanted to work.

Hospitals took a number of steps to resolve their shortage problem. An increasing number recruited nurses abroad, hired contract or "traveling" nurses, employed nurses from supplementary staffing agencies (creating problems of quality and continuity of care), or formed their own pool of nurses who worked per diem (generally with no benefits). The last was sometimes a for-profit venture.[5] Particularly interesting was the variety of techniques used to attract and retain nurses.[6] Most favored were increasing benefit packages, emphasizing retention, reimbursing for tuition, providing bonuses for referral/retention, seeking new hires, and paying interview expenses. Among the benefits were flexible benefits (giving choices); dental, vision, and malpractice insurance; reimbursement for unused sick time; added vacation days (one hospital offered a nine-month year); free educational seminars; added conference days; child care programs; differentials for shift, weekends, education, and certification; longevity bonuses; paid parking; purchasing discounts; health/fitness center discounts; nonmandatory float policies and frequent-floater bonuses; and even maid service.

Probably most dramatic was the increase in wages, rising in some cities on the East and West coasts to a starting salary in the $40,000 range and rising to over $70,000 with longevity. The latter was particularly important, because one negative aspect of nursing salaries has been pay stagnation beyond certain levels no matter how long a nurse has worked in one place. Such large increases (given that the average starting salary just five years earlier was considerably lower) were not universal. The Commonwealth Fund study in 1988 found variation in both turnover and salaries in the cities they surveyed. Because of either the economics of the region or the stability of the nursing population, salary increases in certain areas were more conservative. However, here, too, some efforts toward retention were considered important.[7]

Although hospital administrators have been advised for decades, through many studies on nursing, on what it takes to retain nurses, the advice seemed to fall on deaf ears all too often. By 1990, with a drastic shortage at hand, there was at least some greater inclination to listen. Once salaries, and often benefits, were competitive in most hospitals in a particular commuting area, attention had to turn to improving the environment and the conditions of work where nurses practice. Some changes were elementary and cost little but had been largely ignored, including better communication, with accessibility of administrators, attitude surveys, open forums, nurse-relations programs, newsletters, physician-nurse liaison programs, nurse-recognition and nursing image days, positive stories about nurses and ads praising nurses in local newspapers, employee-of-the-month programs, appreciation of nurses by physicians, directors' letters of commendation, and anniversary/recognition teas or receptions. There were also reward systems, including clinical ladders, clinical-excellence-in-nursing awards, promotions from within, liberal transfer policies, and perfect attendance awards.[8]

Most important, the value of the nurse and the nurse's work was demonstrated by involving nurses in various types of planning; shared governance and nurse empowerment, as in one hospital where nurses determine their own schedules, regulate their own staffing needs, and are accountable for their own productivity; employing assistive personnel under the control of nurses who do the fetching, carrying, transporting, message taking, and other nonnursing tasks often left to nurses; and other reorganizations of staffing (with input from the nurses). Some hospitals have also installed information management systems (computers) that, while not specifically for nurses, have made their work easier.

Another important recruiting/retention factor was flexibility in scheduling. Some innovations are weekend 12-hour days for a full week's salary; 12-hour shifts and shorter work weeks, and top pay for unpopular shifts. There are also signs of better interprofessional relationships between nursing and medicine. Although the AMA did suggest the ill-conceived proposal for registered care technologists (RCTs) as a solution to the nursing shortage,[9] most physicians disowned the idea. Many recognized the need for more collegial relationships and worked in their own settings toward joint practice committees and patient care activities. The lack of such relationships is considered one aspect of nurses' dissatisfaction.[10] In some cases, looking ahead, medical staffs have funded scholarships for nursing students.

As noted earlier, NCNIP's nationwide campaign for attracting potential students to nursing was in part underwritten by groups other than nursing— a sure sign that the shortage is seen as a national emergency. The new federal Commission on the Nursing Shortage, reappointed in 1990, set its goal as finding "doable defined projects" that are both "creative and realistic" without duplicating what was already done.[11] The Commission, in its charter, was also urged to seek commitments from private organizations, as well as state and local governments, to fund some of the specific projects. One example is a Louisiana hospital that provided money to pay nursing faculty in a school that had enough prospective students but not enough faculty. Others have followed.

Clearly, the hospital shortage has received most of the publicity, but other areas of nursing such as home care must deal with shortages also. These agencies try to match the salary and benefit packages of hospitals, as well as many of the communication/service approaches. They also hire per-diem nurses. One practice area of particular concern is long-term care (LTC). Because of fiscal constraints, poor image, and the fact that the federal government mandates only a minimum of RN staff, nurses are even less attracted to nursing homes than they are to hospitals. In various conferences held to consider that problem, it has been recommended (1) that Medicaid, the major payer of LTC, be restructured so that salaries and benefits can be raised; (2) that grass-roots partnerships between LTC facilities and schools of nursing be developed; (3) that LTC facilities redefine the roles for nurses and restructure staffing and compensation accordingly; and (4) that the image of LTC facilities be improved.

The nursing shortage is not expected to vanish in the immediate future or, some say, not in the foreseeable future. Now that nursing enrollments are rising slightly, more women are career oriented, nursing is beginning to be seen as an attractive field by more second-careerists, salaries are becoming competitive, and more places that employ nurses are working at improving nurses' job satisfaction, at least the shortage may become less acute. (On the other hand, there is some concern that the influx of assistive personnel who are carrying out tasks that should only be done by RNs are lowering the quality of care, although theoretically relieving the shortage.) Some hospitals are already noted for their ability to attract and retain nurses,[12] and others are beginning to emulate them. Certainly, the opportunities for nurses today are varied, exciting, and rewarding. Those who see nursing as less attractive than other professions may find that "the grass is not greener."[13] As career opportunities are presented in the succeeding sections, it might be helpful to keep these perspectives in mind.

WHAT EMPLOYERS EXPECT FROM THE NEW GRADUATE

Usually the first job a new graduate takes is a staff position in a hospital. One reason is that most new graduates are a little nervous about how well they can perform the technical skills they learned. They know that most acute care hospitals provide many opportunities to polish techniques, especially with patients being much sicker now during their shortened hospital stay. Since often state board exams are coming up, there is also the opportunity to learn more, or at least to tie in theory with hands-on practice. The fact that more experienced nurses are there to help a newcomer is another advantage.

A natural question is, "What does my employer expect of me?" The competencies shown in Appendix 3 for each type of graduate give some useful information, since nurse administrators were part of the group that developed them. However, there are probably certain basic specific commonalities that can also be identified. These will be described later.

First, it may be useful to look at the way a new graduate enters the work world. There are differences in the hospital settings in relation to staffing patterns (and availability of nurses to supervise a new graduate), staff mix, attitudes about new nurses, and general philosophy. Some of these may have been identified during the interview, as discussed in Chapter 6 and described in more detail later. Some graduates have had an externship program of some kind, that is, an opportunity to ease into a nursing job in a particular place by spending part of their clinical time in the nursing program carrying larger patient assignments under the guidance of an RN in a sort of work-study mode.

There may also be an internship available. Internships come in many forms, but basically the new nurse is gradually oriented to all aspects of nursing care given at that hospital, with partial assignments, good supervision, and the opportunity to get experience in specific tasks as well as in overall care of patients. While this relieves some of the pressure of feeling less than competent in what might be an understaffed, busy unit, the price is a lower salary for that period of time and the possibility that not all the teaching promised will be delivered. Some nurses have felt resentful because they are kept at the intern level longer than they feel necessary and end up participating in care giving without the necessary supervision or protected status. Others have found this a good transitional period.[14]

The internship should not be confused with the regular orientation given by almost every employer. Sometimes the orientation is almost as complete as an internship, but in other cases it can be nothing but a review of policies and a tour of the facility and the assigned patient unit. Sometimes a series of written tests and procedure check-offs are given to see what the new nurse knows or needs. A staff nurse assigned as a preceptor or someone from the in-service education staff may help supervise those practical experiences.

Regardless of whether any or all of these options are available, generally the new nurse is expected to:

1. Know how to write a nursing care plan, using the nursing process, and applying the appropriate theory.
2. Know how to give expert basic care to patients, including supervising aides in their care.

3. Record fully and accurately on the patient's chart, although a particular system may need to be learned.
4. Recognize basic legal responsibilities, beginning with knowing his or her own limitations as well as abilities, asking for help as necessary.
5. Work cooperatively with colleagues and other personnel.
6. Be responsible in personnel relations, such as being on time at the beginning of a shift, after breaks, and meals or not abusing sick leave.
7. Behave ethically with patients, families, and others.
8. Take initiative in learning what is necessary to safely carry a full share of the staff nurse responsibilities as soon as possible.

Chances are that these expectations can be met by any graduate with the motivation and energy.

INSTITUTIONAL NURSING

Hospital Patient Care Positions

Hospitals may differ in size, location, ownership, and kinds of patients, but in addition, an important aspect is how nursing service is structured and the quality of nursing leadership. In an in-depth study of 16 "magnet" hospitals done between 1985 and 1986 as a follow-up to the original Magnet Hospital Study (Appendix 1), two researchers looked at the nursing departments of these hospitals in relation to the qualities of excellence described by Peters and Waterman, who cited "America's best-run companies."[15] They found a good match, because the magnet hospitals also had a bias for action; were close to the customer (had primary concern for the patient); promoted autonomy and entrepreneurship; showed true respect for the individual (a people orientation); created, instilled, and clarified a value system; had a generally simple organizational form and a management team who kept in close touch with staff; and successful coexistence of firm central direction (in terms of values) and optimum individual autonomy.[16] Although the big shortage was beginning and these hospitals had competitive but not top salaries at any level, they still enjoyed a waiting list of applicants. Head nurses chose carefully so that the new employee fit in, with a like attitude of caring and respect for quality. The nurses' statements of how they felt about their place of work are very revealing. As one said, "What is the biggest attraction here? Working someplace where your work has meaning and where you can feel good about your work."[17]

Not all hospitals are magnet hospitals; too many are far from it. However, as noted earlier, many more are finding that, for economic if not altruistic reasons, it is good business to adopt some of the practices and attitudes of the magnet hospitals. Choosing a committed, talented, well-prepared chief nursing executive (CNE) is probably step one, for he or she sets the tone, as shown in both Magnet Hospital studies. Nurses who look for the right place to work soon learn through their networks who those CNEs are.

Another consideration is the organization of nursing care. All the magnet hospitals gave the nurses real autonomy, but the organizational models differed, as they do in other settings. Participation in decision making (PDM) is more difficult to put into action than to talk about, partly because nurses at all levels are not clear about the mechanisms. There are a number of models and sometimes an overlapping of terminology; some models differentiate between participatory management and shared governance.[18] However, it is agreed that significant participation is important, with a free flow of information in all directions.[19] Moreover, it is essential that management and staff both decide to implement PDM, with a clear understanding of what it entails. One proponent calls shared governance a model that offers nurses not just participation but ownership in the organization.[20] In all these models, nurses have not only autonomy but also the corollary responsibility. For instance, in one model, which the participants called *collaborative governance,* day-to-day decision making took place at the unit level. The process required special education for the head nurse, renamed the *clinical manager,* consisting of topics such as decision making, team building, group dynamics, goal development, interviewing skills, budget, discipline, and rewards.[21] Although most hospitals do not have shared governance, a nurse with choices to make needs to consider whether this is how he or she can function best. Some people prefer a more traditional structure.

These various modes of governance affect all levels of nursing personnel. The sections that follow give a *general* description of the different levels and types of nursing positions. The position responsibilities would differ, of course, if one of the models just described were in operation. There would also be differences in specific functions on specialty units.

Positions described in hospital nursing include all those in which the employing agency is a hospital, whether private or voluntary, general or special, and whatever the size. The one element all hospitals have in common is that they are in existence primarily to take care of patients. The greatest differences from an employment point of view are types of responsibility, advancement opportunities, and salaries.

Many hospitals still have fewer than 100 beds, so there may be relatively little separation of specialties, with the exception of obstetrics, pediatrics, and, more frequently now, psychiatric care. Even here, when there is a declining census, hospitals in the same geographic area are beginning to cooperate by sharing such facilities: one may have the only pediatrics unit, another the only cardiac surgery. Therefore, the staff nurse is most often a generalist in these small hospitals. Positions in the emergency room[22] and

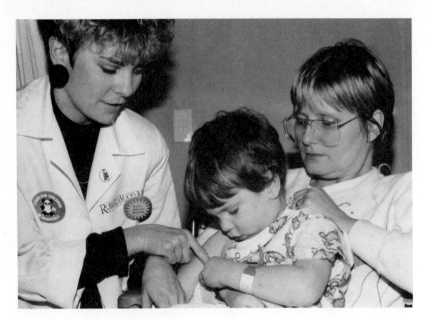

Pediatrics is a nursing specialty that brings many rewards. (*Courtesy of Robert Wood Johnson Medical Center.*)

the outpatient department (which are receiving an increasing number of patient visits), operating room, rehabilitation unit, or ICU[23] may require specialized training, but newly developed settings within the hospital, such as an outpatient surgery unit or "overnight" unit, also present new challenges in nursing care without necessarily mandating more formalized education.

Hospitals with home care services usually require nurses to have had public health experience to function in this area. Nursing roles are changing in all of these clinical areas. In the operating room, for instance, many of the technical tasks are carried out by surgical technicians, whereas the RN has overall responsibility for the safety of the patient, supervision and education of auxiliary nursing personnel, and sometimes support of the patient through pre- and postoperative visits. The increased utilization of NPs and clinical specialists (see Exhibit 7-1), adds another dimension to nursing care in these specialty areas. Although students usually do not have extensive experiences in the areas noted, even limited exposure may attract the nurse to certain kinds of practice. The emergency room and ICU, where quick, life-determining decisions must be made, independent judgments are not unusual, and tension is often high, will probably not attract the same kind of individual as the geriatric or rehabilitation unit, where long-term planning, teaching, and a slower pace are the norm.

Nevertheless, in most hospitals, the variety of experiences is endless. Larger hospitals and those in medical centers may offer a greater variety of specialties, exotic surgery, and rare treatments, as well as the advantages of being in the center of hospital, medical, and nursing research. Smaller hospitals may be less impersonal, are often located in the nurse's own community, and provide the opportunity to be a generalist on smaller patient units (which does not necessarily mean a smaller patient load).

The first-level position for professional nurses is that of general duty or staff nurse and is open to graduates of diploma, AD, and baccalaureate programs in nursing education. Individual assignments within this category will depend on the hospital's needs and policies and the nurse's preferences and ability. Staff nursing includes planning, implementing, and evaluating nursing care through assessment of patient needs; organizing, directing, supervising, teaching, and evaluating other nursing personnel; and coordinating patient care activities, often in the role of team leader. It involves working closely with the health team to accomplish the major goal of nursing—to give the best possible care to all patients.

To help attain this goal, the ANA, in 1973, published standards of practice applicable to all nursing situations. Additional, more specific standards were also developed for medical-surgical, maternal-child, geriatric, community health, psychiatric-mental health nursing practice, and a number of subspecialties. The general standards of practice, which can also be guidelines for practice anywhere were revised in 1991 with the title *Standards of Clinical Nursing Practice*. Standards for advanced or specialty practice are to be developed by the appropriate specialty group.

The *Standards of Clinical Nursing Practice* consist of "Standards of Care" and "Standards of Professional Performance." "Standards of Care" describe a competent level of nursing care as demonstrated by the nursing process of assessment, diagnosis, outcome identification, planning, implementation, and evaluation. "Standards of Professional Performance" describe a competent level of behavior in the professional role, including activities related to quality of care, performance appraisal, education, collegiality, ethics, collaboration, research, and resource utilization.[24] Involved in meeting these standards are literally hundreds of specific nursing tasks, some of which can be carried out by less prepared workers; it is the degree of nursing judgment needed, as well as knowledge and technical expertise, that determines who can best help any patient.

Because the goals of the various kinds of nursing education programs differ, theoretically the responsibilities of each type of nurse should also differ in the staff nurse position. Unfortunately, the tendency is to assign all nurses to the same kinds of tasks and responsibilities, so that differences are not utilized. This is so common that there is even an inclination to praise as innovative those nursing services that do delineate nursing roles and responsibilities at the staff nurse level.

In an informal way, differentiating among nurses based on their competence has existed for many years. However, in the last few years, *differ-*

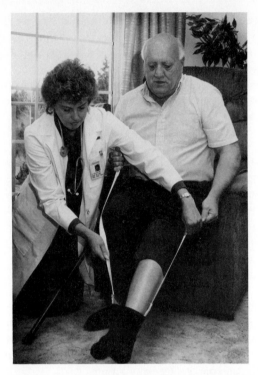

A nurse may act as a case manager to assist patients and their families both in the hospital and in the home. (*Courtesy of the Riverview Medical Center, New Jersey.*)

entiated nursing practice has been defined as structuring of the roles and functions of nurses according to their experience, education, and competence. Although some feel that education is the best basis of such practice, others say that the model should be built on levels of demonstrated competence, that is, the clinical ladder approach. Senior practitioners are then expected to assist the less experienced and less expert to hone their practice skills (in part because middle managers are often bogged down by administrative responsibilities and cannot do so).[25]

There are many variations of the clinical career ladder.[26] Most organizations use a committee composed of the CNE, other representatives of management, and staff nurses to develop and implement a career-ladder plan, but other approaches are also used. Criteria are set, usually including educational levels, experience, and clinical competencies. Positions are categorized as I, II, III, and so on based on these criteria. In some settings, the nursing process is the core of the framework, with added expectations in areas such as patient and family education, leadership and coordination, and research. In others, reaching the role expectations and competencies of primary nursing is the second level, and the nurse may choose to stay there. The lateral mobility or horizontal promotion of the career ladder, as opposed to vertical mobility toward managerial positions, broadens a nurse's existing knowledge and skills and allows him or her to stay at the bedside. It may allow for a change in patient population and in job pressures and expectations. In other words, a nurse may move to another type of nursing, if qualified. Salary increases are given with each change in level. Some nurses may choose realignment (downward mobility), perhaps as they decide to go to school. There are also managerial career ladders. The guiding principle is for nurses to plan and develop their own careers. Through self-assessment, the first step, nurses identify their skills, values, and interests in the context of the practice setting. Included is an evaluation of the nurse's skills as perceived by peers and nurse managers.

As part of the review, the nurse usually prepares for the committee a portfolio that contains information demonstrating the nurse's ability to meet the performance criteria of a particular level of nursing practice. Information may include a case study, a patient-teaching tool, a discharge plan, a nursing data base, or other evidence of the nurse's abilities, as well as evidence of educational advancement (formal course work or CE). The review process should be objective; if it determines that the nurse does not meet the criteria, she or he should have a clear idea of what areas of behavior or practice need to be strengthened. Because both increased salary and prestige are at stake, career ladders must be carefully developed, managed, and explained.

Not everyone likes the clinical career ladder. Some nurses find it time-consuming to develop a portfolio, even with help; some do not want peer evaluation. Others think it really doesn't measure a good nurse. Still others simply don't care and want to stay where they are. However, if their salaries "top out," a number of nurses have said that they would try to "ladder" instead of "level."[27]

Perhaps because of both staff and administrative reluctance about this and other aspects of differentiated practice, even the strongest advocate says that it will not be implemented easily in most settings. However, a number of innovative models have emerged.[28] In the early 1990s the various points of view on this approach have been the topic of considerable discussion, including several high-level conferences.

Regardless of how or if differentiated practice is the underlying philosophy, three basic methods of assignment for patient care in the hospital are functional, team, and case.[29] In *functional nursing,* the emphasis is on the task; jobs are grouped for expediency and supposedly to save time. For instance, one nurse might give all medications, another all treatments; aides might give all the baths. Obviously, the care of the patient is fragmented, and the nurse soon loses any sense of real nursing; patients cannot be treated as individuals or given comprehensive care. Nevertheless, there is a tendency to use this approach in many hospitals, especially on shifts that are understaffed. The work gets done; there is generally little nurse or patient satisfaction.

Team nursing involves a group of nursing personnel, usually RNs, LPNs, and aides, working together to meet patient needs. Team members are under the direction of the team leader (supposedly, but often not, a BSN), who assigns them to certain duties or patients according to their knowledge or skill. She or he has the major responsibility for planning care and coordinates all activities, acting as a resource person for the team. In addition, if there are few or no other RNs on the team, the team leader may perform nursing procedures requiring RN qualifications. Often the team leader is the only nurse directly relating to the physician, but, too often, actual patient contact is infrequent or sporadic. The original concept of the team has been diluted.[30] Planning and evaluation are seldom a team effort; conferences to discuss patient needs are irregular; and too frequently, the team leader does mostly functional nursing, providing treatments and giving medications in an endless cycle. Most hospitals have some version of team nursing, at least to the extent that the RN supervises and directs other nursing personnel in patient care.

Instituted in the 1970s and gaining in popularity is *primary nursing,* a somewhat confusing term for the *case method,* in which total care of the patient is assigned to one nurse, the traditional caregiving pattern. A major difference between primary nursing and other methods of assignment is the accountability of the nurse. The patient has a primary nurse, just as she or he has a primary physician. A nurse is a *primary nurse* when responsible for the care of certain patients throughout their stay and an *associate nurse* when caring for the patients while the primary nurse is off duty. In most places, that nurse is responsible for a group of patients 24 hours a day, even though an associate nurse may assist or take over on other shifts. The primary nurse is in direct contact with the patient, family/significant others, and members of the health team, and plans cooperatively with them for total care and continuity. The head nurse then is chiefly in an administrative and teaching (personnel) role. Almost always the primary nurse is an RN, often with a baccalaureate. Sometimes the nursing team involved in primary nursing is made up of all RNs, with the exception of aides, who are generally limited to "hotel service," dietary tasks, and transportation. There is almost unanimous agreement that the primary pattern is much more satisfying to patients, families, physicians, and nurses and that care is of a highly improved quality. Although there has been some concern over the increased cost of an all-RN staff and the more personalized care, some data show that after the initial start-up time, costs are not greater and are sometimes less than those of other staffing patterns.[31]

Little agreement exists as to which of these methods of assignment is best, based on patient and nurse satisfaction, quality of patient care, cost, and administrative efficiency. Functional assignment may be the most ad-

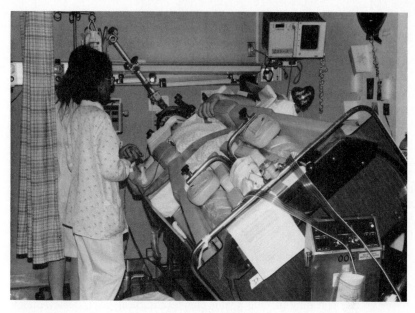

Nursing care in the hospital, which is often high tech, also requires high touch. (*Courtesy of the Robert Wood Johnson Medical Center.*)

ministratively efficient form because of its division of labor according to specific tasks, but almost no one says that either the patient or the nurse finds it preferable to others. Team nursing, when done according to the original concept, may be satisfying to the team who can give their attention to a small group of patients and also develop an esprit de corps that compensates for the time expended in conference and work coordination. It is often considered expensive because of the need for this additional time spent.[32] Primary nursing, often considered the most professional of assignments, also has its detractors; additional stress, role overload, and role ambiguity are cited.[33] The setting and the nurses themselves may also have some effect, as there is some evidence that neither cost nor quality suffers whether team or primary nursing is practiced.[34]

Another approach somewhat between these two is termed *modular nursing*.[35] The utilization of clerical and nonnursing personnel to assume nonnursing tasks is increasing again with the nursing shortage. This frees the nurse for the patient contact for which nurses are prepared. Nurses have long complained that they are required to do an endless number of tasks better carried out by assistants (not necessarily nurses' aides). Such work includes finding supplies and equipment, transporting patients and equipment, cleaning equipment, checking the work of other departments, cleaning up after physicians, and moving furniture.[36] The assistive workers are also considerably less expensive than nurses, especially since nurses' salaries have escalated. Nursing assistants (NAs), once considered a problem because of lack of skills and motivation, are now being welcomed, especially in acute care. However, it has been recommended that these people be carefully trained and that staff be oriented to their responsibilities. Newer graduates who have never worked with NAs may be particularly concerned.[37]

The basic requirement for a staff position (or any other) is graduation from an approved school of nursing and nursing licensure or eligibility for licensure. A graduate nurse (GN) must take and pass the licensure examinations within a specific period of time. A nurse is usually hired for a particular unit, but it is not uncommon to be asked to *float*—replace a nurse on any unit. Floating should not extend to units that require special knowledge and skill unless the nurse is so trained. In some hospitals, there are *float pools* or *resource teams*[38]—highly skilled nurses who never have a regular unit.

In most cases, nurses are required to rotate shifts and work on holidays. For this reason, it is possible to work part time in most hospitals. Usually there are salary differentials for working evenings and nights. In recent years, flexible hours and shifts have become popular.[39] Fringe benefits also vary greatly and may include health plans, retirement plans, arrangements for CE, holidays, sick time, and vacation time.

Another career alternative is employment by a supplemental staffing agency sometimes called a *temporary nursing service (TNS)*. Nurses most commonly using TNSs are some new graduates, nurses enrolled in advanced educational programs, nurses with small children who cannot work full time or all shifts, or nurses who simply prefer the flexibility. The TNS will pay them a salary for the hours worked, with the usual legal deductions, after billing the institutions or the patient/client using the worker's services.[40] There are local and national agencies, and selecting a reputable one is extremely important. Job assignments may be made an hour or a week ahead, but the nurse is not obligated to take them; however, a no-show is usually dismissed. As well as offering a great deal of flexibility and variety, there are also disadvantages, even with a good TNS: no job security, no benefits, sometimes only the minimum rate paid by the area hospitals with no increases, and, of course, the constant reorientation to new nursing units and patients, even to new hospitals, although some nurses limit themselves to one particular hospital. The fact that "agency nurses" are sometimes looked down on by regular staff as incompetent (although they may simply be unfamiliar with that hospital's procedure) also creates problems for these nurses.

A variation of temporary nursing is the *flying* nurse, who accepts short-term contracts directly with a hospital anywhere in the country and sometimes abroad. Arrangements are made through an agency. The hospital usually pays only the benefits required by law, but pays for the nurse's travel and sometimes arranges for or provides housing. The nurse must get a temporary license in each state where he or she is employed. Although the variety is exciting for many nurses, the place of work is seldom ideal.[41]

Depending on the policies a hospital has regarding promotion, a nurse could become a head nurse without further education, but not without experience. *Head nurses* are in charge of the clinical nursing units of a hospital, including the operating room, outpatient department, and emergency room. They may be called *charge nurses* or, more recently, *nursing coordinators*. Head nurses are usually responsible to the next higher person on the scale, usually the supervisor, or, in a smaller hospital, the assistant director of nursing or the director. The head nurse position is the first administrative position most nurses achieve (or perhaps that of assistant head nurse, who may share some of the head nurse functions and substitute for the head nurse in his or her absence).

It is the head nurse's job to manage the nursing care and ensure its quality in a relatively small area of the hospital. This may or may not include supervision of ward clerks in their clerical activities (see Chapter 3). With the trend toward decentralization of nursing authority, the head nurse is expected to give more attention to acting as a consultant and teacher for staff, to following the clinical progress of the patients, and to maintaining communication with physicians and other health personnel.

Head nurses may earn between $500 and $2000 more per year than staff nurses (unless the nurses are unionized); other benefits may vary. In most instances, the head nurse works only the day shift, but may alternate on weekends and holidays with the assistant head nurse.

Other Positions for Nurses in Hospitals

There are a number of other employment opportunities for nurses in hospitals, although they may have only a slight relationship to nursing and are often in a department other than nursing service. Nurses on the intravenous (IV) team are specially trained, and responsible for all the IV infusions given to patients (outside of the operating room and delivery room). They usually bring the appropriate solution to the patient, add ordered drugs, and start and/or restart the IV. In some institutions they are also permitted to start a blood transfusion.

The nurse-epidemiologist or infection control nurse focuses on surveillance, education, and research.[42] The surveillance aspect is designed for the reporting of infections and the establishment, over a period of time, of expected levels of infections for various areas. Patients with infections are checked to see whether the infection was acquired after admission. Reports are used for epidemiologic research, and the staff is educated in the prevention of infection. Nurses have also been trained as epidemiologists in public health agencies, where they perform similar but broader duties that involve the total community. Another challenging role is that of ombudsman, or patient advocate, in which a nurse acts as an intermediary between the patient and the hospital in an attempt to prevent or resolve problems of the patient related to the hospital or hospitalization.

A new professional role is that of director or coordinator of quality assurance (QA), with a variety of titles. Although these persons may have a medical records background, most are nurses. The primary function of QA practitioners is to assess and evaluate indicators of nursing care in actual practice. The position arose from the increasing requirements of the JCAHO, as well as demands on the part of payers and consumers for accountability. Their numbers are estimated to be in the low thousands. Most report to the CNE.

Their primary functions are:

1. Planning, with the clinical staff's full input and approval, areas of nursing to be studied and methods to be used.
2. Gathering, analyzing, ordering, and displaying data in useful and appropriate ways (such as practice profiles).
3. Disseminating this information to those who need it, while taking steps to ensure that it is not lost or ignored.
4. Following up on how the information is used to determine that corrective actions really work and that improvements in care are sustained.[43]

The role is still evolving, but in today's climate the numbers are expected to increase.

Finally, new emphasis on health education in the hospital and community has resulted in the creation of a community health coordinator, who develops and/or coordinates the various aspects of patient teaching, as well as the teaching of outpatients and other interested individuals in the community, on health matters. This nurse may not be a part of the nursing service and is more likely to direct the teaching program than to do the teaching personally.

Nursing in Long-Term Care Facilities

Under Medicare and Medicaid, nursing homes that qualify for reimbursement are called *skilled nursing facilities*. The *intermediate care facility* provides for those who require care beyond room and board but less than that designated as skilled. These include institutions for victims of cerebral palsy or other neurological conditions and mental retardation. The older term *nursing home,* which might apply to either, is still used by most people.

Nurses may have positions in nursing homes similar to those in hospitals. In most nursing homes the pace is slower and the pressure less. (However, with earlier discharge from hospitals, patients are much sicker than they

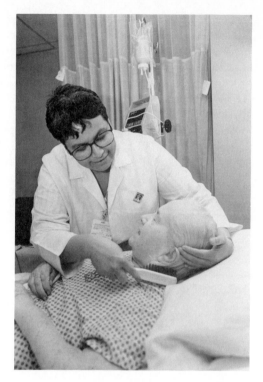

The need for high quality care of elderly patients is a major issue today. (*Courtesy of the Jewish Home and Hospital for Aged, New York; photo by David Grossman.*)

once were.) Nurses interested in nursing home care enjoy the opportunity to know the patient better in the relatively long-term stay and to help the patient maintain or attain the best possible health status.[44] This is not the area of practice for someone impatient for quick results. Both rehabilitative and geriatric nursing require patience and understanding. In rehabilitation, nurses work closely as a team with related health disciplines—occupational therapy, physical therapy, speech therapy, and others. In geriatric nursing, the nurse works to a great extent with nonprofessional nursing personnel and acts as team leader, teacher, and supervisor. It may well be that there is only one professional nurse in a nursing home per shift, with PNs as charge nurses and aides giving much of the day-to-day care.

Because the patients are relatively helpless and often have no family or friends who check on them, the nurse must, in a real sense, be a patient advocate. Physicians make infrequent visits and in some cases, where there are limited or no rehabilitative services, the nurse is the only professional with long-term patient contact. For this reason, geriatric nurse practitioners (GNPs) are considered a tremendous asset in nursing homes. The GNP is responsible for assessing patients and evaluating their progress, sometimes performing certain diagnostic procedures. She or he usually manages medical problems within a general protocol, but a particularly important function is assessing personal and family relationships, patient and staff relationships, and life situations that may affect the patient's health status. In some nursing homes, the GNP is on 24-hour emergency call and also performs the other usual NP functions.

Requirements for employment are similar to those in hospitals for like positions, although often the need for a degree is not emphasized. Benefits and salaries have improved but are not as good as those in hospitals. Because, under Medicare, orientation and in-service education are mandatory, there is an excellent opportunity to learn about long-term care. With an aging population, there are likely to be good job opportunities for some time to come.[45]

COMMUNITY HEALTH NURSING

There is an increasing tendency to refer to *public health nursing (PHN)* and *community health nursing (CHN)* interchangeably. Definitions vary. Some think of this field as focusing on population (the aggregate) and others think in terms of individuals and families. The ANA Division on Community Health Nursing Practice states:

> The community health nurse . . . has responsibility in general and comprehensive areas of health practice for:
>
> a. Determining health needs of the individual, the family, and the community;
> b. Assessing health status;
> c. Implementing health planning;
> d. Evaluating health practices;
> e. Providing primary health care.
>
> The community health nurse needs to be aware of regulations which are developing, as well as new and existing regulations, policies, and laws that directly affect community health nursing practice.[46]

In fulfilling these responsibilities, PHN/CHN nurses practice in many settings. Most are employed by agencies that may carry the title of *public health, community health, home health,* or *visiting nurse.* They differ in both size and ownership.

PHN/CHN employment opportunities are not limited, however, to these agencies. Nurses may also be employed by hospitals to conduct home-care programs or to serve as liaison between the hospital and community facilities, or by other institutions and agencies, private and governmental, in need of the kinds of services the PHN is prepared to provide in schools, industry, outpatient clinics, community health centers, free walk-in clinics for substance abuse and sexually transmitted diseases (STDs), migrant labor camps, and rural poverty areas. PHNs/CHNs may also work for various international agencies assisting less developed countries, because the need for PHN services in these countries is usually urgent.

Although situations differ, nurses in official agencies may make home visits, but their responsibilities are primarily in community health clinics focused on the needs of that agency's population. Traditionally, these have been family planning, maternal-child care, and communicable disease. These needs are increasing, especially with the escalation of TB, STDs, and drug abuse.

Visiting nurses, or home health nurses, regardless of their place of employment, also carry out these functions and may, in addition, give physical care and treatments. With the advent of much earlier discharge from hospitals, patients are quite a bit sicker when they go home, and these nurses are required to know how to care for the acutely ill. If the nurse assessment indicates that such care does not require professional nurse services, home health aides/homemakers may be assigned to a patient/family, with nurse supervision and reassessment. Visiting nurses have also set up clinics that they visit periodically in senior citizen centers or apartments, as well as in the single-room occupancy (SRO) hotels commonly used for welfare clients in large cities. There are also many liaison roles with hospitals, HMOs, clinics, geriatric units, and various residences for the long-term disabled and mentally ill or retarded, primarily to assist in admission and discharge planning, as well as coordinating continuing patient care.

Besides state licensure, and for some agencies, prior nursing experience, one major qualification for PHN work is graduation from a baccalaureate nursing program. Because of the shortage of nurses with the prescribed PHN preparation at the present time, however, graduates of diploma and AD programs can and do find positions in this field, working at the beginning level and under supervision. In some areas they work only in clinics and do not make home visits. Some employers encourage nurses to work toward a baccalaureate degree by providing tuition or scholarship grants.

Pay and advancement at all levels are related to educational and other qualifications. On a national level, salaries are generally competitive, except for the public agencies. Nurses may be promoted as they assume advanced or expanded role functions (NP or CNS) or administrative positions. Many official agencies operate within a civil service system, but in the states with strong labor laws permitting collective bargaining for nurses, nurses may organize through either a union or the SNA and bargain for better salaries

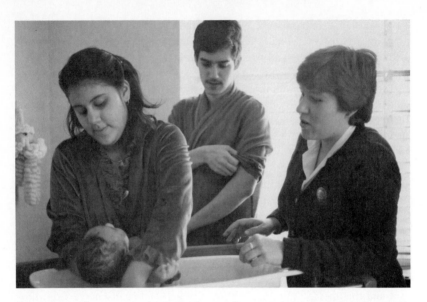

A nurse teaching parents the care of a newborn can be as important as the hi-tech care also part of home health care today. (*Courtesy of the Visiting Nurse Service of New York.*)

and working conditions. In the past, PHN/CHN nurses enjoyed standard daytime hours, with most working Monday through Friday. However, with the move toward more care in the community on a 24-hour basis, rather than in institutions, PHN/CHN nurses are usually expected to rotate shifts and work weekends, much the same as nurses employed in institutions.

A unique and distinct aspect of PHN practice is the autonomy required when working in a setting "without walls." Clinical judgment and clinical decisions are a central part of the nursing practice that demands a high level of knowledge and clinical versatility. PHNs do not generally work in the protected controlling environment of an institution, but rather in the client's setting, where the clients determine who will enter the home, and whether they follow (or even listen to) the health teaching and counseling given. If the setting is a clinic, there is no force that can make a client come to or return to a clinic, or, for that matter, follow any regimen given. Studies have indicated that the poor, especially blacks, may reject health services because they feel a prejudicial attitude among the providers of care, whereas at the same time average middle-class white nurses hold, or feel they hold, different values concerning health care. Even with the best of intentions, nurses (and other health workers in the community) may not be able to convince their clients that certain preventive measures are necessary. Not all nurses can deal with these frustrations or have the skills and personality characteristics that enable them to work and relate effectively with clients who have a different lifestyle and culture.

Professional nurses who select PHN as a career need outstanding ability to adjust to many types of environments with a variety of living conditions, from the well-to-do in a high-rise apartment house to the most poverty-stricken in a ghetto or rural area, and to appreciate a wide range of interests, attitudes, educational backgrounds, and cultural differences. They must be able to accept these variations, to understand the differences, to communicate well so as to avoid misunderstandings and misinterpretations, and to be able to give equally good nursing care to all. PHNs in any position must use excellent judgment and are expected to use their own initiative. They have the opportunity to work with persons in other disciplines and other social agencies to help provide needed services to the clients, services that may include financial counseling, legal aid, housing problems, family planning, marital counseling, and school difficulties. In some instances, PHNs are not only case finders but case coordinators—patient advocates in every sense.[47]

OFFICE NURSING

Office nurses are employed by physicians or dentists to see that their patients receive the nursing they need, usually in the office. Office nurses may give all of this care or assign certain duties to other personnel who work under their direction and supervision. If working for several doctors or dentists in a group practice, the nurse may supervise a staff of several employees. Nurses may be employed in a one-doctor general practitioner's office, which requires general skills, or they may be employed in a specialist's office, which requires special skills. For instance, surgeons may employ nurses who can also act as scrub nurses in surgery done at the hospital or assist them in office surgery.

What the office nurse does in terms of nursing will depend largely upon the employer's type of practice, daily schedule of appointments, and attitude about nurses' scope of practice. Tasks may be as routine as giving medications, chaperoning physical examinations, preparing equipment, and seeing that the patients' records are completed and filed at the end of the day. Better utilization would include observation, communication, teaching, and coordination with community health agencies. A few nurses make hospital patient rounds with or without the physician. Unfortunately, in too many instances the employer expects the nurse to be hostess, secretary, bookkeeper, errand girl, housekeeper, purchasing agent, public relations expert, and laboratory technician as well, tasks that a medical assistant could do. Perhaps one of the most far-reaching effects on office nursing is the development of the NP, who is often part of the physician's private practice and assumes much responsibility for patient care.

Most office nurses do not have a baccalaureate degree but do have considerable experience. Salaries and working conditions in this field are, generally speaking, both flexible and variable, representing private arrangements between the individual office nurse and the employer. Office nurses sometimes say they are willing to make some sacrifices in salary because the hours or responsibilities of office nursing fit their tastes or general life situation. Both salary and fringe benefits are likely to be lower than those for the hospital staff nurse. However, most office nurses seem to enjoy a friendly and congenial relationship with their employing physician or physicians and usually succeed in negotiating mutually satisfactory working conditions and salary. They appear to stay in the job longer than most nurses, an average of nine years.

OCCUPATIONAL HEALTH NURSING

The AAOHN states in its standards of occupational health nursing practice:

Occupational health nursing applies nursing principles in promoting the health of workers and maintaining a safe and healthful environment in occupational settings.

The knowledge is a synthesis of principles from several disciplines in the health sciences including, but not limited to, nursing, medicine, safety, industrial hygiene, toxicology, administration, and public health epidemiology.

Occupational health nursing activities focus on health promotion and protection and maintenance and restoration of health. The occupational health nurse is primarily concerned with the preventive approach to health care, which includes early disease detection, health teaching, and counseling.

Whether the nurse is a sole provider or supervises other professional nurses and paraprofessionals, standards of care are applicable to nursing practice in all types of occupational health settings. Standards focus on nursing practice rather than on the health care provider.

As a professional, the occupational health nurse is accountable for the nursing care provided to the employee first and to the employer second. Standards of nursing practice provide a means for determining quality of care, as well as accountability of the practitioner.

The occupational health unit in which an occupational health nurse (OHN) works may consist of a single room, or it may be a large department with several examining and treatment rooms, x-ray and laboratory facilities, and offices for nurses and physicians. The OHN may work in a multidisciplinary setting or multinurse unit; however, more than 60 percent of OHNs work alone. Physicians are often employed on a contractual basis and provide medical services as needed, but in most cases the OHN is the manager of the unit.

Whether this nurse functions in a sophisticated manner in the delivery of health care depends on his or her education and experience and the policies of the employer. As a prepared NP or nurse clinician, the nurse may assess the worker's condition through health histories, observation, physical examination, and other selected diagnostic measures; review and interpret findings to differentiate the normal from the abnormal; select appropriate action and referral; counsel; and teach.[48] The practitioner must also be concerned with the physical and psychosocial phenomena of the workers and their families, their working environment, community, and even recreation. If the nurse is working in a more conservative environment and/or without the appropriate background, the activities may be limited to first aid and some emergency treatment, keeping records, assisting with physical examinations, and carrying out certain diagnostic procedures. In many cases, most often when the nurse does not function in an expanded role, standing orders or directions, prepared and signed by the medical director, give the necessary authority to care for conditions that develop while the employee is on the job. The nurse may refer employees with nonoccupational illnesses or injuries to their family doctor; however, this type of service is being provided more and more at the work site.

A particularly interesting development that broadens the scope of the OHN's practice is an increased emphasis on workers' health problems that may or may not be directly caused by the job but affect worker performance—alcoholism, emotional problems, stress, drug addiction, and family relations. In many cases, the nurse may be involved in developing employee assistance programs and in counseling and therapy.

In a large occupational health unit in an industry that employs one or more full-time physicians, the OHN may also function as a nursing care coordinator to develop, implement, supervise, and evaluate the delivery of health care to employees, working with professional and nonprofessional staff.

The OHN must know about the laws that govern employee health. This requires interpretation of regulations and the design and implementation of standards to protect worker health. He or she should also be involved in policy decisions affecting worker health and safety. In general, OHN in a health unit of any size means much more than meeting the immediate needs of an ill or injured employee. The nurse uses interviewing, observing, and teaching skills, takes health histories, keeps health records, and is responsible for the operational management. The ability to take and recognize abnormalities in electrocardiograms and to do eye screening, audiometric testing, and certain laboratory tests and x-rays is considered useful. Health promotion and worker safety are particularly important.

Graduation from a state-approved school of professional nursing and current state registration are basic requirements for the OHN. More employers are requiring a college degree, and many find a graduate degree desirable. However, this is still not common. A career OHN will be expected to seek certification by the American Board for Occupational Health Nurses, an independent nursing specialty board authorized to certify qualified OHNs.

Salaries and fringe benefits vary according to the size of the industry or business and its location. Both tend to be somewhat lower than those of other nurses. Some OHNs belong to a union, but this is discouraged by the AAOHN (and by employers). The usual company benefits include vacations, sick leave, pensions, and insurance. Working hours are those of the workers; thus, in an industry with work shifts around the clock, nurses are usually there also. As a professional person, the nurse may have some of the privileges of management, such as temporary absences to attend meetings. Although some industries carry professional liability insurance that supposedly covers the OHN, it may not apply in all cases of possible litigation. It is advisable, therefore, for the nurses to carry their own professional liability insurance.

OPPORTUNITIES IN GOVERNMENT

The U.S. government, with its various departments and agencies including the armed forces, offers excellent career opportunities. Positions range from staff nurse to top executive positions. The settings include hospitals, clinics, classrooms, and administrative offices, with responsibilities similar to those in civilian practice, except, of course, in wartime, when the sites are quite different.[49] There are many benefits not otherwise available.

U.S. Public Health Service (PHS)

The graduate nurse may enter the PHS by appointment to either the Commissioned Corps or the Federal Civil Service. Minimum requirements are U.S. citizenship, at least (generally) 18 and less than 44 years of age, graduation from an approved school of nursing, and physical eligibility. The nurse must have earned a baccalaureate in nursing or a first professional nursing degree from a program NLN accredited at the time of graduation. AD graduates are not eligible for the Commissioned Corps.

The Commissioned Corps is a uniformed service composed of professionals in medical and health-related fields. Pay, allowances, and other privileges are comparable to those of officers of the armed forces. Appointments are generally made at the senior assistant grade, equivalent to lieutenant junior grade in the navy or first lieutenant in the army. The top rank is surgeon general, equivalent to vice admiral and lieutenant general.

Opportunities for collegiate nursing students to become familiar with the careers in the PHS, as well as to further their professional knowledge, are offered through the Commissioned Officer Student Training and Extern Program (COSTEP). In the junior COSTEP, a limited number of carefully selected students are commissioned as reserve officers in the corps and called to active duty for training during "free periods" of the academic year.

The civil service system is considered the basic mode of federal employment and comprises a range of professional and nonprofessional personnel. A civil service examination is not required for RNs before appointment. There is opportunity for advancement through a well-defined merit system. Nurses employed under civil service in the PHS have Social Security benefits. They are eligible for retirement benefits, which they may receive upon resignation, depending on the length of employment.

Included in the areas of employment are the Indian Health Service and the Clinical Center at NIH. For information about job opportunities with the DHHS or the PHS, contact the Federal Job Information Center in your area listed in the telephone directory under "U.S. Government."

Department of Veterans Affairs

The Department of Veterans Affairs (VA) was established in 1930 as a civilian agency of the federal government. Its purpose is to administer national programs that provide benefits for veterans of this country's armed forces.[50] It is the nation's largest organized health care system, with hospitals, clinics, nursing home units, and domiciliaries throughout the United States.

To qualify for an appointment in the VA, a nurse must be a U.S. citizen, a graduate of a state-approved school of professional nursing, currently registered to practice, and must meet required physical standards. Graduates from a professional school of nursing may be appointed pending passing of state board examinations.

There are several salary grades for VA nurses, ranging from junior grade through associate, full, intermediate, senior, chief, assistant director, director, and the executive grade of director, the last reserved for the national leader of the VA Nursing Service. Qualification standards relating to education, experience, and competencies are specified for appointment or promotion to each grade. The VA salary system recognizes excellence in clinical practice, administration, research, and education. Applications and inquiries for full- or part-time employment should be directed to the Personnel Office at the VA Medical Center at the location of interest. A toll-free telephone number (800-368-5629) is available for information about nationwide employment opportunities.

Armed Services

Despite similarities, there are specific differences among the Army Nurse Corps, Navy Nurse Corps, and Air Force Nurse Corps. In recent years there have been a number of changes in qualifications and assignments to meet the changes in society and in the health field. All the armed services have a reserve corps of nurses to provide the additional nurses that are needed to care for members of the services and their families in time of war or other national emergency. Nurses may join the reserve without having joined the regular service; the requirements are similar. A certain amount of training (which is paid) is required, usually one weekend a month and two consecutive weeks a year, at local medical units related to that particular service. There are opportunities for promotion, CE, and fringe benefits such as low-cost insurance, retirement pay, and PX shopping. More information is available from the reserve recruiter of the particular service. In all the services,

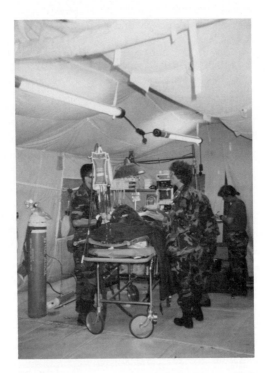

Army nurses are equally skilled in caring for the sick and injured in war and in peace. (*Courtesy of the U.S. Army Nurse Corps.*)

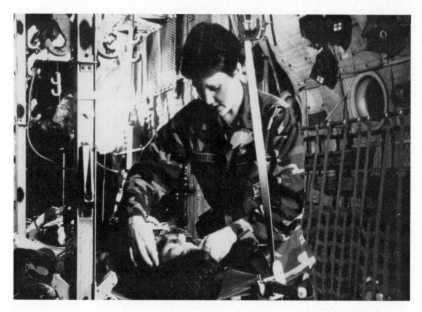

Air Force nurses not only care for patients in hospitals, but also provide expert care during air evacuation. (*Courtesy of the U.S. Air Force.*)

nurses have the economic, social, and health care benefits of all officers, as well as the opportunity for personal travel. After discharge (or retirement, which is possible in 20 years), veterans' benefits are available.[51]

In all the armed services, nurses are commissioned at an officer rank and may advance to a top rank. The basic requirements for a commission are similar: physically qualified, licensed, U.S. citizen (usually), and educationally qualified. However, because of other differences and the fact that these criteria change, it is best to contact the local recruiting stations of the various services for specific information. All three generally send recruiters to nursing conventions, advertise in nursing journals, and are available to speak at schools of nursing. Nurses in the armed services have outstanding opportunities for advancement, further education, and professional nursing experiences throughout the United States and often overseas.

PRIVATE PRACTICE: NURSE ENTREPRENEURS

A private practice is a business, and setting it up and running it must be a businesslike process or it will not survive.[52] There are basic decisions to be made: what kind of organization should be created (corporation, partnership, for-profit, nonprofit); by whom (nurses and other professionals); for whom;

at what fees; what kind and how many employees will be needed; how to get clients (marketing); types of advertising; how to relate to other health professions; where the services will be offered; at what hours; and policies about telephone counseling and/or home visits (house calls).

What kinds of services would these entrepreneurs offer in private practice? If nurses do not have NP training, the usual services offered are any combination of health teaching and health promotion, counseling, home health, professional education (CE programs), and consulting.[53] Some own health-related businesses such as dialysis centers, home health agencies, and equipment rental.

NPs in private practice may have a backup physician, or they may have developed relationships with physicians from whom and to whom referrals are made. (Some NPs are in full partnership in a group practice of physicians.) These NPs do all the things NPs are legally permitted to do in their state, which may or may not include writing prescriptions. Sometimes their practices are in an urban/suburban area, but frequently they are in rural areas with few physicians available, and the nurse is the only health care provider.

Assuming that the nurse does not have legal problems about the scope of practice, a major problem is getting enough patients and reimbursement to earn a living. Many nurses can afford to give only part of their time to the practice because of limited reimbursement, and perhaps hold university teaching positions or are subsidized by some organization.[54] Third-party payment is still uncertain, and most patients cannot or do not choose to pay an independent practitioner if they can get clinic care that is covered.

Another problem has been individual practice privileges in health care institutions, especially hospitals and nursing homes. What this means basically is the privilege of a nurse not employed by that institution to admit patients and/or write orders for their care or participate in any part of his or her patients' care. Some slight progress is being made.

In rural areas where there is no source of health care, the NP may have the same physical, professional, and psychological problems as physicians—isolation, overwork, and some lack of stimulation. Nevertheless, independent practice provides a degree of professional autonomy that many nurses crave.[55] As one of the first acknowledged independent practitioners stated, "in the twenty-fifth year of my nursing career, I have become professionally free and have removed the impediments to my practice of nursing."[56]

Private Duty Nursing

Private duty nursing goes back to the beginning of nursing schools, when students were sent to homes to give patient care and upon graduation continued to do this kind of nursing because there were almost no positions for graduate nurses in hospitals.

Until the last 20 years or so, private duty nursing still attracted many nurses, because they could set their own schedule, often their preferred place of work, and, best of all, could devote their time and nursing skills to one patient. Most now give care in hospitals in 8- or 12-hour shifts, but they are private practitioners, employed by the patient or family. Obviously, this means that they are on their own in terms of retirement plans, Social Security payments, and taxes. They have no paid sick leave, vacation, or other benefits. If they want a day off, they must find a relief nurse. Fees vary but may be quite good. Sometimes nurses going on to school for degrees choose private duty as a way of earning extra money, either by relieving another nurse or by taking short cases. Most private duty nurses are listed in a hospital or other registry where their preferences are noted. Because more LPNs are being employed for less complex cases and the very ill may be in ICUs, there may be times when the private duty nurse cannot get the kind of work he or she prefers.

OTHER CAREER OPPORTUNITIES

It would probably be impossible, or at least extraordinarily lengthy, to give information about every career possibility available for nurses. A list of specific *positions* directly related to nursing, not even including the specialization or subspecialization, runs into the hundreds when the diverse settings in which nursing is practiced are considered.[57] Overall, these are clinical nursing, administration, education, or research (or a combination of all), but the specific setting brings its own particular challenges. Each may require knowledge of another culture and the physical and psychosocial needs of these people, such as nursing in an Indian reservation, or a new orientation to practice such as working in an HMO, or in juvenile court, or the prison system,[58] or even camp nursing. Almost all types of nursing are practiced in international settings[59] for WHO, the Peace Corps, or Project Hope—not easy jobs, but rewarding and often exciting.[60] Some require a baccalaureate.

In some cases, specialization or subspecialization, usually demanding additional education and training, becomes a new career path. There are any number of these, and as each becomes recognized as a distinct subspecialty, involved nurses tend to form a new organization or a subgroup within ANA or some related medical organization to develop standards of practice.

This is not really new; operating room nurses have been practicing since the beginning of American nursing, and coronary care nurses or enterostomal therapists are in their third decade. More recently, there is new emphasis and, consequently, a number of new educational programs in such areas as women's health care, men's health care,[61] family planning, thanatology, and sex education, all of which have an interdisciplinary context that brings additional dimensions to the practice.

When nurses assume positions such as editors of nursing journals or nursing editors in publishing companies, they not only draw on their nursing background but must learn about the publishing field and acquire the necessary skills. In the same way, nurses employed as lobbyists, labor relations specialists, executive directors or staff of nursing associations, nurse consultants for drug or supply companies, or administrative consulting firms and staff for legislators or governmental committees all use their nursing, but must learn from other disciplines not related to nursing and develop new role concepts.

As health care and nursing expand, some nurses will develop new positions themselves. It seems safe to say that opportunities and challenges in nursing today are practically unlimited.

KEY POINTS

1. Nurses have unlimited opportunities within the profession if they continue to develop through formal or continuing education.
2. Nursing positions are available or can be developed in every setting where health care is given.
3. Because of social and economic factors that can create rapid and unexpected demands in health care, it is difficult to predict the number of nurses that would provide a balance of supply and demand.
4. Employers expect new graduates to have at least basic nursing skills, the ability to become proficient in the skills that are more complex, and to apply these by using the nursing process.
5. Employers expect new graduates to be responsible in the employment setting and to practice ethically.
6. Nursing positions that currently do not require advanced education are primarily at the staff level.
7. Nursing positions that generally require further formal education include clinical specialist, NP, student health services, teaching, and administration.

REFERENCES

1. Lewis H. Specialism: The best career path? *RN,* 47:40–47 (June 1984).
2. Gulack R. The main chance. *RN,* 46:35–41 (March 1983).

3. Mattera M. Job security: Will things get any worse? *RN*, 9:36–41 (June 1986).
4. RN shortage suddenly surfaces in many states; hospitals scramble to hire critical care nurses. *Am J Nurs*, 86:851, 860–861 (July 1986).
5. Keith J. A temporary solution to the nursing shortage. *Health Prog*, 70:76–77 (December 1989).
6. Lindquist K, Hart K. How hospitals are responding to the shortage. *Am J Nurs*, 88:1206–1210 (September 1988).
7. Minnick A, et al. What do nurses want? Priorities for action. *Nurs Outlook*, 37:214–218 (September–October 1989).
8. Lindquist and Hart, op. cit.
9. Frels L, et al. RCTs: Not the answer to the nursing shortage. *Nurs Econ*, 7:136–141 (May–June 1989).
10. Aiken L, et al. The nurse shortage: Myth or reality. *N Engl J Med*, 317:641–646 (September 3, 1987).
11. New federal nursing panel tackles the shortage. *Am J Nurs*, 90:118, 122 (June 1990).
12. Scherer P. Hospitals that attract (and keep) nurses. *Am J Nurs*, 88:34–40 (January 1988).
13. Kelly L. The grass is not greener. *Nurs Outlook*, 37:115 (May–June 1989).
14. Kasprisin CA, Young WB. Nurse internship program reduces turnover, raises commitment. *Nurs and Health Care*, 6:137–140 (March 1985).
15. Peters T, Waterman R Jr. *In search of excellence*. New York: Harper and Row, 1982.
16. Kramer M, Schmalenberg C. Magnet hospitals: Institutions of excellence. Part I. *J Nurse Admin*, 18:13–24 (January 1988); Part II, 18:11–19 (February 1988).
17. Ibid., Part II, p. 17.
18. O'Grady TP. Shared governance and new organizational models. *Nurs Econ*, 5:281–286 (November–December 1987).
19. Allen D, et al. Making shared governance work: A conceptual model. *J Nurs Admin*, 18:37–41 (January 1988).
20. O'Grady TP. Shared governance: Reality or sham? *Am J Nurs*, 89:350–351 (March 1989).
21. Jacoby J, Terpstra M. Collaborative governance: Model for professional autonomy. *Nurs Mgt*, 21:42–44 (February 1990).
22. McKay J, Schepers D. Emergency nursing. *Imprint*, 36:47, 49–50 (September–October 1989).
23. Daniels V. Stress and the ICU: Is it for you? *Imprint*, 34:32, 34 (September–October 1987).
24. *Standards of clinical nursing practice*. Kansas City, MO: American Nurses' Association, 1991.
25. McClure ML. Differentiated nursing practice: Concepts and considerations. *Nurs Outlook*, 39:106–110 (May–June 1991).
26. Career ladders: *An approach to professional productivity and job satisfaction*. Kansas City, MO: American Nurses' Association, 1984.

27. Hartley P, Cunningham D. Staff nurses rate clinical ladder program. *Am Nurse,* 20:13 (September 1988).

28. Moritz P. Innovative nursing practice models and patient outcomes. *Nurs Outlook,* 39:111–114 (May–June 1991).

29. Stevens B. *The nurse as executive,* 3rd ed. Rockville, MD: Aspen Systems Corporation, 1985, pp. 106–110.

30. Fassel GE. A courageous voice for nursing. *Nurs Outlook,* 39:115–119 (May–June 1991).

31. Fairbanks J. Primary nursing: What's so exciting about it? *Nurs 80,* 10:55–57 (November 1980).

32. Stevens, op. cit., pp. 106–110.

33. Betz M, O'Connell L. Primary nursing: Panacea or problem? *Nurs and Health Care,* 8:457–460 (October 1987).

34. Chavigny K, Lewis A. Team or primary nursing care? *Nurs Outlook,* 32:322–326 (November–December 1984).

35. Bennett M, Hylton J. Modular nursing: Partners in professional practice. *Nurs Mgt,* 21:20–24 (March 1990).

36. Survey of nonnursing functions spots time wasters. *Am J Nurs,* 88:429 (April 1988).

37. Morse G. Resurgence of nurse assistants in acute care. *Nurs Mgt,* 21:34–36 (March 1990).

38. Stenske J, et al. Resource teams: Their structure and use. *J Nurs Admin,* 18:34–38 (April 1988).

39. The demise of the traditional 5–40 work-week? *Am J Nurs,* 81:1138–1143 (June 1981).

40. Kehrer B, et al. The temporary nursing service RN. *Nurs Outlook,* 32:212–217 (July–August 1984).

41. Hoffer W. A high-flying career for footloose nurses. *RN,* 7:96–99 (May 1984).

42. Nadolny MD. What does the infection control nurse do? *Am J Nurs,* 80:430–434 (March 1980).

43. Kibbee P. An emerging professional: The quality assurance nurse. *J Nurs Admin,* 18:30–33 (April 1988).

44. Strumpf NE, Knibbe KK. Long-term care; Fulfilling promises to the old among us. In McCloskey JC, Grace HK, eds. *Current issues in nursing,* 3rd ed. St. Louis: C.V. Mosby Company, 1990, pp. 217–225.

45. Selby TL. Opportunities in long-term care. *Am Nurse,* 22:10 (April 1990).

46. *Standards: Community health nursing practice.* Kansas City, MO: American Nurses' Association, 1980.

47. Almost the entire September 1990 issue of *American Nurse* is devoted to public health nursing.

48. Murphy D. The primary care role in occupational health nursing. *AAOHN J,* 37:470–473 (November 1989).

49. Boulay DM. A Vietnam tour of duty. *Nurs Outlook,* 37:271–273 (November–December 1989).

50. Parsons M, DeLoor R . . . to care for him who shall have borne the battle . . . The Veterans Administration today. *Nurs and Health Care,* 3:127–131 (March 1982).

51. Owen D. Reserve nursing. *Imprint,* 35:19–22 (September–October 1988).

52. Dickerson P, Nash B. The business of nursing: Development of a private practice. *Nurs and Health Care,* 6:327–329 (June 1985).

53. Welton J. Going into business as a nurse. *Am J Nurs,* 89:1639–1641 (December 1989).

54. Aydelotte M, et al. *Nurses in private practice.* Kansas City, MO: American Nurses' Foundation, 1988.

55. Dayani E, Holtmeier P. Formula for success: A company of nurse entrepreneurs. *Nurs Econ,* 2:376–381 (November–December 1984).

56. Kinlein ML. Independent nurse practitioner. *Nurs Outlook,* 20:22–25 (January 1972).

57. Smith GR. Alternative careers in nursing. *Imprint,* 30:23–24 (December 1983–January 1984).

58. Alexander-Rodriguez T. Prison health—A role for professional nursing. *Nurs Outlook,* 31:115–118 (March–April 1983).

59. Malone RE. The challenge of third world nursing. *Am J Nurs,* 90:32–37 (July 1990).

60. Rodgers S. International opportunities for nurses. *Imprint,* 35:136–142 (April 1988).

61. Bozert F, Forrester DA. A proposal for a men's health practitioner. *Image,* 21:158–161 (Fall 1989).

CHAPTER 8

POWER, AUTONOMY, INFLUENCE

OBJECTIVES

After studying this chapter, you will be able to:

1. Define autonomy and describe how a nurse functions autonomously in patient care.
2. Compare two different approaches to leadership and power.
3. Identify three obstacles to nurse influence.
4. Give examples of how nurses can be risk takers and role breakers.
5. Describe how the peer pal system works and its relationship to networking and collegiality.
6. Describe how nurses can prepare to influence health policy in their community.
7. Explain how you can market a positive nursing image.

Why bother to concern yourself with issues of power, autonomy, and influence? Maybe you don't care whether nursing is considered a profession. Maybe, right now, you plan to do your nursing job, do it well, and not get involved in issues of politics and power. Leave that to those who enjoy it. It's not as easy as that. "Right now" will become the future, and unless

278

you're unlike most people, you'll want a part in deciding the future. Chances are that you will be in the workforce for as long as 45 years. (Even if you started your nursing program late in life, you probably expect to work for at least 15 or 20 years.) Chances are also that you will be an employee most of that time, with all the constraints a bureaucracy can put on you. Without doubt you're going to want, at the least, some say about how you do your job, how best to care for your patients or clients. You won't be alone. Every survey and study done about nurses' job satisfaction comes up with autonomy as a major factor. And with autonomy, there is accountability—to the public.

If nurses do have the ability and responsibility to control their practice so that they can give the best possible care, then they have to use their knowledge, talents, and numbers to influence health care, either directly or through leaders they choose. They need to develop collegial relations that provide a support system; they need to help one another. Too often nurses have discovered this too late and have had to scramble to catch up in a health care system where the power figures started their influence training early. As a nurse, you can't divorce yourself from what your profession is; its influence or lack thereof will affect your working life in every way. A strong profession can make your practice more rewarding. Whether or not you choose to be an activist now or see that role only as part of the dim future, it's not too early to know where nursing is now in the power game and who the players are.

NURSING AUTONOMY

Professional *autonomy* has been defined as the right of self-determination and governance without external control. Identified as components of autonomy are control of the profession's education, legal recognition (licensure), and a code of ethics that persuades the public to grant autonomy. A distinction has been made between "job content" autonomy, the freedom to determine the methods and procedures to be used to deal with a given problem, and "job context" autonomy, the freedom to name and define the boundaries of the problem and the price to be paid for dealing with it.[1] The keys to autonomy as applied to nursing are that no other profession or administrative force can control nursing practice, and that the nurse has freedom of action in making judgments in patient care within the scope of nursing practice defined by the profession. Brown, referring particularly to primary nurses, described the autonomous nurse as one who

- is responsible to patient and family for total, individualized care
- is capable of independent decision making that need not be physician ratified

- has a thorough command of nursing practice
- provides direct care to patients and families, providing opportunities for their participation
- serves as consultant to patients and families, helping them to make informed decisions
- has professional parity with physicians and participates in providing patient care as a fully accountable member of the team
- provides the "complete professional model of service, education, consultation, and research."[2]

This model can apply equally to nurses in all settings.

POWER, INFLUENCE, AND LEADERSHIP

Power and influence are sometimes equated, because both affect or change the behavior of others; however, when they are separated, it is on the theory that power is the potential that must be tapped and converted to influence. Almost all authorities agree that a person or group must be valued in order to have power or influence.

All of the classic definitions of *power* include the concepts of influence, control, and strength—for instance, "the ability of a person, group, or system to use their concerted strategies, energy, or strength to influence the behavior or actions of others."[3] Power is usually seen as a social relationship, not necessarily the attribute of a person or group; it is given, maintained, or lost within those relationships.

To some, power has a negative tone of force and domination. Jacobs sees it as "essentially coercive in nature," with one person able to punish or reward according to the other's compliance; one person is, in a sense, dependent on another to gratify or deny his or her needs.[4] This concept has made power seem bad or corrupt, in the mode of Lord Acton's famous remark, "Power tends to corrupt and absolute power corrupts absolutely." Many women and nurses shy away from being identified with such a concept. (On the other hand, there is a lot of evidence that powerlessness corrupts and impotence corrupts totally.) Power can be a positive and reciprocal process in which people are motivated to invest their time and effort to achieve goals without coercion or threats. While probably closer to the preferred nursing self-image, this type of power is much more complex and less easily achieved. It requires that power be used wisely, including clear identification of goals. "Effective use of power is associated with a high degree of responsibility, accountability, the ability to form alliances and procure resources, and the courage to take action, often in a competitive mode, in the face of obstacles and outside power."[5]

A particularly interesting concept is *reputational power,* in which power is equated with a person's reputation for being influential. Thus, reputational power is equated with real power: if people think you have power, then you have power. This theory, too, has an opposite; it says that no one individual or group necessarily dominates, but that power is diffused in the community. Power may be tied to issues and shift accordingly.[6] Here we see what might be considered nursing power at a national level. Almost all authorities agree that a person or group must be valued in order to have power or influence. French and Raven have described six sources of such power: reward power and coercive power, which seem self-explanatory; legitimate power (power derived from certain cultural values that are held or form a legitimizing act such as an election); referent power (liking or identifying with another); expert power (based on the knowledge, abilities, and credibility of the person or group); and informational power (arising from the communication activity of the person/group exerting influence).[7]

Does nursing have power? Considering these and other generally accepted concepts,[8] it is clear that nursing has the *potential* for power with its overwhelming numbers, its special knowledge and skill, and its place in public trust and is, in fact, already beginning to exercise that power, especially since the new nursing shortage has made the value of nurses much more visible. Nursing leaders also have power of various kinds, including positional power in high government policy-making positions. But what of nurses themselves? They are still complaining of lack of power on the job—the lack of autonomy and of involvement in budget setting and in policymaking. Don't they already have power?

That staff nurses have power has been demonstrated frequently when a nurse administrator has been the type of power figure who is willing to work to achieve the goals of a group or organization without using coercive/reward power and who derives satisfaction from seeing others achieve. Power is shared, and both the organization's goals and, indirectly, the individual's goals are met. The followership role of staff nurses has a definite element of power since they can affect the opinions and behaviors of others in the group. However, the power is based on how their peers and supervisors view their professional credibility, their competence, and their ability to relate to, and communicate to, others. Power, in this case, has its source in competence. When administration and staff work together to solve problems, everyone benefits.[9]

Another benefit is that nurses who work in such an environment are more satisfied with their jobs and more inclined to stay. The Magnet Hospital Study sponsored by the American Academy of Nursing showed this very clearly (see Appendix 1). Hospitals that were able to attract and hold nurses during the wildly competitive nursing shortage of the early 1980s were studied. What the staff nurses found so attractive, besides reasonable salary and benefits, were opportunities for professional practice, participatory management, nurse-nurse and physician-nurse mutual respect, and the visibility, accessibility, and support of a strong, knowledgeable director of nursing. Similar findings came out of a follow-up study.[10]

LEADERS: HOW, WHY, WHO

If the leader in the work setting is so important, it's small wonder that nursing seems to have joined the universal cry for leadership. Just what makes a leader has been the subject of both myth and science. No one really knows whether leadership occurs because an individual has or acquires certain traits; whether leaders are born, not made; whether the key is charisma, which arouses a special kind of popular loyalty and enthusiasm; or whether leadership is simply situational, so that a person can be a leader in one situation and a follower in another. Probably all of these theories have some truth. While the qualities of leadership are hard to define, they are not hard to identify. Everyone has a list of characteristics, attitudes, or behaviors that they want in a leader.

Yura et al.,[11] in their long-term research on leadership, have developed a process of leadership, which, they say, can be learned, just as the nursing process, research process, and teaching-learning process are learned (thus belying the "leaders are born, not made" myth). Noting that nursing is an interpersonal process and that a shortage of nursing leadership behavior exists, they flatly state, "Leaders in nursing can be deliberately prepared." The theoretical considerations underlying their work are based primarily on the work of Tannenbaum et al.,[12] who consider interpersonal influence to be the essence of leadership, with the leader trying to affect the behavior of followers through communications. The goals may be organizational, group, or personal for both leader and follower. To meet organizational goals, which may have little or no motivational importance, the leader may use inducements relative to the needs of the followers. Group goals evolve through interaction of group members and reflect what the group decides. The follower's personal goals are met when the leader "uses his influence to establish an atmosphere of warmth, security and acceptance, and when, through interpersonal techniques, the leader helps another to reach ends that could not possibly be reached alone."[13] The leader's personal goals may be met primarily through his or her influence and may coexist with organizational or group goals. To function successfully, the leader particularly needs sensitivity, for influence is exerted through communication. Leadership, in this concept, is a "cyclical process in that events at any step may be fed back to the leader so that modification in behavior may be made and parts of the sequence can be altered"[14] (if not successful).

These concepts are very similar to what has been called *transformational leadership,* linked to a "paradigm shift of world view," characterized by "mutuality and affiliation, acknowledging complexity and ambiguity, cooperation versus competition; an emphasis on human relations, process versus task, acceptance of feelings, networking versus hierarchy, and recognition of the value of intuition."[15] Another similarity is shared power, which tends to be a feminine style of leadership since women have been socialized to operate from an interpersonal focus. This beta-style leadership is more complex and more open than alpha style. There is emphasis on interdependence in relationships and human interaction as a source of power, differing from the male-oriented alpha-style of leadership, which is direct, aggressive, and competitive, striving for all or nothing, clear win-or-lose, and zero-sum solutions.

People do have definite feelings about what they want in leaders. Kouzes and Posner state that leadership is in the eye of the follower, and that credibility and a sense of direction are the essence of leadership. They report that the most often cited attributes that followers expect of their leaders are integrity, competence, forward looking, inspiring, intelligence, fair-minded, broad-minded, straightforward, imaginative, and dependable.[16] Exhibit 8-1 describes other qualities of leadership.

Are similar traits important in nursing leadership? Who are nursing's leaders? Some studies on nursing leadership have, of course, been done, although many are simply first-level studies at the master's level. One topic that has particular potential is leadership styles. Commonly identified styles are autocratic, democratic, and bureaucratic, but new concepts have emerged: *multicratic* (moving flexibly back and forth along the continuum of leadership behaviors as the situation demands) and *professional* (basically a democratic style with much adaptability).[17]

Other nursing research on leadership has taken a people-oriented tack. In the last decade, there has been a new interest in learning about contemporary leaders. Safier's oral history gives an exciting insight into the lives and ideas of nurses who attained leadership during and after World War II, a crucial time of change for nursing.[18,19] A more recent publication presents the autobiographies of 48 nursing leaders (including the editors).[20] Various journal articles, cited in the Bibliography, also give insight into nursing's leadership.

Vance's doctoral study probably made available the first profile of contemporary nursing leaders, her so-called nursing influentials.[21] An interesting comparison can be made between the leadership traits described earlier and what these nursing leaders identified as their source of influence. In order of importance, those traits and characteristics cited as highly important by at least half of the respondents were communication skills, intellectual ability, willingness to take risks, interpersonal skills, creativity in thinking, ability to mobilize groups, recognized expertise in an area of the profession, charisma, and innovativeness. Having academic credentials, collegial sup-

Exhibit 8-1

On Leadership

What is leadership?
Its qualities are difficult to define.
But they are not so difficult to
identify.

Leaders don't *force* other
people to go along with them.
They *bring* them along. Leaders
get commitment from others by
giving it themselves, by building
an environment that encourages
creativity, and by operating with
honesty and fairness.

Leaders demand much of
themselves. They are ambitious—
not only for themselves, but also
for those who work with them.
They seek to attract, retain, and
develop other people to their full
abilities.

Good leaders aren't "lone
rangers." They recognize that an
organization's strategies for
success require the combined
talents and efforts of many
people. Leadership is the catalyst
for transforming those talents
into results.

Leaders know that when there
are two opinions on an issue,
one is not bound to be wrong.
They recognize that hustle and
rush are the allies of superficial-
ity. They are open to new ideas,
but they explore their ramifications thoroughly.

Successful leaders are emotionally and intellectually oriented
to the future—not wedded
to the past. They have a hunger
to take responsibility, to innovate,
and to initiate. They are not
content with merely taking care
of what's already there. They
want to move forward to create
something new.

Leaders provide answers as
well as direction, offer strength
as well as dedication, and speak
from experience as well as
understanding of the problems
they face and the people they
work with.

Leaders are flexible rather than
dogmatic. They believe in unity
rather than conformity. And they
strive to achieve consensus out of
conflict.

Leadership is all about getting
people consistently to give their
best, helping them to grow to
their fullest potential, and motivating them to work toward a
common good. Leaders make the
right things happen when they're
supposed to.

A good leader, an effective
leader, is one who has respect.
Respect is something you have to
have in order to get. A leader
who has respect for other people
at all levels of an organization,
for the work they do, and for
their abilities, aspirations, and
needs, will find that respect is
returned. And all concerned will
be motivated to work together.

Courtesy of United Technologies Corporation.

port, and a professional work position of power/prestige were also considered important. Traits listed as most important for future leaders were scholarship, intelligence, courage, humanism, sense of self, vision, communication abilities, commitment, political abilities, competence, adaptability, drive, and integrity.

About 10 years later, Kinsey replicated the study.[22] Kinsey's subjects numbered 42 (compared to Vance's 71), the top 25 percent of the 10 nurse influentials identified by each positional nursing leader who was queried. Sixty-two percent (26) of these nurse influentials had also been included in Vance's study. (While the emergence of new influentials is inevitable, one wonders what, other than death or retirement, took the other 45 off the new list. As it is, 9 percent of Kinsey's subjects reported retirement.)

There were many similarities between the two studies, with no real difference shown in the influentials' occupations, clinical specialty, geographic location, or sources of influence. The average age was a little younger, and one more man was added. (Vance had only one.) These studies give some interesting information and raise some questions. Were these the kinds of leaders we needed at this stage of nursing's development? Should we now look to a new breed?

For instance, one observation about these studies is that they show a phenomenon different from other professions, at least according to one educator. Houle notes that a profession's influentials, those who develop and apply new knowledge, are as likely to be drawn from the ranks of the practitioners as from the leadership elite. The latter he identified as *positional leaders,* with a slightly different connotation than that usually applied to this term. They are seen as facilitators—persons who maintain career identification but do not practice their profession directly. Instead, they "teach, do research, organize, administer, regulate, coordinate, and engage in other activities that advance the profession."[23] In nursing the influentials also tend to be the positional leaders, as opposed to clinicians.

What are a nursing leader's responsibilities? In the nursing literature, suggestions have been made over the years, many of them related to strengthening nursing, guiding nurses to greater autonomy, and speaking for nursing to other disciplines and to the public. More than 20 years ago, a respected nurse offered four major tasks to which nursing leaders must devote themselves, tasks not yet accomplished:

1. Advancing knowledge through research;
2. Making plans for and preparing personnel in sufficient numbers to meet the nursing needs of society;
3. Creating social systems in which exemplary nursing care, excellent nursing education, and significant scientific inquiry are demonstrated and can flourish; and

4. Identifying and developing nurse leaders who vitalize nursing itself and who utilize their very substantial talents toward identifying and promoting worthwhile and cherished values of the larger society of which nursing is a vital part.[24]

Changes are beginning to happen slowly. Although having the leadership qualities discussed earlier, and even charisma, may be distinct advantages, aspects of leadership can be taught early on—and the earlier, the better. Suggestions to help novice nurses assess and develop their leadership potential have been made.[25] Every student, every nurse, soon finds that there are things that need improvement—in nursing, health care, and society. More are serious about acting to make changes. Becoming a leader at any level is the way to do it.

OBSTACLES TO POWER AND INFLUENCE

Nursing and Sexism

When it is asked why nurses, with so much potential for influence, do not seem to be able to or want to use it, there is inevitable reference to the fact that nursing is still about 97 percent a woman's profession. Even with changing legislation and attitudes, women as a whole are still subject to discrimination and are still often victims of female socialization.

For many years, most women nurses looked at nursing as a useful way to earn a living until they were married, a job to which they could return if circumstances required. Most nurses did marry, and most married nurses did drop out to raise families, working only part time, if at all. Unmarried nurses (like male nurses) were more inclined to stay in nursing but, unlike men, frequently did not plot an orderly path to positions of authority and influence. This is similar to the career patterns of other women. In business, most women have traditionally been in their thirties or forties before they realized that they either wanted to or would be forced to continue working, and by then they were often frozen in dead-end, low-prestige (but productive) jobs. When they decided to compete for power positions in management, they were up against an "old boy" network that prevented or held back their progress, the "glass ceiling." Moreover, they had to overcome their own reluctance to be aggressive and to reject traditional female social goals.

Nurses have tended to move into the administrative hierarchy more through default than intent, perhaps gathering credentials on the way. But until the last few decades, relatively few had attained power *outside* nursing, either as recognized expert practitioners within a practice setting or as representatives of nursing in health policy determination. Why? Maraldo notes: "Nurses lack the most basic fundamental source of power, self-confidence. Projection of a powerful image of the sort that emanates from a sturdy self-image escapes nursing."[26]

There is ongoing speculation about just why nurses do not seem to seek power. Is it their historical pattern of obedience to authority, which has been transmitted by education and practice? Is it their social, cultural, or economic background? Is it because, according to personality tests, nurses have a low power motive? Is it because they think they don't have what it takes to be powerful and influential—for whatever reason? This situation, too, may be changing. Women nurses now entering the field are generally more comfortable with the beliefs of feminism and see no need to take an inferior role in a profession they have chosen to make a career.

Has the women's movement had an impact on this situation? As noted in Chapter 6, despite many obstacles still in the path of women on the way up (and even of those who aren't interested in this path), the women's movement has had a tremendous influence in improving many aspects of women's lives. Yet, nurses have had an uneasy relationship with feminists as a group, in part because many feminists have incorrect knowledge about nursing and were more interested early on in encouraging women to move into the powerful male bastions of law, medicine, and business. On the other hand, many of the issues concerning nurses, such as comparable worth and child care, are also feminist issues.

Feminism can be defined as a world view that values women and confronts systematic injustices based on gender. There are a number of feminist theories and ideologies, but Chinn and Wheeler maintain that none are antimale, but are simply opposed to the "male-defined systems and ideologies that oppress women."[27] These feminists point out that, even now, women believe that they must choose between the "stifling male-defined feminine role and the more interesting male role." Overall, they feel that nursing, with its largely female component, follows "oppressed group behavior" and also tries to emulate what it sees as powerful, that is, male. Shea agrees that nursing tends to identify with the oppressor (administration? medicine?) and is sometimes self-aggressive. The fact that nurses blame themselves and each other for failure to solve the complex dilemmas of the profession is seen as another form of antifeminist self-aggression.[28] Gordon, a journalist, takes a slightly different tack. She says that women have lost the battle for equality because they have adapted to men's goals, rather than bringing women's goals, such as caring and cooperation, into the marketplace. She uses nursing as an example of the devaluation of caring.[29]

Although nurses have not always been supportive of the women's rights movement, there is general agreement that the consciousness raising that helps women to see their worth, and to love and value themselves, has not only affected individual nurses who were involved but has also made nurses in general more aware of and resistant to discrimination, whether against men or women.

The Dilemma of Nurses in a Bureaucracy

One of the major constraints to nursing autonomy and professionalism is the status of most nurses as employees in bureaucratic organizations (especially hospitals) where nursing, unlike medicine, is a department in the institutional hierarchy. The nurse executive (whatever the title) usually reports to the hospital administrator. Most decision making occurs at the top hierarchical level, and the goals of the bureaucracy are those that receive first priority. If, in the care of patients, those goals conflict with the nurse's professional goals, the nurse is in a dilemma that may result in the nurse's leaving the job or even the profession.

The other alternative has been, too often, accepting goals not necessarily in the patient's best interest: getting the work done to suit the hospital's schedule, not nursing to meet the patient's needs—a transformation from nurse professional to nurse bureaucrat. When a nurse is rewarded for this behavioral shift, there is inevitably a slow drift to a survival mentality that prevents creative risk taking. As Nightingale said, "A good nurse does not like to waste herself," and lack of adequate resources and apparent lack of respect by administrators and others for *professional* nursing practice not only creates great job dissatisfaction but may make the nurse's work "slovenly."

Job satisfaction surveys of staff nurses almost inevitably reflect two major dissatisfactions: lack of professional autonomy and the perception that they are not respected, or at least not listened to, as professionals. Some agency administrators are extremely controlling and some nurse administrators are not strong, all of which has an extremely limiting effect on nurse autonomy. Such a combination of factors has in recent years brought about a number of job actions in which the right of nurses to be involved in patient care decisions was a key issue, and nurses have won. There are also a few instances of nursing staff organizations similar to those of physicians described in Chapter 3.

This notion that shared power is loss of power has been a deterrent in nursing administration–staff relationships, but shared power can actually enhance the power of the sharers. For example, one group of nurses worked with the support of their directors of nursing to resolve specific problems that prevented them from fully utilizing their nursing knowledge. Not only were the situations improved, but the nursing staff as a whole (not just the doers) and the director both found that their power was enhanced by this exercise of shared power.[30] A newer dimension of nurse autonomy is the process by which clinical privileges are granted to NPs. This trend, too, is limited, but growing. When hospital physicians decide that they don't want to give certain nurses clinical privileges, it may turn into a court case.[31]

Physician-Nurse Relationships

Physician-nurse relationships are a large, if not major, factor in nurse autonomy. There is necessarily a fine line between overstating and understating the problems, or, as some would have it, between paranoia and servility. Physicians' recognition of nurses as coprofessionals and colleagues has been present almost since the beginning of nursing, but a hard core of physicians who see and prefer a nurse-handmaiden role, although less common than even a decade ago, still exists.

Some physicians and, to some extent, a part of organized medicine seem to have limited, stereotypic images of nurses and resist nurse autonomy—either because they honestly doubt nurses' ability to cope with certain problems (bolstered, unfortunately, by the behavior of some nurses they work with) or because they are threatened by the expansion of nursing roles. The latter is demonstrated by the periodic action of certain medical societies and boards to restrict expanded nursing practice by lobbying against the newer expanded definitions of practice in nurse practice acts, by opposing reimbursement for nursing services unless there is physician supervision, or by using their power to limit nursing practice in a particular community or health care setting.

The reasons for problems in nurse-physician relationships have been examined repeatedly. One reason given is that physician education tends to impress on the medical student a captain-of-the-ship mentality and a need for both omniscience and omnipotence (Aesculapian authority), whereas nursing education often does not develop nurses as independent and fearless thinkers. This is also seen as one cause of the doctor-nurse game in which the nurse must communicate information and advice to the physician without seeming to do so, and the physician acts on it without acknowledging the source.[32]

Other reasons include the different socioeconomic and educational status of doctors and nurses; the physicians' lack of accurate knowledge about nursing education and practice, and vice versa, which enables them to work side by side without really understanding each other or communicating adequately; different orientations to practice; nurses' lack of control over their practice, particularly in hospitals; and physicians' exploitation of nurses.

With more nurses looking toward expanded practice, the fact that many physicians surveyed do not seem comfortable with having nurses carry out responsibilities that were traditionally medicine has caused considerable misunderstanding. This is particularly true when nurses feel that they must prove themselves to be accepted in new roles and that a "role challenge" has been thrown out by physicians.

On the other hand, an increasing number of physicians encourage and promote nurse-physician collegial relationships and see them as inevitable and necessary for good health care. Joint practice and other collaboration, both at the unit level and in various manifestations of physician-nurse practitioner practice, are evidence of this cooperation.[33,34]

That doctors and nurses are willing to work together, that is, to collaborate, has a more serious meaning than symbolism. Over the years, an impressive amount of data has been gathered to show that nurse-physician collaboration has a significant outcome for patient well-being. The critical attributes of collaboration have been identified as "sharing in planning, making decisions, solving problems, setting goals and assuming responsibility; working together cooperatively; coordinating; and communicating openly."[35]

In a number of studies, it was shown that this kind of collaboration had positive results by improving the conditions of geriatric patients in several settings, including lowering mortality; lowering costs; increasing patient satisfaction; improving professional nurse-physician relationships; decreasing the hospital stay of patients; and, most dramatic, being the key factor in the life or death of ICU patients.[36]

Does the doctor-nurse game still exist? Stein is convinced that there have been major changes in the two decades since his first observations. He admits that in some places the game still functions as described in 1967, but he predicts that the changes visible elsewhere will spread. One factor is that "the image of nurses as handmaidens is giving way to that of specialty-trained and certified advanced practitioners with independent duties and responsibilities to their patients."[37] Physicians depend on this special expertise. Interdisciplinary models have also been shown to improve care in specialty areas. Stein adds that the many other influential roles nurses take in utilization review and quality assurance may threaten doctors' authority in clinical decision making. In explaining how and why the physician-nurse interaction has changed, he stresses the nurses' goal of becoming autonomous practitioners; changes such as the civil rights and women's movements and the nursing shortage; nurses' education, in terms of both content and socialization of nursing students to relate to physicians differently than in the past; the success of the National Joint Practice Commission; and the improved environment of some hospitals.

Is Stein too optimistic? Given his caveat that the doctor-nurse game still exists and realizing that everything takes time, probably not. In recent years, there have been many more reports of health care settings where the new interdependent mode prevails. Resolving the overall issue is a part of the challenge that both medicine and nursing must face.[38]

STRATEGIES FOR ACTION

Yes, nursing does have influence. Yes, nursing does have power. This is evident in areas of politics and power. It is evident in the increased status of nursing and in the expansion of nursing practice to every possible setting. It is probably a healthy sign that so many nurses are saying, "But compared to what we can do and should do, it's not enough." And they're right. The major problems within nursing are caused by the lack of cohesiveness, the lack of agreement on professional goals, the lack of planned leadership development, the diversity of nurses in background, education, and position, the lack of internal support systems, and the divisiveness of nursing subcultures, all coping with a rapidly changing society. If nursing is to have the full autonomy of a profession, there must be unity of purpose and action on major issues. Leadership is vital, but grass-roots nurses must be a part of the final decision, or achievement of the goals will continue to be an uphill struggle. Therefore, the strategies that are suggested in the following sections are the responsibility not just of nursing leaders but of all nurses.

Mentors, Networks, Collegiality: The Great Potential

The term *mentoring* is usually defined as a formal or informal relationship between an established older person and a younger one, wherein the older guides, counsels, and critiques the younger, teaching him or her (the protégé) survival and advancement in a particular field. The system has been described as the *patron system,* a continuum of advisory support relationships that make access to positions of leadership, authority, or power easier.

At the far end of the continuum is the mentor, a very powerful, influential individual. Here the relationship with the protégé is the most intense (and perhaps the most stressful). Sheehy[39] says that a mentor supports a younger adult's dreams and helps him or her to make them a reality, and is a protector and supporter who provides the extra confidence needed to take on new responsibilities, new tests of competence, and new positions. (Emphasis on competence is of paramount importance; the mentor teaches, supports, advises, and criticizes.) She also notes that the presence or absence of a mentor is enormously important in professional development.

Protégés are carefully selected. True, someone who wants another for a mentor can bring himself or herself to that person's attention, but the protégé must be seen as worthy. One group of executives cited certain qualities that they looked for in potential protégés: has depth, integrity, a curious mind, good interpersonal skills; wants to impress; has an extra dose of commitment; has a capacity to care; can communicate; understands ideas; can identify problems and help find solutions; ambitious; hard-working; willing to do things beyond the call of duty; someone looking for new avenues and new challenges; someone dedicated to a purpose; and always—someone who would be a good representative of the profession. Usually the individual is also expected to be well groomed and appropriately dressed.

Interest in mentoring in nursing has been rising in terms of preparation for scholarliness,[40] development of minority nurses,[41] and leadership in general. In relation to this last item, it is particularly important to note several pieces of extensive research, all of which point to the importance of mentors in the development of today's nursing leaders.[42–44] However, although almost everyone says that being mentored is a key to success, even quick success, others disagree.[45] After all, there are not enough true mentors for every ambitious person, and yet many succeed with no mentor at all. There is now much literature on mentoring, particularly in business and education and in research studies. A selected list is found in the Bibliography.

The sponsor—a strong patron, but less powerful than a mentor in shaping or promoting the protégé's career—is seen as next in the patron continuum, followed by the guide, less able than either of the other two to serve as benefactor or champion, but capable of providing invaluable intelligence and explaining the system, the shortcuts, and the pitfalls. (Any of these can also act as role models, although role models may also be more distant figures that are admired.) At the beginning of the continuum are the *peer pals,* peers who help each other to succeed and progress. The first step is seen as being more like the feminist concept of women helping women, less intense and exclusionary, and therefore more democratic, by allowing access to a large number of young professionals.[46]

Peer pals can create their own networks. There is a male corollary—the "good old boy" networks—which, through an informal system of relationships, provide advice, information, guidance, contact, protection, and any other support that helps a member of the group, an insider, to achieve his goals, goals obviously not in conflict with those of the group. The good old boys frequently share the same educational, cultural, or geographic background, but whatever the basis of their commonalities, mutual support is the name of the game. It could be group pressure; it could be a word to the right person at the right time; it could be simply access to information sources, but it exists. You can count on it; you can take risks; you won't be alone. (And you don't necessarily have to like each other or agree on everything.) Could this work for nurses? Why not? What is needed is a network that promotes support *of* nurses *for* nurses, men or women. A network that provides backup for the risk takers until all can become risk takers for a purpose. A network that shows unified strength on issues that can be generally agreed upon, so that the profession as well as the individual practitioner can put into practice the principles of care to which both voice commitment. A network that avoids destructive competition and instead develops new leaders at all levels through peer pals, mentors, and role models. A network that encourages differences of opinion but provides an atmosphere for reasonable compromise. In essence, a network that develops and uses the essential abilities of nurses to share, to trust, to depend on one another.

Puetz describes how to start a network in a formal sense, almost like a new organization, and offers a number of practical tips on networking, as well as other good advice about networking given by Welch:

- Learn how to ask questions.
- Try to give as much as you get.
- Follow up on contacts.
- Keep in touch with contacts.
- Report back to contacts.
- Be businesslike as you network.
- Don't be afraid to ask for what you need.
- Don't pass up any opportunities.[47]

Because networking is "in" and is sometimes seen as what one writer called a "quick fix for moving up," and because it is also new to many women, it is being abused by some. Besides the warnings noted above, networkers are advised to observe both common and uncommon courtesies: don't make excessive requests; be appreciative; be sensitive to your contacts' situation; and be helpful to others.[48]

There are already formal nurse networks in operation, often initiated by a nursing organization or subgroup made up of nurses with common interests, clinical or otherwise. The participants help each other make contacts when they relocate, or they supply needed information or suggest someone else who would know. They alert one another to job opportunities and suggest their colleagues for appointments, presentations, or awards. They give visibility to nurses and boost and praise one another, instead of being unnecessarily critical.

Could this also be called collegiality? In a sense, yes. A *colleague* is usually defined as an associate, particularly in a profession. In a thesaurus, we also find ally, aider, collaborator, helper, partner, peer, friend, cooperator, coworker, co-helper, fellow worker, teammate, or even right-hand man and buddy. The implications are great. Colleagues may be called upon confidently for advice and assistance, and will give it. Colleagues share knowledge with one another, together rounding out the necessary information to improve patient care. Colleagues challenge one another to think in new ways and to try new ideas. Colleagues encourage risk taking when the situation requires daring. Colleagues provide a support system when the risk taker needs it. Colleagues are equal, yet different—that is, they may have varying educational preparation, experience, and positions, perhaps even belong to another profession, but when they work together for a particular purpose, that work is bettered by their cooperation.

Nurses as Risk Takers

Role breakers and risk takers have been identified as essential to changing the nursing image and to acquiring autonomy. This involves personal and professional behavior on an individual level, being assertive, taking a stand on an issue, and laying claim to the part of health care that is nursing. It also means making a concerted effort to identify and change those aspects of the nursing image that are incorrect or negative to help the public understand what nursing is and does. One aspect of this new recognition is the effort made by ANA to get third-party reimbursement for nurses. Maraldo believes that this is essential if nurses are to have a power base.[49] Nursing services in institutions are frequently lumped in with the hotel services provided, and the distinct professional nursing services are not winnowed out. Thus, the public often has no idea what nursing care involves. Third-party reimbursement could provide nurses sufficient economic leverage to demand nurse-patient ratios appropriate for rendering of professional services, but nursing must also be able to justify expensive professional nurses in preference to less prepared personnel. And reimbursement of NPs would give the public greater choice in access to the health care system (and frequently much better care).[50,51]

Another aspect of role breaking is to reinforce the budding colleague relationship between nurses and other health professionals, especially physicians. This should be focused on all aspects of patient care in all places where professional nurses function. NPs and clinical specialists may, because of their specialized knowledge and skills, be quickly identified as colleagues. It has already been shown that primary nurses in hospitals and public health nurses who have full responsibility for nursing care of a group of patients are equally able to function effectively in collegial relationships. Changes are already occurring as more nurses see nursing as a career, not just a job.

Nurses as Change Agents

Nurses, the only health professionals in contact with every facet of the health care system, are in key positions to bring about change. However, planned change involves problem-solving and decision-making skills, as well as the ability to work well with others.

Why do nurses (and others) resist change? There are a number of reasons, some quite understandable: satisfaction with the current situation; a lack of clarity about what the change is; a feeling of threat from the change agent;

a feeling that the process and the result of the change have not been thought through; selective perception and retention (hearing and remembering only what you wish); too much work involved; fear of failure or disorganization; lack of two-way communication; and the belief that the change seems to benefit the change agent, not necessarily the group. It is obvious that some of these objections could be quite valid and, if not solved, would weaken the proposed change. If recognized by the change agent, they can be overcome—if the project is worthwhile and the change agent is good in human relations. If not all participants are won over, the decision must be made to stop or go ahead, trying to anticipate the negative aspects of what may become covert resistance if the resister is outvoted.

Conflicts of some kind are probably inevitable. It is important that the change agent develop effective methods of dealing with conflict. Action, rather than reaction, is the better course, but a compromise might quite realistically result. Key steps include keeping the issue in focus, clarifying the problems, encouraging two-way communication, creating dialogue that involves group members in full participation, and always remaining responsive. How a nurse handles resistance may be a matter of individual style and the particular situation.

Being a change agent is part of the leadership role, but it is also a role that can be legitimately and effectively taken by a nurse not yet at that stage of professional development. Whether working as an insider or an outsider, each of which has advantages and disadvantages, knowing the process of change, planning carefully and thoroughly, and acting strategically and with an appropriate sense of timing are essential.

Political Action

Politics may be defined as the art or science of influencing policy. There is a legitimate tendency to think of politics in the context of government, but affecting policy and operations at the institutional level is often just as important in the work life of a nurse. The term *in-house law* has been used to describe the power nurses can have if they can determine policies and procedures that affect daily practice. An example is a policy stating that nurses may (or should or must) develop and implement teaching plans for patients or arrange for referrals to the visiting nurse, all of which have been blocked by physicians or administrators in some hospitals.

It is vital that nurses participate actively in the agencies or community groups where decisions are being made, such as local or state planning agencies.[52] The strategy used to gain input may vary. A basic principle is applicable: before, during, and after gaining entree, nurses must show that they are knowledgeable, that they have something to offer, and that they can put it all together into an action package. There are many places to start, for most community groups are looking for members who work and

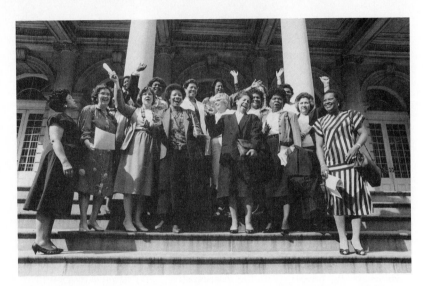

By using their political power, New York City nurses are able to celebrate a victory for better patient care. (*Courtesy of the New York State Nurses' Association.*)

are willing to hold office (for example, church groups, charity groups, and PTAs). These activities may be seen as (1) a way of getting experience on boards, using parliamentary procedure to advantage, politicking, gaining some sophistication in influencing decisions, and (2) being visible to other groups and the public. Many community groups interlock, and by being active in some, nurses come in contact with others. It also helps to gain the support of women other than nurses. Organized women are becoming more successful in getting representation on policymaking groups. It pays for them to have someone who is ready and able to assume such responsibilities. But participating nurses must be capable; there is nothing worse than having an incompetent as the first nurse on a major board or committee. That could do the profession more damage than having a nonnurse, for it appears that women (and nurses) still have to be better than those already in power to gain initial respect.

Another aspect to consider and use is the potential economic power of nurses. A nurse executive who controls a multimillion-dollar budget wields power in determining how that money is spent. This kind of status enables these nurses to move in power circles where they can cultivate individuals who influence public and private decision making. Community nurses are also particularly good resources, because most make strong community contacts. Today the participation of the consumer in health care decisions is increasing. An activated consumer who supports nursing has impact on local decision making, as well as on state and national legislation. A legislator is more inclined to hear the consumer who presumably is a neutral participant, as opposed to an obvious interest group. But nursing must sell that consumer the profession's point of view, and must balance consumer needs and nursing goals.

Although it is often through the influence of consumer groups and the community's traditional power figures that nurses get on decision-making committees, boards, and similar groups, after that, they're on their own and must be prepared, perceptive, articulate, and under control.[53] In meetings and at coffee breaks, the politicking and the formation of coalitions may well influence which way a decision goes. Nurses who haven't learned to play that game had better take lessons: using role play, assertiveness training, group therapy, group process, speech lessons—whatever is necessary. As Stevens advises power seekers:

- Pay the entry fee
- Have a voice
- Have something to say
- Look upward and outward (not just at nursing)
- Act like a powerful person[54]

This kind of political participation will be particularly important as the cost control mentality gains momentum.

On the level of governmental politics, nurses not only can and have influenced such issues as Social Security, quality assurance, patients' rights, and care of the long-term patient, but have a vital interest in such issues as reimbursement for nursing services, use of technology, children's services, nurse licensure, funds for nursing education, and a national health plan. The specifics of the legislative process and guidelines for action are described in Chapter 10. However, in addition, there is no reason that nurses should not run for office. They are intelligent, frequently well educated, and know a lot about human relations. Those who have won office are not only effective, but often offer extraordinary insight into health issues.[55] Some have been responsible for major legislative breakthroughs for nursing and health care. This is equally true of the dynamic group in regulatory agencies and congressional offices.[56,57] Profiles of some of these nurses are presented in Chapter 4. These women always point out the importance of nurse involvement in health policy formation.[58]

Regardless of the setting, there are some basic guidelines for effective political action. The first is to know the social and technical aspects of professional practice; second, to know the current professional issues and the implications for various alternative actions; third, to be aware of emerging social and political issues and trends that will affect health care and nursing; fourth, to learn others' points of view (those of potential supporters or opponents) and come to terms with what policy changes are possible, as well as desirable; and fifth, to seek allies who can espouse or at least see the desirability of a particular course of action.

Accountability and Professionalism

Without demonstrating accountability for practice, nursing will never be or be considered an autonomous profession. Standard setting, peer review, continued competence, and protection of patients' rights all indicate that nursing is taking on the responsibilities to see that the public is protected. However, more nurses must also recognize that for nurses to be professional, the majority of practitioners must consider nursing a career and make the time, effort, and commitment necessary to participate in the key decision making.

Fagin says that "the higher chronicity, the increased percentage of aged persons in the population, the public's recognition of the importance of leading healthier lives and taking steps to prevent illness, and everyone's interest in keeping costs down—force us to take a new look at our profession."[59] She points out the importance of blending our concern with quality with a concern for gaining autonomy, recognition, and suitable compensation. She notes elsewhere that nursing has delivered cost-effective care that can be substituted for physician services, has provided new services in long-term care, and has continued to provide high-level services in hospitals, showing cost savings through their productivity.[60]

As to the nursing shortage, beside the recruitment and retention activities, is it not important to see how nursing service could be managed better, as there will not be enough nurses for some time? New models are being developed, both for this purpose and to improve patient care.[61]

These are only a few of the issues that require professional nursing input, but there are many others, such as the ethical/legal dilemmas that can only increase in the coming years. All are aspects of nurses' accountability and professionalism.

Professional Unity, Professional Pride

It is a political fact that the most powerful groups are those that are united. Almost always this means that an organization speaks for that group, and that is one of the purposes of a professional organization. Nursing has many organizations representing various interest groups (see Chapter 14). At times they cooperate, but too often they are at odds or simply act separately. Fortunately, more serious efforts are being made by most groups to form political coalitions in relation to important issues for nurses. This trend may or may not overcome the fact that only about 10 percent of nurses belong to the largest nursing organization, ANA. Yet almost everyone agrees that support of the professional organization, where unity and a resolution of internal problems must occur, is crucial if nursing is to be an autonomous, influential power group.

Unity is hard to achieve, however, if you're not proud of yourself and your profession and what it stands for; if you're embarrassed by nursing's image or if, worse yet, you believe it. Because then, nurses are not a group with whom you want to be identified. Unity is not important because it doesn't seem worth the effort. The feeling of powerlessness is a comfort, in a sense, because it excuses you from taking action. That action *can* be taken is illustrated in the preceding pages. To look at the image of nursing is to see what you want to see. A nurse is not one kind of person, good or bad, handmaiden or entrepreneur. Nursing, like its components, has various images at various times. When you are that reflection, it should be what you want nursing to be.

A small point—or, perhaps, a large one: the fashionable image might be woman as slob, but nurse as slob is not attractive. Thirty years ago, how to dress was taught in nursing schools to young working-class women. A sloppy uniform was cause for a reprimand. The same was true for the RN. Then that was no longer considered appropriate; modern women knew how to dress and behave in a socially correct manner without needing grammar school lessons. Are the results evident today? But perhaps we've come full circle. The business literature aimed at men and women is full of advice on "dressing for success," and now it might be nursing's turn. What is nursing's image when a patient is cared for by an unkempt nurse in nondescript clothes with long hair sweeping across the patient's body?[62] Yes, the public does notice. One individual being treated in a college health clinic reported, "I wondered who that person was in blue jeans and a top like men's underwear." A noted editor said at a meeting, "If you nurses are so worried about your image, you'd better clean up your nurses." Not you? Then perhaps a little peer pressure would help—a little direct or indirect action. Personal image and nonverbal behavior do convey a message—possibly a message of "no pride, no interest." Now, both nurses and their employees are taking a second look at this state of affairs and making changes. So are students.[63] A positive image creates power. Who better than the nurses can shape that image?

It is time to look at what nursing has accomplished and is continuing to accomplish. It is a career of unlimited opportunities. It has produced documented evidence that its practitioners make major contributions to health care. And they are reaping some rewards. For instance, another change that is evolving is legal approval for third-party reimbursement. In 1990, 23 states had already given approval; in 8, there was direct reimbursement from insurance companies without legislative mandate; and in 25, they received direct Medicaid reimbursement.[64]

Although the focus is on NPs, all these activities include nurse-midwives and nurse anesthetists and, perhaps later, other kinds of nurse specialists. Moreover, nursing has exercised political power for the good of the public.

There's a lot to be legitimately proud of, even if there is unfinished business. Power and autonomy do not come to the spineless, the indifferent or downtrodden, or those who think they are.

Everyone has his or her own concerns, but individuals acting in isolation are vulnerable. In this era of social revolution, more and more individuals are uniting to secure their legitimate rights and privileges. Why would nursing want less? As Edith Draper, one of nursing's leaders, said in 1893, "To advance, we must unite."

KEY POINTS

1. Professional autonomy is one of the most crucial aspects of satisfying practice in nursing.
2. Power can be coercive, but a more effective approach is shared power that strengthens both leader and follower.
3. Staff nurses have real power that can be used positively.
4. Nurses who are women must overcome some of the stereotypes others have of what women can and can't do.
5. Physician-nurse relationships can be problems or assets, depending on how the two professions understand each other and whether each sees the other as rival or colleague.
6. Peers as colleagues enhance one another's practice.
7. Networking is an effective way to broaden professional opportunities.
8. Nurses can have a strong impact on health policymaking by their effective participation in community groups.
9. Nurses who have pride in nursing and themselves and, with others, work together to strengthen it will be major factors in moving nursing forward.

REFERENCES

1. Dachelet C, Sullivan J. Autonomy in practice. *Nurse Practitioner,* 4:15 (March–April 1979).
2. Brown B. The autonomous nurse and primary nursing. *Nurs Admin Q,* 1:33 (Fall 1976).
3. *Webster's new collegiate dictionary.* Springfield, MA: G.&C. Merriam Company, 1975.
4. Jacobs T. *Leadership and exchange in formal organizations.* Alexandria, VA: Human Resources Research Organization, 1970, p. 4.

5. Wynd C. Packing a punch! Female nurses and the effective use of power. *Nurs Success Today,* 2:1520 (September 1985).
6. Tatano C. The conceptualization of power. *Adv Nurs Sci,* 4:2–17 (January 1982).
7. French J, Raven B. The base of social power. In Cartwright D, ed. *Studies in social power.* Ann Arbor: Institute of Social Research, University of Michigan, 1959, pp. 150–167.
8. Harsanyi J. Measurement of social power, opportunity, costs, and the theory of two-person bargaining games. In Belle R, et al., eds. *Political power.* New York: Free Press, 1969, p. 226.
9. Cipriani P. Staff nurse power can solve problems. *Nurs Success Today,* 2:13–16 (May 1985).
10. Kramer M. Trends to watch at the magnet hospitals. *Nurs 90,* 20:67–74 (June 1990).
11. Yura H, et al. *Nursing leadership: Theory and process,* 2nd ed. New York: Appleton-Century-Crofts, 1981.
12. Tannenbaum R, et al. *Leadership and organization.* New York: McGraw-Hill Book Company, 1961.
13. Yura et al., op. cit., p. 88.
14. Ibid., p. 90.
15. Barker AM. An emerging leadership paradigm: Transformational leadership. *Nurs and Health Care,* 12:204–207 (April 1991).
16. Kouzes J, Posner B. *The leadership challenge.* San Francisco: Jossey-Bass Publishers, 1988, pp. 15–27.
17. Brooten D. *Managerial leadership in nursing.* New York: J.B. Lippincott Company, 1984, pp. 34–35.
18. Safier G. Leaders among contemporary U.S. nurses: An oral history. In Chaska N, ed. *The nursing profession: Views through the mist.* New York: McGraw-Hill Book Company, 1978.
19. Safier G. *Contemporary American leaders in nursing: An oral history.* New York: McGraw-Hill Book Company, 1977.
20. Schorr T, Zimmerman A. *Making choices, taking chances.* St. Louis: C.V. Mosby Company, 1988.
21. Vance C. A group profile of contemporary influentials in American nursing. Unpublished EdD dissertation, Teachers College, Columbia University, 1977. A detailed review of this and Kinsey's study is found in Kelly LY. *Dimensions of professional nursing,* 5th ed. New York: Macmillan Publishing Company, 1985, pp. 364–365.
22. Kinsey D. The new nurse influentials. *Nurs Outlook,* 34:238–240 (September–October 1986).
23. O'Connor A. Continuing education for nursing's leaders. In Chaska N, ed. *The nursing profession: A time to speak.* New York: McGraw-Hill Book Company, 1983, pp. 156–165.
24. Schlotfeldt R. Knowledge, leaders and progress. *Image,* 2:2–5 (February 1968).
25. Lee J. Leadership in practice. *Imprint,* 34:57–59 (April–May 1987).
26. Maraldo P. The illusion of power. In Wieczorek R, ed. *Power, politics*

and policy in nursing. New York: Springer Publishing Company, 1985, p. 71.

27. Chinn P, Wheeler C. Feminism and nursing. *Nurs Outlook,* 33:74 (March–April 1985).

28. Shea C. Feminism: A failure in nursing? In McCloskey J, Grace H, eds. *Current issues in nursing.* St. Louis: C.V. Mosby Company, 1990, pp. 448–453.

29. Gordon S. *Prisoners of men's dreams.* Boston: Little, Brown and Company, 1991.

30. Gorman S, Clark N. Power and effective nursing practice. *Nurs Outlook,* 34:129–134 (May–June 1986).

31. Jenkins S. Exercising nurses' right to fight for clinical privileges. *Nurs and Health Care,* 7:477–482 (November 1986).

32. Stein L. The doctor-nurse game. *Arch Gen Psychiatry,* 16:699–703 (June 1967). Reprinted in *Am J Nurs,* 68:101–105 (January 1968).

33. Devereux P. Essential elements of nurse-physician collaboration. *J Nurs Admin,* 11:19–23 (May 1981).

34. Alt-White A, et al. Personal, organizational and managerial factors related to nurse-physician collaboration. *Nurs Admin Q,* 8:8–18 (Fall 1983).

35. Baggs J, Schmitt M. Collaboration between nurses and physicians. *Image,* 20:145–148 (Fall 1988).

36. Kelly L. A matter of life and death. *Nurse Outlook,* 34:175 (July–August 1986).

37. Stein L, et al. The doctor-nurse game revisited. *N Engl J Med,* 322:546–549 (February 22, 1990). Reprinted in *Nurs Outlook,* 38:264–268 (November–December 1990).

38. Mariano C. The case for interdisciplinary collaboration. *Nurs Outlook,* 37:285–288 (November–December 1989).

39. Sheehy G. *Passages: Predictable crises of adult life.* New York: E.P. Dutton & Co., 1976.

40. May K, et al. Mentorship for scholarliness: Opportunities and dilemmas. *Nurs Outlook,* 30:22–28 (January 1982).

41. Weekes DL. Mentor-protégé relationships: A critical element in affirmative action. *Nurs Outlook,* 37:156–157 (July–August 1989).

42. Vance, op. cit.

43. Kinsey, op. cit.

44. Spengler C. Mentor-protégé relationships: A study of career development among female nurse doctorates. Unpublished PhD dissertation. University of Missouri-Columbia, 1982.

45. Hagerty B. A second look at mentors. *Nurs Outlook,* 34:16–19 (January–February 1986).

46. Shapiro E, et al. Moving up: Role models, mentors, and the patron system. *Sloan Mgt Rev,* 19:51 (Spring 1978).

47. Puetz B. *Networking for nurses.* Rockville, MD: Aspen Systems Corporation, 1983, pp. 63–80.

48. Handler J. Networking: The rules of the game. *Savvy,* 5:90–91 (April 1984).

49. Maraldo, op. cit., p. 71.
50. Diers D, Molde S. Nurses in primary care: The new gatekeepers? *Am J Nurs*, 83:742–745 (May 1983).
51. *Nurse practitioners, physician assistants, and certified nurse-midwives: A policy analysis*. Washington, DC: Office of Technology Assessment, 1986.
52. Donaho BA. Creating wider circles of influence. *Nurs Outlook*, 38:134–135 (May–June 1990).
53. Porter-O'Grady T. A nurse on the board. *J Nurs Admin*, 21:40–46 (January 1991).
54. Stevens B. Power and politics for the nurse executive. *Nurs and Health Care*, 1:208–212 (November 1980).
55. McCarty P. Nursing is political asset, say four RNs. *Am Nurse*, 21:15 (January 1989).
56. Barry C. Profiles of nurses professionally involved in public policy. *Nurs Econ*, 8:174–176 (May–June 1990).
57. Clark L. The advice of an expert: Making a difference on Capitol Hill. *Nurs and Health Care*, 9:291–293 (June 1988).
58. Senate outlook: An interview with Sheila Burke. *Nurs and Health Care*, 6:245–249 (May 1985).
59. Fagin C. Opening the door on nursing's cost advantage. *Nurs and Health Care*, 7:353–357 (September 1986).
60. Fagin C. Nursing's value proves itself. *Am J Nurs*, 90:17–18, 22, 25, 29, 30 (October 1990).
61. Moritz P. Innovative nursing practice models and patient outcomes. *Nurs Outlook*, 39:111–114 (May–June 1991).
62. Little D. The "strip tease" of nurse symbols or nurse dress code: No code. *Imprint*, 31:49–52 (February–March 1984).
63. Smith B, Nerone BJ. Marketing a profitable nursing image: Recognizing image is power. *Imprint*, 33:26–30 (March–April 1986).
64. 1990–1991 Update: How each state stands on legislative issues affecting advanced nursing practice. *Nurse Practitioner*, 16:11–18 (January 1991).

PART IV

NURSING ETHICS AND LAW

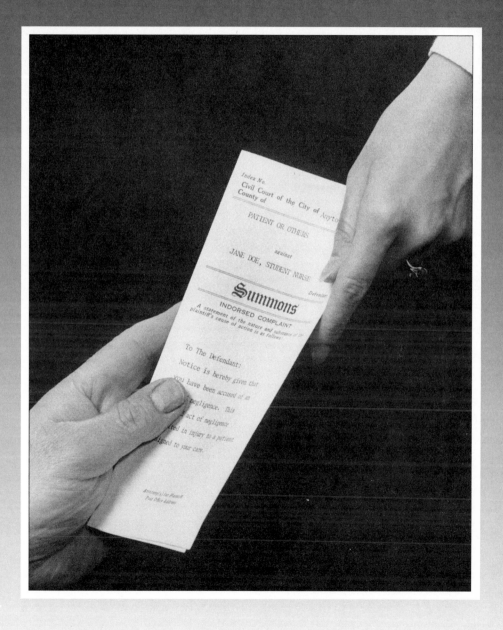

CHAPTER 9

ETHICAL ISSUES IN NURSING AND HEALTH CARE

OBJECTIVES

After studying this chapter, you will be able to:

1. Differentiate between the concepts of morals and ethics.
2. Recognize the kinds of dilemmas nurses and others face in health care.
3. List factors that create these dilemmas.
4. List factors that influence the way you react to ethical problems.
5. Develop a way of assessing and dealing with ethical concerns.
6. Relate and apply the ANA Code for Nursing to your professional life.
7. List two ways in which nurses can demonstrate accountability in practice.

Most people who decide to enter nursing are aware that there are times that they will be dealing with life and death. If they think about it to any extent, they probably assume that they would do their best to help the patient to live or keep him or her comfortable until death. Asked whether they expected to have a conflict with the law or with other colleagues or even a conflict within themselves at such a time, they would probably react with astonishment. How could this happen? If you asked whether they expected to have any trouble behaving ethically in these situations, the reply might well be, "Why would I?"

Is that the way you felt? Is that the way you feel now? It's quite possible that the shock of dealing with ethical questions is not as great now as it might have been even a few years ago. Movies, plays, television, books, magazines, and even newspaper reports are beginning to recognize that the ethical dilemmas in health care faced every day by those in the field must also be faced by the public.

WHAT CREATES ETHICAL DILEMMAS?

Why are things different now? One simple answer is that it is a much more complex world, with many conflicting pressures on both consumers and providers. For instance:

1. Technology in the form of transplants, artificial parts, and machinery can keep alive young and old patients who would once have died, **but** the cost of surviving after such intervention may be so high financially that either the government must pay for both the treatment and lifelong care, or only the rich can afford it. An average family would become impoverished. In some cases, the public pays to keep alive a nonfunctioning human being and then has to deny resources to someone with the possibility of a productive life. And people's notions are changing about whether the quality of life made possible by technology, or its sanctity, is most important.
2. People are beginning to recognize their right to make decisions about their medical treatment even if the decision would lead to death; **but** even though family and significant others agree with the individual, his or her wish may be thwarted after the individual becomes technically "incompetent," because the health professionals and/or institutions are afraid of lawsuits, and the law does not clearly define how or whether such wishes can be carried out.
3. The law does cover certain rights, such as abortion, **but** groups with their own religious or moral agendas try to prevent people from exercising those rights.
4. In general, the public accepts the idea that everyone has a right to health care, **but** there are limited resources and no one ways to pay for the reality of equal access.

These situations may not only create conflict between professionals and family but pit colleague against colleague, health professional against administration, family against courts, lawyer against lawyer, church against individuals, and any variation of these. Yet, almost everyone wants to do what is right. What is "right"? It's not easy to decide. Look at these not uncommon ethical dilemmas.

- A fragile man in his eighties, riddled with cancer, is admitted to the hospital. When his heart stops, he is resuscitated and awakens with tubes in every orifice. He begs to be allowed to die but is repeatedly resuscitated.
- A 26-year-old quadriplegic woman with cerebral palsy has herself admitted to a hospital and then asks to be kept comfortable, but allowed to die by starvation because she finds life unbearable. The hospital force-feeds her.
- An 85-year-old man with many illnesses has been fasting in a nursing home to hasten his death. His daughter supports his decision, and he dies in a few days.
- Two physicians terminate intravenous feeding of a comatose man, with the consent of the family. They are reported by nurses and criminally prosecuted.
- A baby is born with Down's syndrome and various other congenital defects, one of which requires immediate surgery in order to save the infant's life. The parents refuse permission because they believe that the child, if she survives, will not have a reasonable quality of life and they will not be able to care for her.
- Another baby with similar defects undergoes surgery, but the mother, an unwed teenager, cannot keep the child. It is in a public institution, requiring total care for all of its five years of life.
- A depressed patient admitted to a mental hospital refuses electroshock therapy after several treatments because he thinks it will kill him even though he is improving with treatment. He cannot care for himself at home, and his wife cannot manage his erratic behavior. He is committed, under the state's laws, given the treatment, and recovers.
- A retarded 15-year-old boy in the county home refuses kidney dialysis because he fears it. No effort is made to relieve his anxiety, and others on the hospital's waiting list are moved forward into therapy. The boy dies.
- Two men on the same hospital unit have a cardiac arrest within several minutes of each other. The first to arrest is an alcoholic street person with various other conditions; the other is a businessman with a wife and four children. There is one cardiopulmonary resuscitation cart. The resident says, "First come, first served" and resuscitates the alcoholic; the businessman dies.
- A young couple with two boys decides that they can afford only one

more child and want a girl. If amniocentesis indicates a boy, the mother wants an abortion.

• A couple has been advised that they are carriers of a hereditary disease. Two of their teenage children have it, and one does not. When the mother becomes pregnant again, she decides on an abortion, but both parents decide not to "spoil the children's lives" by telling them they may later manifest the disease.

• A patient about to undergo surgery clearly does not understand the risks or the available alternatives. The nurse tells the physician, but he replies that he did explain, that patients seldom understand these explanations, and that the patient should be prepared for surgery.

• A patient with cancer is on an experimental drug. Although hospital policy states that the physician must get an informed consent before the drug is administered, the patient's very prestigious physician calls in and tells the nurse to start the drug because it is important to begin at once; he will be in later to get the consent. When the nurse hesitates, her supervisor tells her to go ahead.

If you were the nurse involved in any of these situations, what would you do? Whose rights are or might be violated? The patient's? The family's? The nurse's? The doctor's? Society's? Nobody's? How much would you be affected by your own moral beliefs? If your action was contrary to what the hospital administrators, the physicians involved, or even some of your colleagues thought best (for whatever reason), would you be willing to face the consequences? What if your concept of "right" collided with a legal ruling? What if the patient or family asked you to help them?

All of these cases cited are real, but not always made public. A nurse somewhere faced one of these difficult situations (and probably others) and had to make the decision to act or not to act. How that decision was arrived at is the essence of ethics.

Almost every day, some situation that has presented an ethical dilemma to family, friends, health care professionals, and health care institutions is reported in the media, often because it is no longer in the arena of unofficial voluntary action but has become a legal battle. One that got months of attention is the case of Nancy Cruzan, who after a car accident remained in a permanent vegetative state (PVS) for years. When her parents wanted her gastric tube feeding discontinued so that she could die peaceably, objections by others eventually took the case to the U.S. Supreme Court.[1] (This is discussed in Chapter 13.) The aftermath of this decision had legal implications for what might once have been a private matter, decided according to the ethical beliefs of the family and the quiet cooperation of like-minded health professionals. In fact, it has been estimated that some 75 percent of those who die in hospitals die because some potential life-prolonging treatment is willingly withheld. Once, these issues would not have come up at all. People got sick and died, probably at home. Grossly malformed infants were quietly allowed to die. There was no technology to keep these people alive, and except in very rare circumstances, available life-prolonging techniques like feeding tubes were not used. Dying was a natural act—sad, perhaps, but inevitable.

There was also a quiet understanding that a dying patient in pain could be helped to die, perhaps by giving a larger dose of a narcotic than usual. Doctors ordered it; nurses gave it. Yet, one of the big ethical issues evolving is *doctor-assisted suicide*. An opinion piece by a physician was published in a respected medical journal, describing how he had prescribed barbiturates for a patient dying of cancer, at her request. He knew her well and knew she had asked because this was an essential ingredient in Hemlock Society (a right-to-die group) suicide.[2] The article created some furor but no legal prosecution, as opposed to the reaction to another physician who helped a woman with early Alzheimer's disease to commit suicide with a "death machine." Even that case was eventually dismissed, and he helped others to die later. Just how many dying or PVS patients are helped to die will never be known. But to some nurses and others, *not* to help them would be unethical; to others, to do so would be both unethical and worthy of legal action.

On a much larger scale is the ethical question of access to care when limited access could well result in death. Not a nursing problem? But it is: every time a nursing unit is short-staffed and a nurse must make continuous decisions on priorities, the possibility of some patients being neglected and even dying becomes a reality.[3] In fact, nurses have admitted that this is exactly what happens, because they have no other choice.[4] Moreover, the very fact that nurses are the largest group of health professionals makes them important players in resolving issues of access to care, difficult though this is. An example is the national health plan developed by the Tri-Council, which represented much of nursing on this issue; this is described in Chapter 3.

True, there has never been equal access to health care. True, ethical dilemmas have always existed in health care. But in recent years, just as the focus on the more dramatic right-to-live/right-to-die ethical issues have become more visible, the problem of access to care for the poor and those 37 million or so individuals with little or no health insurance is being seen as not only a political issue, but an ethical one. For instance, new technology has created many new opportunities to save lives. Yet, almost inevitably, these therapies are extremely expensive both initially and in follow-up care. Should those who cannot pay for such care be denied? If not, who will pay for it? The government?

In an era of limited resources that will probably never change, what other funding should be cut? Education? Environment? Housing? Social services?

Transportation? Civil rights enforcement? Drug enforcement? Police? Defense? Not only is the decision not a simple one, it is highly political. Every one of the other areas that exists primarily through public funding is important, one way or another, to the public's well-being. Every legislator has one or more constituencies that demand attention to their needs or wishes. Therefore, it's not surprising that legislative action is slow in coming, seldom satisfactory, and, unfortunately, hardly enacted before it is evident that the action taken is not enough, too much, or already out of date. Moreover, the cost factor will undoubtedly increase, not decrease, and new, expensive technology continues to develop.

So, what happens? Except in rare instances, limits are set by default. What standards, if any, should be used to determine who gets what? There has been considerable discussion about age as a criterion, especially in terms of prolonging the life of an elderly patient. In part, this is because a large percentage of Medicare funds is used for life-prolonging care in the last few months of an elderly patient's life. (The fact that such a person may not wish such care, but is given no choice, is another issue.) Clearly it is not easy to use age as an indicator. However, there *have* been suggestions that certain limits be set on care for those who have "lived out a natural life span."[5]

In the case of transplants, there are additional questions related to the number any one person should get, use of experimental techniques,[6] "harvesting" organs from an irrevocably damaged newborn,[7] using the tissues of aborted fetuses,[8] using mechanical hearts,[9] and—what used to be a private issue—having a baby on the chance that its tissues or bone marrow might save a sibling.[10]

These questions, all relating to real situations, do not necessarily call for a negative response. The point is that there are so many questions, seldom clear-cut answers, and never easy answers. Overall, putting aside the legal ramifications, the health care provider simply acts according to his or her own moral beliefs or sometimes in accordance with the needs or attitude of the health care institution. For instance, in a study on how people were selected for kidney transplants, there clearly were unwritten criteria, none of which were reported as being age or race.[11] Another study showed that white men were more likely to receive kidney transplants than white women or blacks of either sex.[12] There is also some evidence that patients with AIDS were much more likely to have "do not resuscitate (DNR)" orders.

What should be done about these access issues? Many suggestions have been made, but little agreement has been reached. Some ask "Can we any longer afford the moral price of inequity in health care?"[13] and maintain that although it might prove costly, a universal system of health insurance and government- and employer-based programs are the only answer. Others say that we must set limits for new technology if it is too costly.[14] Ideas for national health plans (insurance?) are discussed endlessly in Congress and in the media, as well as in the health care literature (see the Bibliography). Still others have simply concluded that overt, orderly rationing of health care is inevitable.

Oregon has taken such a step,[15] but the philosophy is that this actually *increases* access to health care.[16] In 1990, the state government approved a plan to "insure equitable access without excessive burdens to an adequate level of health care for all, including all not currently covered by some form of health insurance and extend Medicaid coverage to the maximum allowed by the Federal government." A commission, including a public health nurse, set priorities after a series of community meetings. Prevention, quality of life, and cost effectiveness headed the list of community values elicited at these meetings. Of course, not everyone agreed;[17] people often seem to prefer silent to overt rationing. Yet the priority of, for instance, primary care for all, especially children and pregnant women, as opposed to access to certain life-prolonging treatments, seemed sensible to others. The list is still in revision, but it includes preventive care for children, burn treatment, chronic disorders of the back, and comfort care for cancer and AIDS patients. Oregon does require approval of the federal government to make changes in Medicaid. This situation is still in limbo.

As mentioned earlier, the rapid spread of AIDS has created new ethical dilemmas. Some health professionals refuse to treat or even interact with patients with AIDS.[18] Do they have that right?[19] Although nurses have been applauded for the quality of personalized care they have given to AIDS patients, a number of studies have shown that the majority of nurses feel that nurses should have a right to refuse to care for AIDS patients, especially if the nurse is pregnant. The majority, also given the choice, would prefer not to care for AIDS patients.[20] However, the reason appears to be fear of infection, not matters of morality or prejudices. (This raises the questions of whether all patients should be tested for AIDS; doctors and nurses think so. What then of testing health professionals?) In addition, the issue of confidentiality is at the forefront. Do families of AIDS patients have the right to know the patient's diagnosis if the patient doesn't want them to know?[21] Should health professionals reveal whether they are infected? They think not.

As you read the sections on morality and the various theories of ethics, as well as the nursing code of ethics, consider the ethical problems given as examples and note how your decisions depend on your ethical or, perhaps, moral beliefs.

Even if you are not in a position to make a direct decision, you will be in that environment where such dilemmas will continue to occur, and you will have to come to some understanding about how you can deal with them, directly or indirectly. There is no such thing as "no decision."

FACTORS THAT INFLUENCE ETHICAL DECISION MAKING

Morals and Ethics

There is a tendency to use the words *moral* and *ethical* interchangeably in the literature of health professions. However, in the last few years, the need to differentiate between the two terms has become more evident. One simple explanation is:

> Morality is generally defined as behavior according to custom or tradition. Ethics, by contrast, is the free, rational assessment of courses of actions in relation to precepts, rules, conduct. . . . To be ethical a person must take the additional step of exercising critical, rational judgment in his decisions.[22]

Kohlberg, structuring a theory of moral development, used the term *stages* for individual phases of moral thinking.[23] Although his theory is still widely used when discussing moral development, there is some disagreement with his approach, in part because of certain limitations in his study, including the fact that he had only male subjects.

Gilligan[24] was particularly disturbed that Kohlberg did not acknowledge the concerns and experience of women in moral development. She carried out a study designed to clarify the nature of women's moral judgment as they faced the moral dilemma of whether to continue or abort a pregnancy. Results showed that women's moral judgment differs from that of men. For women, the worst problem was defined in terms of exercising care and avoiding hurt. The infliction of hurt was seen as selfish and immoral. "Women's moral judgment proceeded from initial concern for survival, to focus on goodness, to a principled understanding of care."[25]

The whole issue of ethics versus morals may seem to be purely philosophical; however, given the differentiation described, the code of ethics of professional nurses may require action that goes beyond what their immediate associates see as necessary. It is also possible that individuals must struggle with what seems to be a conflict between ethical behavior and personal religious beliefs.

Theories

There are a number of theories on which ethical decision making is based. Using the cases mentioned earlier as examples, some of these theories will now be described.[26]

The *egoism* theory says that a decision is right because the doer or "agent," in this case the nurse, desires it; it is the most comfortable one for that person, without consideration for how the decision might affect others. For example, the nurse may simply prepare the patient for surgery, accepting the doctor's statement that the patient was given an adequate explanation.

The theory of *deontology* (formalism) asserts that rightness or wrongness must be considered in terms of its moral significance. *Act deontology* considers the agent's own moral values. *Rule deontology* suggests that there are rules or standards for judging morally, often a command by God. Thus, a nurse may oppose abortion because of either personal moral beliefs or religious beliefs.

Utilitarianism defines right as the greatest good and the least amount of harm for the greatest number of people. For instance, deformed babies might be allowed to die rather than be a burden on society for many years.

Justice as fairness—the distribution of benefits (good) or harm (evil) to society—is Rawls's theory. The two principles of justice are equal rights for everyone and the greatest benefit given to the least advantaged. With this reasoning, the retarded boy would take precedence over others for the kidney dialysis, and efforts would be made to persuade him into therapy.

These theories, which have been presented very briefly, and others, are often complex and sometimes appear more philosophical than practical. However, they provide an interesting framework for ethical decision making.[27]

Code of Ethics

Another guide to ethical behavior is a professional code of ethics. In the last several years, ethical behavior has been increasingly a topic of discussion in almost every field—business, politics, law, and, perhaps most of all, health. One sign of this focus is the new interest in codes of ethics. Codes of ethics, by whatever name, have been common in professions for some time. It is generally conceded that medicine was the first profession in the United States to adopt a code of ethics, but law, pharmacy, and veterinary medicine were also early comers. However, in the last decade or so, one interesting phenomenon has occurred: ethics has become fashionable, and codes have been newly adopted by organizations representing business and industry.

A code of ethics is considered an essential characteristic of a profession, providing one means whereby professional standards may be established, maintained, and improved. It indicates the profession's acceptance of the trust and responsibility with which society has invested it. The public has granted the professionals certain privileges, with certain expectations in return. Nevertheless, one ethicist stated, "There is a fair degree of public and professional cynicism about codes and a wide range of complaints about them—that they are self-serving, pious, or public relation devices."[28] It is perhaps because of the influence of changing times that the self-serving aspects of ethical codes have diminished considerably over the last few years, and recent revisions of most codes are beginning to show more concern for protecting society than for protecting the profession.

Nursing's code of ethics has also changed over the years.[29] The 1976 version of the code, with interpretive statements, was developed by an ad hoc committee of the ANA's Congress for Nursing Practice and is available from the American Nurses' Association (Exhibit 9-1). The interpretive statements are especially valuable because they not only enlarge upon and explain the code in more detail, but also provide more focus and direction on how the nurse can carry out the code. Particularly important is the first statement, which sets the tone of the nurse-client relationship as partners:

> Whenever possible, clients should be fully involved in the planning
> and implementation of their own health care. Each client has the moral
> right to determine what will be done with his/her person.

Key areas in the interpretations deal with the nurse as patient advocate, nurse participation in political decision making and public affairs, and nurse involvement in advertising of products. Nurse accountability is a major issue and is considered important enough to require a separate statement; the code now has 11 instead of 10 statements.

Overall, the code was intended to express nursing's moral concerns, goals, and values, rather than announcing a set of laws dictating nurses' behavior. However, in 1988, the ANA published *Ethics in Nursing: Position Statements and Guidelines* because of nurses' stated need for help in applying the code to newly complex situations. Included are "Guideline on Withdrawing or Withholding Food and Fluid," which emphasized the need to respect the competent patient's autonomy but added many caveats as to when such action was not appropriate. In a statement examining at what point it ceases to be a nurse's duty to undergo risk for the benefit of the patient, probably in response to the care of AIDS patients, responsibility to the patient is stressed, but the conclusion is that there are limits to the moral obligation of the nurse to benefit patients. Examples are given. Other statements emphasize the importance of nurses' participation in institutional ethics committees, a prohibition of nurses' participation in capital punishment, and the "nonnegotiable nature" of the Code. A number of ANA resources on ethics are also listed.[30]

The International Council of Nursing (ICN) also has a code of ethics. The 1973 version was presented as "useful to nurses in many cultures but able also to stand the tests of time and social change." (Exhibit 9-2.) A striking change from the 1965 code is one that makes explicit the nurse's responsibility and accountability for nursing care, deleting statements in the

Exhibit 9-1

American Nurses' Association Code for Nurses (1976)

PREAMBLE

The Code for Nurses is based on belief about the nature of individuals, nursing, health, and society. Recipients and providers of nursing services are viewed as individuals and groups who possess basic rights and responsibilities, and whose values and circumstances command respect at all times. Nursing encompasses the promotion and restoration of health, the prevention of illness, and the alleviation of suffering. The statements of the Code and their interpretation provide guidance for conduct and relationships in carrying out nursing responsibilities consistent with the ethical obligations of the profession and quality in nursing care.

1. The nurse provides services with respect for human dignity and the uniqueness of the client unrestricted by considerations of social or economic status, personal attributes, or the nature of health problems.
2. The nurse safeguards the client's right to privacy by judiciously protecting information of a confidential nature.
3. The nurse acts to safeguard the client and the public when health care and safety are affected by the incompetent, unethical, or illegal practice of any person.
4. The nurse assumes responsibility and accountability for individual nursing judgments and actions.
5. The nurse maintains competence in nursing.
6. The nurse exercises informed judgment and uses individual competence and qualifications as criteria in seeking consultation, accepting responsibilities, and delegating nursing activities to others.
7. The nurse participates in activities that contribute to the ongoing development of the profession's body of knowledge.
8. The nurse participates in the profession's efforts to implement and improve standards of nursing.
9. The nurse participates in the profession's efforts to establish and maintain conditions of employment conducive to high quality nursing care.
10. The nurse participates in the profession's effort to protect the public from misinformation and misrepresentation and to maintain the integrity of nursing.
11. The nurse collaborates with members of the health professions and other citizens in promoting community and national efforts to meet the health needs of the public.

Source: Reprinted with permission of the American Nurses' Association.

Exhibit 9-2

International Council of Nurses' Code for Nurses (1973)

Ethical Concepts Applied to Nursing

The fundamental responsibility of the nurse is fourfold: to promote health, to prevent illness, to restore health, and to alleviate suffering.

The need for nursing is universal. Inherent in nursing is respect for life, dignity, and rights of man. It is unrestricted by considerations of nationality, race, creed, colour, age, sex, politics, or social status.

Nurses render health services to the individual, the family, and the community and coordinate their services with those of related groups.

NURSES AND PEOPLE
The nurse's primary responsibility is to those people who require nursing care.

The nurse, in providing care, promotes an environment in which the values, customs, and spiritual beliefs of the individual are respected.

The nurse holds in confidence personal information and uses judgment in sharing this information.

NURSES AND PRACTICE
The nurse carries personal responsibility for nursing practice and for maintaining competence by continual learning.

The nurse maintains the highest standards of nursing care possible within the reality of a specific situation.

The nurse uses judgment in relation to individual competence when accepting and delegating responsibilities.

The nurse when acting in a professional capacity should at all times maintain standards of personal conduct that would reflect credit upon the profession.

NURSES AND SOCIETY
The nurse shares with other citizens the responsibility for initiating and supporting action to meet the health and social needs of the public.

NURSES AND CO-WORKERS
The nurse sustains a cooperative relationship with co-workers in nursing and other fields.

The nurse takes appropriate action to safeguard the individual when his care is endangered by a co-worker or any other person.

NURSES AND THE PROFESSION
The nurse plays the major role in determining and implementing desirable standards of nursing practice and nursing education.

The nurse is active in developing a core of professional knowledge.

The nurse, acting through the professional organization, participates in establishing and maintaining equitable social and economic working conditions in nursing.

Source: Reprinted with permission of the International Council of Nurses.

1965 code that had ignored the nurse's judgment and personal responsibility and showed dependency on the physician that nurses worldwide no longer see as appropriate. This code was reaffirmed in 1989.

Using the ANA Code

The ANA Code of Ethics, like other professional codes, has no legal force, as opposed to the licensure laws, enforced by state boards of nursing (not the nurses' associations). However, the requirements of the Code often exceed, but are never less than, the requirements of the law. Violations of the Code should be reported to constituent associations of ANA, which may reprimand, censure, suspend, or expel members. Most state nurses' associations (SNAs) have a procedure for considering reported violations that also gives the accused due process. Even if the nurse is not an SNA member, an ethical violation, at the least, results in the loss of respect of colleagues and the public, which is a serious sanction. All nurses should be familiar with the profession's ethical code. It is a professional obligation to uphold and abide by the code and ensure that nursing colleagues do likewise. (Not all ethical problems deal with patient care; some relate to the behavior and actions of nursing and other colleagues.)

Implementation of the code is at two levels. The nurse may be involved in resolving ethical issues on a broad policy level, participating with other groups in decision making to formulate guidelines or laws. But the more common situation is ethical decision making in daily practice, on a one-to-one basis, on issues that are probably not a matter of life and death but must be resolved on the spot. The Code, and particularly its interpretations, is useful as a guideline here, but more than likely in specific incidents, personal reactions will be both intellectual and emotional and strongly influenced by the nurse's own cultural background, education, and experience.

Specific guidelines for nurses involved in any research or caring for research patients are found in the 1968 publication *The Nurse in Research: ANA Guidelines on Ethical Values*. A more recent ANA statement on the ethical issues of research is *Human Rights Guidelines for Nurses in Clinical and Other Research* (1975), developed by two nurse researchers and accepted as a position statement on human rights for research nurses. These principles are generally accepted.[31] The legal/ethical rights of human subjects in research are discussed in more detail in Chapter 13.

There have been a number of scandals that involve physicians and even governmental agencies concerning research done on prisoners, the mentally retarded, or others who simply weren't properly informed. Some experiments caused serious harm; all violated patients' rights. Therefore, there is special importance in nurses observing the basic principles outlined in the ANA Guidelines and elsewhere.[32] With so much data being computerized

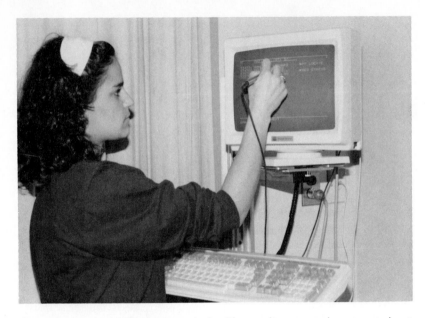

The widespread use of computers in health care has aroused concerns about patient privacy and confidentiality. (*Courtesy of the Robert Wood Johnson Medical Center.*)

now, the security of these systems is another issue.[33] Finally, the increase in scientific misconduct defined as fabrication, falsification, plagiarism, or other practices that seriously deviate from those commonly accepted within the scientific community,[34] although thus far only involving physicians, also has implications for nursing research.

GUIDELINES FOR ETHICAL DECISION MAKING

How can you tell if you're facing an ethical issue? Some ethicists maintain that because all of professional nursing is ethical, "all decisions made with, for, or about patients or clients or other human beings have an ethical dimension."[35] Theoretically, then, there are ethical decisions that do not create a problem. However, in reality, everyone involved may agree on an action, but it could still be considered unethical by someone's standards. What creates most crises is the ethical dilemma—a situation involving a choice between equally satisfactory (good) or unsatisfactory (bad) alternatives or a problem that seems to have no satisfactory solution. Curtin argues

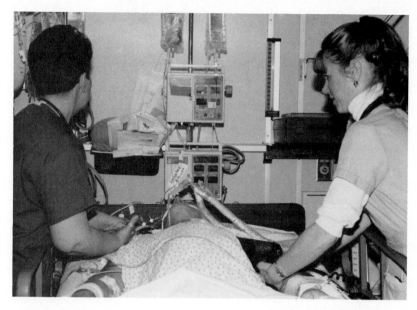

Nurses caring for comatose patients must be supportive of families who face the ethical dilemma of life or death. (*Courtesy of the Robert Wood Johnson Medical Center.*)

that a true dilemma is relatively rare because often, if there is adequate information and time, there are clearer guidelines for action. But, she says:

> A dilemma may not be solvable, but it is resolvable. Even though there is no right or wrong between two *equally* unfavorable actions, taking no action may be even worse than making the choice.[36]

Models and Ethics Rounds

Making that choice, whether or not it can be made by the nurse as an individual or as part of a group, is not easy. To make ethical decisions, it is sometimes useful to use a structured format. A number of bioethical decision models have been presented over the years;[37,38] most include the steps found in Exhibit 9-3 or variations of them. (Having some educational background on the issues, including a course in which these frameworks are explained and used, is also important.)[39]

While going through these steps does not permit snap decisions, there are many ethical dilemmas in which the nurse can take time for thought and discussion with others. Even if the situation does not allow this kind of thoughtful decision making (such as the case in which the doctor made an instant decision as to whom he would resuscitate), later analysis can help

---

Exhibit 9-3

A Bioethical Decision Model

1. Identify the health problem.
2. List the relevant facts needed to understand the situation.
3. Identify the ethical problem or issues.
4. Determine who's involved in making the decision (the nurse, the doctor, the patient, the patient's family).
5. Identify your own role. (Quite possibly, your role may not require a decision at all.)
6. Define your own moral/ethical position, the profession's (code of ethics), and, as much as possible, that of the key individuals involved.
7. Consider as many possible alternative decisions as you can.
8. Try to identify value conflicts.
9. Consider the long- and short-range consequences of each alternative decision.
10. Reach your decision and act on it.
11. Follow the situation until you can see the actual results of your decision, and evaluate it.
12. Use this information to help in making future decisions.

---

in future situations. The nurse can also gain insight into others' thinking and reasoning.

Another useful way to learn to make ethical decisions is to initiate or participate in "ethics rounds." The format is the same as that of most rounds—discussing a case in an organized fashion—but this time the clinical aspects are background. The case could be hypothetical, a recently discharged or deceased patient, or a current patient. The key is open and free discussion with no blame-laying.[40]

Ethics Committees

It is also helpful to consult with or discuss ethical concerns in an interdisciplinary meeting. Nurses are not the only health providers who are recognizing the need to provide procedures to promote effective decision making. A number of institutions have formed ethics committees made up of doctors, nurses, other health professionals, a minister and/or rabbi and priest, representatives from administration, and sometimes an ethicist and members of the public. Ethics committees were assigned an important role in making right-to-die decisions by a variety of court decisions and federal regulations, as described in Chapter 13. However, they also have nonlegal roles: providing nonbinding consultation to the families of incapacitated patients and physicians; educating professionals on ethical issues; and providing a setting for people in medical institutions to become "knowledgeable and comfortable about relating ethical principles to specific decisions."[41]

There is still only a small (but growing) number of ethics committees, but about half of these set ethical and social policies for the care of critically ill persons. Some are actual decision makers about issues of life support, although many feel that this should be the prerogative of the family and physician. One general purpose is to provide a forum in which professionals can discuss their views regarding a particular case. Participating in such a committee is a two-way street; nurses contribute a great deal and they also learn a lot.

Sources of Information

Learning as much as possible about ethical issues in health care is helpful because then the nurse can be somewhat prepared when dealing with them personally. There are, of course, many books, journals, articles, and even videotapes and movies, on ethics in health care and nursing. A particularly interesting series of reports came out of the President's Commission for the Study of Ethical Problems in Medicine and Biomedical Behavioral Research, which is still quite pertinent. The Commission's 1983 reports covered such issues as informed consent, the right to die, whistle blowing in biomedical research, protecting human subjects, implementing human research regulations, genetic engineering, and access to health care. The reports were decidedly pro-public and pro-patient. Among other things, they included results of polls and surveys taken on crucial ethical issues and extensive searches of literature, which resulted in quite valuable and otherwise unavailable information. The reports should be available at most libraries.

Other good resources are organizations with an ethical focus. Their publications and meetings are usually directed at both the public and the professional. Among these are the Hastings Center (Institute of Society, Ethics, and the Life Sciences) in Hastings-on-the-Hudson, New York, and Choice in Dying, the newly merged Concern for Dying and Society for the Right to Die, in New York City. The latter is particularly involved with the living will, a voluntary statement of a person's wishes in the event of incapacity. (See Chapter 13.) Concern has had interdisciplinary sessions with students in nursing, medicine, and law through their professional student organizations, which are expected to continue. These and similar worldwide organizations are often on the cutting edge of emerging ethical issues, and since they all have an educational function, they make available such information.

DEALING WITH ETHICAL CONCERNS

The major ethical issues for those in the health professions today have been identified as the quality of life versus the sanctity of life; the right to live versus the right to die; informed consent; confidentiality; rights of children; unethical behavior of other practitioners; role conflict (who's responsible?); and the allocation of scarce resources (who shall live?). Increasingly, these issues have become subjects of legislation or court decisions (as discussed in later chapters), but even this does not lessen your potential conflicts. Not only must you confront the distinct possibility that your personal value systems may be different from that of the profession, but you may also be caught in the value system of your employing institution.

In the first situation, you must come to terms with your responsibility to the patient or client, regardless of your personal beliefs. For instance, nurses today are faced constantly with the need to make decisions about their roles in euthanasia or abortion. The decision for action may not be easy. When it comes to ending the life of a terminally ill patient or participating in an abortion, you may choose not to participate if the action is against your moral principles. But what about caring for responding, reacting patients? There have been reports of health professionals neglecting or even abusing (mentally if not physically) patients about whom they have moral reservations, such as homosexuals, criminals, alcoholics, or women having abortions. Clearly, this situation is intolerable and violates any professional code of ethics.[42]

Still, there is no question that nurses may experience what has been termed *moral distress,* painful feelings that occur because they or someone else performs an action they believe to be immoral but are powerless to stop. If it is someone else, the feeling escalates to one of *moral outrage.* An example is the repeated resuscitation of an elderly patient with a terminal illness who does not want to be resuscitated. Fear of sanctions often restrains the nurse from acting, even though the sanction is an unlikely one, such as loss of the license. The results are often a feeling of loss of self-worth, a negative effect on personal relationships, psychological effects (depression), behavioral manifestations (nightmares), and even physical symptoms (headache, diarrhea). Some nurses even leave the workplace or nursing altogether because they feel that they "can't fight the system." The ones who are not upset are generally those who hold the same values as the institution and the physician. Moral distress and moral outrage are felt by nurses across the age range. An interesting sidelight is that nurses see the nurse administrator as an enemy in these situations and feel that they have no support.[43]

There are many specific patient-related ethical issues that may cause the nurse distress, anxiety, or confusion beyond the classic right-to-die/right-to-live issues involving both newborns,[44] and the elderly.[45,46] One is the questionable use of invasive technology, which nurses at the bedside 24 hours a day certainly recognize. Yet they often find themselves at a disadvantage in arguing with a physician.[47] The use of mechanical restraints when there is uncertainty about their safety or effectiveness is another.[48] As in a number of other situations, the law is becoming involved in the latter issue, particularly in relation to the elderly. Unfortunately, as described in Chapter 12, a nurse may be sued if a patient is hurt with or without such restraints. At times, it is difficult to untangle ethical and legal responsibilities; indeed, there are times when the law or the legal decision in a case does not seem ethical in itself.

Other Surveys and Studies

The conflicts nurses often face come from another source: the physician or employer. In one survey of nurses on ethical behavior, despite the feeling of the respondents that they and other colleagues were ethical, 83 percent said that they had had to compromise their ethical values for some reason. Hospital policy, self-protection, a patient's request or demand, and a doctor's request were the chief reasons, although supervisor and peer pressures were also mentioned. Nurses over 50 years of age tended to feel more pressured by hospital policy and younger nurses by doctors' requests. Nurses who compromised their ethical standards worried most about harming their patients or feeling ashamed, but one-fourth were also worried about getting into legal trouble. Nevertheless, the majority had either kept information from patients or had deceived them about their medications. They were more honest with doctors than with patients and their families.[49,50] Bureaucratic pressure is known to be a factor for students and RNs in such cases.[51–53]

A particularly interesting survey is one involving RNs and LPNs in LTC facilities.[54] One problem they faced was that difficult decisions were complicated by multiple decision makers, including doctors and anxious families, with the result that patients/residents felt pressured to agree with them. About one-third of the respondents said that physicians seldom discussed the treatment and prognosis with the residents, and they wished this could be done while the person was still able to participate in the decision-making process. What disturbed them most, besides the decision on whether or not to use restraints, were disputes with physicians and their own colleagues on how aggressive treatment should be, whether to hospitalize the resident, value conflicts with staff and family about a resident's quality of life, and what to do when a competent resident opposed the treatment plan. Ninety-six percent felt that treatment should be stopped when the resident requests. They also said that they would give pain medication to a dying resident even if hastening death was unavoidable. They themselves, by a vast majority, indicated that if *they* were critically ill, with no chance of recovery, they would not want CPR, mechanical ventilation, renal dialysis, hyperalimentation, or food and water per nasogastric or gastrostomy tube.

Problems with Colleagues

The theme of loyalty to the doctor seems to have diminished, according to the ethics surveys, although nurses expressed frustration because they felt they could not act against incompetent physicians. Younger nurses were more inclined to report them than older nurses, but a general response was that reporting at the hospital level was almost useless. Yet, whether on the basis of ethical principles or, in some states, the law, such physicians must be reported (see Chapter 11). There are also intraprofessional problems of ethics that nurses must face. Some are actually criminal, as when nurses steal from patients or, for that matter, take even small items from the employer. *Pilfering,* as the latter is called, is both unethical and illegal. A serious issue is the number of nurses impaired by dependence on drugs or other addictions. In the last few years, both state nurses' associations and individual employers have developed plans for helping these nurses and for protecting the public from them.[55] In addition, nurses are taking more responsibility for dealing with incompetent nurses. However, much remains to be done. All of these issues have serious legal complications related to licensure (Chapter 11).

NURSES AS PATIENT ADVOCATES

Over time, it appears that nurses themselves, and others, have come to see nurses as natural patient advocates.[56,57] In a sense, this has been manifested by the fact that long before the American Hospital Association published its Patient's Bill of Rights (see Chapter 13), the National League for Nursing (NLN) had drafted a statement on what the patient might expect from the nurse.[58] (This was done at a time when no one told patients what their caregivers should be doing.) The statement coincided closely with the statements in the ANA Code for Nurses. Then in 1977, the NLN released a new document on patients' rights (Exhibit 9-4). Again, this clearly spelled out nursing's support for patients' rights.

Despite nurses' desire to search for ethical solutions and to act accordingly, despite their desire to act as patient advocates, there are still some concerns. Suppose that the nurse does carry out his or her ethical and legal responsibilities, such as being sure that a patient has given an informed consent before receiving a particular kind of treatment. What if this action comes into conflict with what the doctor or the hospital sees as a limit to the nurse's role? Will the nurse's job be in jeopardy? Will he or she be subtly punished? How does the nurse handle a neglectful family?[59] What if the nurse reports unethical or illegal behavior on the part of another practitioner? Again, what happens? Who provides backup support—nursing

Exhibit 9-4

Nursing's Role in Patients' Rights (1977)

NLN believes the following are patient's rights which nurses have a responsibility to uphold:

- People have the right to health care that is accessible and that meets professional standards, regardless of the setting.
- Patients have the right to courteous and individualized health care that is equitable, humane, and given without discrimination as to race, color, creed, sex, national origin, source of payment, or ethical or political beliefs.
- Patients have the right to information about their diagnosis, prognosis, and treatment—including alternatives to care and risks involved—in terms they and their families can readily understand, so that they can give their informed consent.
- Patients have the legal right to informed participation in all decisions concerning their health care.
- Patients have the right to information about the qualifications, names, and titles of personnel responsible for providing their health care.
- Patients have the right to refuse observation by those not directly involved in their care.
- Patients have the right to privacy during interview, examination, and treatment.
- Patients have the right to privacy in communicating and visiting with persons of their choice.
- Patients have the right to refuse treatments, medications, or participation in research and experimentation, without punitive action being taken against them.
- Patients have the right to coordination and continuity of health care.
- Patients have the right to appropriate instruction or education from health care personnel so that they can achieve an optimal level of wellness and an understanding of their basic health needs.
- Patients have the right to confidentiality of all records (except as otherwise provided for by law or third-party payer contracts) and all communications, written or oral, between patients and health care providers.

Source: Reprinted with permission of the National League for Nursing.

administration? nursing peers? What of dealing with physicians who are incompetents, drug abusers, or alcoholics? Does the profession protect the co-professional or the public? Unlike personal ethical conflicts, these are real dilemmas that may have serious economic repercussions for the nurse, and it is quite possible that a nurse cannot resolve them alone.[60] Instead, nursing must develop a support system for individual nurses who experience conflict in the employment setting with respect to implementation of the ANA code, and the precepts of the code must be widely publicized so that not only nurses, but also the public and others in health care, understand the ethical basis of nursing practice.[61]

ACCOUNTABILITY

Accountability is a concept that has been discussed widely in nursing literature. Nursing students have been told that they must have it in order to be professional; practicing nurses are said to be accountable because they are licensed; and primary nursing, a system for delivering care, identifies it as a basic component of practice. Feelings of accountability are much like feelings of patriotism; most of us have them but do not find means of expressing them on a day-to-day basis. Still, whether or not a person feels accountable should not determine the level of accountability of a professional group, such as nursing; rather, the profession has an obligation to ensure accountability on the part of its members.

Accountability, as a professional characteristic and responsibility, is discussed by Parsons.[62] "Professional groups must, to some essential degree, be self-regulating, taking responsibility for the technical standards of their profession and for their integrity in serving societal functions." He continues: "where a division of labor is involved . . . this will always have to include the legitimation of the functions of the groups and types of activity in question, of the ways in which the standards of performance of those functions are upheld, and of the protection or enhancement of the rights and interests of those outside the groups of performers of the functions on whom the actions of such groups impinge."

Accountability, as defined by *Webster's* dictionary, means "subject to giving an account: answerable." There is a clear distinction between the reality of being answerable and feeling answerable, and being answerable is essential to nursing's professionalization and viability. Showing accountability in nursing practice provides the opportunity to evaluate nursing's contribution within health care and is a means of clarifying the significance of nursing to society. As accountability is discussed in relation to professional nursing, two questions consistently arise: Accountable for what? and Accountable to whom?

Accountable for What?

Accountability for what is perhaps the more important of the two questions. The history of nursing is filled with the need to answer for things for which it was not accountable, such as why the medication prescribed by the physician was not received from the pharmacy; why the laboratory failed to draw blood for an ordered test; why the patient received the incorrect diet; why housekeeping did not clean a patient's room; and why the radiology department did not perform an ordered x-ray before noon. This type of answering is not accountability; rather, according to Lewis and Batey, it is "recounting."[63] You can only be accountable for that for which you are responsible, and you can only be responsible for those things that are clearly designated and accepted as your responsibility. In addition, you must have authority to act and be expected to use judgment based on a body of knowledge in order to fulfill your responsibilities as a professional. Then, and only then, can accountability be expressed. Accountability is not a vague feeling or an obscure concept. It is a clear obligation that must be a definable part of nursing practice.

Nursing is accountable for those professional responsibilities that are allocated and accepted. Those responsibilities change as knowledge expands and roles evolve; however, at any point in time, nursing must clearly understand the scope and specificity of those responsibilities for which it is accountable. Responsibilities are delineated in nursing through practice acts of individual states, standards of care developed by recognized professional nursing groups such as ANA, and position descriptions of institutions and agencies where nurses work. Also, responsibilities may be individually negotiated between a nurse and a client.

Responsibilities in nursing should be consistent with and reflective of current knowledge and role definitions. Clearly defined responsibility is a component and the basis of professional accountability. Although the terms *responsibility* and *accountability* are often used interchangeably, they are not the same. Batey and Lewis define responsibility as "a charge for which one is answerable," whereas accountability consists of answering in relation to the fulfillment of defined responsibility.[64] Broad responsibilities of nursing are contained in ANA's Social Policy Statement,[65] and it is these responsibilities and those in the licensure law, for which nursing as a profession must answer. Professional nurses must be expected to exercise autonomy and must be willing to make independent and interdependent decisions as part of every phase of their practice.

Accountable to Whom?

The Social Policy Statement also states that "nursing can be said to be owned by society, in the sense that nursing's professional interest must be, and must be perceived as, serving the interests of the larger whole of which it is a part."[66] Because traditional nursing practice has evolved primarily within the hierarchical structure of organizations such as hospitals, it has often been unclear to nurses to whom they are answerable. Nurses have frequently interpreted the object of accountability as being the physician or the institution in which they are employed. In reality, the traditional role of the nurse consisted of performing delegated tasks or carrying out policies of the institution. In this sense, nurses were answerable to physicians and institutions for these functions. As nursing's body of knowledge has expanded and its roles have been delineated, the traditional object of answerability has changed. Nurses, physicians, and institutions are equally accountable for their specific functions within health care delivery, and there is now a sharing of accountability to society and the recipients of care. An increasing number of malpractice suits recognize this difference as physicians, nurses, and administrative personnel, as well as other providers of care, are listed as defendants.

Nurses cannot claim immunity or justification for inadequate or inappropriate nursing care because they followed a physician's orders or an institution's policies. Consumers are demanding individual and collective accountability. They also demand that nursing critically evaluate the quality and quantity of its contribution. Peer review is one tool used for evaluation and accountability. The ANA has defined *peer review* as "the process by which registered nurses, actively engaged in the practice of nursing, appraise the quality of nursing care in a given situation in accordance with established standards of nursing practice." Four major purposes for peer review are given: (1) to evaluate the quality and quantity of nursing care; (2) to determine the strengths and weaknesses of nursing care; (3) to provide evidence to utilize as the basis of recommendations for new or altered policies and procedures to improve nursing care; and (4) to identify those areas where practice patterns indicate more knowledge is needed.[67]

There are two types of peer review. The first is a system that focuses on clients and recipients of care. Most peer reviews that focus on clients are done as a nursing audit. The JCAHO requires the existence of such a structure in hospitals. This type of peer review includes both retrospective and process audits. Committees and subcommittees develop criteria against which past or present documentation of care is compared. Although the standards set for peer review are generally those determined by nursing in the setting where the evaluation is done, the ANA Standards of Clinical Nursing Practice, made more explicit for evaluation purposes, are frequently considered a logical starting point.

The second type of peer review focuses on individual practitioners and theoretically gets to the essence of individual and collective accountability. Some recent efforts have been made with clinical career ladder review procedures to incorporate peer review as a part of consideration for promotion. However, most nursing care delivery systems are designed in such a way that individual excellence or incompetence is masked by collective responsibility. This situation may be changing. Some nursing organizations have structured their practice setting's governance in such a way that nurses involved in clinical practice have the right and responsibility to participate in its governance activities. Such activities include the development of policies and procedures, evaluation and selection of equipment and supplies used in patient care, recruitment and retention activities, and quality assurance and primary nursing committees. All of these activities have a role to play in the fulfillment of responsibilities to clients and offer a means of demonstrating accountability for nursing practice.

We are in an "era of accountability" that demands that one be answerable for those things for which one assumes responsibility. Nursing as a profession and nurses as individuals must justify outcomes of nursing care in relation to their defined responsibilities with regard to the quality, appropriateness, and affordability of care. In order to fulfill this professional obligation, each nurse must understand and operationalize the concept.

Avoid taking on responsibilities that are not clearly within the domain of nursing. Be sure that actions are documented at all levels of practice. Acquire the authority of knowledge and position for each responsibility. Be sure that it is understood that professional nurses exercise independent judgment and participate in interdependent decision making based on a specific body of knowledge. Be willing to take the risks of collaboration. Then evaluate the outcomes in relation to responsibilities in individual practice and within the profession, and answer to society for nursing practice. Then and only then will the questions of whether or not nursing is a profession or what its significance is within society will subside. Accountability in every aspect of practice is the challenge facing nursing.

KEY POINTS

1. Ethics requires a degree of decision making beyond morality, which relates to custom, tradition, and religion.
2. Technology, economies, and changes in attitudes about life and death have helped to create some of the ethical dilemmas in health care.
3. A code of ethics is an essential element in professionalism, but if the practitioners violate it, society may take away their special status and privileges.
4. Nurses can use the ANA Code as guidelines for ethical practice, in conjunction with decision-making models.
5. Other useful ways to learn to deal with ethical concerns are ethics rounds, ethics committees, and self-study to become familiar with the issues.

6. Nurses are accountable for those professional responsibilities that are allocated and accepted, and must evaluate their own and their colleagues' practice.

REFERENCES

1. Aroskar MA. The aftermath of the Cruzan decision: Dying in a twilight zone. *Nurs Outlook,* 38:256–257 (November–December 1991).
2. Quill TE. Death and dignity: A case of individualized decision making. *N Engl J Med,* 324:691–694 (March 7, 1991).
3. Kelly L. When nurses ration patient care. *Nurs Outlook,* 33:123 (May–June 1985).
4. The right to die. *Nurs Life,* 4:47–53 (May–June 1984).
5. Callahan D. Terminating treatment: Age as a standard. *Hastings Center Rep,* 17:21–25 (October–November 1987).
6. Altman L. The limits of transplantation: How far should surgeons go? *New York Times.* (December 19, 1989), p. C3.
7. Fry S. Brave new world: Removing body parts from infants. *Nurs Outlook,* 38:152 (May–June 1990).
8. Robertson J. Rights, symbolism, and public policy in fetal tissue transplants. *Hastings Center Rep,* 18:5–11 (December 1988).
9. Vaughn-Cole B, Kee H. A heart decision. *Am J Nurs,* 85:535–536 (May 1985).
10. Morrow L. When one body can save another. *Time,* 137:54–58 (June 17, 1991).
11. Kilner J. Selecting patients when resources are limited.: A study of U.S. medical directors of kidney dialysis and transplantation facilities. *Am J Pub Health,* 78:144–147 (February 1988).
12. Blakeslee S. Studies find unequal access to kidney transplants. *New York Times* (January 24, 1989), pp. C1, C9.
13. Bayer R, et al. Toward justice in health care. *Am J Pub Health,* 78:583–588 (May 1988).
14. Callahan D. Rationing medical progress. *N Engl J Med* 322:1810–1813 (June 21, 1990).
15. Rooks J. Let's admit we ration health care—then set priorities. *Am J Nurs,* 90:38–43 (June 1990).
16. Capuzzi C, Garland M. The Oregon plan: Increasing access to health care. *Nurs Outlook,* 38:260–263, 286 (November–December 1990).
17. Dougherty CJ. Setting health care priorities: Oregon's next steps. Conference report. *Hastings Center Rep,* 21:1–10 (May–June 1991).
18. Kelly J, et al. Stigmatization of AIDS patients by physicians. *Am J Pub Health,* 77:798–791 (July 1987).
19. Daniels N. Duty to treat or right to refuse. *Hastings Center Rep,* 21:36–46 (March–April 1991).

20. Wiley K, et al. Care of HIV-infected patients: Nurses' concerns, opinions, and precautions. *Appl Nurs Res,* 3:27–33 (February 1990).
21. Laufman J. AIDS, ethics, and the truth. *Am J Nurs,* 89:924–925 (July 1989).
22. Churchill L. Ethical issues of a profession in transition. *Am J Nurs,* 77:873 (May 1977).
23. Chally P. Theory derivation in moral development. *Nurs and Health Care,* 11:302–306 (June 1990).
24. Gilligan C. *In a different voice.* Cambridge, MA: Harvard University Press, 1982.
25. Chally, op. cit.
26. Davis A, Aroskar M. *Ethical dilemmas and nursing practice.* New York: Appleton-Century-Crofts, 1978.
27. Smurl J. Making hard choices: Finding solutions to everyday ethical problems. *Nurs 88,* 18:105–108 (June 1988).
28. Revising the United States Senate code of ethics. *Special Supplement, Hastings Center Rep,* 11:1–28 (February 1981).
29. Kelly LY. *Dimensions of professional nursing.* Elmsford, NY: Pergamon Press, 1991, pp. 209–213.
30. *Ethics in nursing: Position statements and guidelines.* Kansas City, MO: American Nurses' Association, 1988, pp. 2–7, 9–16.
31. Rogers B. Ethical considerations in research. *AAOHN J,* 10:456–457 (October 1987).
32. Miya P. An ethical dilemma. *Image,* 16:105–108 (Fall 1984).
33. Romano C. Privacy, confidentiality, and security of computerized systems: The nursing responsibility. *Computers in Nurs,* 5:99–104 (May–June 1987).
34. Abdellah F. Scientific misconduct: Myth or reality. *J Prof Nurs,* 6:6, 63 (January–February 1990).
35. Thompson J, Thompson H. *Bioethical decision making for nurses.* Norwalk, CT: Appleton-Century-Crofts, 1985.
36. Curtin L, Flaherty MJ, eds. *Nursing ethics: Theories and pragmatics.* Bowie, MD: Robert J. Brady Company, 1982, p. 39.
37. Thompson and Thompson, op. cit.
38. Murphy M, Murphy J. Making ethical decisions systematically. *Nurs 76,* 6:CG13 (May 1976).
39. Fry S. Ethical decision-making part I: Selecting a framework. *Nurs Outlook,* 37:248 (September–October 1989).
40. Davis AJ. Helping your staff address ethical dilemmas. *J Nurs Admin,* 12:9–13 (February 1982).
41. President's Commission for the Study of Ethical Problems in Medicine and Biomedical and Behavioral Research. *Deciding to forego life-sustaining treatment.* Washington, DC: U.S. Government Printing Office, 1983, pp. 161–163.
42. Davis AJ. Professional obligations, personal values in conflict. *Am Nurse,* 22:7 (May 1990).
43. Wilkenson JM. Moral distress in nursing practice: Experience and effect. *Nurs Forum,* 23(1):17–29 (1987–1988).

44. Smith J. Ethical issues raised by new treatment options. *MCN*, 14:183–187 (May–June 1989).

45. Wilson VC. How can we dignify death in the ICU? *Am J Nurs*, 90:38–42 (May 1990).

46. Wurzbach ME. The dilemma of withholding or withdrawing nutrition. *Image*, 22:226–230 (Winter 1990).

47. Pauly-O'Neill S. Questioning the use of invasive technology. *Am J Nurse*, 91:19–20 (January 1991).

48. Moss RJ, La Puma J. The ethics of mechanical restraints. *Hastings Center Rep*, 21:22–24 (January–February 1991).

49. How ethical are you? Part 1. *Nurs Life*, 3:25–33 (January–February 1983).

50. How ethical are you? Part 2. *Nurs Life*, 3:46–56 (March–April 1983).

51. Swider S, et al. Ethical decision making in a bureaucratic context by senior nursing students. *Nurs Res*, 34:108–112 (March–April 1985).

52. Mayberry MA. Ethical decision making: A response of hospital nurses. *Nurs Admin Q*, 10(3):75–81 (1986).

53. Davis A. Clinical nurses' ethical decision making in situations of informed consent. *Adv in Nurs Sci*. 11:63–69 (April 1989).

54. Lund M, Wei FF. Speaking out on ethics. *Ger Nurs*, 11:223–227 (September–October 1990).

55. Miller H. Addiction in a coworker—getting past the denial. *Am J Nurs*, 90:72–75 (May 1990).

56. Winslow G. From loyalty to advocacy: A new metaphor for nursing. *Hastings Center Rep*, 14:32–40 (June 1984).

57. Nelson M. Advocacy in nursing. *Nurs Outlook*, 36:136–141 (May–June 1988).

58. National League for Nursing: *What people can expect of modern nursing service*. New York: National League for Nursing, 1959. Also found in Kelly L. *Dimensions of professional nursing*, 4th ed. New York: Macmillan Publishing Company, 1981.

59. Kayser-Jones J, et al. An ethical analysis of an elder's treatment. *Nurs Outlook*, 37:267–270 (November–December 1989).

60. Fry S. Whistle-blowing by nurses: A matter of ethics. *Nurs Outlook*, 37:56 (January–February 1989).

61. Robinson M. Patient advocacy and the nurse: Is there a conflict of interest? *Nurs Forum*, 22(2):58–63 (1985).

62. Parsons T. *Action theory and the human condition*. New York: Free Press, 1978.

63. Lewis F, Batey M. Clarifying autonomy and accountability in nursing service: Part II. *Nurs Admin*, 12:10–15 (October 1982).

64. Batey M, Lewis F. Clarifying autonomy and accountability in nursing service: Part I. *Nurs Admin*, 12:14 (September 1982).

65. American Nurses' Association. *Nursing: A social policy statement*. Kansas City, MO: The Association, 1980.

66. Ibid., p. 3.

67. American Nurses' Association. Peer review guidelines proposed. *Am Nurse*, 5:1, 5 (July 1973).

CHAPTER 10

LAW AND LEGISLATION

OBJECTIVES

After studying this chapter, you will be able to:

1. Define statutory law, regulatory law, judicial law, criminal law, and civil law.
2. Explain two basic elements of the judicial system.
3. Explain how a bill becomes a law.
4. List ways in which you can get information about legislation.
5. Describe how nurses and others can influence the legislative process.
6. Name and explain briefly four federal laws that have a major effect on nurses.

Every nurse today needs to know something about law and legislation because there is so much in health care and nursing that is affected by law. Some federal laws influence how health care is given and how it is reimbursed. On a more personal level, other laws have to do with the rights and privileges of individuals, whether they are providers or consumers. State laws regulate our practice. Court decisions also outline certain rights, and they pinpoint liability in cases of negligence or other malpractice. Few nurses set out to break the law or violate anyone's rights, but there are so many complex situations in health care today that there is a tendency to feel helpless about knowing what's *legal*. Yes, you can always consult with your employing institution's attorney, but that isn't very practical on a day-to-day basis. Worse yet, everyone dealing with the law knows that there is no final or absolute answer—something that is quite frustrating for those who want to know exactly what they can or cannot do. Yet, there are certain principles that may serve as guidelines to avoid problems and as a basis of understanding American law and influencing it. Providing this basic, practical know-how is the focus of this and the following chapters. [For more details, read any nursing law book or Chapter 17 in Lucie Kelly, *Dimensions of Professional Nursing*, 6th ed. (New York: Pergamon Press, 1991). Chapter 18 discusses legislation in considerable detail.]

INTRODUCTION TO LAW

As the American colonies were founded one by one, the way in which they would be governed was a primary consideration. Gradually, a system similar to that of the common law then in effect in England was adopted. However, the problems within the colonies varied so widely that each eventually developed its own procedures and laws, both common and statutory, based on its own needs.

From this evolved the concept of *states' rights,* which has played an important role in the history of the United States. Any infringement of these rights, either by the federal government or by other states, is usually strongly opposed. States do adopt the same or similar laws as others, such as voting age, seat belt use, and drinking age. However, a state can retain, revise, or repeal its own laws without interference from other states or the federal government. Variance in state laws creates a great deal of confusion, misunderstanding, and red tape. How much simpler it would be, for example, if the laws regulating the practice of nursing were uniform throughout the country.

Federal law is based on the U.S. Constitution, ratified in 1789. Since then, the volume and complexity of problems facing the legislature have increased tremendously, but the Constitution always guides the action.

The Constitution has been amended 26 times. The first 10 Amendments, known as the Bill of Rights, were adopted within three years of the Constitution's ratification. These amendments guarantee certain freedoms, such as freedom of speech, press, religion, assembly, and due process. They are the basis of the civil rights we hear so much about. In recent years, the Bill of Rights has had relevance to health care issues, such as when the Fourteenth

Amendment's protection of personal liberty is used in defense of a woman's right to choose to have an abortion or when the right to assemble allows nurses and others to rally as an expression of concern over labor issues. It is interesting to note that the Constitution does not specify access to health care as a guaranteed right. Nor do state constitutions.

UNITED STATES LEGAL SYSTEM

Under the U.S. government, the law is carried out at a number of levels. The Constitution is the highest law of the land. Whatever the Constitution (federal law) does not spell out, the states retain for themselves (Tenth Amendment). Because they can create political subdivisions, units of local government—counties, cities, towns, townships, boroughs, and villages—all have certain legal powers within their geographic boundaries. On all levels, but most obviously on the federal and state levels, there is a separation of power: legislative, executive, and judicial. The first makes the laws, the second carries them out, and the third reviews them, a system that the founders of the United States believed would create a balance of power.

There are three basic sources of law: statutory law, executive or regulatory law, and judicial law.

Statutory law refers to enactments of legislative bodies declaring, commanding, or prohibiting something. Statutes are always written, are firmly established, and can be altered only by amendment or repeal. They are published in *codes*. The Nurse Education Act is one example of a federal law. The Social Security Act, which includes Medicare as Title XVIII and Medicaid as Title XIX, is another. Statutory laws also exist at the state level. Licensing laws for professional nurses, requiring them to be licensed before they can legally practice nursing, are examples of a state statute.

Executive, administrative, or *regulatory law* refers to the rules, regulations, and decisions of administrative bodies.[1] In a sense, they spell out the specifics of a statutory law. For example, the DHHS Division of Nursing develops the regulations that determine the requirements for the various programs in the Nurse Education Act; the State Board of Nursing spells out the requirements for a nursing school; a city health code may adopt a patients' bill of rights as a requirement for all hospitals in the city. All have the effect of law but are more easily changed than statutory law.

Judicial law, also called *decisional, case,* or *common law,* is a body of legal principles and rules of action that derive their authority from usage and custom or from judgments and decrees of courts. Courts are agencies established by the government to decide disputes. (The term *court* is also sometimes used to refer to the person or persons hearing a case). *Superior, supreme, common pleas, district,* and *circuit courts* are all courts of appeal (appellate). The kind of court in which a case is brought depends on the offense or complaint.

Federal courts established in all states hear cases related to the Constitution. With the introduction of written decisions, one of the most important principles known in the law was born, the principle of *stare decisis,* which means to stand as decided, or "let the decision stand." This means that if a case with similar facts has been decided finally in that particular jurisdiction, the court will probably make the same decision on a like case, citing the *precedent* of the previous case. If the precedent is out of date or not applicable, a new rule will be made.[2]

THE LEGISLATIVE PROCESS

It is not unusual for hundreds of health-related bills to be introduced during a legislative term. If nurses want to have some control over the laws that affect their practice, it is important that they learn how to influence the legislative process. The first step is to get the necessary information, as discussed in the next section.

The Legislative Setting

Even with the best intentions, no legislators can be experts on all the issues that come up. For instance, in one two-year session in Congress, 25,000 or so bills were introduced. Not all are acted on, but even reading them all is almost impossible. Therefore, all senators and congressmen and most state legislators have staffs of varying size, depending on seniority and other factors. Some staffs are in the capital; others are in home offices in the legislator's district in order to keep in touch with and help constituents. Some perform administrative duties, and others act as legislative aides, assistants, and/or researchers. These are individuals who summarize background material on key bills and brief the legislator on specific issues and on constituents' feedback. The legislator generally uses this information to decide how he will vote. (In order to avoid constant repetition of the phrase "his or her," the masculine pronoun is used in this chapter when referring to legislators, most of whom are men.) The administrative assistants share the power of the legislators, if not the glory. Committee staff do the preparatory work that comes before committees and subcommittees, drafting bills, writing amendments to bills, arranging and preparing for public hearings, consulting with people in the areas about which the committee is concerned, providing information, and frequently writing speeches for the chairman.

Because these assistants get information from numerous sources, it is a good idea to become acquainted with them, maintain good relations, and provide accurate, pertinent information about the issues in which you are interested. Do not ignore them; they are very influential.

A measure of the prestige a legislator has is his placement on committees, where most of the preliminary action on bills occurs. Appointments are influenced or made by party leaders in the House of Representatives or the Senate. Chairmanships of committees, extremely powerful positions, are awarded to members of the majority party, usually senior members of the House or Senate. Some committee assignments are more prestigious than others and are eagerly sought. Although there are cases in which the chairmen of some of these committees, particularly on the national level, have remained for years, the makeup of a committee may change with each new session. It is important to know on which committee your legislators sit, because the action of committees affects the future of a bill.

How a Bill Becomes a Law[3]

A lot of compromise goes into the legislative process, and often there is behind-the-scenes negotiating that is never seen in the open committee hearings or on the floor of the House or Senate. Nevertheless there is a formal process by which a bill becomes a law. This is charted in Figure 10-1. Here the bill starts in the House, but it could just as well be the Senate. Note particularly the steps at which you can influence the process by the various lobbying techniques described later. Some important details follow.

1. Anyone can initiate a bill. Common sources include the President and his administration; a group or organization, such as ANA; and private citizens who can convince a legislator about a need. The bill is put in the appropriate format by legal specialists.

2. One or more lawmakers sponsor the bill, with the major sponsor (the author) introducing the bill and guiding it through the legislative process. The more powerful that sponsor, the better. Bipartisan sponsorship is also desirable, because then it does not become a party issue.

3. The bill is introduced (commonly referred to as "put in the hopper") and given a number. Numbers are consecutive within each two-year session and begin with "HR" in the House or "S" in the Senate. If the bill does not become law, it can be reintroduced the following session and is given a new bill number.

4. After the bill is introduced and printed in the *Congressional Record* (*first reading*), it is assigned to one or more committees that have responsibility for that subject. You can obtain a copy of a federal bill from your representative or, preferably, from the House or Senate Documents Room. State legislatures also have document or bill rooms.

How a Bill Becomes a Law at the Federal Level

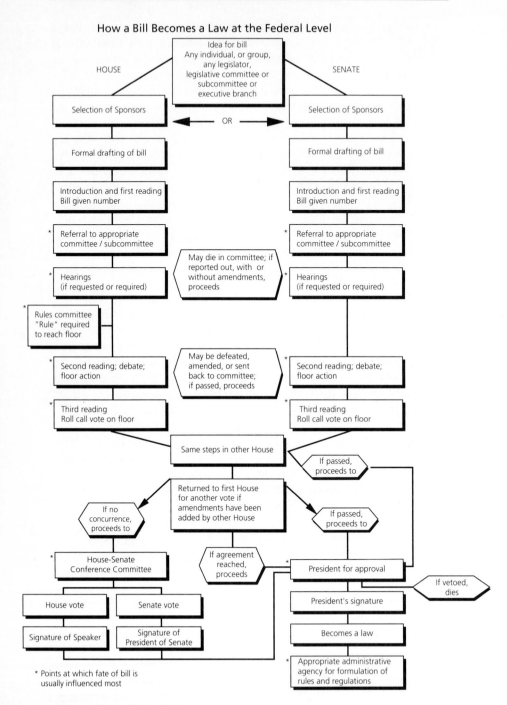

Figure 10-1 The legislative process.

Addresses for Document Rooms can be obtained from your representative. It is a good idea to call the Documents Room first to verify the proper procedure. Be sure to have the bill number whenever requesting information. A section-by-section analysis of the bill is usually easier to understand than the bill itself, and can be obtained from your congressman or from the *Congressional Record,* which is available in many libraries.

5. Legislators spend a lot of time in committees. The committee chairman is very powerful and can influence the fate of a bill by introducing it for discussion very quickly or by keeping it off the agenda for the entire session. Committees also conduct hearings, which are usually open to the public. Often nurses testify on health care issues by representing professional nursing organizations or appearing as individual witnesses. When a committee decides on a bill, it is either killed or passed with amendments or as a new bill. The process of deliberating and voting on a bill is called *mark-up*.

6. If the bill is passed, the Director of the Congressional Budget Office submits an estimate of the cost of the measure, and this is included in the Committee Report.

7. The bill then goes to the full House for action on the floor *(second reading)*. Visitors can watch from the gallery but may not speak during floor deliberations. If you want to know when a particular bill will be brought to the floor, it is best to contact the leadership of the appropriate house. A bill is usually brought to the chamber of one house independent of events in the other.

8. At the end of floor action, the *third reading* is called for and the vote taken. Amendments added in committee or on the floor are a big factor in determining the fate of the bill. Adding amendments to a bill that seems sure to pass is a technique for putting through some action that might not succeed on its own and that may be only remotely or not at all connected to the content of the original bill. On the other hand, amendments that are totally unacceptable to the bill's sponsors may be added as a mechanism to force withdrawal or defeat of the bill. In general, amendments are introduced to strengthen, broaden, or curtail the intent of the original bill or law. If passed, they may change its character considerably. When debate is closed, the vote is taken by roll call and recorded. Passage usually requires a majority vote of the total House.

9. If the bill is passed, it goes to the Senate for a complete repetition of the process it went through in the House, and with the same opportunities to influence its passage. A bill introduced in the Senate follows the same general route, with certain procedural differences. Also, the President of the Senate is the Vice-President of the United States. Filibustering is a unique senatorial process whereby senators opposed

to a motion to consider a bill may speak to it for extensive periods, thus preventing or defeating action by long delays.

10. At times, the same or a similar bill is introduced in both houses on certain important issues. If these bills are not the same when passed by each house, or if another single bill has been amended by the second house after passing the first and the first does not agree on the amendments, the bill is sent to a conference committee consisting of an equal number of members of each house. The conference committee tries to work out a compromise that will be accepted by both houses. Usually an agreement is reached.

11. After passing both houses and being signed by each presider, the bill goes to the President, who may obtain opinions from various sources. If he signs it or fails to take action within 10 days, the bill becomes law. He may also veto the bill and return it to the house of origin with his objections. A two-thirds affirmative vote in both houses for re-passage is necessary to override the veto. Because voting on a veto is often along party lines, overriding a veto in both houses is difficult. However, the National Center for Nursing Research was established in 1985 through a veto override of the NIH reauthorization bill, demonstrating the political strength of nurses and others who lobbied for the bill. If the Congress adjourns before the 10 days in which the President should sign the bill, it does not become law. This is known as a *pocket veto*.

12. Another type of legislation is a resolution. Joint resolutions originating in either house are, for all practical purposes, treated as a bill but have the whereas-resolved format. They are identified as *HJ Res.* or *SJ Res.*

13. All bills that become law are assigned numbers, beginning with "PL" (different from their original number), and then are printed and attached to the proper volume of statutes.

14. The last step is sending the new law to the appropriate administrative agency for rules on implementing the law. This is another juncture at which nurses can have input. Proposed and final rules are published in the *Federal Register,* which is available in many libraries.

15. It is important to keep in mind that the federal government's fiscal year is designated by the calendar year in which it ends. Thus, the period from October 1, 1990, to September 30, 1991, is fiscal year 1991 (FY91).

INFLUENCING THE LEGISLATIVE PROCESS

There are many factors to be considered before a legislative body or even individual legislators make a final decision on how to vote on a piece of

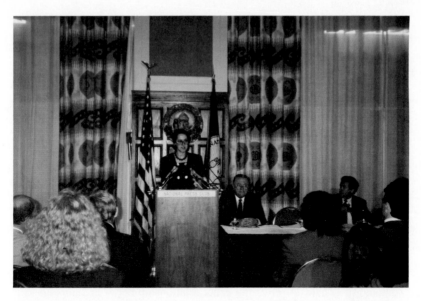

Nurses testify at congressional hearings and may hold news conferences to present the ANA viewpoint on legislative issues. (*Courtesy of the American Nurses' Association.*)

legislation. Some are probably personal—how the legislator feels about an issue. Some are internally political—support of the party leadership or a favor owed to a colleague. But likely to be the most influential is the voice of the legislator's constituency, "the folks back home." Most legislators want to be reelected to the same or a higher office. If their constituents are not pleased with them, their voting record, or their attitude, they are replaced.

Just who are these powerful constituents? Actually, they range from the ordinary householder to the powerful conglomerate, and include individuals as well as interest groups. Kalisch and Kalisch define an *interest group* as "an association of people concerned with protecting and promoting shared values through the use of the political process."[4] Their purpose is basically to represent and promote the policy preferences of their constituents and use the power of the group to influence public decisions that affect them. In recent years, nurses have become increasingly influential with their legislators. Professional organizations at all three levels of government, as well as individual nurses with expertise in various aspects of health care, have knowledge of the health care system and patients' needs that make them valuable resources to legislators.

One method used to influence legislation is to support a candidate, either for election or for reelection. For many decades, making political contributions has been illegal for certain incorporated groups such as ANA, and more recently, tighter constraints have been placed on contributions and spending. Because the law requires that campaign contributions be kept as a separate fund and that no organizational money may be used for this purpose, many groups have created separate organizations for political activity. These are known as *political action committees (PACs)*. They may be located in the same office as an organization, such as ANA-PAC in ANA's Washington office, but by law funding activities are carefully separated from the rest of the organization's activities.

Many nurses have formed state PACs based on the ANA model. They have endorsed candidates, contributed to campaigns, and encouraged fellow nurses to run for office. It is important to remember that the success of any nurse PAC depends on the input and support of individual nurses. You can always start by volunteering a small amount of time, and, in so doing, have a voice in advancing the political strength of nursing. State professional nursing organizations are a good source of information on PACs and political groups at the state level. (ANA-PAC is described in Chapter 14.)

In recent years, many political participants have criticized PACs, claiming that they make it easy for certain groups to "buy" legislators and their votes. Although it is hard to prove the exact relationship between campaign contributions and voting patterns, there is no doubt that substantial contributions "ensure easy access to public officials and create an unhealthy atmosphere of familiarity."[5] Furthermore, the high costs of campaigns and politicians' dependence on PACs have led many legislators and consumer groups to call for campaign reform laws. Even with limits on spending, the average amount spent by winners of congressional and Senate races in 1988 reached $400,000 and $3.5 million, respectively. Thus, in the late 1980s and early 1990s, there have been several legislative proposals to revise presidential and congressional campaign financing laws. However, getting Congress to reach a consensus is difficult.

Another important, if unofficial, component of lawmaking is lobbying. *Lobbying* is generally defined as an attempt to influence a decision of a legislature or other governmental body. Since it is a type of petition for redress of grievances, lobbying is constitutionally guaranteed. Lobbying exists at several levels, from a single individual who contacts a legislator about a particular issue of personal importance to the interest groups that carefully (and often expensively) organize systems for monitoring legislation, initiating action, or blocking action on matters that concern them.

Professional lobbyists must be registered with Congress, and there are regulations concerning the types of organizations that may employ lobbyists. They spend all or part of their time representing the interests of a particular group or groups. Lobbyists provide information to legislators and their staffs (not necessarily objectively) and introduce resource people to them. Lobbyists are knowledgeable in the ways of legislation and are often familiar with legislators' personalities and idiosyncracies. They keep their interest group informed about any pertinent legislation and the problems involved, and help them to take effective action.

This organized approach to lobbying, effective though it is, should not overshadow the efforts of the individual who, in effect, lobbies when she or he contacts the appropriate legislator about an issue. Groups such as nurses have proved to be very effective in lobbying by coordinating the efforts of individuals for unified action.

NURSES AND POLITICAL ACTION

Organizations such as the ANA, NLN, and various specialty groups have taken leadership roles in mobilizing nurses in grass-roots lobbying. They have started educational programs and political consciousness-raising sessions, both to teach nurses techniques and strategies and to make them aware of issues. Networks have been set up whereby the lobbyist or a monitoring group in the state or national capital alerts the organization about the status of a bill at a crucial time, and an action plan begins. Usually not all members are mobilized, only certain volunteer activists. Some are experts on a particular topic, or they may be from some social, ethnic, or age group that the legislator is most inclined to listen to.

Using these strategies, nursing has had quite a good track record in Washington and is increasingly seen as influential in health policy. The action of individual nurses is especially effective.

Grass-Roots Lobbying

There are certain ways to lobby that give a better chance of success than if you approach it with good will but little organization. One of the first steps is making personal contact. It is sensible to become acquainted with your legislators before a legislative crisis occurs. This gives you the advantage of having made personal contact and shown general interest, and gives the legislator or staff member the advantage of a reference point. In small communities, legislators often know many of their constituents on a first-name basis through frequent contacts at town meetings or as other opportunities arise. This personal relationship may be more difficult to manage in large areas, but the effort to meet and talk with legislators is never wasted.

Having identified and located the legislator, call for an appointment or find out when the legislator is available in his local office (or in his capital office if this is convenient for both). Before the visit, it is helpful to know the following:

1. The geography of his legislative district and district number.
2. His present or past leadership in civic, cultural, or other community affairs.
3. How he voted on major controversial issues recently under consideration.
4. How he has voted in the past on major bills of interest to nurses.
5. The subject areas of his special interest, such as health, consumer affairs, and so on.
6. His political party affiliation and committee assignments.
7. His previous occupation or profession, with which he may still have some involvement.
8. What bills of major importance he has authored or co-authored.
9. Previous contacts with nursing organizations in the area.
10. Nursing organizations' endorsements of him or his opponents in past elections.

This information may be available from the SNA, political action groups, or literature from the legislator's office.

No one can say how such a visit should be conducted—it is obviously a matter of personal style—but generally it is wise to be dressed appropriately, to be friendly, to keep the visit short, to identify yourself as a nurse and, depending on your level of expertise, to offer to be a resource. Comment on any of his bills or votes of which you approve. If the first visit coincides with pending health legislation, ask whether he has taken a stand and perhaps add a few pertinent comments. Probably not more than three major issues should be discussed. A *brief* written account of the key points and/or documentation of facts can be left, along with an offer to provide additional information if he wants it. Legislators respond best if what is discussed is within the context of what their other constituents might want. In other words, is it good for the public and not just for nursing?

It is important to be prompt for the visit, but be ready to accept the fact that the legislator may be late or not able to keep the appointment. The administrative assistant who substitutes will probably be knowledgeable and attentive, and the time will not be wasted. If distance and time make visiting difficult, a telephone call is a good approach. The same general guidelines can be followed, and here also, speaking to the legislator's administrative assistant serves as good a purpose as speaking to the legislator directly.

Although personal visits and calls are considered useful in trying to influence a legislator, letter writing is also effective, especially if an initial introductory visit has already been made. It is also the most frequent way to communicate. Legislators are particularly sensitive to communications from constituents. They give far less attention to correspondence from outside their state or district and are often annoyed by it. If you don't know the legislator's local address, address the letter to the state or federal house or senate. However, addresses should be on hand before the need arises, and some say that mail received in the local office is apt to get more attention, since the letters don't compete with other mail at the capital. Accepted ways of addressing public officials are found in Exhibit 10-1. Then, follow these guidelines:

Do:

1. Identify yourself as a nurse and a constituent.
2. State the specific reason for the letter.
3. Be brief and to the point.
4. Use local examples (legislators like to use these anecdotes in their speeches).
5. Give reasons for your objections or support.
6. Use correct spelling and grammar and a typed business letter format.
7. Include the bill number and title or at least its popular name, for instance, the Nurse Education Bill.

Don't:

1. Be trivial.
2. Be insulting, sarcastic, or threatening.
3. Use a form letter.

If speed is important, as when a vote is pending, use the telephone, a fax, or a telegram. Night letters are generous in the number of words allowed and inexpensive; a 20-word public interest telegram can be sent to any congressman, or to the President or Vice-President, for a minimal cost.

If you support the legislator (or any candidate), then it is politically smart to contribute to his election campaign and/or volunteer your services in the campaign. These might include house-to-house canvassing to check voter registration or to register votes; supplying transportation to the polls; making telephone calls to stimulate registration and voting; acting as registration clerk and watcher, poll clerk and watcher, block leader, or precinct captain; raising funds; preparing mailing pieces; planning publicity; writing and distributing news releases; making speeches; answering telephones; staffing information booths; planning campaign events; or having "coffees" to meet the candidate.

Nurses who are knowledgeable about a particular issue are sometimes asked by ANA or another group to testify before a congressional committee. This requires both know-how and assurance but it can be a very interesting and satisfying experience. However it is important to be properly prepared

Exhibit 10-1
How to Address Public Officials

Official	Address	Official	Address
President	The President of the United States The White House Washington, DC 20500 Dear Mr. President:	Assemblywoman	The Hon. Mary Doe The State House Trenton, NJ 08625 Dear Ms. Doe:
Governor	The Hon. John Doe Executive Chamber Albany, NY 12224 Dear Governor Doe:	Mayor	The Hon. John Doe City Hall New York, NY 10007 Dear Mayor Doe:
U.S. Senator	Senator John Doe Senate Office Building Washington, DC 20510 Dear Senator Doe:	City Councilman	The Hon. John Doe City Council New York, NY 10007 Dear Mr. Doe:
Congressman	The Hon. John Doe House Office Building Washington, DC 20515 Dear Mr. Doe: or Dear Congressman:	Judge	The Hon. Mary Doe (Address of Court) Dear Judge Doe:
State Senator	The Hon. John Doe Senate Chambers Albany, NY 12224 Dear Senator:	Other officials	(Not included above) The Hon. John Doe Dear Mr. Doe:

Note: Addresses for state and local officials vary by locale.

and do it right. [For details on how to testify, see Lucie Kelly, *Dimensions of Professional Nursing,* 6th ed. (New York: Pergamon Press, 1991), pp. 407–408.]

OVERVIEW OF THE FEDERAL GOVERNMENT

To understand the politics of health care legislation at the federal level, it is important to know the government's organizational structure. The federal agencies with responsibility for health care are primarily within DHHS, although certain health-related programs are administered by other departments. An example is the Food Stamps program, which the Department of Agriculture administers. Within DHHS, there are four major health-related divisions: the Office of Human Development Services, the Social Security Administration (SSA), the Public Health Service (PHS), and the Health Care Financing Administration (HCFA) (see Figure 10-2). Most of the programs discussed in this chapter come under the HCFA or the PHS.

The HCFA administers the Medicare and Medicaid programs. The PHS includes the following agencies: Centers for Disease Control (CDC), Food and Drug Administration (FDA), Health Resources and Services Administration (HRSA), National Institutes of Health (NIH), Alcohol, Drug Abuse, and Mental Health Administration (ADAMA), and the new Agency for Health Care Policy and Research (AHCPR). The Division of Nursing within the HRSA and the National Center for Nursing Research (NCNR) at the NIH are focal points for nursing initiatives at the federal level. However, nurses are involved in every agency listed, and the activities of each agency have an impact on nursing practice. It behooves nursing students and faculty to be knowledgeable about them and provide input whenever possible.

MAJOR LEGISLATION AFFECTING NURSING

Both federal and state laws have a major impact on nursing practice and education. At the state level, nurses need to know about their own nursing practice acts and should be acquainted with the licensure laws of other health practitioners. These are discussed in Chapter 11. Other state legislation affecting the health and welfare of nurses may be equally important, and you should keep abreast of both proposed and enacted legislation.

In this section, the focus is on federal legislation that affects the practice of nursing and the rights of nurses; occasionally, state laws that are almost universal or closely related to federal laws are included. Obviously, all

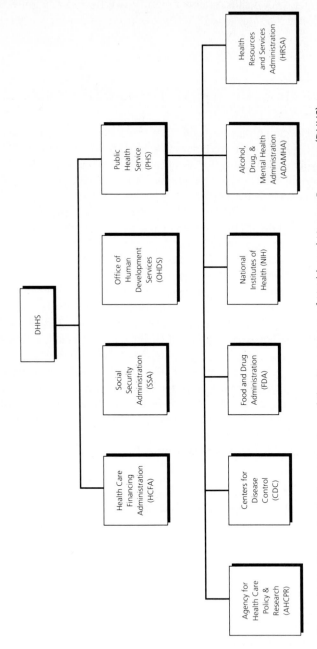

Figure 10-2 The organizational structure of the Department of Health and Human Resources (DHHS).

health legislation fits into that category, but those laws that seem to have particular significance are highlighted here.

Social Security

The *Social Security Act,* passed in 1935 and amended many times since, is the origin of most health and social welfare legislation in this country. Programs under the act are administered by the DHHS. Each title (or component) covers a specific social program. The average person who talks about Social Security benefits is usually referring to the federal Old-Age and Survivors' Insurance (OASI) program. It provides individuals with a monthly payment from the government after retirement age. Contributions to OASI (as well as to disability and hospital insurance) are made from employees' earnings. They are withheld from wage and salary payments and matched by employers. Deductions appear on employees' paycheck stubs under the category "FICA" *(Federal Insurance Contributions Act),* which is the tax law mandating employees' and employers' contributions. Self-employed individuals are also required to contribute. In recent years, the aging of the U.S. population has raised concerns about the solvency of the Social Security Trust Fund. In response, Congress has periodically enacted legislation to protect the program while ensuring that beneficiaries receive adequate payments.

Medicare

Medicare, authorized under Title XVIII of the Social Security Act, is a nationwide health insurance program for the aged and certain disabled persons. In both of the two parts (A and B) of Medicare, the benefits are limited to those who are 65 years of age or older and some disabled persons under 65.

Most Americans are automatically eligible for Part A, which consists of hospital insurance (HI), upon turning 65. Others, who are disabled or in need of kidney dialysis, qualify regardless of age. Under Part A, the patient pays a small deductible (which has been increasing) for hospital care, and the federal government pays the rest. Part A also covers skilled nursing facilities, home health care, and hospice care, with certain limits in each category.

Part B of Medicare is an optional supplemental medical insurance (SMI) program available to those over 65 upon payment of a monthly premium. SMI is financed through these premiums, along with general government funds. Most Part A beneficiaries are also enrolled in Part B. Part B pays 80 percent of the individual's cost for physicians' services in excess of an annual deductible. Services covered include the physician's care in the hospital, home, or office; laboratory and other diagnostic tests; outpatient services at a hospital; therapeutic equipment such as braces; home health services; mammograms; and respite care for caretakers of homebound Medicare beneficiaries. Certain services, such as long-term and preventive care that the elderly often need, are still unavailable under Medicare. Long-term care, in particular, is likely to be an area to which Congress will devote more attention in the near future as the demand for such services increases and the costs escalate.

The Medicare program is the responsibility of HCFA. HCFA enters into contracts with Blue Cross-Blue Shield, commercial carriers, and group practice prepayment plans to serve as administrative agents.

The term *intermediaries* is used for those handling claims from hospitals, home health agencies, and skilled nursing facilities; *carriers* is used for those handling claims from doctors and other suppliers of services covered. This arrangement is considered by some not only as adding another layer of bureaucracy, but also as increasing costs.

Medicare Legislation

Since 1966, Congress has enacted a number of Medicare amendments aimed primarily at controlling the soaring costs of the program. There are now rigid regulations regarding the length of the institutional stay that will be reimbursed and payment for specific services. Another major concern, quality of care, has also resulted in amendments.

The most far-reaching legislative changes were the provisions of the *Tax Equity and Fiscal Responsibility Act (TEFRA)* of 1982 (PL 97-248). This legislation required the Secretary of DHHS and certain congressional committees to develop Medicare prospective reimbursement legislative proposals for hospitals, skilled nursing facilities (SNFs), and, to the extent feasible, other providers. Other cost-cutting mechanisms affecting health care facilities and providers were also included.

The work on the prospective payment mechanisms resulted in enactment of PL 98-21, variously called the *Social Security Amendments of 1983,* the *Social Security Rescue Plan,* or simply the *DRG law.* This legislation established a "prospective payment system based on 467 Diagnostic Related Groups (DRGs) categories that allow pretreatment diagnosis billing categories for almost all United States hospitals reimbursed by Medicare."[6]

What DRGs mean to a hospital is that if a patient is kept more than the number of days designated by the patient's DRG category, the extra costs must be absorbed. If the patient goes home early, the amount designated for the scheduled days is the hospital's clear profit.

Needless to say, the DRG system had a direct effect on nursing. (See the References for specific articles on how nurses work within the DRG system.) In some cases, hospitals desperate to cut costs chose to retain lower-paid nursing personnel, rather than RNs. Others chose to turn to all-RN staffs that could actually save money by teaching patients or by anticipating potential complications, so that the patient would be discharged before the DRG-set time. As noted in Chapter 7, the job market for nurses also became tighter for a while. However, some nurses felt that this was also a good time to identify nursing services so that they could be separated from general daily charges. Others identified ways of determining the acuity of nursing care so that these could be considered in the DRG system.[7,8] In general, the Medicare prospective payment system has encouraged all health care providers, including nurses, to be more aware of the cost components in health care. For nursing, this has often been an advantage. Increasingly, nurse researchers have been able to document the cost effectiveness of nurse providers. This, in turn, has facilitated the enactment of legislation providing for reimbursement of nurses under federal and state health programs. Prospective payment also resulted in hospitals discharging patients "quicker and sicker." This led hospital administrators to appreciate, more than they previously did, the indispensable role that nurses have in caring for patients with higher levels of acuity in all types of health care settings.

The 1983 Medicare legislation also mandated the formation of peer review organizations (PROs) to replace the then existing professional standards review organizations (PSROs). The intent of the legislation was to establish mechanisms for local practicing physicians to review and evaluate the medical care rendered under Medicare. In general, each state has one PRO. However, some larger states have subcontracts with regional units. Nurses have been involved with PROs as staff and as members of PRO review boards. Consumers also play a significant role in PROs, because the 1983 law mandated that a certain proportion of the members of the PRO boards be composed of consumers. PROs are organized through the American Medical Peer Review Organization (AMPRO), based in Washington, D.C.

Since the enactment of prospective payment in 1983, there have been a series of revisions in Medicare through legislation and regulation. Many of the new laws deal with prospective payment rates, based on recommendations of the Prospective Payment Assessment Commission (ProPAC). Nursing has had an impact on these deliberations through the nurse representatives on the Commission, through studies of the costing out of nursing services under DRGs, and through the lobbying of major nursing organizations. Congress has also approved changes in the scope of services provided under Medicare. In 1990, Pap smears, mammography, and expansion of hospice benefits were added.

In addition to increasing the scope of services provided, Medicare revisions have included reimbursement for specific health care providers. In recent years, nurses have successfully lobbied for Medicare reimbursement of various types of nursing services. The year 1989 was a major one for legislation on nursing and physician reform under Medicare. First, certified registered nurse anesthetists (CRNAs) succeeded in obtaining legislation (PL 99-509) that authorized direct reimbursement under Medicare to CRNAs for anesthesia services that they are legally authorized to perform in the state.

Second, the 1989 reconciliation bill authorized nurse practitioners (NPs) and clinical nurse specialists (CNSs), working in collaboration with a physician, to certify and recertify the need for care under Medicare.

Third, the reconciliation bill mandated a Physician Payment Review Commission (PPRC) study of nonphysician providers, to be submitted to Congress by July 1, 1991. Nurses had input to the call for this study through their representatives on the PPRC and the lobbying of ANA and other nursing organizations.

The PPRC's work, in general, became the focus of attention when Congress began to reevaluate the system under which Medicare pays physicians' fees. Some of this concern was due to the dramatically rising costs of Medicare Part B, especially compared to the steadier increases in Part A. The 1989 bill revamped the system of paying doctors on the basis of "customary, prevailing, and reasonable fees" and replaced it with a "standard based on the total costs of the services provided, including the costs of a doctor's training and equipment and the relative value of the technical skills needed."

The new system is based on a resource-based relative value schedule (RBRVS) that places emphasis on time spent with patients, instead of the traditional way of allocating fees according to the type of specialty care of service rendered.[9] These changes in physician reimbursement under Medicare have provided incentives for review of nonphysician and noninstitutional reimbursement, including reimbursement for nurses.[10,11]

In 1991, the PPRC recommended that nonphysician practitioners (including certain nurses) under Medicare should also be paid based on RBRVS, taking into account the differences in education and training between physicians and nonphysician providers.[12]

Medicaid

Medicaid was authorized in 1965 as Title XIX of the Social Security Act to pay for medical services in behalf of certain groups of low-income persons. It is a federal-state means-tested entitlement program, which HCFA also administers. Certain groups of persons (i.e., the aged, blind, disabled, members of families with dependent children, and certain other children and pregnant women) qualify for coverage if their incomes and resources are sufficiently low. Each state designs and administers its own Medicaid program, setting eligibility and coverage standards within broad federal guidelines. As a result, substantial variation exists among the states in terms of persons covered, types and scope of benefits offered, and amount of payments for services. On the average, the federal government pays 56 percent of the benefit costs and states pay the rest. Until 1986, Medicaid eligibility was tied to welfare. In that year, Medicaid was extended to include certain women and children with low incomes who were not covered by the Aid to Families with Dependent Children (AFDC) program. This change was important because state poverty levels are considerably lower than the federal poverty level and were used as AFDC eligibility criteria, thus keeping many poor women and children from receiving necessary health care.

The expansion of Medicaid in recent years has occurred incrementally, with intense deliberations at state and federal levels of government. The discussions focused on what states were required and had the option to provide under Medicaid. The changes have had a significant impact on access to and financing of health care for America's women and children.[13] However, the escalating costs have caused states to cut back services. Some, such as Oregon, have set up plans that will allow more primary care and preventive services and limit more expensive services that are seen as less necessary (see Chapters 3 and 9).

In 1989, nurses reached another milestone when Congress enacted legislation providing for coverage of family nurse practitioner and pediatric nurse practitioner services under Medicaid, as long as they are practicing within the scope of state law. Since July 1990, states have been required to cover the services of these two types of NPs, regardless of whether they are under the supervision of or associated with a physician.

Block Grants

The block grant approach consolidates categorical programs into blocks and turns over control of money to the states, with little accounting to the federal government as to how the funds are spent. Block grants are funded through federal and state-matched funds. They shift much of the political and administrative accountability to the states, without subsequent increases in state funding, and they intensify inequities among states in terms of the populations covered by the programs. The major advantage of block grants is the streamlining they provide at the federal level by consolidating programs into clusters for legislative and programmatic purposes.

In 1981, three health block grants were formed: maternal and child health, preventive services, and mental health (including alcohol and drug abuse). Congress originally designated a primary care block grant that consisted of community and migrant health center programs, but it was never officially made a block grant, and today it remains a categorical program.

The Alcohol, Drug Abuse, and Mental Health Administration (ADAMHA) Block Grant is a high priority because it includes the drug abuse prevention programs that are part of the "war on drugs." The Maternal and Child Health Block Grant continues to gain support because of the country's unacceptably high infant mortality rate. The Prevention Block Grant is considered important because of the growing evidence that disease prevention and health promotion initiatives are cost effective and improve health status in many ways.

Health Services Legislation

Various other laws providing health care programs and services of interest to nurses include the following: *The Health Maintenance Organization Act of 1973* authorized the spending of $375 million during the next five years to help set up and evaluate HMOs in communities throughout the country. The concept is an arrangement in which subscribers pay a predetermined flat fee monthly or yearly that entitles them to basic health care services as needed. Emphasis is on preventive care and health teaching (see Chapter 3). The federal government continues to support HMOs through legislation that provides incentives to patients and providers for Medicare and Medicaid enrollees to use HMOs.

During the 1980s, federal funding for AIDS became a hot topic. The federal AIDS policies are extremely fragmented, lacking well-coordinated programs in health care or education. Nonetheless, the government supports a wide range of programs, which many AIDS advocates believe is still insufficient given the needs for research, community-based alternatives, and support for health professionals.

Across all agencies in the PHS, funding for AIDS rose to almost $1.6 million in 1990. Most went to the NIH, CDC, and ADAMHA. Elsewhere in the PHS, the HRSA received over $100 million for grants to provide home health and subacute care to AIDS patients, funds for training people who counsel or care for HIV-infected persons and AIDS patients, and demonstration activities for intermediate and long-term care facilities and children with AIDS.

The AIDS Commission appointed by President Reagan urged broad, comprehensive plans to fight the epidemic. Since its inception, nurses on the AIDS Commission have represented the concerns of nurses nationwide who are pivotal in providing AIDS treatment and outreach.

Also in the 1980s, one of Congress's attempts to combine concerns about the cost and quality of health care was the establishment of the Agency for Health Care Policy and Research (AHCPR) within the PHS. The agency was authorized under OBRA 1989 (PL 101-239), replacing what had been the National Center for Health Services Research and Health Care Technology Assessment. The mission of the AHCPR includes conducting research on the quality and effectiveness of health care services, developing practice guidelines, and assessing technology. The agency has the primary responsibility for implementing the Medical Treatment Effectiveness Program (MedTEP) within the DHHS. The purpose of MedTEP is to improve the effectiveness and appropriateness of health care services through better understanding of the effects of health care practices—including nursing—

on patient outcomes. The effectiveness initiatives are of particular importance because many policymakers look to effectiveness research as a way of controlling health care costs and streamlining medical practice. The AHCPR convened a Nursing Advisory Panel on Guideline Development to provide input to effectiveness research as it pertains to nursing. It is important for nurses to understand and contribute to the agency's programs as much as possible, because its recommendations will affect nursing practice.[14]

Nursing Education and Research

In the 1960s, as the federal government urged the enactment of legislation to provide health care for the aged under Social Security, health facilities and personnel became matters of urgency to Washington. More and more funds were channeled into health and education projects. At the same time, nurses were becoming more vocal, and their organizations stronger, more self-assured, and more convincing, when their representatives met with legislators and appeared before legislative committees. As a result of these and other factors, several new laws were enacted in the early 1960s that supported nursing and the individual nurse.

Most significant among these was the *Nurse Training Act* of 1964 (Title VIII of the Public Health Service Act). (For more details on federal funding of nursing education, see Chapter 19 in the fifth edition of *Dimensions of Professional Nursing*). The purpose of this law was to increase the number of nurses through financial assistance to diploma, associate AD, and baccalaureate degree nursing schools, students, and graduates taking advanced courses, and thus to help ensure more and better schools of nursing, more carefully selected students, a high standard of teaching, and better health care for the people.

Renewal of the law has had its ups and downs over two decades, especially during the era of retrenchment in the early 1980s. However, due to the successful lobbying of nursing organizations and individuals across the country, the program remained on the books. In 1985, federal legislation for nursing education was renamed the *Nurse Education Act* (*NEA*). That year was also a landmark year for nurses because it marked the establishment of the National Center for Nursing Research (NCNR) at NIH. Nurses claimed victory on November 20, when the Senate voted 89 to 7 to override President Reagan's veto of the NIH bill. The House had already supported the bill in its 380 to 32 vote to override the veto the previous week. The bill culminated several years of negotiations among various interest groups, legislative chambers, and branches of government. Within a short time, the center was up and running under the dynamic leadership of a distinguished nurse scientist,[15] Ada Sue Hinshaw, RN, PhD, FAAN. Since its inception, the center has begun collaborative intramural research (within NIH) on topics such as the frail elderly, extramural grants to schools of nursing, a research program in bioethics and clinical practice, and research initiatives for low-birthweight infants and patients with HIV infections.

The *Nursing Shortage Reduction and Extension Act* of 1988 increased the authorization level for nursing education to $119.5 million in 1991. However, appropriations have been lower than authorizations, mostly because of the budget deficit. For 1991, Congress funded the NEA at almost $60 million.

Nursing education legislation was due for reauthorization in 1991, and as Congress raced towards adjournment, nurse lobbyists were optimistic that nursing education would be authorized again, despite the administration's continued lack of support. In the House bill, Congress combined nursing with other health professions creating the *Health Professions Education Act of 1991*. The Senate was working on a similar bill with much higher funding for nursing. On the appropriations side, Congress allocated $61.4 million. After the expected conference committee compromise in early 1992, funding for nursing education was reauthorized.

In general, federal funding for nursing research seems to have fared better than funding for nursing education. By 1992, funding for nursing research had increased to $45 million (from $10 million in 1985). It may be that the significance of nursing research is catching on and the findings of nursing studies are being disseminated in the right circles. Nonetheless, given the overall multibillion-dollar NIH funding and the competition within NIH for these dollars, it is clear that nurses need to continue lobbying for funds to support nursing education and research and to muster all their political savvy in the process. Updates on the status of the NEA and NCNR legislation can be obtained from SNAs and nursing specialty organizations, as well as from the ANA's Washington office.

Support for other health professions education (medicine, osteopathy, dentistry, veterinary medicine, optometry, podiatry, and pharmacy), known by its acronym, MODVOPP, has been supported by such early laws as the *Health Professions Education Assistance Act* of 1963 and its successors. This law has a funding history similar to that of the NEA.

Workmen's Compensation

Workmen's compensation is becoming ever more important to nurses as the hazards of their work and workplace increase. These include exposure to environmental hazards, some of which are described in Chapter 3, and potentially fatal diseases such as AIDS and hepatitis B. The first such insurance to be held constitutional was the *Workmen's Compensation Act,* enacted by the state of Washington in 1911. Today all states require employers in industry to carry workmen's compensation, but in some states, nonprofit organizations, including hospitals, are exempt. However, most nurses are covered by some version of this type of insurance. Federal employees are usually covered by the *Federal Employees' Compensation Act,* enacted in 1952.

Workmen's compensation insurance, the cost of which is carried entirely by the employer, pays to employees who are injured on the job a proportion of their regular salaries for the time they are unable to work because of their injuries. If they are permanently disabled, they are entitled to additional compensation. Workmen's compensation insurance laws do away with the requirement of proof that the employer was negligent or that the employee was free from contributory negligence. They also prevent court action for injuries and provide instead an administrative procedure for securing awards of compensation.

Many states have extended the coverage provided by workmen's compensation laws to include occupational diseases; other states have enacted separate occupational disease acts, some of which cover all types of occupational disease; others specify which ones are covered.

The major breakthrough on the federal level was the enactment of the *Occupational Safety and Health Act* of 1970 (also discussed in Chapter 3), which established administrative machinery for the development and enforcement of standards of occupational health and safety. There are still no standards for the health care industry, which means, according to the law, that state safety rules remain in effect. These vary from state to state and even among specific communities. Of course, in case of negligence, the employer is liable to employee suits. This is important to nurses[16,17] who may acquire a disease, infection, or other illness on the job, for which they might be entitled to benefits under the state law.

Civil Rights, Employment, and Labor Relations

Beginning in the 1960s, a number of laws were passed to prohibit discrimination based on sex as well as race, color, religion, and national origin. Many of these are particularly important to women and are referred to in Chapter 13. Some of the most important ones are discussed below. (Comparable worth issues and other rights are discussed in Chapter 13 and are also mentioned in Chapter 3.)

Title VII of the *Civil Rights Act* of 1964 (Equal Employment Opportunity Law) has affected the job status of nurses because it includes a section forbidding discrimination against women in job hiring and job promotion among private employers of more than 25 persons. Executive Order No. 11246, as amended, extended the law to include federal contractors and subcontractors. Hospitals and colleges are subject to this order because of their acceptance of federal grants of various kinds.

Among other civil rights that have been given new protection are the rights of patients, children, the mentally ill, prisoners, the elderly, and the handicapped. Actions to protect these rights have come through a variety of legal means at state and national levels. Protection has increasingly been specified through regulations of various laws such as the amendments and subsequent regulations of the Social Security Act. Another is the *Rehabilitation Act* of 1973. Section 504 of that law reads, "no otherwise qualified handicapped individual in the United States shall, solely by reason of his handicap, be excluded from the participation in, be denied the benefit of, or be subjected to discrimination under any program or activity receiving federal financial assistance." The definition of *handicapped* includes drug addicts and alcoholics, as well as those having an overt physical impairment such as blindness, deafness, or paralysis of some kind. A major issue now is whether and under what circumstances AIDS patients and HIV-infected people come under this law. Some state and local jurisdictions have ruled that AIDS-related illness does come under their laws as a protected handicap. Those that do not consider communicable diseases as protected have ruled differently. In recent years, there have been two types of renewed civil rights activities. First, the *Americans with Disabilities Act* was enacted in 1990 with the intent of barring firms from denying jobs to individuals solely on the basis of disability, as long as reasonable accommodations can be made. The legislation is aimed at protecting the nearly 43 million disabled Americans, including people infected with HIV. Discrimination is prohibited in areas such as public accommodations, transportation, and private employment. This did not prevent an applicant to a nursing school who was hearing impaired from being refused. The Supreme Court upheld the decision.

In 1991, following a veto the previous year, President Bush signed the *Civil Rights Act of 1991*. The legislation was in response to 1989 Supreme Court rulings that shifted the burden of proof from employer to employee in cases where employees experience discrimination. The 1991 bill restored the previous standard by requiring employers to prove that the hiring practice is required for the job in question. The bill pertains mostly to women and minority members who claim to have experienced discrimination in job hiring situations. Its enactment was an important step in sustaining the civil rights of all Americans.

The right to privacy also affects nurses. One of the most important federal laws in this area is the *Freedom of Information Act* (FOIA) of 1966 and the *Privacy Act* of 1974. The purpose of the FOIA is to give the public access to files maintained by the executive branch of government. Recognizing that there are valid reasons for withholding certain records, the law exempts broad categories of records from compulsory public inspection, including medical records. It also gives access to their hospital records to patients in federal hospitals.

Another step in providing access to the individual's own records was enactment of the *Family Educational Rights and Privacy Act* of 1974, also known as the *Buckley Amendment*. The basic intent of this law was to provide students, their parents, and guardians with easier access to and control over the information contained in academic records. Educational records are defined broadly and include files, documents, and other materials containing information about the student and maintained by a school. Students must be allowed to inspect these records within 45 days of their request. They need not be allowed access to confidential letters of reference preceding January 1975, records about students made by teachers and administrators for their own use and not shown to others, certain campus police records, certain parental financial records, and certain psychiatric treatment records (if not available to anyone else). Students may challenge the content, secure the correction of inaccurate information, and insert a written explanation regarding the content of their records.

The law also specifies who has access to the records (teachers, educational administrators, organizations such as testing services, state and other officials to whom certain information must be reported according to the law). Otherwise, the records cannot be released without the student's consent. The law applies to nursing education programs as well as others.

The rights of research subjects have also been incorporated in diverse federal laws, especially in the last decade. PL 93-348, the *National Research Act* of 1974, not only provided some funds for nursing research but also set controls on research, including the establishment of a committee to identify requirements for informed consent, and required an institutional committee to review a research project to protect the patient's rights. The 1974 *Privacy Act* required a clear, informed consent for those participating in research. The 1971 *Food and Drug Act* also gave some protection in regulating the use of experimental drugs, including notification to the patient that a drug is experimental. The *Drug Regulation Reform Act* of 1978 took further steps to protect the patient receiving research drugs. Other drug and narcotics laws also affect nursing.

The *Comprehensive Drug Abuse Prevention and Control Act* of 1970 (Controlled Substance Act) replaced virtually all other federal laws dealing with narcotics, depressants, stimulants, and hallucinogens. It controls the handling of drugs by providers, including hospitals. The *Drug Regulation Reform Act* of 1978 took further steps in protecting the patient; at the same time, the FDA set requirements about sharing product information on drugs with consumers.

Also within the broad categories of rights are those laws related to labor relations. The first was the *National Labor Relations Act* (*NLRA*), one of several laws enacted to pull the country out of the Great Depression. The thesis, according to Werther and Lockhart,[18] was that labor unions could prevent employers from lowering wages, resulting in higher incomes and more spending. To achieve the growth of unions, employers had to be limited; for instance, they could no longer legally fire employees who tried to unionize. The National Labor Relations Board (NLRB), created by law, was empowered to investigate and initiate administrative proceedings against those employers who violated the law. (If these administrative actions did not curtail the illegal acts, court action followed. Only employers' violations were listed.)

In 1947, the NLRA was substantially amended, and the amended law, entitled the *Labor Management Relations Act* (or *Taft-Hartley Act*), listed prohibitions for unions. Section 14(b), for instance, contained the so-called right-to-work clause, which authorizes states to enact more stringent union security provisions than those contained in the federal laws.

In 1959, a third major modification was made. One of the purposes of the law, the *Labor-Management Reporting and Disclosure Act* or *Landrum-Griffin Act,* was to curb documented abuses such as corrupt financial and election procedures. For this reason, it is sometimes called the union members' Bill of Rights. The result is a series of rights and responsibilities of members of a union or a professional organization, such as ANA, that engages in collective bargaining. Required are reporting and disclosure of certain financial transactions and administrative practices and the use of democratic election procedures. That is, every member in good standing must be able to nominate candidates and run for election and must be allowed to vote and support candidates; there must be secret ballot elections; union funds must not be used to assist the candidacy of an individual seeking union office; candidates must have access to the membership list; records of the election must be preserved for one year; and elections must be conducted according to the procedures specified in the bylaws.[19]

Highly significant for nurses is the 1974 law that again amended the Taft-Hartley Act, PL 93-360, the *Nonprofit Health Care Amendments*. This law made private nonprofit health care facilities that had, through considerable lobbying, been excluded in the 1947 law, subject to national labor laws. These employees were now free to join or not join a union without employer retribution, a right previously denied to them unless they worked in a state that had its own law allowing them to unionize. It also created special notification procedures that must precede any strike action. The definition of *health care facility* included a broad range of acute care and community health care facilities.[20]

In 1988, the NLRB issued rules regarding the appropriate bargaining units for various types of facilities in the health care industry. The Board determined that RNs constitute a separate bargaining unit and have a strong desire for separate representation. Also, "the Board found LPNs to be appropriately included with technical employees in light of their skill level and licensure requirement."[21] In 1991, the Supreme Court ruled against the American Hospital Association and unanimously upheld the 1988 NLRB rules sanctioning the separate bargaining unit for RNs. This victory gave a strong impetus to SNAs across the country as they strove to increase the collective bargaining strength of RNs.[22]

Another recent piece of nursing legislation in the labor arena was the *Nurse Pay Act of 1990*. It was intended to enhance recruitment and retention of nurses in the Veteran's Administration (VA). Since the bill was implemented in April 1991, recruitment of VA nurses has improved. However, retention has been difficult due to the unintended salary compression of certain nurses, especially those earning a mid-range salary.

Another right that should be reported is the revision of the *Copyright Law,* amended in 1976 to supersede the 1909 law. The categories of work covered include writings, works of art, music, and pantomimes. The owner is given exclusive rights to reproduce the copyrighted work. The new law has some significance in this time of photocopying from journals and books; there are certain limits and need for permission to copy anything beyond certain minimums. Libraries can provide the appropriate information. Some books and journals specify their copying permission requirements.[23]

National Health Insurance (NHI)

Our patchwork system of health care delivery and insurance has resulted in approximately 37 million individuals lacking health insurance, one-third of whom are children. Furthermore, contrary to popular belief, the majority of uninsured people are working or dependents of people who are working.

In the 1980s and 1990s, policymakers discussed various proposals to provide health coverage for the uninsured. The major obstacles to all of these proposals were that the burden of cost would fall on different groups, depending on the policy scheme, and that invariably the plans involved increased costs and spending. In addition, each plan targeted a different group and, unless Congress accepted some form of national health insurance, there was no way to provide coverage for everyone.

Underlying all of these proposals are unanswered questions about health care as a right or a privilege. If one assumes that access to affordable health care is a right, then which level of government is responsible for it? The issue of equity needs to be addressed. Are all individuals entitled to the same level and quality of health care, regardless of their ability to pay for their care? Or can we accept a two-tiered system of care wherein those who can afford to pay more are entitled to the better quality and quantity of services their money can buy? Although the answers to these questions seem elusive, they raise important issues for nurses to consider as they become increasingly involved with the health care system.

In 1989, Congress took action to alleviate the burden of health insurance on the disabled by passing a law extending the period in which employers must let former workers who are disabled keep the group rate. The period was extended from 18 to 29 months, and the law is expected to protect the disabled, including individuals infected with HIV.

In 1990, the U.S. Bipartisan Commission on Comprehensive Health Care (renamed the Pepper Commission after its chairman, the late Congressman Claude Pepper) issued one of the most noteworthy reports. It called for extensions of job-based insurance, a national health insurance plan for those not covered by an employer, and a proposal for long-term care including a nursing home plan that was a catalyst for discussion on these issues.[24]

In the fall of 1990, for the first time in years, the Senate Committee on Labor and Health, chaired by Senator Edward M. Kennedy, approved health reform legislation. The following year, proponents of health care reform seemed to have more support, especially as they focused on the needs of the uninsured. Legislators talked seriously about "pay or play" options, whereby employers with a minimum number of employees would have to provide health insurance ("play") or "pay" a fee that would go to a national fund to cover the costs of insuring the unemployed. By the early 1990s, most health care organizations had designed or endorsed at least one plan for health care reform. In 1991, many nursing organizations supported *Nursing's Agenda for Health Care Reform,* calling for a "basic 'core' of essential health care services to be available to everyone."[26]

These activities were accompanied, or perhaps inspired, by two important developments that altered the political landscape. First, the business community became increasingly vocal about the financial burden of health care costs. Second, organized medicine, traditionally opposed to major social reform in medicine, shed its inhibitions and called for changes in the current health care system. With congressional leadership also pushing for health care reform and with public opinion polls pointing to the growing concern about rising health care costs, there is no doubt that health care will be an increasingly visible political and campaign issue. However, the political obstacles involved in health care reform could delay serious changes in the near future. Meanwhile, in the absence of a national policy for the uninsured, states have launched programs of their own (see Chapters 3 and 9). In addition, many health care policy analysts are looking to the Canadian system of national health insurance as a potential model for the United States. It is important that participants in these discussions differentiate between national health *service* and national health *insurance.* NHS would make all health workers government employees, and all care would be provided in government hospitals and health centers (as in many European countries). Financing is mainly by general revenues, but some insurance funds are used. In NHI plans such as Canada's, the crucial feature is that all health providers, including institutions, are independent entrepreneurs who contract with the government to provide services.[25] Throughout all of these deliberations, it is important to keep in mind the strengths and weaknesses of health care systems in other countries and to formulate one for the United States that best serves the distinctiveness of our political culture, diverse population, and economic realities.

OTHER LEGISLATION

Even a cursory look at *The American Nurse* or *The Nation's Health* makes it clear that there is a tremendous amount of legislation that is of interest to nurses, in relation both to their own profession and to their role in health care or as individuals. While some of these laws have been reviewed in this chapter, Chapter 13, concerned with the rights of people, also points out how judicial rulings affect them. For instance, after the Supreme Court ruled (*Rust v. Sullivan*) that regulations preventing doctors and others from discussing abortion in clinics receiving Title X federal funds were constitutional, the House and Senate immediately went to work to write a bill (or section of a bill) that would invalidate the decision. They could do this since the regulation that forbade such discussions was an administrative interpretation of a law they had passed, which some legislators said was a misinterpretation of what they intended. (Although such a bill did pass, it was vetoed by President Bush, and Congress was not able to override the veto.) Previously, a number of laws had been passed both supporting and limiting access to abortion in Congress and state legislatures. This is likely to be an ongoing issue.

In addition to abortion, there are several other family-related issues that Congress and interest groups such as nurses have been discussing. Two that received considerable attention during the late 1980s and early 1990s are family leave and child care. Several times during that period, Congress came close to enacting legislation on family and medical leave that would have required employers to give unpaid time off to parents of newborn or sick children or dependents. Women's rights groups and organized labor supported the bill. However, business groups opposed any type of parental leave bill that makes benefits mandatory. Congress did pass the Family and Medical Leave Act in 1990 and 1991, but failed to override President Bush's veto in both years. Legislation on the health of children is also expected.

In terms of child care, Congress enacted landmark legislation as part of the 1990 budget reconciliation act. The law includes tax credits for child care and grants to states that target low-income families. The administration's willingness to sign it is seen by many as a hopeful sign of more activism in social policy in the years ahead.[27] At the other end of the age spectrum, some action on long-term care may evolve.

Agencies and Regulations

Follow-up of federal legislation requires close attention. It is not just the law itself that affects the public, but the proliferating federal regulations. Legislators have charged that regulations have been used specifically to circumvent the intent of the law; at the least, regulations often shape the legislation they are intended to carry out.

Equally important are the agencies created by the various laws, such as the FDA and Federal Trade Commission (FTC). The FTC, for instance, goes back to 1914, when the Federal Trade Commission Act was passed. It has extensive power; it can represent itself in court, enforce its own orders, and conduct its own litigation in civil courts, and it seems to have relative freedom from the executive branch of government. Its forays into the health field, with rulings on professional advertising, licensure, and other aspects of health care delivery never thought of in 1914, may indicate a direction for other administrative agencies such as FDA. On the other hand, some subjects of the FTC rulings have banded together to lobby for limitation of FTC powers. This occurred, for instance, in 1982, when attached to the FTC reauthorization bill was an amendment exempting state-licensed professionals from its jurisdiction. A major supporter was AMA; an opponent was ANA.

WHAT NEXT?

Pressure to enact legislation for the uninsured and to hold down the spiraling health care costs of this country will dominate the political scene in the next few years. These problems will be compounded by complex bioethical issues raised by new technologies and the need to meet all of these demands in an era of continued budget deficits. Family concerns will also play an important role. Lawmakers will view health care policy within the context of broad social and environmental issues, both nationally and internationally. Without doubt, nurses will want to have a role in making these decisions.

KEY POINTS

1. The balance of power in the U.S. legal system is due to the fact that statutory law, executive law, and judicial law all have separate functions.
2. The judicial system is made up of courts at national, state, and local levels, each handling different kinds of cases, with appeals courts providing further legal options.
3. Important aspects of the legislative process include committee hearings and decisions, debate, amendments, possible conference committee agreements, final vote, administrative signature, and assignment to an administrative agency.

4. Information needed to influence legislation can be acquired from many sources, including consumer organizations, nursing organizations, governmental offices at various levels, and many publications.
5. Nurses can influence legislation in many ways by keeping legislators informed of their opinions and by supporting PACs in which they are interested.
6. Federal laws influence both the education and the practice of nurses, as well as their early professional lives, through social legislation.

REFERENCES

1. Northrop C, Kelly M. *Legal issues in nursing*. St. Louis: C.V. Mosby Company, 1987, pp. 3–35.
2. Creighton H. *Law every nurse should know*, 5th ed. Philadelphia: W.B. Saunders Company, 1986, p. 7.
3. The legislative process is described in full detail in many political action handbooks and pamphlets from organizations, as well as in the introduction to annual issues of the *Congressional Quarterly Almanac*.
4. Kalisch B, Kalisch P. *Politics of nursing*. Philadelphia: J.B. Lippincott Company, 1982.
5. Common Cause: Money talks on health issues. *Nation's Health*, 8:5 (December 1978).
6. Shaffer F. DRGs: History and overview. *Nurs and Health Care*, 4:388 (September 1983).
7. Hamilton J. Nursing and DRGs: Proactive responses to prospective reimbursements. *Nurs and Health Care*, 5:155–159 (March 1984).
8. Joel L. DRGs and RIMs: Implications for nursing. *Nurs Outlook*, 32:42–49 (January–February 1984).
9. Mittelstadt P. Medicare fee schedule recommended. *Am Nurse*, 22:8 (May 1991).
10. Harrington C., Culbertson RA. Nurses left out of health care reimbursement reform. *Nurs Outlook*, 38:156–158 (July–August 1990).
11. Burke SP. Reflections on the 100th Congress. *Nurs Economics*, 8:15–16 (January 1990).
12. Mittelstadt, op. cit.
13. Cohen SS. The politics of Medicaid. *Nurs Outlook*, 38:229–233 (September–October 1990).
14. Joel L. Seizing an exceptional moment: The effectiveness initiative. *Am Nurse*, 22:6 (April 1990).
15. Hinshaw AS. The National Center for Nursing Research: Challenges and initiatives. *Nurs Outlook*, 36:54–56 (March–April 1988).
16. Creighton H. Recovery for on-the-job injuries or illness. *Nurs Mgt*, 15:70–71 (March 1984).
17. Rosenthal T. Understanding Workers' Compensation: When you get hurt, who will help? *Nurs Life*, 2:39–42 (May–June 1982).

18. Werther W, Lockhart CA. *Labor relations in the health professions*. Boston: Little, Brown and Company, 1976, pp. 6–8.
19. Ibid., pp. 22–27.
20. Northrop and Kelly, op. cit., pp. 502–508.
21. National labor relations board. *Capital Update*, 6:5 (November 25, 1988).
22. Supreme Court okays all-RN unit. *Am Nurse*, 23:1 (June 1991).
23. Fay M. Borrower beware . . . ! *Nurs Success Today*, 1:16–18 (January 1985).
24. Commission calls for job-based national health insurance. *Nation's Health*, 20:1 (March 1990).
25. Schell E. Lessons from the Canadian health care system. *Nurs Economics*, 7:306–309 (November–December 1989).
26. American Nurses' Association. Nursing agenda for health care reform. *Am Nurse*, 23(Suppl):2 (June 1991).
27. Oda DS. The imperative of a national health strategy for children. *Nurs Outlook*, 37:206–208 (September–October 1989).

CHAPTER 11

HEALTH CARE CREDENTIALING AND NURSING LICENSURE

OBJECTIVES

After studying this chapter, you will be able to:

1. Define licensure, certification, registration, and accreditation.
2. List three criticisms of licensure.
3. Describe the major controversies about institutional licensure.
4. Explain the difference between mandatory and permissive licensure.
5. Explain the meaning of a "grandfather clause."
6. List the key components of a nurse practice act.
7. List four reasons for which a license may be revoked or suspended.
8. Describe two current problems related to nursing certification.
9. Differentiate among the various ways of legalizing advanced practice.
10. Explain the meaning of "sunset legislation."
11. Identify the problems related to proving continuing competence.

For most nurses, licensure after graduation is a primary goal. For some this will be the only credential they will hold after the diploma or degree they earned from their educational program. To both the nurse and the public, being licensed is something special and important—and they're right. However, licensure is not the only credentialing mechanism in health care. (See Exhibit 11-1 for definitions.) Nor is it (or the others) without problems. Health manpower credentialing has been blamed by consumers and the government as being one of the factors responsible for some of the serious problems in health care: fragmentation of services, accelerating costs, and poor use and distribution of health manpower.

In the 1970s health manpower credentialing was the object of considerable attention, especially by the federal government. The strong recommendations of the various reports created an uproar among both health practitioners and

Exhibit 11-1

Definitions

Accreditation:[a] The process by which an agency or organization evaluates and recognizes an institution or program of study as meeting certain predetermined criteria or standards.

Licensure:[a] The process by which an agency of government grants permission to persons to engage in a given profession or occupation by certifying that those licensed have attained the minimal degree of competency necessary to ensure that the public health, safety, and welfare will be reasonably well protected.

Registration:[b] The process by which individuals are assessed and given status on a registry attesting to the individual's ability and current competency. Its purpose is to keep a continuous record of the past and current achievements of an individual.

Certification:[a] The process by which a nongovernmental agency or association grants recognition to an individual who has met certain predetermined qualifications specified by that agency or association. Such qualifications may include (1) graduation from an accredited or approved program; (2) acceptable performance on a qualifying examination or series of examinations; and/or (3) completion of a given amount of work experience.

[a]U.S. Department of Health, Education, and Welfare, *Report on Licensure and Related Health Personnel Credentializing* [DHEW Publ. No. (HSM) 72–11], 1971.

[b]*The Study of Credentialing in Nursing: A New Approach,* Vol. 1. The Report of the Committee (Milwaukee, Wisc.: 1979).

employers, for there was the implied threat that if the credentialing problems were not resolved, the federal government would step in and take control away from the professions. What resulted was both internal and external scrutiny, with some changes that improved the system to some extent.[1] Action on the federal level has almost died out, since more conservative administrations have shifted responsibility to the states. Because the credentialing issues are not resolved, the states have responded with actions that affect every health care practitioner, including nurses. Therefore, knowing about the pros and cons of licensure and other credentialing options can help you think through some of these issues before they come to the inevitable crisis stage.

LICENSURE AND OTHER TYPES OF CREDENTIALING

Licensure is a police power of the state; that is, the state legislative process determines what group is licensed, and with what limits. It is the responsibility of a specific part of the state government to see that that law is carried out, including punishment for its violation. Although licensure laws differ somewhat in format from state to state, the elements of each are similar. For instance, in the health professions laws, there are sections on definition of the profession that describe broadly the scope of practice; requirements for licensure, such as education; exemptions from licensure; grounds for revocation of a license; creation of a licensing board, including members' qualifications and responsibilities; and penalties for practicing without a license.

Licensure laws are either mandatory (compulsory) or permissive (voluntary). If mandatory, the law forbids anyone to practice that profession or occupation without a license or face a fine or imprisonment. If permissive, the law allows anyone to practice as long as she or he does not claim to hold the title of the practitioner (such as RN).

Licensing of the health occupations was advocated in the early nineteenth century, but it was not until the early 1900s that a significant number of licensing laws were enacted. They were generally initiated by the associations of practitioners that were interested in raising standards and establishing codes for ethical behavior. Because they could not count on voluntary compliance, the associations tried to get regulatory legislation. To some critics, this movement is also seen as a way of giving members of an occupation or profession as much status, control, and compensation as the community is willing to give. It is true that as the health occupations proliferate, each group begins to organize and seek licensure. Because many of these occupations are subgroups of the major health professions or are highly specialized, licensure creates problems of further fragmentation and increased cost in health care—according to the critics.

In all of the proposals for changes in health manpower credentialing, criticism of individual licensure is implicit or explicit. Particularly in the last 15 years, the evils were cited; changes (often slow in coming) were dismissed as too little and too late. Some of the key criticisms were (and are) as follows:

1. The minimal standards of safety, theoretically guaranteed by granting the initial license, are often no longer met by some (perhaps many) practitioners because there is no organized system of monitoring continued competence. There is even the question of whether any written exam can determine safe practice in the actual work setting.
2. There is too much rigidity in the rules and regulations in relation to curriculum, so that minimal standards may lag behind the times and educational innovations are stifled.
3. Definitions of practice are so general that, when challenged, allocation of specific tasks may be determined by legal opinions or interpretations by lay people who cannot make an accurate judgment about what is or should be done in practice.
4. Definitions may be so limiting that impractical or unrealistic boundaries are established between practitioners of different kinds.
5. Too many licensing boards are still composed of members of that particular profession (or, in some cases, the professional superior of that group), without representation by competent lay members or allied health professions. This is seen as allowing these professionals to control the kind and number of individuals who may enter their field, with the possibility of shutting out other health workers climbing the occupational ladder and limiting the number of practitioners for economic reasons.
6. There are always some licensed practitioners who are unsafe, and even if they lose their license in their own state, boards in other states are not notified, and the individual simply crosses a state line and continues to practice.

Of the licensed occupations, only 14 are licensed in every state (but not every territory): chiropractors, dental hygienists, dentists, nursing home administrators, optometrists, pharmacists, physical therapists, physicians (MD and DO), podiatrists, professional and practical nurses, psychologists, and veterinarians. Other practitioners find their mobility restricted as they discover that they must be licensed in one state but not another. Even those licensed in all states may need to take licensing exams again when they relocate. Each state controls its own licensing exam. Nursing, with its state board examinations, now called the *National Council Licensure Examination*

(*NCLEX*), is accepted in every state. This allows for licensure by endorsement. That is, assuming that other criteria for licensure are met, a nurse need not take another examination when relocating to another state.

Despite these problems, it seems that almost all of the established or fledgling health occupations, more than 250 at last count, consider licensing as a primary means of credentialing. The licensure problems of one health occupation obviously are not necessarily the same as those of all the others.

Institutional Licensure

Because the majority of all kinds of health workers function in institutional settings, one suggested alternative to individual licensure is institutional licensure. *Institutional licensure* is a process by which a state government regulates health institutions; it has existed for more than 35 years. Usually, requirements for establishing and operating a health facility have been concerned primarily with such matters as administration, accounting requirements, equipment specifications, structural integrity, sanitation, and fire safety. In some cases, there are also minimal standards of square footage per bed and minimal nursing staff requirements. The issue in the "new" institutional licensure dispute is whether personnel credentialing or licensing should be part of the institution's responsibility under general guidelines of the state licensing authority.[2]

There are various interpretations of just what institutional licensing means and how it could or should be implemented. The general idea, according to Nathan Hershey, who originated the concept, is that since health care institutions are held accountable for the actions of their employees, they should be given the responsibility of regulating them. The state licensing agency would establish certain basic standards of education and experience, but the institution's administrators would decide just what kind of position that individual could hold. An example given was that of a nurse returning to work after 10 or more years. Her RN licensure would not count. Instead, she would be placed first in an aide position, then an LPN position, and gradually raised to a staff nurse level when she "regained her skills and became familiar with professional and technological advances through inservice programs"[3] Hershey was, then and later, rather evasive as to the place of the physician in this new credentialing picture, implying that the current practice of hospital staff review was a pioneer effort along the same lines and might as well continue to function. However, he did list as sites all institutions and agencies providing health services, such as hospitals, nursing homes, physicians' offices, clinics, and the all-inclusive "et cetera."

The advantages for the employer are obvious: financial savings and almost total control, including the ability to place employees where and when they would be most useful, without needing to consider individual licensing laws. For instance, an aide trained on the job might do procedures that now only

RNs are permitted to do. This may or may not give the public cheaper care, but it certainly won't be better. The disadvantages for the licensed person are great. Particularly for nursing, it raises the specter of a return to the corrupted apprentice system of early hospital nursing in the United States. Probably a hospital's own personnel would be used as teacher-preceptors. Who then would do their job? How would they be compensated? How long would "students" be expected to function in their current positions with their current salaries while they "practice" the new role? And with what kind of supervision? What kind of testing programs would exist for each level? Testing by whom? With what kinds of standards? Such sliding positions might well cut personnel costs, but might they not also indenture workers instead of freeing them with new mobility?

Problems of criteria for standards are obvious. If 50 states cannot now agree on criteria for individual licensure, why would institutional licensure be any different? Instead of making interstate mobility easier, institutional licensure would more likely limit even interinstitutional mobility. A worker could qualify for position X in institution A, with absolutely no guarantee that this would be acceptable to institution B.

It is true that many of these practices already exist in hospitals, but it hardly seems progressive to make an unsatisfactory system legal. Expecting the state licensing agency to prevent abuse is overly optimistic. The number of inadequate and even dangerous caregiving facilities, supposedly inspected by the state but still in existence, is evidence of the problems in controlling even minimum quality. Checking who does what how well will be almost impossible, resulting in one more paper tiger—inspection by paperwork.

In the late 1970s the leadership of ANA pointed out these problems to other health professionals and the public. The resulting furor forced the federal government to stop encouraging the institutional licensure approach. Does this eliminate the threat of institutional licensure? Not really, for it seems now that the concept is reappearing, if it ever disappeared, without its label.[4] In some states, overt attempts to legislate institutional licensure (which had been kept in committee or killed primarily through the efforts of organized nursing) keep emerging. One expert in the field predicts that with the trend toward multi-institutional ownership, especially by for-profit groups, and the concomitant trend for physicians to become employees, "corporate-wide credentialing" would be sought by the corporate giants. He speculated on whether the professional groups would have the political clout to prevent it.[5]

Certification

Certification was and is attracting considerable attention as a substitute for, or an adjunct to, licensure; in the latter case, it is a means of identifying specialists within a field. For instance, many of the health occupations described in Chapter 3 are only certified, but physicians with all-encompassing licensure increasingly use certification to differentiate specialists. Nurses are also starting to do so.

Still, certification is not a clearly understood credentialing mechanism. Two points are essential for understanding: (1) certification is voluntary on the part of the individual, and (2) the organization or agency that certifies is nongovernmental and is usually made up of experts or peers in that particular field. This "private credentialing" differs fundamentally from "public credentialing" (licensure) in that the latter can legally prohibit unlicensed practice. Those who lack private credentials "still possess a legal right to practice, although they may be disadvantaged in the marketplace because independent decision-makers such as consumers, hospitals, and public or private financing plans value their services less highly."[6] Private credentialing can be described as serving solely informational purposes, a sort of "seal of approval" from the professional association or nongovernmental board that grants it.[7] It gives the consumer an opportunity to make more informed decisions, in that certification indicates that the certified person has voluntarily met certain standards that similar caregivers have not.

In general, criticisms of certification are remarkably like those of licensure. First, the validity of written examinations is challenged. Second, there is the question of grandfathering, also a licensure problem. Usually those who practiced a specialty before certification existed are "grandfathered in," that is, permitted to hold certification without fulfilling the usual requirements. Thus, the information given the public—that these persons fulfill certain criteria—is not accurate. Here the answer may lie in requirements to demonstrate ongoing competence for recertification—providing that that measure is valid. More certifying groups now have a recertification mechanism.

Finally, there is the concern that certification is done by the professional organization that also accredits the educational program from which the candidate must graduate in order to qualify for certification. Clearly, that mechanism provides complete control by the occupation and can also shut out potential candidates. This problem was resolved, to a large extent, by the FTC rulings that such arrangements were illegal restraint of trade.[8] Professions then gradually separated these functions into independent entities. Two examples are the nurse-midwives and nurse anesthetists, whose organizations are described in Chapter 14. They are also the first nursing specialties to have certification.

Despite these criticisms, certification is generally advocated as a way to help the consumer make choices. Certification rather than specialized licensure is the route preferred by ANA to identify nurse specialists/practitioners. (ANA certification is described in Chapter 14, and the specialty organizations that have certification mechanisms are noted in Appendix 5).

Because the public needs to know that the certifying group and its standards have some legitimacy, there is a second-tier credentialing organization (to certify the certifiers) that can be either voluntary or governmental. A number of these organizations exist, such as the National Commission of Certifying Agencies, and they do set certification standards, to which most legitimate certifying groups adhere. Nursing attempted to set up a central organization to establish guidelines and approve existing and future specialty nursing certification programs in 1990. This was part of a project funded by the Josiah M. Macy Foundation to establish a National Board of Nursing Specialties (NBNS). It had been the consensus of a group of nursing leaders meeting with the Foundation that the quality of nursing care in the United States was not consistent and that perhaps some link between national standards for certification and quality of nursing care could be drawn. (The standards for certification by ANA and those of other specialty organization certification groups may differ considerably.) When the committee formed to create NBNS presented its ideas to the National Federation of Specialty Nursing Organizations (NFSNO), the 28 member organizations seemed to receive the concept positively. However, when it came to commitment to such an organization, a considerable number refused. It was almost a replay of the 1982 action when some of the same organizations plus NLN agreed, *in principle,* to a national credentialing center but ultimately balked at central control.[9]

What were the objections to the NBNS? In the fall of 1990, seven of the largest specialty organizations released a public statement that the proposed NBNS Board would not be suitable because, in part, certain delineations of responsibilities were not clear and because the BSN was being set as a criterion. The latter was probably a major sticking point, because many of those certified by these groups do not have BSNs. With such large and powerful nursing organizations unwilling to participate in the proposed NBNS, whether it can became a meaningful entity is not clear. Nevertheless, eight other nursing groups that did support the NBNS concept joined together to establish the American Board of Nursing Specialties (ABNS). They hoped to persuade others to join them and also to find additional funding, perhaps from a foundation.[10]

Probably, one of the problems in certification of nursing, the fact that both ANA and certain specialty organizations each certify the same specialists with different criteria, will not change immediately.[11] Both the nurse and the consumer, then, must decide which, if either, is more reliable. However, now the organizations are making more positive efforts either to coordinate their certification activities into single tests or to accept one another's certification. (Information about specific certification procedures can be obtained from each organization.)

Accreditation

Accreditation, another voluntary nongovernmental method of credentialing, occurs on an institutional, not an individual, basis. Both educational programs and institutions and health care institutions often seek accreditation because it is presumably a mark of excellence, that is, it indicates that higher standards than are required by a government entity are met.[12] Quite often, accreditation is necessary for hospitals, for instance, to have medical residency programs and for educational institutions to receive federal or state funds for scholarships or other purposes. (However, in 1991, the Secretary of Education recommended that the link between federal aid and accreditation be cut.) As with certification, there has been a great deal of criticism, with questions about the standards and procedures as well as the cost. In 1991, one regional accreditation group was under fire from the federal government because of a standard that required an educational institution to have a "sufficient" number of minority faculty, although this governmental "interference" drew an angry response from the American Council on Education, which represents many colleges and universities. The rigidity of accreditation standards was also seen to stifle creativity. Most of all, the lack of public representation on accrediting bodies (which has been rectified somewhat), and the lack of scientific development and validation of accreditation criteria, are still seen as serious problems.

In nursing, accreditation has also been a controversial issue. All nursing programs, including PN programs, are eligible for NLN accreditation, which is seen as an important asset. It is not a simple process.[13] Certain fees are required, and the program must complete a self-study report. If the report indicates that NLN criteria have been met, a site visit by a team of nurse educators from the same level of program is made. After consideration by a board, recommendations are made to accredit for a certain period of time or not, a decision that may be appealed. (This is a very brief overview; changes in procedure are made periodically.) Besides the criticisms of accreditation in general, another in nursing is that a university or college already goes through a regional accreditation process and that NLN accreditation is duplicative and costly, a point that is being made by academic administrators about other kinds of specialty accreditation, too. A unique issue is just which nursing organization should be accrediting. Both ANA and the American Association of Colleges of Nursing (AACN) think that this is their role, although neither has made any progress in wresting accreditation from NLN.

As noted in Chapter 3, the JCAHO accredits a number of health care institutions and agencies. Whereas once it was involved only in hospital accreditation, its expanded activities now clash with nursing in at least one area. An independent subsidiary of the NLN, the Community Health Accreditation Program (CHAP), has been involved with accreditation of home health care agencies for some time. CHAP also provides management consultation to assist agencies in meeting its high standards for accreditation. Both groups require a self-study report and send a team for a site visit, but CHAP's visits are unannounced. CHAP, considered by many as the only consumer-oriented health care accreditation body, has an interdisciplinary board. Perhaps because of this, and its high standards, in 1992, CHAP was the first home care accrediting group to be awarded "deemed status" by DHHS. This means that HCFA grants CHAP authority to determine home care agencies' eligibility for Medicare reimbursement. The JCAHO has membership by organizations, with AMA and AHA having the majority of the 21 corporate seats, with fewer from the American College of Physicians, the American College of Surgeons, and the American Dental Association. There are three public members. ANA has consistently been denied a seat on the JCAHO board, although nurses are on some committees and are usually on a site-visit team. Like certification, accreditation is not likely to disappear, but issues will continue to be raised.

Sunset Laws and Other Public Actions

Besides considering alternatives, improving the licensure process has become a national mandate. Although the speed of the action taken has varied from state to state, steps taken almost universally at one level or another include adding consumers and sometimes other functionally related health professionals to each board, giving more attention to disciplinary procedures, and gradually developing proficiency and equivalency examinations. In a number of states, boards have been consolidated, sometimes under committees of lay people (or at least a majority of consumers), who make the decisions about licensing, with the individual boards acting in an advisory capacity. Although one reason given is improved efficiency, some nurses fear that this is an indirect approach to institutional licensure because these reorganizations tend to weaken nursing's control over its practice.

For some professions, improving the licensure laws to protect the public was a new experience. A motivating factor was the enactment of "sunset laws" that require the periodic reexamination of licensing agencies to determine whether particular boards or activities should be eliminated. Most of the states have now enacted such laws, a result of a lobbying campaign by Common Cause, a consumer group, to bring about legislative and executive branch oversight of regulating boards and agencies of all kinds. Common Cause identified 10 principles to be followed, including a time schedule. An important component was that an evaluation was to allow for public input, as well as that of the boards and occupations involved. Consolidation and "responsible pruning" were encouraged. Although the review would be done by appropriate legislative and executive committees, safeguards were to be built in to prevent arbitrary termination of boards and agencies.[14] These principles are generally adhered to, but states do vary in their management of sunset reviews. If a sunset law is in effect, the data and justification for existence are a joint staff-board responsibility, although the professional organizations are also usually helpful.

Nursing was no more ready for sunset review than other disciplines, but nurses learned, sometimes the hard way.[15,16] Both Grobe and Thomas suggest specific strategies.

By 1985, most nursing boards had undergone sunset reviews, and the new or amended laws usually reflected changes in practice and society. Most practice acts have broadened the scope of practice, added consumers to their boards, and sometimes required evidence of current competence through various means, including CE. State boards have given increased attention to removing and/or rehabilitating incompetent nurses. Meanwhile, educators are working seriously on equivalency and proficiency examinations and other methods of providing flexibility and upward mobility for nursing candidates. Nurses in the field have continued to improve techniques of peer evaluation, implement standards of practice, and encourage voluntary CE.

OVERVIEW OF NURSING LICENSURE

Mandatory and Permissive Laws

Enactment of nurse licensure laws was one of the primary purposes of ANA at its inception (as described in Chapter 2). In every instance, the original state law was permissive. The first mandatory nursing practice act was enacted in New York in 1938, but it was not put into effect until 1947. One of the dangers of permissive licensing is that schools with poor curricula and inadequate clinical experience produce workers who can legally nurse, although they are potentially dangerous practitioners.

As of 1991, all states had mandatory licensure laws for professional and practical nurses. However, some states are loose in their interpretation of *mandatory*. States that have global exemption clauses in licensure laws stating that almost anyone can be a nurse, providing that there is some kind of supervision, are sometimes seen as permissive states regardless of a mandatory clause.

The Grandfather Clause

One concern about mandatory laws is that those already practicing in the field will be abruptly removed and deprived of their livelihood. This is, however, untrue because mandatory laws are forced, for political and constitutional reasons, to include a grandfather clause. A *grandfather* or *waiver clause* is a standard feature when a licensure law is enacted or a current law is repealed and a new law enacted.

The grandfather clause allows persons to continue to practice the profession/occupation when new qualifications are made law. Although the concept goes back to post–Civil War days, it is also related to the Fifth and Fourteenth Amendments of the Constitution. The U.S. Supreme Court has repeatedly ruled that the license to practice a profession/occupation is a property right and that the Fourteenth Amendment extends the due process requirement to state laws. Many nurses currently licensed were protected by the grandfather clause when a new law was passed or new requirements were made, although most probably never realized it. For instance, when various states began to require psychiatric nursing as a condition of licensure, those who had not had those courses in their educational programs did not forfeit licensure.[17]

When the grandfather clause is enacted in relation to mandatory licensure, those who can produce evidence that they practiced as, say, a PN, if applying for LPN status, must be granted a license. However, grandfathering does not guarantee employment. Thus, some employers chose not to employ "waivered" LPNs, just a they had not employed them as unlicensed practitioners.

ANA and NCSBN

Over the years, it was generally accepted that the professional organization ANA developed model practice acts that SNAs used as a model when introducing new practice acts (licensure laws). This was when a Council of State Boards with representatives from state boards was more or less a part of ANA. When the group broke off to become an independent organization, the National Council of State Boards of Nursing (NCSBN), there was limited coordination between the two groups. In a way, the National Council was establishing its own power base. Therefore, when in 1980 an ANA committee developed guidelines for state legislation to replace the 1976 Model Practice Act, NCSBN chose to go its own way and published a Model Practice Act in 1982. Despite months of negotiating, the two organizations could not agree on a similar philosophy or even a common language. Why? Each group has its own constituents: NCSBN, with its representatives from all the state boards of nursing, who deal with state officials and legislatures on a day-to-day basis; and ANA, with its diverse group of nurses committed to setting standards for nursing. The new ANA document *Suggested State Legislation* is intended as a policy guide for "nurses, state nurses' associations, state boards of nursing, and state officials who are considering changes to their state nursing practice act or overall health regulatory legislation."[18] NCSBN's revised Model Practice Act is intended "to serve as a guide to states in considering revisions to their Nursing Practice Acts."[19] There are useful elements in each document, but one radical change in the new ANA *Suggested State Legislation* is that although now both organizations call for only one broad statement defining nursing (and one board), ANA refers only to professional nursing practice and technical nursing practice; the NCSBN Model Practice Act refers only to registered nursing and practical nursing. Perhaps ANA is oriented to a philosophy that expects its definitions to become reality in the future, and NCSBN is dealing with current reality. The other major difference is that ANA specifies a separate act for prescriptive authority and another for "disciplinary diversion," which means that nurses with addictions or mental health problems are treated differently from others with problems in professional discipline. NCSBN does not mention either. An analysis of the two documents shows other differences.[20] Some will be pointed out in the following sections. Neither document has any legal clout, but their titles do have different meanings:

> A model bill is a piece of legislation, which seeks to address, in comprehensive fashion, a determined need. Model bills are often reform legislation intended to provide order in an area where existing legislation is out of date, internally inconsistent, too broad or too narrow, or for some other reason inadequate to implement current state policy.
>
> On the other hand, suggested legislation, although in appropriate legislative form, is designed to bring to the attention of policymakers some of the critical issues which need to be addressed.[21]

The differences in the two nursing documents are seen as not very helpful for legislation or for anyone trying to speak for nursing, and the emphasis on states' rights makes conformity difficult. For instance, in 1986, the North Dakota Board of Nursing put into effect revised administrative rules for nursing education programs. Graduates entering programs after January 1, 1987, must have completed an approved nursing program that awards the appropriate academic degree in order to be eligible for licensure. For the RN, this is the baccalaureate; for the LPN, the associate degree. The North Dakota law does not allow equivalency preparation in determining eligibility for licensure, so licensing for out-of-state graduates not fulfilling those criteria has had to be worked out.

CONTENT OF NURSING PRACTICE ACTS

Because each state law differs to a degree in its content, it is important to have available a copy of the law of the state in which you practice and, if possible, the regulations that spell out how the law is carried out. You can get these from the state board or agency in the state government that has copies of laws for distribution. The language in all laws often seems stilted because the laws are written in legal terms, but the following sections can help you understand the key points.

Most nursing practice acts have basically the same major components, although not necessarily in the same order: definition of nursing, requirements for licensure, exemption from licensure, grounds for revocation of the license, provision for reciprocity (or endorsement) for persons licensed in other states, creation of a board of nursing, responsibilities of the board, and penalties for practicing without a license. Only the RN (not the LPN) licensure law or component of the nursing practice act is discussed in the following sections.

Definition and Scope of Practice

The definition of *nursing* in the licensure law determines both the legal responsibilities and the scope of practice of nurses. Inevitably, the definition of nursing in all nursing practice acts is stated in terms that are quite broad. This is generally frustrating to nurses who turn to the definition to find out if they are practicing legally, because it does not spell out specific procedures or activities. Often such activities are not even spelled out in the regulations of the laws. However, a broad definition is usually preferable because of the problems of including specific activities in a law. Changes in health care and nursing practice often occur more rapidly than a law can be changed, and the amending process can be long and complex. If particular activities were named, the nurse would be limited to those listed. Not only would the list be overwhelmingly long, but it is possible that any new technique easily and, perhaps necessarily, performed by a nurse would require an amendment to the law. An occasional state law does specify certain procedures but always includes the phrase "not limited to."

Until 1974 the nursing practice acts of most states had as their definition of nursing one similar to a model suggested by ANA in 1955. The definition distinguished between independent acts that the nurse might perform, but also identified certain dependent acts and prohibited diagnosis and treatment (not preceded by the word *medical*). In the 1970s, with expanded functions being assumed by nursing, SNAs increasingly became concerned about the adequacy of this definition. Therefore, the first states to change their laws concentrated on broadening the definition to encompass these roles. Then the ANA counsel suggested that a new clause be added to the ANA model definition:

> A professional nurse may also perform such additional acts, under emergency or other special conditions, which may include special training, as are recognized by the medical and nursing professions as proper to be performed by a professional nurse under such conditions, even though such acts might otherwise be considered diagnosis and prescription.

In 1976, after various states had amended their laws with this phrase or changed it altogether, with varying success, an ANA ad hoc committee revised the definition entirely. This model law, recommending one nursing practice law with provisions for licensing practitioners of nursing, used the terms *registered nurse* and *practical/vocational nurse*. The new definition differentiated between the independence of the RN's functions and the dependence of the LPN/LVN. It also placed the responsibility for what the RN can legally do in the hands of the nursing profession, always considered a hallmark of professionalism.[22]

Exhibit 11-2 shows the difference between the ways ANA and NCSBN currently conceive of what may be the most important aspect of a nursing practice act: the definition of nursing. There are clearly many similarities, although the language is different. AD nurses or students may find the ANA definition confusing (or insulting) in relation to "technical nursing practice." However, the intent was to use this description for what is now the LPN position. Current AD nurses holding an RN license would be grandfathered into the "professional component." NCSBN does not address that possibility, staying with the current status of licensure laws (except for North Dakota).

Although definitions vary from state to state, what most nurses are concerned about is whether the care expected in the employment situation is legal or in the domain of another health profession. Many of the activities in health care overlap. A common example is the administration of drugs, which may be done by the physician, RN, LPN, or various technicians in other hospital departments if related to a diagnostic procedure or treatment. Yet dispensing a drug from the hospital pharmacy, commonly done by some hospital nursing supervisors at night when no pharmacist is on duty, is in most states a violation of the pharmacy licensing law.

Obviously, one of the greatest concerns for nurses is the possible violation of the Medical Practice Act. Nurses have gradually come to perform more and more of the technical procedures that once belonged exclusively to medicine, but often these are delegated willingly by physicians. Whether nurses are always properly prepared to understand and perform them well is seldom questioned. However, as some nurses have assumed more comprehensive overall responsibilities in patient care, questions have been raised

Exhibit 11-2

Comparison of ANA and NCSBN Suggested Definitions of Nursing in Licensure Law

ANA

The "practice of nursing" means the performance of services for compensation in the provision of diagnosis and treatment of human responses to health or illness; "professional nursing practice" encompasses the full scope of nursing practice and includes all its specialties and consists of application of nursing theory to the development, implementation, and evaluation of plans of nursing care for individuals, families, and communities. Professional nursing practice requires substantial knowledge of nursing theory and related scientific, behavioral, and humanistic disciplines. Professional nursing practice includes, but is not limited to:

1. assessment, diagnosis, planning, intervention, and evaluation of human responses to health or illness;
2. the provision of direct nursing care to individuals to restore optimum function or to achieve a dignified death;
3. the procurement, coordination, and management of essential client resources;
4. the provision of health counseling and education;
5. the establishment of standards of practice for nursing care in all settings, including the development of nursing policies, procedures, and protocols for a specific setting;
6. the direction of nursing practice, including delegation to those practicing technical nursing;

NCSBN

The "Practice of Nursing" means assisting individuals or groups to maintain or attain optimal health, implementing a strategy of care to accomplish defined goals, and evaluating responses to care and treatment. This practice includes, but is not limited to, initiating and maintaining comfort measures, promoting and supporting human functions and responses, establishing an environment conducive to well-being, providing health counseling and teaching, and collaborating on certain aspects of the health regimen. This practice is based on understanding the human condition across the lifespan and understanding the relationship of the individual within the environment.

"Registered Nursing" means the practice of the full scope of nursing which includes but is not limited to:

a) Assessing the health status of individuals and groups;
b) Establishing a nursing diagnosis;
c) Establishing goals to meet identified health care needs;
d) Planning a strategy of care;
e) Prescribing nursing intervention to implement the strategy of care;
f) Implementing the strategy of care;
g) Delegating nursing interventions that may be performed by others and that do not conflict with this act;
h) Maintaining safe and effective nursing care rendered directly or indirectly;

7. the supervision of those who assist in the practice of nursing;

8. collaboration with other independently licensed health care professionals in case finding and the clinical management and execution of intervention as identified to be appropriate in a plan of care; and

9. the administration of medication and treatments as prescribed by those professionals qualified to prescribe under the provision of (*cite state statute[s]*);

    e) "technical nursing practice" includes the skilled application of nursing principles in the delivery of direct care to individuals and families within organized nursing services. Technical nursing practice requires the study of nursing within the context of the applied sciences. Technical nursing practice includes, but is not limited to:

      (1) participation in the development, evaluation, and modification of a plan of care;

      (2) the provision of direct care to individuals to restore optimum function or to achieve a dignified death;

      (3) patient teaching;

      (4) the supervision of those who assist in the practice of nursing;

      (5) the administration of medications and treatments as prescribed by those professionals qualified to prescribe under the provisions of (*cite state statute[s]*).

i) Evaluating responses to interventions;

j) Teaching the theory and practice of nursing;

k) Managing and supervising the practice of nursing;

l) Collaborating with other health professionals in the management of health care; and

m) Practicing advanced clinical nursing in accordance with knowledge skills acquired through graduate nursing education.

Licensed Practical Nursing means practice of a directed scope of nursing practice which includes, but is not limited to:

a) Contributing to the assessment of the health status of individuals and groups;

b) Participating in the development and modification of the strategy of care;

c) Implementing the appropriate aspects of the strategy of care as defined by the Board;

d) Maintaining safe and effective nursing care rendered directly or indirectly;

e) Participating in the evaluation of responses to interventions, and;

f) Delegating nursing interventions that may be performed by others and that do not conflict with this Act.

The Licensed Practical Nurse functions at the direction of the Registered Nurse, licensed physician, or licensed dentist in the performance of activities delegated by that health care professional.

Source: American Nurses' Association, 1990. *Suggested State Legislation: Nursing Practice Act, Nursing Disciplinary Diversion Act, Prescriptive Authority Act.* Kansas City, MO: The Association. Reprinted with permission.

Source: Model Nursing Practice Act, 1988. Reprinted by permission of the National Council of State Boards of Nursing, Inc.

by both nurses and physicians. Some are resistant to such changes; others are supportive but worry about the legality of such acts. Therefore it is useful to know how states have legislated for advanced nursing practice, which is related to both definition and regulations. This was reported in 1983 in considerable detail, including the practice of nurse-midwives and nurse anesthetists.[23] Surprisingly, this has not changed very much, according to a survey first done in 1990 and repeated yearly.[24]

Up to now, state legislatures have chosen three general means of dealing with expanded nursing practice in the legal definition of the licensure law.[25] All have their advantages and disadvantages. The first trend, and by far the largest (35 in 1990), is the use of administrative statutes. These permit nurses to perform expanded duties (additional acts), as authorized by the professional licensing boards: nursing alone, nursing and medicine, or medicine alone. Regulations are an important part of that mechanism.

Whether or not the additional acts clause is part of the law, the majority of state boards have now been granted the right to develop administrative rules and regulations for the NP, and most have developed such rules. The primary regulatory method of authorizing advanced practice is accepting certification by an organization approved by the state board. (In a sense, this makes voluntary certification a mandatory legal process.) Separate licensure, using a term such as *advanced nurse practitioner*, is also favored by some states. With the exception of nurse-midwives and nurse anesthetists, this identification and the specific requirements are part of the general nursing practice act, with, of course, appropriate regulations. The second approach could be called the use of nonamended statutes. These states either have made no changes from the 1955 ANA model and allow a liberal interpretation of the definition by the state board or have made minor changes. In some, the word *medical* has been inserted to describe prohibited acts. Thus, certain acts of diagnosis and treatment would presumably be identified as nursing. Other states have retained portions of the traditional definition but have omitted or substituted certain other phrases. Although all these states maintain that their acts allow expanded practice, interpretation is the key, so a change in attitude or political/medical pressures could bring a rapid about-face.

The last category of nursing definitions is termed *authorization,* which also has problems of interpretation. These states have developed a new definition of nursing that is intended to cover expanded or advanced practice as well as what might be considered ordinary practice at this time. The first of these states was New York (1972), which pioneered the use of the phrase "diagnosing and treating human responses to actual or potential health problems." A number of other states copied this terminology almost verbatim. However, New York NPs had difficulty in practicing "legally," and in 1988, legislation was enacted to authorize NPs certified by the State Education Department, to "engage in the performance of primary health care services well beyond the scope of practice of nursing," using the NP title. In 1990, only seven states authorized NP practice under a broad practice act, with no specific title protection.

A breakthrough may have occurred when the Missouri Supreme Court ruled in 1983 that that particular general definition did indeed allow advanced nurse practice.[26] This landmark case, *Sermchief v. Gonzales,* was the outcome of a threat by the Missouri Board of Registration for the Healing Arts, which licenses physicians and osteopaths, to initiate proceedings against nurses in a family planning clinic. (Physicians in the area had lodged a complaint.) The nurses, working under standing orders and protocols signed by the clinic physicians, performed a variety of diagnostic and treatment functions. The trial court judgment was that the nurses were practicing medicine without a license, but the Missouri Supreme Court ruled that the acts of the nurses were "precisely the types of acts the legislature had contemplated when it granted nurses the right to make assessments and nursing diagnoses." The 1975 Missouri law was similar to the earlier ANA guidelines and used the phrase "including, but not limited to." The nursing board had not developed any rules and regulations regarding advanced practice, so the case stood on the interpretation of the definition alone. Although the judgment is limited to Missouri, it is considered a victory for NP practice, with the focus on how clearly a general definition can legally determine whether a nurse is practicing nursing in performing what was once considered the exclusive function of medicine.[27] On the other hand, there is a question as to whether the case was a good example, since Missouri had been open to NP practice for some time, which is not true of other states.

It is clear that advanced NP practice is still in legal flux. (Nurse-midwives and nurse anesthetists may be included within a nursing practice act, a medical practice act, separately, or totally ignored legislatively. If mentioned, certification is usually a prerequisite for legal practice.) Short of a state supreme court ruling, the legality of certain practices can change in that state with attorney general appointments, the attitude of a judge, or simply the political climate. Health care facility lawyers can only advise on how they interpret the practice act (and they may be influenced by physicians' attitudes or advice). A strong statement for or against advanced practice made by a voluntary professional association (medicine or nursing, for instance) is quite common but has no legal authority; it *can* help mold public opinion.

The doctrines of common practice or custom and usage may also be invoked. This means basically that the act is performed in that particular community or at that current time and is accepted as being within the responsibility of the nurse by the individuals' employer and/or physicians in the area. It usually assumes appropriate training for that function. Although this has been considered acceptable in some courts, it has been denied in others. Practically speaking, statues cannot be changed informally by mass violation, although they may be changed through the legislative process eventually, because of evidence that a nurse has been taught to perform such a function and is capable of carrying it out safely.

Creation of a Board of Nursing

The name of the state administrative agency varies from state to state, as does the number of members. *Board of Nursing* is used by the NCSBN. The majority of states now have consumers or other professionals, as well as nurses, as members. These are appointed by the governor, with or without nursing input. Board size ranges from 5 to 19 appointed members, who make policy. Staff employed by the board carry out the day-to-day activities.

Responsibilities of the Board of Nursing

The major responsibility of a board is to see that the nursing practice act is carried out. This involves establishing rules and regulations to implement the broad terms in the law itself and setting minimum standards of practice and education. Among specific responsibilities are issuing licenses to qualified applicants; disciplining those who violate the law or are found to be unfit to practice nursing; and collecting data.

Other responsibilities include developing standards for continuing competency of licensed practitioners and issuing a limited license (for someone who cannot practice the full scope of nursing, perhaps due to a handicap). Nursing boards may also offer educational programs, collect certain data, and cooperate in various ways with other nursing boards or the boards of other disciplines. If they operate under an overall board, certain administrative responsibilities will be carried out on a central level.

The power of the board should not be underestimated. For instance, it was simply by changing their regulations that the North Dakota Board changed its requirements for RN and LPN licensure.

Requirements for Licensure

Licensure is based on fulfilling certain requirements. The following points are usually included:

1. The applicant must have completed an educational program in a state-approved school of nursing and received a diploma or degree from that program; usually the school must send the student's transcript. Some states ask for evidence of high school education. There is some legislative pressure that the applicant not be required to have completed the program, particularly if the uncompleted courses are in a nonnursing area such as liberal arts. Neither ANA nor NCSBN approves of this.

2. The applicant must pass an examination given by the board. This examination is currently the NCLEX-RN, developed under the direction of the NCSBN and given in every state.
3. Some states require evidence of good physical and mental health, but this is not recommended by either ANA or NCSBN. Actual practice varies a great deal from state to state. Handicapped students have been admitted, have graduated, and have taken state boards in some states; in others, this opportunity has been denied. Court cases often result.[28]
4. Most states maintain a statement that the applicant must be of good moral character, as determined by the licensing board, but this, too, is impractical. The Model Act suggests terminology that refers to acts that are grounds for board disciplinary action if the nurse is licensed.
5. A fee must be paid for admission to the examination. This varies considerably among states.
6. A temporary license may be issued to a graduate of an approved program pending the results of the first licensure exam.
7. Demonstrating competence in English is the newest recommendation.

It has been declared unconstitutional to make requirements of age, citizenship, and residence.

Provisions for Endorsement

Nurses have more mobility than any other licensed health professionals because of the use of a national standardized examination. However, usually the nurse must still fulfill the other requirements in the state in which licensure is sought and must submit proof that the license has not been revoked.

If all requirements are satisfactorily fulfilled, the nurse is granted a license without retaking the state board examination. A fee is also required for this process of endorsement. Endorsement is not the same as *reciprocity;* the latter means acceptance of a licensee by one state only if the other state does likewise.

Renewal of the License

Until the early 1970s, nursing licenses were renewed simply by sending the renewal fee when notified, usually every two years. For nurses licensed in more than one state, as long as the license was not revoked in any state, the process was the same. Usually the form asked for information about employment and the highest degree (and still does), but no attempt was made to determine if the nurse was competent. At about that time (also the time of the credentialing reports), there was increased concern about the current competency of practicing health professionals, and an estimate was made that perhaps 5 percent of all health professionals were not competent for some reason. One outcome was the enactment of a mandatory CE clause in a number of licensure laws; that is, a practitioner's license would not be renewed unless she or he showed evidence of CE. A number of health disciplines have such legislation, but not all requirements are well enforced.

Forms of CE accepted by states include various formal academic studies in institutions of higher learning converted to CEU credit; college extension courses and studies; grand rounds in the health care setting; home study programs; in-service education; institutes; lectures; seminars; workshops; audiovisual learning systems, including educational television, audiovisual cassettes, tapes, and records with self-study packets; challenge examinations for a course or program; self-learning systems such as community service, controlled independent study, delivery of a paper, or preparation and participation in a panel; preparation and publication of articles, monographs, books, and so on; and special research. The required number of hours of CE or CEUs varies considerably among states. *No law requires formal education directed toward advanced degrees.* In fact, although additional formal education is acceptable, the emphasis is on continuous, *updated competence in practice*.

Objections to mandatory CE focus on the difficulty of assessing true learning; the question of whether learning can be forced (attendance does not mean retention of knowledge or change in behavior); the danger of breeding mediocrity; the lack of research on the effectiveness of CE in relation to performance; limitation of resources, particularly in rural areas; the cost to nurses; the cost to government; the usual rigidity of governmental regulations; the problems in record keeping; and the lack of accreditation or evaluation procedures for many CE programs.

The issue is far from resolved. The trend toward mandatory CE slowed considerably in the 1980s for all occupations, although the call for continued competence did not. It is possible that another trend, peer evaluation, and other kinds of performance evaluation may provide a more effective answer to continued competence.

Exemptions from Licensure

This may also be called an *exception clause*. Generally exempted from RN licensure are basic students in a nursing program; anyone furnishing nursing assistance in an emergency; anyone licensed in another state and caring for a patient temporarily in the state involved; anyone employed by the U.S. government as a nurse (Veterans Administration, public health, or armed services); any legally qualified nurse recruited by the Red Cross during a disaster; anyone caring for the sick if care is performed in connection with the practice of religious tenets of any church; anyone giving incidental care in a family (home) situation; and any RN or LPN from another state engaged in consultation as long as no direct care is given.

In all these cases, the person cannot claim to be an RN of the state concerned. Over strong nursing protests, some states have also incorporated in the exemptions nursing services of attendants in state institutions, if supervised by nurses or doctors, as well as other kinds of nursing assistants under various circumstances. This, of course, weakens the mandatory aspect of the law.

An interesting development is that the NCSBN model act suggests for this clause statements that permit the establishment of an independent practice and fee-for-service reimbursement.

Grounds for Revocation of Licensure

The board has the right to revoke or suspend any nurse's license or otherwise discipline the licensee. The reasons most commonly found in practice acts for revoking a license are acts that might directly endanger the public, such as practicing while one's ability is impaired by alcohol, drugs, or physical or mental disability; being addicted to or dependent on alcohol or other habit-forming drugs or being a habitual user of certain drugs; and practicing with incompetence or negligence or beyond the scope of practice. Other reasons are obtaining a license fraudulently; being convicted of a felony or crime involving moral turpitude (or accepting a plea of *nolo contendere*); practicing while the license is suspended or revoked; aiding and abetting a nonlicensed person to perform activities requiring a license; and committing unprofessional conduct or immoral acts as defined by the board. The refusal to provide service to a person because of race, color, creed, or national origin has also been added in some states.

The most common reasons that nurses lose their licenses are the same as those that apply to physicians—drug use, abuse, or theft.

Nurses' drug use and abuse may be on the increase, since this is also a trend in society, but certainly it has gotten considerably more attention in recent years, with many reports in nursing and lay publications and other media. At one time, given sufficient evidence, boards suspended or revoked nurses' licenses readily for drug abuse. (In a recent survey, it was found that nurses impaired by drug abuse are more likely to be the target of disciplinary action than mentally or physically impaired nurses.[29]) Criteria for reinstatement are based on a written statement from a physician that the nurse is cured and can function in the workplace or is under treatment and can function in the workplace or that board evaluation shows that the nurse is able to function.[30] A number of boards have had the legal freedom to take no action but to provide information or recommend rehabilitative programs for the nurse to get treatment.[31] Almost none did so. Eventually SNAs recognized this is a professional responsibility and made such arrangements, along with counseling and support. (Alcohol abuse or intemperance interfering with safe practice may also be part of what is considered substance abuse). Seeing the need for official action, the ANA has suggested a separate law (Nursing Disciplinary Diversion Act) that mandates that the board of nursing will seek ways to rehabilitate impaired nurses and to "establish a voluntary alternative to traditional disciplinary actions."[32] Only nurses who request such diversion and supervision by a committee are permitted to participate in the program. The NCSBN Model Act does not include such a provision.

As is true in obtaining or renewing licenses, a nurse can also lose his or her license because of physical or mental impairment. Legal blindness is the most common physical condition involved, but there are many exceptions, especially since the passage of the Rehabilitation Act described in Chapter 10. It is possible that none of these conditions are specifically cited in the statutes, but if the nurse's practice is affected in any way, discipline is authorized by the ubiquitous "unprofessional conduct" clause. Depending on the seriousness of the situation, nurses may also be given limited licenses in some jurisdictions, which restrict nursing practice to certain parameters.[33]

Unprofessional conduct "as defined by the board" was at one time seldom defined in public rules and regulations. A turning point was the Tuma case. In Idaho in 1977, Jolene Tuma, an instructor in an AD program, went with a student to the bedside of a terminally ill woman to start chemotherapy after obtaining the patient's informed consent. When the patient asked Ms. Tuma about alternative treatments for cancer, she was told about several. Her son, upset because his mother stopped the chemotherapy, told the physician, who brought charges against Ms. Tuma. Subsequently, she was not only fired, but her license was suspended for six months by the Idaho Board of Nursing for unprofessional conduct, because her actions "disrupted the physician-patient relationship."[34] The case aroused a national nursing furor.[35] Ms. Tuma took her case through the courts, and on April 17, 1979, the Idaho Supreme Court handed down the decision that Ms. Tuma could not be found guilty of unprofessional conduct because the Idaho Nurse Practice Act neither defined unprofessional conduct nor set guidelines for providing warnings. The judge also questioned the ability of the hearing officer, who lacked "personal knowledge and experience" of nursing, to determine if Ms. Tuma's behavior was unprofessional.[36] Unfortunately, the court did not address itself to Ms. Tuma's actions, which leaves the nurse's right to inform the patient in some question—at least in Idaho.

While a number of states already had regulations defining unprofessional conduct, this court ruling spurred on those that did not. Statements in the various laws are pretty much alike, but the focus is on behavior that fails to conform to the accepted standards of the nursing profession and that could jeopardize the health and welfare of the people. Many of the statements relate to competence, patient abuse, falsifying records, delegating improperly, and failing to report incompetent practitioners.[37] A useful definition of *unprofessional conduct* that emerged is "nursing behavior that fails to conform to the accepted standards of the nursing profession and which could jeopardize the health and welfare of the people."

Regulatory language concerning unprofessional conduct is not always specific and is almost never so in the statutes, because this might foreclose action in unanticipated types of behavior. This problem is sometimes resolved by using the phrase "not limited to," but if the legislature has a particular concern, this may be written into the law. Some states have also adopted the ANA standards of practice as criteria for incompetence.[38] Another interesting point is the possibility of unprofessional kinds of nursing conduct once considered specific to medicine, such as fee splitting.

A particular problem in both statutory and regulating language relates to such terms as *moral, ethical,* and *moral turpitude,* since these can be interpreted in various ways. The model act uses phrases such as "has engaged in any act inconsistent with standards of nursing practice as defined by Board Rules and Regulations" and "a crime in any jurisdiction that relates adversely to the practice of nursing or to the ability to practice nursing."

Although the law seems to protect the public, data show that relatively few nurses have had their licenses revoked or suspended. In part, the reason is believed to be the reluctance of other nurses to report and consequently testify to these acts by their colleagues before either the nursing board or a court of law.[39] Nursing associations and state boards are now emphasizing the responsibility of professional nurses to report incompetent practice. The Model Act makes nonreporting a disciplinary offense.

When a report is filed with the state board, charging a nurse with violation of any of the grounds of disciplinary action, he or she is entitled to certain procedural safeguards (due process). After investigation, the nurse must receive notice of the charges and be given time to prepare a defense. A hearing is set and subpoenas are issued (by the board, the attorney general, or a hearing officer). The accused has the right to appear personally or be represented by counsel, who may cross-examine witnesses. If the license is revoked or suspended, it may be reissued at the discretion of the board. (Sometimes the individual is only censured or reprimanded.)

As pointed out earlier, one of the complaints about licensure is that incompetent practitioners so seldom lose their licenses, and if they do, they may simply go to another state, applying for a new license to practice. All too frequently, the license has been granted with inadequate checking to see whether the person had a record of incompetence. Another aspect of this problem in relation to physicians was that they could lose their hospital clinical privileges for incompetence, substance abuse, or similar reasons, and other hospitals at which they had or would seek privileges would be unaware of this situation. In all cases, patients were endangered, and the professions involved were accused of failing to police, rehabilitate, or remove their own. Therefore, as often happens, legislation follows. The Health

Care Quality Improvement Act of 1986 (PL 99-660) mandated a National Practitioner Data Bank (NPDB), later enlarged by the Medicare and Medicaid Patient and Program Protection Act of 1987 (PL 100-93). Although it did not go into effect until September 1990, it will eventually influence all health care professionals.[40] The intent of the law is to "collect and release certain information" relating to the professional competence and conduct of physicians, dentists, and other health care practitioners. Reporting requirements vary among professional groups. However, adverse licensure actions and reporting of payments resulting from a written claim or judgment on the part of malpractice insurers is mandatory for all health professionals. Copies are sent to state licensing boards. If a claim is settled on behalf of several named individuals, as often happens to nurses in hospital-related incidents, a separate report must be filed for each. NPs, nurse-midwives, and nurse anesthetists are particularly affected by another provision, although optional, that hospital-level professional disciplinary actions affecting clinical privileges or "action by professional societies" be reported. Institutions must check with the NPDB about new applicants and make an inquiry every two years about nurses with clinical privileges. Although there is limited access to the Data Bank—licensing boards, hospitals, professional societies, and health care entities involved in peer review—obviously any error in the information or leak in confidentiality can have a serious affect on a nurse's career. Therefore, nurses are advised to check their NPDB record, to which they also have access, to make sure that it is accurate.[41]

Penalties for Practicing Without a License

Penalties for practicing without a license are included only in the mandatory laws. Penalties vary from a minimum fine to a large fine and/or imprisonment. Usually legal action is taken. Penalties are being strengthened to deter illegal practice.

PROCEDURE FOR OBTAINING A LICENSE

Almost all new graduates of a nursing program apply for RN licensure, because it is otherwise impossible to practice. Although there is nothing to prohibit you from postponing licensure, it is generally more difficult, both psychologically and because of lack of clinical practice, to take the state board examination (NCLEX) much later.

As a rule, your school makes available all the data and even the application forms necessary for beginning the licensure procedure. Should you wish to become licensed in another state because of planned relocation, request an application from that nursing board (see Appendix 4). Current titles and addresses of the nursing boards of all states are found in the directory issue of the *American Journal of Nursing,* usually April. The board advises you of the proper procedure, the cost, and the data needed. For this initial licensing, you must take the state board examination in the state where licensure is sought.

After receiving the completed necessary data, fee, and application, the appropriate state board notifies you of the time and place of the examination. These exams are given twice a year simultaneously throughout the country.

In 1979, NCSBN voted to adopt a new test plan, effective July 1982. The new examination, titled NCLEX (RN), was based on the nursing process and was intended to test primarily for application of knowledge, not just recall of facts. The new test plan states that

> nursing is perceived as deliberate action of a personal and assisting nature. The practice of nursing requires knowledge of: (1) normal growth and development; (2) basic human needs; (3) coping mechanisms; (4) actual or potential health problems; (5) effects of age, sex, culture, ethnicity and/or religion on health needs; and (6) ways by which nursing can assist individuals to maintain health and cope with health problems. Embodied in these six categories of nursing knowledge are concepts considered relevant to nursing practice, including management, accountability, life cycle, and client environment.[42]

Since that time, a number of changes have occurred including the use of a simple pass/fail score, and others are to come. However, both NCLEX (RN) and NCLEX (LPN) will continue to be based on periodic job analyses. The tests are the same for all nurses seeking an RN, whether graduating from a diploma, AD, or baccalaureate program. This has been the subject of considerable criticism, because the stated goals of all three programs are different. However, proponents of a single licensing exam state that the purpose is to determine safe and effective practice at a minimal level, and that this criterion applies to all levels of RN.

Great precautions are taken to preserve the security of the tests. Teachers in schools of nursing do not know the specific questions on the examination, but they are familiar with the types of questions with which the applicant will be confronted, and this type of test is often used in the classroom. Although review books and special review classes or courses are available to assist you to study for the examinations, the best preparation is, of course, a sound educational background. Currently, there are no "practical" examinations, that is, tests of proficiency in real patient care situations or laboratories. Computerized clinical simulation tests (CST) are being tested by the NCSBN and appear to be a viable alternative.[43]

When you pass the licensing examination, you receive a certificate bearing a registration number that remains the same as long as you are registered in that state. The certificate (or registration card) will also carry the expiration date, which is usually one, two, or three years hence.

To become licensed or registered by endorsement, you must already be registered in one state, territory, or foreign country. You then apply to the state board of nursing in the new state and present credentials, as requested, to prove that you have completed preparation equal to that required. A temporary permit is usually issued to allow you to work until the new license is issued.

Should you wish to be reregistered after allowing your license(s) to lapse, it's best to contact the state board for directions. If you wish to practice nursing in another country, investigate its legal requirements for practice. Members of the armed forces or the Peace Corps, or those under the auspices of an organization such as the World Health Organization or a religious denomination, will be advised by the sponsoring group. Licensure in one state is usually sufficient.

Nurses educated in other countries are expected to meet the same qualifications for licensure as graduates of schools of nursing in the United States. The procedure for obtaining a license is the same as for graduates of schools here. However, generally nurses from other countries are now expected to take the Commission on Graduates of Foreign Nursing Schools (CGFNS) Qualifying Examination, which screens and examines foreign nursing school graduates while they are still in their own countries to determine their eligibility for professional practice in the United States.[44] The one-day examination covers proficiency in both nursing practice and English comprehension; both exams are given in English. If the applicant passes, she or he is given a CGFNS certificate, which is presented to the U.S. embassy or consulate when applying for a visa and to the state board in the state where the nurse wishes to practice. The nurse still must take the state board examination and otherwise fulfill the licensing requirements for that state. Because of the nursing shortage, some states are considering dropping the CGFNS requirement preceding NCLEX, although it would still be necessary in order to receive a temporary permit to practice. However, California's experience with this pointed out the problem: the vast majority who had not taken or passed CGFNS failed NCLEX, even after several repetitions. Specific information about requirements for licensure must be obtained directly from the board of nursing in the state in which the foreign nurse wishes to be licensed.

ISSUES, DEVELOPMENTS, AND PREDICTIONS

It seems that almost every month brings information about changes in nurse practice acts or challenges as to what they permit. The scope-of-practice issue will not be resolved for quite a while. Many changes relating to NPs are already occurring in nurse practice acts. For instance, in 1983, 18 states had formally given prescription-writing authority to certain categories of nurses. By 1990 the number had reached 35, with more pending.[45] (NPs in states without this authority still manage to get prescriptions for their patients by other means.)

Because of the hodgepodge of regulations and other legal means of giving nurses prescriptive authority, ANA has proposed separate legislation with the purpose of regulating "the authority of nurses licensed to practice professional nursing to prescribe."[46]

Certification for specialties will certainly grow, possibly, but not probably, with an overview organization certifying the certifying groups. Whether there might be a battle about which group has the authority or whether all will work together is another question. The growth in the number of certifying groups, sometimes overlapping in functions, is astounding.

At the other end of the educational scale is the growing concern about the competence of nurses' aides. New positions are growing for aides in hospitals, LTC facilities, and home care; 433,000 *new* jobs are predicted for the year 2000. As the least expensive and least prepared nursing person, the aide is still expected to detect behavioral changes that may signal a serious health problem—and isn't trained to do so. Although the need for national training standards has been recognized, just who will implement them is still undecided. Some states, such as New Jersey, now regulate homemaker-home health aides. How can nurses who are ultimately responsible for nurses' aides ascertain that they are safe and competent?[47] Will the state boards have a role? The NCSBN has developed standards for the regulation of nurses' aides called the National Council's Nurse Aide Competency Evaluation Program (NACEP). It is intended for use by state agencies charged with the responsibility of evaluating the competence of nurses' aides, as required by the Nursing Home Reform Act (OBRA, 1987), and is also used by agencies wishing to test their aides.

Equal concern can be directed at the growing responsibilities of LPNs. Many state boards are put under tremendous pressure by employers to approve procedures for LPNs that are not in their curricula, such as venipuncture. Some boards approve and demand that PN programs include these procedures in their curricula. Schools say that there is already enough to cover in one year.[48] The impact of this problem is uncertain. Will patients be endangered? What of the responsibility of nurses who supervise LPNs? Might these new demands, partially due to the nursing shortage, escalate the move toward AD education for LPNs?

Another problem is that nurse disciplinary problems are likely to increase. In part, this is also due to the nursing shortage and the extra stress for caring for sicker patients better, with fewer people. Stress has been seen to cause substance abuse, and nurses are not exceptions. It may be that there will be more state board programs to help addicted nurses to recover and return to work. This seems to work.[49] A research project to evaluate the efficacy of the different approaches used by state boards has been developed. Still another concern is nurse involvement in right-to-die issues, where their own moral/ethical philosophy is to let patients discontinue treatment if they wish and to help them to do so. The reality is that nurses can, at the least, lose their licenses in such circumstances, depending on the attitudes of the members of the state board involved.

Nursing state boards have some challenging years ahead. For one thing, the licensure examinations are expected to change radically. A new form of testing, Computerized Adaptive Testing (CAT), began field testing in 1990 and was expected to be in full use by November 1993. With CAT, each candidate's test is unique; it is assembled interactively as the individual is tested. The computer calculates a competence estimate based on earlier answers. A final score is available immediately.[50] And, of course, CST is another breakthrough.

Other issues about licensure will include concerns about item bias related to culture and gender; developing a mechanism to ensure competence, including that of returning nurses; the great diversity of definitions of nursing and scope of practice; what to do about temporary licenses for foreign nurses during the nursing shortage; and developing better means of verifying licensure across state lines.

Finally, the credentialing issues in health care in general are not expected to improve greatly because they are so disorganized now. More health occupations will continue to seek licensure or other legal status.[51] Turf battles will continue. (An interesting issue here is the growth of lay midwifery and the attempts of legislatures to either prohibit or legalize their practice.[52]) All these groups will have problems similar to nursing with definition, scope, discipline, and testing methods. And what of the uncredentialed health worker? How can we best guarantee at least safe care for the public? Resolution of the problems posed here could help to resolve some of the other problems of health care delivery.

KEY POINTS

---

1. There are a variety of mechanisms for credentialing nurses and other health care workers, all of which have some problems.
2. Mandatory licensure means that an individual cannot practice without a license and safeguards the public more than permissive licensure.
3. Among the criticisms of licensure are too much control by the profession or occupation, a tendency for practice requirements to be rigid

and out of date, and primarily that the public has no guarantee of competence.

4. Institutional licensure, although favored by administrators for economic and other reasons, would not guarantee improved care but would limit the autonomy and mobility of nurses who now have individual licenses.

5. Nurse practice acts may vary from state to state, but they generally have the same components that define and control practice.

6. Nurse practice acts must change with the times, but the current practitioner is protected by a grandfather clause.

7. The most common reasons for revocation of a license are drug abuse or misuse, or other failure to meet the standards of the profession.

8. One purpose of nursing certification is to recognize advanced practice, but because there is not yet coordination among certifying groups, the public may be confused.

9. The most common approaches to authorizing advanced nursing practice are interpreting current statutes to include advanced practice, writing regulations, or developing a totally new definition.

10. Sunset legislation, which requires a review of existing agencies to determine if they are fulfilling their purpose, has resulted in some good revisions of nurse practice acts.

11. A major problem with CE as a requirement for relicensure is that there is little evidence that it results in improved competence.

12. Many changes are occurring in the testing of individuals for nurse licensure.

REFERENCES

1. Kelly LY. *Dimensions of professional nursing,* 5th ed. New York: Macmillan Publishing Company, 1985, pp. 439–447.
2. Tollett J. The issue of licensure—institutional vs. individual. *Nurs Leadership,* 5:8–31 (September 1982).
3. Hershey N. Alternative to mandatory licensure of health professionals. *Hosp Prog,* 50:73 (March 1969).
4. Kelly LY. Oh no, not again: An old ghost rises. *Nurs Outlook,* 38:121 (May–June 1990).
5. Shimberg B. Licensing in the year 2000. *Issues* 5:1, 8 (Summer 1984).
6. Havighurst C, King N. Private credentialing of health care personnel: An antitrust perspective. Part One, *Am J Law and Med,* 9:131–201 (Summer 1983).
7. Havighurst C, King N. Private credentialing of health care personnel: An antitrust perspective. Part Two, *Am J Law and Med,* 9:263–334 (Fall 1983).

8. Ibid.
9. Kelly LY. *Dimensions of professional nursing*, 6th ed. Elmsford, NY: Pergamon Press, 1991, pp. 74–76.
10. Hartshorn J. A national board for nursing certification. *Nurs Outlook*, 39:226–229 (September–October 1991).
11. Fickeissen JL. 56 ways to get certified. *Am J Nurs*, 90:50–57 (March 1990).
12. Moccia P. Accreditation: Quality for all to see. *Nurs and Health Care*, 11:362, 364 (September 1990).
13. Strutz R, Gilje F. How to prepare for an NLN self study. *Nurs and Health Care*, 11:363, 365–367.
14. Grobe S. Sunset laws. *Am J Nurs*, 81:1355–1359 (July 1981).
15. Thomas C. Sunset: What and why. *Nurse Practitioner*, 7:10 (March 1982).
16. Thomas C. Sunset: How and when. *Nurse Practitioner*, 7:10–11 (April 1982).
17. Bouchaird J, Montueffel C. Constitutional issues related to grandfather clauses. *Issues*, 8(1):5–6 (1987).
18. *Suggested state legislation: Nursing practice act, nursing disciplinary diversion act, prescriptive authority act*. Kansas City, MO: American Nurses' Association, 1990, p. 1.
19. *Model nursing practice act*. Chicago: National Council of State Boards of Nursing, Inc., 1988, p. 1.
20. Kelly (1991), op. cit., pp. 454–457.
21. Council of State Governments, National Task Force on State Dental Policies. *State regulatory policies: Dentistry and the health professions*. Lexington, KY: The Council, 1979, p. 3.
22. Kelly (1991), op. cit., pp. 451–455.
23. LaBar C. *The regulation of advanced nursing practice as provided for in nursing practice acts and administrative rules*. Kansas City, MO: American Nurses' Association, 1983.
24. How each state stands on legislative issues affecting advanced nursing practice. *Nurse Practitioner*, 15:11–18 (January 1991).
25. Trandel-Korenchuk D, Trandel-Korenchuk K. How state laws recognize advanced nursing practice. *Nurs Outlook*, 66:713–719 (November 1978).
26. Wolff M. Court upholds expanded practice roles for nurses. *Law, Med and Health Care*, 12:26–29 (February 1984).
27. Greenlaw J, Sermchief V. Gonzales and the debate over advanced nursing practice legislation. *Law, Med and Health Care*, 12:30–31, 36 (February 1984).
28. Champagne M, et al. State board criteria for licensure and disciplinary procedures regarding impaired nurses. *Nurs Outlook*, 35:54–57, 101 (March–April 1987).
29. Swenson I, et al. State board members' perceptions of impaired nurses. *Nurs Outlook*, 35:154–155 (July–August 1987).
30. Swenson I, et al. State boards and impaired nurses. *Nurs Outlook*, 37:94–96 (March–April 1989).

31. Champagne et al., op. cit.
32. *Suggested state legislation,* op. cit. pp. 29–30.
33. Swenson I, et al. Interpretations of state board criteria and disciplinary procedures regarding impaired nurses. *Nurs Outlook,* 35:108–110, 145 (May–June 1987).
34. Professional misconduct? Letters. *Nurs Outlook,* 25:546 (September 1977). See also the editorial, p. 561.
35. Follow-up letters in the December 1977 issue, *Nurs Outlook*, pp. 738–743; January 1978 issue, pp. 8–9; February 1978 issue, p. 78; and March 1978 issue, pp. 142–143.
36. Jolene Tuma wins: Court rules practice act did not define unprofessional conduct. *Nurs Outlook,* 27:376 (June 1979).
37. Kelly (1991), op. cit., pp. 464–465.
38. Northrop C. Unprofessional conduct and licensure revocation. *Nurs Outlook,* 34:45 (January–February 1986).
39. Price D, Murphy P. How—and when—to blow the whistle on unsafe practices. *Nurs Life,* 3:51–54 (January–February 1983).
40. Birkholz G. The National Practitioner Data Bank. *Am J Nurse,* 90:49–51 (September 1990).
41. Culbertson RA. National Practitioner Data Bank has implications for nursing. *Nurs Outlook,* 39:102–103, 142 (May–June 1991).
42. A new licensing exam for nurses. *Am J Nurs,* 80:723–725 (April 1980).
43. Wendt AL, et al. Computer simulation: The time is now. *Issues,* 12(1): 5 (1991).
44. Kelly (1991), op. cit., p. 611.
45. How each state stands, op. cit.
46. *Suggested state legislation,* op. cit. p. 35.
47. Reinhard S. Jurisdictional control: The regulation of nurses' aides. *Nurs and Health Care,* 9:373–375 (September 1988).
48. LPNs widen their role; disagreement grows. *Am J Nurs,* 90:16, 17 (February 1990).
49. Penny J. Spotlight on support for impaired nurses. *Am J Nurs,* 86:688–691 (June 1986).
50. 1990 marks start of field testing for computerized adaptive testing project. *Issues,* 10(5):2, 4, 5, 11 (1989).
51. De Vries R. The contest for control: Regulating new and expanding health occupations. *Am J Pub Health,* 76:1147–1150 (September 1986).
52. Butter I, Kay B. State laws and the practice of lay midwifery. *Am J Pub Health,* 71:1161–1169 (September 1988).

CHAPTER 12

LEGAL ASPECTS OF NURSING PRACTICE

OBJECTIVES

After studying this chapter, you will be able to:

1. Define basic legal terms.
2. Explain the elements of the standard of care as it might be applied in a court of law.
3. Give examples of legal problems nurses may encounter in caring for patients.
4. Present specific ways in which nurses may avoid malpractice suits.
5. Name three charting errors that may cause problems for the nurse in a malpractice suit.
6. Identify key points in selecting liability insurance.
7. Give examples of criminal activities for which nurses can be held responsible in their practice.
8. Explain how best to handle a situation calling for a critical incident report.
9. Explain the usual steps in a trial.
10. List the main points a nurse should know about testifying.

It appears that today a quick reaction to a grievance of any kind is to file a civil suit. Comments about the litigious tendencies of the American public are widespread. For some years, the situation has been particularly acute in the health field, with the news media reporting multimillion-dollar awards for patients and families who have suffered injury. Sometimes the case seems clear-cut, for example when a child is paralyzed and brain-damaged for life because anesthesia was improperly given. "What price do you put on a ruined life and the burden and sorrow of the family?" juries are asked. In other cases, the damage is less evident, with a lot of emphasis on mental and emotional trauma. The idea seems to be: sue if possible; I'm entitled. For physicians, particularly, this has resulted in a sometimes dramatic escalation in the cost of malpractice insurance, to the point where some have retired early and others have abandoned litigation-prone practice, such as obstetrics. (This also affects nurse-midwives.)[1] In obstetrics, if an infant is injured, whether or not the doctor is at fault, it is becoming more common to sue years afterward; the *long tail* of malpractice suits. The *statute of limitations* is the legal limit of time a person has to file a suit in a civil matter. The statutory period usually begins when an injury occurs, but in some cases, it starts when the injured person discovers the injury. In the case of a minor, the statute will not "toll" and begin to run until the child has reached age 18. Nurses are often held to longer limits than doctors.[2] On the other hand, lawyers contend that the primary reason for malpractice suits is malpractice.

What does this have to do with nursing? Once people were reluctant to sue nurses or even doctors and nonprofit hospitals, either out of respect for their "services to humanity" or because they felt that none of them had any money. As doctors became more conspicuously affluent, health care became big business, and both became somewhat more impersonal, those feelings were discarded. Once hospitals had *charitable immunity,* which granted them freedom from liability, but like the *sovereign immunity* that does the same for the government, this is gradually being wiped out in the courts. Nurses are included, too. Everyone assumes that nurses are either covered by their employer's insurance or their own, or are making enough money that if they hurt a patient, they, as well as any other health care provider, should pay. Moreover, as patients are sicker, care is more complex and nurses, who must know more, are also more overburdened, the chances of a patient's being hurt by a nurse's carelessness, lack of knowledge, or even an unavoidable error are much greater. And nurses *are* being sued, sometimes as one of a whole list of caregivers who are included in a suit (the *fishnet theory* of naming every possible defendant) or as individuals. A *defendant* is the person being sued; a *plaintiff* is the one seeking damages or other legal relief.

It is only common sense, then, to know (1) the kinds of situations that lead to litigation, (2) steps to take to avoid being sued, and (3) what to do if a patient is hurt. This chapter gives an overview of the legal problems in which nurses can be involved in their practice within the common law of *torts,* that is, an intentional or unintentional civil wrong. Criminal problems that are common are reviewed more briefly.

Some of the cases cited later are classic cases that are repeatedly cited in nursing law; others are more recent. At times, when two similar cases are judged in quite different ways, both are given. The findings may change with the changing role of the nurse and a court's concept of what a nurse is and does. For instance, one attorney who has handled nurse liability cases for 40 years reflects that 35 years ago a nurse client was not held responsible when she gave a wrong medication that had been ordered by the physician. She should have known it was wrong; yet she blindly administered it anyhow. But she was "just following the doctor's orders." Then, in recent years, he defended a nurse who followed routine orders for a tetanus injection without checking for patient allergy. She was judged liable because she didn't use her nursing judgment.[3]

APPLICATION OF LEGAL PRINCIPLES

The majority of incidents leading to legal action in which nurses are involved occur in an employment situation, generally the hospital. That is to be expected because that is where most nurses work and where patients are usually sickest and most helpless. When a person is injured, chances are that the hospital will be sued, even when an employee or a doctor has done the actual damage. In the case of the employee, the hospital is sued under the legal principle of *respondeat superior*: "let the master answer" or be responsible for the actions of the employees.[4]

This does not prevent the employee from being sued, since the rule or doctrine of personal liability says that everyone is legally responsible for his or her acts, even though someone else may also be held legally liable under another rule of law such as *respondeat superior*. The latter is called *vicarious* liability, imposed without personal fault or without a causal relationship between the actions of the one held liable and in injury.

At one time, physicians were held directly responsible for any error of personnel who worked with them in a patient care situation (*borrowed servant*) on the basis of the "*captain of the ship*" doctrine, but this has been overturned by most courts. The institution, however, can be held accountable for physicians' acts, even if they are not employees, under the principle of *corporate negligence*. A classic example is the 1965 landmark decision of *Darling v. Charleston Community Memorial Hospital,* which has set several precedents. It also illustrates the elements that must be present in order to have cause for action based on malpractice or negligence.

1. A duty was owed to the plaintiff by the defendant to use *due care* (reasonable care under the circumstances).
2. *The duty was breached* (the defendant did not behave in a reasonable manner).
3. The plaintiff was injured or damaged in some way.
4. The plaintiff's injury was caused directly by the defendant's negligence (*proximate cause*).

No matter how negligent the health provider was, if there was no injury, there is no case. The plaintiff must also establish that a health practitioner-patient relationship existed and that the practitioner violated the standard of care.

CASE

A minor broke his leg playing football and was taken to Charleston Community Memorial Hospital, a JCAH-accredited hospital. There a cast was put on the leg in the emergency room, and he was sent to a regular nursing unit. The nurses noted and charted that the toes became cold and blue. They called the physician, who did not come. Over a period of days, they continued to note and chart deterioration of the condition of the exposed toes and continually notified the physician, who came once but did not remedy the situation. The mother then took the boy to another hospital, where an orthopedist was forced to amputate the leg because of advanced gangrene. The family sued the first doctor, the hospital, and the nurses involved.

The physician settled out of court; he admitted that he had set few legs and had not looked at a book on orthopedics in 40 years. The hospital's defense was that the care provided was in accordance with the standard practice of like hospitals, that it had no control over the physician, and that it was not liable for the nurses' conduct because they were acting under the orders of the physician.

The appellate court, upholding the decision of the lower court, said that the hospital could be found liable either for breach of its own duty or for breach of duty of its nurses. The new hospital standards of care set by that ruling were in reference to the hospital by-laws, regulations based on state statutes governing hospital licensure and criteria for JCAH accreditation. The court reasoned that these constituted a commitment that the hospital did not fulfill. In addition, the court held that the hospital had failed in its duties to review the work of the physician or to require consultation when the patient's condition clearly indicated the necessity for such action.

NURSING IMPLICATIONS

You must be persistent in reporting inadequate care. It is not enough to observe and record. For nurses, the crucial point in the court decision was the newly defined duty to inform the hospital administration of any deviation from proper medical care that poses a threat to the well-being of the patients. Specifically, the court said:

skilled nurses would have promptly recognized the conditions that signalled a dangerous impairment of circulation in the plaintiff's leg, and would have known that the condition would become irreversible in a matter of hours. At that point, it became the nurses' duty to inform the attending physician, and if he failed to act, to advise the hospital authorities so that appropriate action might be taken (211 N.E. 2d at 258).

(The hospital was also expected to have a sufficient number of trained nurses capable of recognizing unattended problems in a patient's condition and reporting them.)

Two terms used here and almost inevitably in most suits are *malpractice* and *negligence*.

Negligence means failing to conduct oneself in a prescribed manner, with due care, thereby doing harm to another or doing something that a reasonably prudent person would not do in like circumstances. *Criminal negligence* and *gross negligence* are sometimes used interchangeably and refer to the commission or omission of an act, lawfully or unlawfully, in which such a degree of negligence exists as may cause a serious wrong to another. Almost any act of negligence resulting in the death of a patient would be considered criminal negligence.

Contributory negligence is the rather misleading expression used when the plaintiff has contributed to his or her own injury through personal negligence. This may have been done accidentally or deliberately. Some authorities assert that a plaintiff who is guilty of contributory negligence cannot collect damages; others state that he or she may collect under certain conditions. As in most legal matters, decisions vary widely. Because contributory negligence must be proven by the defendant, as much written evidence as possible is needed.

Malpractice is any *professional* misconduct, unreasonable lack of skill, or lack of fidelity in professional duties. (Note that malpractice refers only to professionals.) Another classic case illustrates these definitions. It is another example of the *fishnet* theory and the various kinds of liability of a student and teacher, even though the equipment used may now be considered outmoded by most.

CASE

A first-year student nurse in Pennsylvania was assigned by the instructor to care for a patient who later went into shock. Among other things, the student applied hot water bottles around the patient. The patient survived but was badly burned and sued the doctor, hospital, head nurse, faculty members, and school of nursing.

NURSING IMPLICATIONS

Be sure you know what you're doing. The student was clearly negligent, perhaps grossly negligent, because she should have known the correct temperature and procedure for applying a hot water bottle to anyone and should have taken special precautions with an unconscious patient. (Whether the hot water bottle was ordered by the doctor or not was immaterial, for the action, properly carried out, was appropriate for a patient in shock.) The student is held to the standards of care (*standards of reasonableness*) of an RN if he or she is performing RN functions. If the student is not capable of functioning safely unsupervised, he or she should not be carrying out those functions. The doctor may or may not be held liable, depending on that court's notion of the *captain-of-the-ship doctrine,* or perhaps on whether the doctor saw and/or felt the hot water bottles. The hospital will probably be held liable under *respondeat superior,* because students, even if not employed, are usually treated legally as employees. In addition, because the head nurse is responsible for all patients on the floor and presumably should have been involved in or should have assigned an RN in such an emergency, she, too, would be liable (and again, so would the hospital, under *respondeat superior*).

The instructor might be found liable on the basis of inadequate supervision or improper assignment. The school might be found liable in the case of the student if the court believed the director had not used good judgment in employing or assigning the faculty member carrying out those teaching responsibilities.

The captain-of-the-ship doctrine, less commonly accepted now, was negated in a case that cost the hospital $5 million (*Nelson v. Trinity Medical Center,* 1988). The physician of a woman in active labor ordered assessment of fetal heart tones, an IV, and analgesia. Standing orders in that labor unit called for continuous fetal heart monitoring, but the nurse, without checking, assumed that the monitors were all in use and did not place one on the patient until an hour later. It indicated fetal distress, and despite an immediate cesarean, the infant was born with severe brain damage. According to the expert who testified, the damage was caused by placental separation, which could have been diagnosed by earlier fetal monitoring. The defendant hospital tried to invoke the captain-of-the-ship doctrine to cover the nurse's negligence. The court ruled that even though the doctor was in charge of the case, he had no direct control over what the nurse did (as opposed to an operating room situation) and that the nurse was performing a routine act.[5]

Another incident illustrates *contributory* and *comparative negligence*.

CASE

A student gave an electric heating pad, per the doctor's order, to a patient who was alert and mentally competent and who demonstrated to the nurse her ability to adjust the temperature and her knowledge of the potential hazards. The patient fell asleep on the pad, set at a high temperature, and burned her abdomen.

NURSING IMPLICATIONS

No matter how simple and safe a treatment seems, check back with the patient. In this case, there would seem to be sufficient evidence of *contributory negligence* on the part of the patient, with the student having good reason to assume that the patient was capable of managing the heating pad. Therefore, even if the patient sued, her case would be weak. However, if the court used the doctrine of *comparative negligence,* some liability might be assigned to the student if, for instance, she or he did not check on the patient in a reasonable time. If the heating paid was faulty, the hospital would probably be liable, not the nurse, providing there was no evidence that the heating pad was faulty and it was used anyway. In some situations, nurses have been held responsible for not checking equipment properly.

An important legal concept is *res ipsa loquitor* ("the thing speaks for itself"), a legal doctrine that gets around the need for expert testimony or the need for the plaintiff to prove the defendant's liability because the situation (harm) is self-evident to even a lay person. The defendant must prove, instead, that he or she is not responsible for the harm done. Before the rule of *res ipsa loquitor* can be applied, three conditions must be present: the injury would not ordinarily have occurred unless there was negligence; whatever caused the injury at the time was under the exclusive control of the defendant; the injured person had not contributed to the negligence or voluntarily assumed the risk.[6]

The cases above are examples of this concept; another occurs in the operating room.

CASE

A pregnant woman was admitted to a hospital in Texas, where she underwent a cesarean section. Nursing service policy required that both the scrub nurse and the circulating nurse be responsible for opening and counting the sponges before and after surgery. After the section, the scrub nurse reported the count as being correct and the doctor did not check further. After the incision was closed, the scrub nurse reported one sponge missing. It could not be found, and x-rays were ordered. The films were not clear, but the doctor read them as showing no sponge. Some time later the patient returned to the hospital with various complaints, the sponge was located in the abdomen and removed surgically. The hospital, doctor, and nurses were sued. All were found liable—the hospital for having faulty x-ray equipment and, under *respondeat superior,* the physician for not following through and the nurses for carelessness.

Dangerous mistakes can be made when you are careless or hurried in doing simple, frequently performed tasks.[7] The court particularly noted that the nurses had not exercised the ordinary *due care* that they owed to the plaintiff. They shared the burden of negligent conduct that was the *proximate cause* of the patient's injuries and could have been prevented.

Another case of *res ipsa loquitor,* reported in 1987, resulted in an award of over $2 million.[8] A 4-day-old infant suffered trauma to her head as a result of being dropped or mishandled by the nursing staff. The hospital and staff denied responsibility, although the baby had been under the exclusive control of the hospital staff throughout her stay. Even when the parents visited, staff was present. It appears that whoever caused the injury chose to cover up the incident. The hospital paid under the *respondeat superior* doctrine, since all the staff members were employees.

MAJOR CAUSES OF LITIGATION

Certain practices are more likely than others to result in nurses being sued or included in a malpractice case. Sometimes legal problems are caused by lack of knowledge, as when a nurse simply does not know the most current use or dangers of a drug or treatment or how to respond to a complication. For instance, in a 1987 case, $7.3 million was awarded to a husband in Illinois when his wife died because nurses did not recognize or handle an emergency correctly. A central venous pressure line, which had been inserted through the patient's internal jugular vein during surgery, perforated the wall of her heart, allowing fluid to accumulate in the pericardial sac. Even though in the first five postoperative hours the blood pressure became undetectable and her heart rate rose, the nurses failed to call the physician. The suit alleged inadequate postoperative care because of the nurses' failure to act.[9]

Often problems result from poor nursing judgment, as when a nurse in the emergency room sends away a patient without consulting with or calling a physician,[10] or does not question a doctor's order or behavior, despite having doubts that the action is correct.[11] A large number of cases are the result of poor physician-nurse communication.

Communication Problems

Do you have a responsibility to take action when a doctor writes an order that you think is incorrect or unclear? When he or she does not respond to a patient's worsening condition? When he or she does not come to see a patient even if you think it's urgent? When he or she does not follow accepted precautions in giving a treatment? What if the physician becomes angry and abusive? What if he or she was right? According to court decisions in the last few years, the answer to all these questions is that it *is* the nurse's responsibility to take action. Medications seem to be a major problem. When an order is incomplete or written illegibly and the nurse does not question it, the results can be tragic.

CASE

A nursing manager thought she would help out in a pediatrics unit when it was short-staffed, even though she was not familiar with current pediatric nursing practice. An order for a medication for an infant did not state the appropriate route of administration and, after asking nearby physicians whether the dose was appropriate (not the route), the nurse gave it by injection. By this route, the amount given was a massive overdose and the child died. The nurse was not aware that the drug came in an oral solution and had not called the physician who wrote the order. Both were found liable.[12]

NURSING IMPLICATIONS

Don't follow orders blindly. A nurse who follows a physician's orders is just as liable as the physician if the patient is injured because, for instance, a medication was the wrong dose, given by the wrong route, or was actually the wrong drug.[13] If the order is illegible or incomplete, clarify that order with the physician who wrote it. If you doubt its appropriateness, check with a reference source or the pharmacist, and always with the physician who wrote the order.

You have a right to question the physician when in doubt about any aspect of an order, and the nursing service administration should support you. In fact, there should be a written policy on the nurse's rights and responsibility in such matters, so that there is no confusion on anyone's part and no danger of retribution for justifiable questioning when faced with an irate physician. What if the physician refuses to change the order? You should not simply refuse to carry out an order, for you may not have the most recent medical information and could injure the patient by *not* following the order. You should report your concern promptly to your administrative supervisor and record your action on the chart. The supervisor or other nurse administrator is often expected to act as an intermediary if there is a problem. However, a good collegial relationship and mutual courtesy can prevent or ease a doctor-nurse confrontation.

Verbal or telephone orders are another part of this problem.[14] Although they are considered legal, the dangers are evident. In case of patient injury, either the doctor, or the nurse, or both will be held responsible. There frequently are or should be hospital, sometimes legal, policies to serve as guides. If telephone orders are forbidden and a patient is injured through confused orders, the situation could be considered negligence. If telephone orders are acceptable, precautions should be taken to ensure that they are clearly understood (and questioned if necessary), with the doctor required to confirm the orders in writing as soon as possible. Some hospital policies require a repetition of the order; it is not unheard of to have two nurses listen together to a telephone order. In states where PAs' orders have been declared legal (as an extension of the physician), the same precautions must be taken, with the physician again confirming the order as quickly as possible.

Other common problems in doctor-nurse communications involve nurses who do not inform doctors about observations or requests, such as the nurse who did not tell a doctor that two children had been exposed to ticks, and they died from Rocky Mountain spotted fever.[15] A common situation is the need to observe and report problems with IVs that may cause a hematoma or other serious injury. Neglecting to anticipate danger from early symptoms has also led to suits.[16] Poor nurse-nurse communication can be just as deadly to the patient.

CASE

On the morning of surgery for a laminectomy, a woman in California had an atrial catheter inserted into a vein in her left arm until it entered the upper right atrium of her heart. Her postoperative course in the recovery room was without problems, and she was transferred to a postoperative unit. No evaluation of her condition was done, nor was her chart reviewed. She developed a number of problems, which were not attended to by the nurse and resulted in a cardiac arrest during a vomiting episode. Panic-stricken, the staff did not check her airway or start cardiopulmonary resuscitation (CPR). When a doctor arrived, all medications were given through the atrial catheter because no one knew what it was and assumed it was a regular IV line. The patient died after two months of being in a persistent vegetative states (PVS). Her four minor children sued, and the jury awarded $400,000, which was affirmed on appeal.[17]

NURSING IMPLICATIONS

When patients move from the care of one nurse to that of another, in the same or different units or institutions, share full pertinent information together. Read the record! Sometimes patients are transferred rapidly and no time is allowed for lengthy conferences, but it does not take long to share key points.

Another incident that repeatedly shows up in litigation is the failure of a physician to see a patient either on the unit or in the emergency room.[18] Often the nurse is held liable for not following through. More and more often, it is suggested that a system (or a policy) be set up specifying who the nurse then contacts.[19] If you neglect to call a doctor when the patient needs help or simply because you are not aware of the seriousness of the patient's condition, simply charting is not enough. Nurses in a Veterans Administration hospital were found liable because they failed to recognize the emergency condition of a postoperative patient and failed to take prompt steps to notify attending physicians. When the physicians were slow to respond, the nurse on duty made no effort to call another physician or anyone else because she said she thought no one else was capable of handling the situation (which was not so). Moreover, the nurses did not observe the patient carefully postoperatively, causing further delay in treatment. This case also points out the importance of a patient's chart, which the judge called "a mess"—sketchy and unreliable, with important data missing. The court stated that the lack of charting contributed to the decision against the nurses. Actually, because physicians and nurses working in a VA hospital cannot be sued separately, under the Federal Tort Claims Act, the United States was the defendant.[20] In another frequently cited case, the nurse did not call the physician when a pregnant woman continued to bleed excessively, "because he wouldn't come."[21] The patient died, and the hospital was held vicariously liable because of the nurse's negligence.

Another failure in communication occurs when a nurse does not report a situation because she or he doesn't fully investigate or fully assess it.[22] Still other judgments against the nurse have been given when a doctor has not followed through on appropriate technical procedures, such as the timely removal of an endotracheal tube.[23] If you know that a particular procedure is being done incorrectly (because it's within the scope of your knowledge) and do nothing about it, you, as well as the physician, can be held liable.

Nurses have also been held liable in cases involving the suicide of psychiatric patients, a frequent cause for suits. For instance, although a psychiatrist and a psychologist declared that suicide precautions were not necessary for a patient who showed suicidal tendencies, the nurse was held responsible when the patient drowned herself. She had not used nursing judgment and had not supervised the patient closely enough.[24]

These examples reinforce the need for nurses to recognize their accountability to the patient, even if it means disagreeing with physicians and reporting them if the patient appears to be endangered. Some hospitals that appreciate how difficult the nurse's situation can be in such a potential confrontation have set policies that clarify everyone's responsibilities.[25]

Nurses need to take precautions anyway. There are a number of actions you can take. Don't hesitate to call a physician; be persistent in tracing down the attending or substitute physician; stay on the phone until you get the information you need (use nursing judgment).[26] Be especially careful about telephone orders. Make sure you're both talking about the same patient. Make certain you understand what the doctor is saying even if it requires repetition. Repeat the order. Document the order, noting the physician's name, the time and date, and the name of the third party if there was a witness.[27]

Legal Problems in Record Keeping

It is almost impossible to overemphasize the importance of records in legal action, especially nurses' notes. They are the only evidence that orders were carried out and what the results were; they are the only notes written with both the time and date in chronological order; they offer the most detailed information on the patient. Nurses' notes, like the rest of the chart, can be subpoenaed. No matter how skillfully you practice, if your actions and observations are not documented accurately and completely, the jury can judge only by what is recorded. If you are subpoenaed, comprehensive notes will not only give weight to your testimony, but will help you remember what happened. A case may not come up for years, and unless there was a severe problem at the time, it is difficult to remember exact details about one patient. General, broad phrases such as "resting comfortably," "good night," and "feeling better" are totally inadequate. How could a jury interpret them? How could even another professional who did not know that patient interpret them?

Some of the most serious problems arising from poor charting concern lack of data, which have resulted in liability judgments against nurses and hospitals, although in each case it was contended that the right thing had been done.[28] Moreover, there are instances when a patient might be legally harmed by inaccurate reporting, as in child or adult abuse or rape.[29–31]

The correct way to chart, with legal aspects in mind, is probably to chart as you were taught and to follow good nursing practice.[32]

Do:

1. Be objective: write what you see, hear, smell, and feel.
2. Be complete[33]: for medications, record what, where, and how.
3. Be accurate: if a mistake is made, recopy or cross out, with the original copy attached; never use white-out.[34]
4. Be specific.
5. Record the patient's progress and any change in condition.
6. Record abnormal patient behavior.
7. Document any patient teaching.
8. Write legibly.
9. Use only standard abbreviations.
10. Be careful about how statements read. ("Bathed in wheelchair in lounge" can cause a legal problem.)
11. Record the time and date of entries.
12. Sign every entry.

Don't:

1. Use a pencil.
2. Make flip, derogatory, critical, or extraneous remarks about anyone.
3. Omit data such as amounts and kind of fluids, oxygen, or the physician's visits.
4. Guess at such things as output and vital signs.
5. *Ever* lie or cover up for anyone.[35] *Never* alter a record other than as described above; this has been shown to influence a jury negatively. Every good malpractice attorney calls on experts to examine charts for alterations, erasures, and additions. This can also lead to criminal charges.
6. Let anyone chart for you or change what you have charted.
7. Chart for anyone else. When you must chart what an aide says he or she did or what occurred when you have not personally seen it, add a statement that clarifies the fact to protect yourself.

Checking doctors' orders and following through might seem to be ordinary acts, but when they are neglected, they can have dire consequences. Nurses failed to pick up and transcribe a surgeon's postoperative order to remove rectal packing four hours after insertion. Two days later, noting that this had not been done, the surgeon removed it himself, but it was too late.

The patient had become septic and later died. When the surgeon and hospital were sued, the hospital paid the bulk of the settlement because of nursing negligence.[36]

Medication Errors

Medication errors are a particularly serious problem. Studies have shown that drugs were the major cause of illness and injury to patients in hospitals, caused by the treatment given by physicians and others. Twenty percent caused a serious disability. The major errors, in order, are wrong dose, wrong drug, omission of a dose, wrong rate of administration, wrong route, and wrong time.[37] Nurses who take unsafe shortcuts or otherwise fail to follow what they know is competent nursing practice are being negligent. If harm to a patient or coworker can be traced to a nurse, and it often can, she or he may be held liable. Negligence tends to involve carelessness as much as lack of knowledge.

Carelessness in giving an injection can cause serious injury. A patient who had received several injections contracted an infection, eventually re-

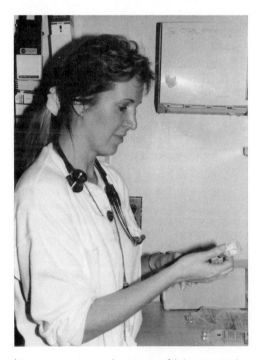

Because medication errors are a major cause of injury to patients, nurses must follow the appropriate procedure carefully. (*Courtesy of the Robert Wood Johnson Medical Center.*)

quiring plastic surgery. In the resulting trial, a nurse expert witness testified that the cause was improper sterile technique (*Tripp v. Humana Inc.*, 1985.)[38]

Another example of carelessness and haste is demonstrated in *Breit v. St. Luke's Memorial Hospital* (1987). A patient had had a laminectomy; by the next day he had full use of his extremities and could walk. When the patient complained of pain, the nurse took an unwise shortcut: she gave him the injection when he was in an upright position. Soon he lost all sensory and motor function and became an invalid. Two expert nurse witnesses testified that the morphine should not have been given in that way, because it could cause hypotension and the pooling of blood in the legs could precipitate a stroke. The nurse admitted that she knew this. She was found liable.[39]

Other Common Acts of Negligence

Among the acts of negligence a nurse is most likely to commit in the practice of nursing are the following (not in order of importance):

1. *Abandoning a patient.* Abandonment simply means leaving a patient when your duty is to be with him. One example would be leaving a child or incompetent adult without the protection you would have offered. This may include leaving a patient in the bathroom or on a chair or stretcher while attending to something else. Falls often bring on suits. The results of abandonment can be more serious than a broken bone.

CASE

A circulating nurse went, at a doctor's demand, to assist in another operating room while the OR technician was removing the surgical drapes at the end of a patient's surgery. No one else was in that OR, and when the patient went into cardiac arrest, the technician could not handle the situation alone. The patient became permanently paralyzed and semicomatose. Although the physician and the anesthesiologist were also held liable, the court focused on the duty of the circulating nurse, as spelled out in the hospital procedure book. The jury concluded that the nurse was negligent for leaving the unconscious patient's side.[40]

NURSING IMPLICATIONS

Your first responsibility is to the patient. Use your nursing judgment to decide whether a patient can be safely left alone or with a less prepared person.

2. *Improper delegation and supervision.* Unless you work in a place that has all-RN staffing, you probably will be delegating certain patient assignments to an LPN or aide. Theoretically you can look to the LPN's licensure as evidence that this person is qualified to perform certain tasks. However, it is your responsibility to know an individual's competence before assigning an LPN or aide to patient care. In other words you can't simply say "You take the patients on that side of the hall" if any one of those patients requires the care of an RN. Should a patient be injured, you can be held responsible.

3. *Failure to use adequate precautions to protect the patient against injury.* As a nurse, you are expected to know that drugs, or hot liquids, or potentially harmful implements, such as scissors, must be kept out of the reach of a young child or a delirious or confused patient. You know the danger of falls or slips when weak, elderly, or disabled patients are walking or left alone. Patients often fall when trying to get out of bed when their call light isn't answered or they are confused. To use or not use siderails in these situations is an ongoing dilemma. As shown here, there is no clear-cut answer from the courts.

CASE

In a hospital in Massachusetts, an 80-year-old woman received Dalmane at bedtime. An hour later, when getting out of bed, she fell and was injured. The bedrails at her head were up; those at her legs were down. Some of the side effects of the medication were known to be dizziness, light-headedness, and staggering. Hospital policy required that the bed be down and the bedrails up for all confused patients. The patient sued, and the nurse was found liable.[41]

NURSING IMPLICATIONS

As a nurse, you are expected to use your nursing judgment to anticipate risks for patients. Even if the patient in this case was not confused, the medication could cause a condition in which she could get hurt if she got out of bed (which old people often do at night). The judge ruled that under these circumstances and in the presence of the hospital policy, the nurse should have anticipated the risk to the patient. (This is also called *foreseeability*.) Yet it is not good enough simply to depend on a policy, since patients do not respond according to rules. For instance, in another case, a 78-year-old man who had gotten to the bathroom without any problems for several nights requested that the siderails be left down. The next night he fell and was injured. Although sued, the nurses were not held liable.[42]

4. *Failure to respond or to ask someone else to respond promptly to a patient's call light or signal* if, because of such failure, a patient attempts to take care of his or her own needs and is injured. This might happen when the patient attempts to get out of bed to go to the bathroom or reaches for a bedpan in the bedside stand. Sometimes the bedpan or urinal is not even at hand. After prostate surgery, a 79-year-old man rang to go to the bathroom. The nurse said that an orderly would help him. Despite the flashing call light, no one came. The patient got out of bed, fell, and injured himself. The court faulted the nurse; she had not left a urinal, and she did not see to it that he got help. It was deemed her responsibility, even though the orderly didn't come.[43] This is also an example of not supervising properly someone to whom you have delegated care.

5. *Inadequate or dated nursing knowledge.* Since having current knowledge is a professional responsibility, there seems to be little excuse for this kind of negligence. However, on occasion, even the most competent nurse has a problem. If an entirely new type of treatment or piece of equipment is introduced on your unit, it is your responsibility, as well as that of the head nurse or supervisor, to get the appropriate information.

6. *Failure to teach a patient.* Nurses sometimes neglect to teach a patient in preparation for discharge, either because of the time it takes or because the physician objects. An increasing number of suits are being filed because such teaching was not done or not done thoroughly or understandably. Written instructions are often considered necessary to help the patient and family remember the information.[44]

7. *Failure to make sure that faulty equipment is removed* from use, that crowded corridors or hallways adjacent to the nursing unit are cleared, that slippery or unclean floors are taken care of, and that fire hazards are eliminated.

   This is an area of negligence that, in most instances, would implicate others just as much as, or more than, the professional nurse. For example, the hospital administration would certainly share responsibility for fire hazards and dangerously crowded corridors, and the housekeeping and maintenance departments would not be blameless either. This does not lessen your responsibility for reporting unsafe conditions and following up on them or for checking equipment you use.[45] Report persistent hazards in writing and keep a copy for personal protection.

THE PROBLEM OF SHORT STAFFING

Can an injury to a patient be excused on the basis of short staffing? Not really. Even if there is a staff shortage, nurses have a responsibility to use good judgment. A man was admitted with a serious case of pneumonia; he was confused, uncoordinated, and weak. He was placed in a room with a balcony. His wife stayed with him, but when she left, he was seen on the balcony calling to workers below to bring a ladder. The nurses restrained him and called the wife to sit with him. She asked them to call her mother, who lived only five minutes away, to come until she could get there and asked that someone sit with him until her mother arrived. The nurses said that they were short-staffed and couldn't. By the time the mother arrived the patient was on the ground below. In part because an aide had been sent to supper and other staff were performing routine duties that could have waited, the court ruled in favor of the plaintiff.[46]

Further problems can come from "floating." In these cases, you may be placed in a specialty area with which you are not familiar, with or without a more experienced nurse. There is no clear answer to this dilemma, since some courts have ruled that shifting staff is the employer's privilege and refusal can be considered insubordination. The supervisor, of course, is also responsible for any damage done because he or she is supposed to delegate safely. The float nurse must be especially careful and report any change in a patient's condition. Cushing notes that perhaps the best defense if injury occurs is to be able to document that you recognized your knowledge gap, but did not know that speciality and had asked for help.[47] Meanwhile, some union contracts and some individual agreements in hospitals specify that a nurse is not to be floated to an unfamiliar unit without some training in that specialty.

SPECIALTY NURSING

As nurses assume more responsibility in nursing, particularly in specialty areas, they often seek help in determining their legal status. Frequently their concern has to do with the scope of practice: are they performing within legal bounds? Negligence, whether in a highly specialized unit, an emergency, or a self-care unit, is still a question of what the reasonably prudent nurse would do. Therefore, although a nurse might look for a specific answer to a specific question, the legal dangers lie in the same set of instances described earlier, simply transposed to another setting.[48-52]

STANDARD OF CARE

The standard of care basically determines nurses' liability for negligent acts.[53] This standard requires an individual to perform a task as any "reasonably prudent man of ordinary prudence, with comparable education, skills, and training under similar circumstances" would perform that same function. It is often described as requiring a person of ordinary sense to use ordinary care and skill. Who makes that judgment on what the "reasonably prudent" nurse would do?

In litigation, it is the judge or jury, based on testimony that could include the following:

1. *Expert witnesses*. Did the nurse do what was necessary? A nurse with special or appropriate knowledge testifies on what would be expected of a nurse in the defendant's position in like circumstances. The expert witness would have the credentials to validate his or her expertise, but because the opposing side would produce an equally prestigious expert witness to say what was useful to them, the credibility of that witness on testifying is critical. A nurse would generally be judged by an expert in his or her particular kind of nursing.[54]

2. *Professional literature*. Was the nurse's practice current? The *most current* nursing literature would be examined and perhaps quoted to validate (or invalidate) whether the nurse's practice in the situation was totally up-to-date.

3. *Hospital or agency policies*. Were hospital policies, especially nursing policies (in-house law), followed? For example, if restraints were or were not used, was the nurse's action according to hospital policy? On the other hand, if a nurse followed an outdated policy or followed policy without using nursing judgment (according to the expert witness), it could be held against her or him.)

4. *Manuals or procedure books*. Did the nurse follow the usual procedure accurately? Example: If the nurse gave an injection that was alleged to have injured the patient, was it given correctly according to the procedure manual? If the procedure book is not up-to-date and the nurse followed it, she or he might still be liable on the basis of needing to be aware of current practice.

5. *Drug enclosures or drug reference books*. Did the nurse check for the latest information? For example, if the patient suffered from a drug reaction that the nurse did not perceive, was the information about the potential reaction in a drug reference book, such as the *Physicians' Desk Reference (PDR)* or a drug insert?[55]

6. *The profession's standards*. Did the nurse behave according to the published ANA standards, both general and in the specialty, if any?[56]

7. *Licensure*. Did the nurse fulfill her responsibilities according to the legal definition of nursing in the licensure law or the law's rules and regulations? For example, did she teach a diabetic patient about foot care?

If the judge or jury is satisfied that the standards were met satisfactorily, even if the patient has been injured, the injury that occurred would not be considered the result of the nurse's negligence. Different judgments in different jurisdictions must be expected. For instance, in one case, an occupational health nurse, not recognizing the signs and symptoms of a coronary occlusion, sent the patient home unattended. When he died and she was sued, she was found not liable because having such knowledge was not seen as being a nursing responsibility. In an almost identical situation elsewhere, the nurse was found liable.

INCIDENT REPORTS

In case of patient injury, most hospitals and health agencies require completion of an *incident report*. The purpose is to document the incident accurately for remedial and correctional use by the hospital or agency, for insurance information, and sometimes for legal reasons. The wording should be chosen to avoid the implication of blame and should be totally objective and complete: what happened to the patient; what was done; what his or her condition is.[57] The incident report may or may not be *discoverable* (used as part of evidence), depending on the state's law. It is considered a business record, not a part of the patient's chart, but some courts rule that it is not privileged information.[58] The incident *must* be just as accurately recorded in the patient's chart; omission casts doubt on the nurse's honesty if litigation occurs. However, the fact that an incident report was filed should not be charted.

Appropriate behavior by nurses and other personnel is often a key factor in whether or not the patient or family sues after an incident, regardless of injury. Maintaining good rapport and giving honest explanations as needed are very important. It has been shown that often patients do not sue the nurses, or at all, because nurses were caring and concerned.[60]

OTHER TORTS AND CRIMES

The average nurse probably will not get involved in criminal offenses, although in the last few years, a number of nurses have been accused of murder.[61] Nurses, like anyone else, may steal, murder, or break other laws. Crimes most often committed are criminal assault and battery (striking or otherwise physically mistreating or threatening a patient); murder (sometimes in relation to right-to-live principles); and drug offenses. If found guilty of a felony, the nurse will probably also lose her or his license.

Whether the nurse is a perpetrator or victim, or simply has to deal with people who are, it is useful to know the definition and scope of the most common criminal offenses. These can be found in most nursing law texts. Several are discussed here. Not discussed but worth mentioning are some torts and crimes in which nurses occasionally are involved in their professional lives: *forgery*—fraudulently making or altering a written document or item, such as a will, chart, or check; *kidnapping*—stealing and carrying off a human being; *rape*—illegal or forcible sexual intercourse; and *bribery*—an offer of a reward for doing wrong or for influencing conduct.

Assault and Battery

Any attempt to use force and violence with an intent to injure, or put one in fear of injury, constitutes an *assault,* such as striking at a person with or without a weapon; holding up a fist in a threatening way near enough to be able to strike; or advancing with a hand uplifted in a threatening way with intent to strike or put someone in fear of being struck, even if the person is stopped before he or she gets near enough to carry out the intended action.

Battery, as distinguished from assault, is the actual striking or touching of a person's body in a violent, angry, rude, or insolent manner. Every laying on of hands is not a battery: the person's intention must be considered. To constitute a battery, intent to injure or put one in fear of injury must be accompanied by "unlawful violence." However, the slightest degree of force may constitute violence in the eyes of the law. Legal action can result from any of these acts unless they can be justified or excused.[62]

Defamation, Slander, and Libel

As is true of so many legal terms, there is some overlapping of meaning and interpretation of the terms *defamation, slander,* and *libel.* In general, however, it is correct to consider *defamation* as the most inclusive term because it covers any communication that is seriously detrimental to another person's reputation. If the communication is oral, it is technically called *slander;* if written or shown in pictures, effigies, or signs (without just cause or excuse), it is called *libel.* All three are considered wrongful acts (torts) under the law, and a person convicted in court is ordered to make amends, usually by paying the defamed person a compensatory fee.

In both slander and libel, a third person must be involved. For example, one person can make all kinds of derogatory statements directly to another without getting in trouble with the law *unless* overheard and understood by a third person. Then the remarks become slanderous. Likewise a person can write anything she or he wishes to another, and the communication will not be considered libelous unless it is read and understood by a third person. A malicious and false statement made by one person to another about a third person also comprises slander.[63]

Uncomplimentary statements are not necessarily slanderous or libelous. They must be false, damaging to the offended person's reputation, and tending to subject him or her to public contempt and ridicule. The best and often the only defense allowed under the law is proof that she or he told the truth in whatever type of communication used.

Given the many "ifs," "ands," and "buts" associated with defamation, slander, and libel, it's better to avoid becoming embroiled in such litigations. Be careful in what you say or write about anyone. Also, proceed with caution when you are the victim of slander or libel. Litigation is expensive and time-consuming and, in many instances, hardly worth the trouble. On the other hand, don't be overly meek in accepting unfair and untrue statements about yourself that are likely to adversely affect your reputation. There have been documented cases in which nurses were slandered by a physician, for instance, and collected damages.

Homicide and Suicide

Homicide means killing a person by any means whatsoever. It is not necessarily a crime. If it is unquestionably an accident, it is called *excusable homicide*. If it is done in self-defense or in discharging a legal duty, it is termed *justifiable homicide*. The accused must be able to prove justification, however. *Criminal homicide* is either murder or manslaughter; murder is usually with intent.

Suicide is considered criminal if the person is sane and of an age of discretion at the time of his or her action. A person who encourages another to commit suicide is guilty of murder if the suicide is successful. Statutes vary from state to state.

As a professional person, it is not unusual for a nurse to become involved in cases of murder and suicide, usually associated with patients. Following are a few suggestions for keeping as free of legal involvement as possible:

1. Take seriously any indication on the part of any patient or employee that she or he has suicidal tendencies. Report this to the appropriate person.
2. Generally, don't leave a patient with known suicidal inclinations alone unless completely protected from self-harm by restraints or confinement.
3. Keep items that a depressed person might use for suicidal purposes out of reach.
4. Make and report observations accurately on the patient's chart.
5. Try to get help for individuals or their families immediately upon becoming aware of suicidal tendencies.

6. Cooperate with the police and hospital authorities guarding a patient who is accused of homicide.
7. Avoid unethical discussions of a homicide case involving a patient or employee.
8. Keep complete and accurate records of all facts that might have a bearing on the legal aspects of a case.

DRUG CONTROL

In 1914, the United States adopted an antinarcotic law, the *Harrison Narcotic Act,* to be administered by a bureau of narcotics within the Department of the Treasury. It was amended frequently to meet the demands of changing times. As noted in Chapter 10, the *Comprehensive Drug Abuse and Control Act* of 1970 (*Controlled Substance Act*) replaced virtually all earlier federal laws dealing with narcotics, stimulants, depressants, and hallucinogens. Sections of this law prohibit nurses from prescribing controlled substances, but they may administer drugs at the direction of legalized practitioners (who are registered). All registrants must follow strict controls and procedures against theft and diversion of controlled substances.[64] New state laws are based on the federal law, although there are variations. Controlled substances are identified as such in health care delivery sites. New drugs are also being given closer scrutiny because of misuse and consequent dangerous effects.

Knowledge of the laws controlling the use of drugs will help you to understand the reasons for the policies and procedures established by an institution or agency for the mutual welfare of the employer, employee, and patient. It will also help you to keep free of legal involvements and to direct and advise intelligently others whom you may supervise or who may look to you for guidance in such matters. Be alert to changes in drug laws at either the state or the national level.

GOOD SAMARITAN LAWS

The enactment of Good Samaritan laws in many states exempts doctors and nurses (and sometimes others) from civil liability when they give emergency care in "good faith" with "due care" or without "gross negligence." All states and the District of Columbia have Good Samaritan laws, but not all include nurses in their coverage. No court has yet interpreted these statutes, and prior to their enactment, no case held a doctor or nurse liable for negligence in giving care at the site of an emergency. The law is intended to encourage assistance without fear of legal liability. As far as the law is concerned, there is no obligation or duty to render aid or assistance in an emergency. Only by statutory law can the rendering of such assistance be required. Emergency treatment in a health care setting is not covered under the Good Samaritan laws.

Because of the lack of clarity of terms and the many differences in the law from state to state, many health professionals are still reluctant to give emergency assistance.[65] One lawyer gives this advice:

- Don't give aid unless you know what you're doing.
- Stick to the basics of first aid.
- Offer to help, but make it clear that you won't interfere if the victim or family prefers to wait for other help.
- Don't draw any medical or diagnostic conclusions.
- Don't leave a victim you've begun to assist until you can turn his or her care over to an equally competent person.
- Whether you do or do not volunteer your services, be absolutely certain to call or have someone else call for a physician or emergency medical service immediately.[66]

MALPRACTICE (PROFESSIONAL LIABILITY) INSURANCE

Almost all lawyers in the health field now agree that nurses should carry their own malpractice or, as it is increasingly called, *professional liability* insurance, whether or not their employer's insurance includes them. The employer's insurance is intended primarily to protect the employer; the nurse is protected only to the extent needed for that primary purpose. It is quite possible that the employer might settle out of court, without consulting the nurse, to the nurse's disadvantage. The nurse has no control and no choice of lawyer.[67]

There are a number of other limitations. The nurse is not covered for anything beyond the job in the place of employment during the hours of employment. If the nurse alone is sued and the hospital is not, the hospital has no obligation to provide legal protection (and may choose not to). Moreover, if the nurse carries no personal liability insurance, there is the possibility of subrogation.[68] *Subrogation* means that the employer can sue the employee for the amount of damages paid because of the employee's negligence. Should there be criminal charges, the employer or insurance carrier may choose to deny legal assistance, or the kind offered could be inadequate.[69] Remember that no matter how trivial or how unfounded a charge might be, a legal defense is necessary and often costly, aside from the possibility of being found liable and having to pay damages.

Malpractice insurance should be bought with some care so that adequate coverage is provided. Certain features are optional. Decide which coverage meets your needs, but don't necessarily choose the least expensive. For instance, the most important distinction to be made in selecting insurance is whether it has an *occurrence based coverage* or a *claims made coverage*. If the insurance policy is allowed to lapse, an incident that occurred at the time of coverage will be covered in an occurrence based policy but not in a claims made policy. The latter may be less expensive but will require almost continuous coverage, which might be a problem for a nurse planning to interrupt practice for any reason or for one close to retirement.

Before deciding on a policy, check:[70]

1.   What kinds of acts are covered on the job.
2.   What kinds of acts are covered off the job.
3.   Whether personal liability is covered.
4.   Under what circumstances a lawyer will be provided.
5.   Whether you have any choice of lawyer.
6.   Whether a settlement can be made without your approval.
7.   The term of the policy.
8.   What affects renewability.
9.   The cost.

Benefits usually include paying any sum awarded as damages, including medical costs, paying the cost of attorneys, and paying the bond required if appealing an adverse decision. Some policies also pay damages for injury arising out of acts of the insured as a member of an accreditation board or committee of a hospital or professional society, personal liability (such as slander, assault, or libel), and personal injury and medical payments (not related to the individual's professional practice).[71]

Generally speaking, an ANA or SNA policy is the best buy. Until a few years ago, nurse-midwives and NPs had no difficulty buying malpractice insurance. Then, in 1985, in response to the general malpractice crisis, the American College of Nurse-Midwives, (ACNM) was notified by its insurer that its members would no longer be covered. Actually, there were no data to justify this action, even though it would effectively put nurse-midwives out of business. Finally, after intense efforts, a consortium of insurance companies and ACNM began to provide the insurance. Insurance journals noted that the claims experience was very favorable. In like fashion, this kind of action was threatened against NPs, who also have had few claims against them. In response, ANA made arrangements with a new insurance carrier that covers all nurses, including NPs and nurses in private practice (the only one that does). Premiums depend on the position of the nurse. Only nurse anesthetists and nurse-midwives are not covered. In 1990, ANA also expanded its coverage to include students.

Most malpractice cases are settled out of court (although this still requires a lawyer) and multimillion-dollar awards are not as common as the newspapers may imply. However, for the careful nurse, professional liability insurance is a good investment, as well as being tax deductible.

IN COURT: THE DUE PROCESS OF LAW

Yes, you can be sued. What happens if you become involved in litigation? What steps should you take to try to make sure that the case will be handled to your best advantage throughout? The answers to these questions will depend on (1) whether you are accused of committing the tort or crime; (2) whether you are an accessory, through actual participation or observance; (3) whether you are the person against whom the act was committed; or (4) whether you appear as an expert witness.

Assuming that this is a civil case, five distinct steps are taken:

(1) the filing of a document called a *complaint* by a person called the *plaintiff* who contends that his legal rights have been infringed by the conduct of one or more other persons called *defendents*; (2) the written response of the defendants accused of having violated the legal rights of the plaintiff, termed an *answer*; (3) pretrial activities of both parties designed to elicit all the facts of the situation, termed *discovery*;[72] (4) the *trial* of the case, in which all the relevant facts are presented to the judge or jury for decision; and (5) *appeal* from a decision by a party who contends that the decision was wrongly made.[73]

The majority of persons who are asked to appear as witnesses during a hearing accept voluntarily. Others refuse and must be subpoenaed. A *subpoena* is a writ or order in the name of the court, referee, or another person authorized by law to issue the same, which requires the attendance of a witness at a trial or hearing under a penalty for failure. Cases involving the care of patients often necessitate producing hospital records, x-rays, and photographs as evidence. A subpoena requiring a witness to bring this type of evidence to court contains a clause to that effect and is termed a *subpoena duces tecum*.

The plaintiff, defendant, and witnesses may be asked to make a *deposition,* an oral interrogation answering various questions about the issue concerned. It is given under oath and taken in writing before a judicial officer or attorney. Tips given by experts on how to handle yourself at a deposition are basically the same as for testifying.[74] You may be cross-examined by the opposing lawyer; the only limitation on the scope of questioning is that the inquiry must be relevant to the subject under suit. Since the primary purpose is *discovery,* the procedure is sometimes referred to as a "fishing expedition."[75]

A witness has certain rights, including the right to refuse to testify as to privileged communication (extended to the nurse in only a few states) and the protection against self-incrimination afforded by the Fifth Amendment to the Constitution. The judge and jury usually do not expect a person on trial or serving as a witness to remember all the details of a situation. Witnesses in malpractice suits are permitted to refer to the patient's record, which, of course, they should have reviewed with the attorney before the trial. Only under serious circumstances is someone accused (and convicted) of *perjury,* which means making a false statement under oath or one that the person neither knows nor believes to be true.

There are certain guidelines on testifying that are the same whether serving as an expert or other witness or if the nurse is the defendant:[76]

1. Be prepared; review the deposition, the chart, technical and clinical knowledge of the disease or condition; discuss with the lawyer potential questions; educate the lawyer as to what points should be made. Trials are adversary procedures that are intended to probe, question, and explore all aspects of the issue.
2. Dress appropriately; appearance is important.
3. Behave appropriately: keep calm, be courteous, even if insulted; don't be sarcastic or angry; take your time (a cross-examiner attorney may try to put you in a poor light).
4. Give adequate and appropriate information: if you can't remember, notes or the data source, such as the chart, can be checked. Answer fully, but don't volunteer additional information not asked for.
5. Don't use technical terminology, or, if use is necessary, translate it into lay terms. Enunciate clearly.
6. Don't feel incompetent; don't get on the defensive; be decisive.
7. Don't be obviously partisan (unless you're the defendant).
8. Keep all materials; the decision may be appealed.

In the expert witness role,[77,78] the same suggestions hold, but in addition, the nurse should present her or his credentials, degrees, research, honors, and whatever else is pertinent, without modesty; the opposing expert witness will certainly do so.

Expert witnesses are paid for preparation time, pretrial conferences, consultations, and testifying. Nurses are just beginning to act officially in this capacity, and several SNAs accept applications for those interested in placement on an expert witness panel, screen applicants in a given field for a specific case, submit a choice of names to attorneys requesting such information, and have developed guidelines and CE for nurse expert witnesses.

Should you be sued, here are some tips for defending yourself:

- Cut off all communication with the claimant; simply tell whoever contacts you that your insurer will be in touch. (Then find out why they haven't already done so.)
- Educate the insurer; claims adjusters may know little about nursing.
- Keep tabs on the claim. Don't be afraid to ask questions.
- Be sure that your claim is supervised adequately. You have a right to ask that it be handled by an experienced and attentive professional.
- Seek input on settlement decisions. You may not have the right, but you can ask your insurer to check with you before making an offer.
- Remember that the defense attorney is *your* attorney. If you really think his or her qualifications are inadequate, ask for a change.
- Dictate all memories of the patient to the attorney. Do it as soon as possible, but not until an attorney has been assigned to your case, or your information may not be considered "privileged."
- Retrieve medical records. You have access if you still work at the same place and can get access before the attorney does.
- Review the records.
- Compile a list of experts; the case may hinge on getting the best. (Although in some courts physicians have been allowed as expert witnesses on a nursing case, ordinarily it should be the nurse(s) who are most knowledgeable about the type of situation involved.)
- Have a reference list available.
- Speak up in court; you must project self-confidence.[79]

Other attorneys also point out that you shouldn't talk to anyone about the case at your hospital except the risk manager, or with anyone involved in any way with the plaintiff, or to reporters. Certainly don't hide any information from your attorney, and *never* alter the patient's record.[80]

AVOIDING LEGAL PROBLEMS

Malpractice continues to be an issue in health care from the point of view of both patient endangerment and cost. Physicians are said to practice "defensive medicine," that is, ordering every possible test to make sure that nothing was neglected that may eventually result in litigation. That and the rising cost of malpractice insurance adds to the overall cost of health care.

The possibilities of pretrial arbitration and no-fault insurance have been considered. Some states use an arbitration procedure that makes preliminary recommendations on the viability of a suit. The attraction of no-fault in-

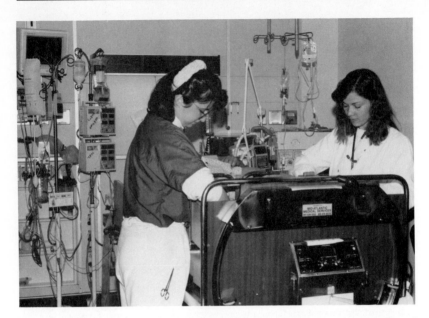

The complexity of care in hospitals today and the increased responsibility of nurses require nurses to be knowledgeable and careful in order to avoid malpractice suits. (*Courtesy of the Robert Wood Johnson Medical Center.*)

surance is the increasing public tendency to believe that if someone is hurt, someone must pay, whether or not negligence is clearly evident; but the cost may be prohibitive. To get to the root of the problem—quality of care— government and health providers are looking at the impact of quality assurance techniques. It has also been noted that physicians are more stringently controlling the practice of their peers.

In addition, many hospitals have now adopted *risk management* programs in which nurses are very much involved, focusing on the review and improvement of employee guidelines, personnel policies, incident reports, physician-nurse relationships, safety policies, patient records, research guidelines, and anything else that might be a factor in legal suits.[81]

Risk management initiatives are now required by JCAHO and more and more by state legislation. The purpose is not only to protect the interest of the hospital and its personnel but also to improve the quality of patient care. Risk management means taking steps to control the possibility that a patient will complain and minimizing any risks *before* complaints are filed.

All of this involves nurses, especially since the likelihood of their being in potentially litigious situations is increasing. Because of the various legal doctrines, explained earlier, the aggrieved patient has the option of suing multiple defendants. The *deep pocket* theory of naming those who can pay has become traditional tort law strategy, as has the *fishnet theory* of suing every defendant available. Thus, the likelihood of recovery from one or more defendants is greater, and a favorite defense of admitting negligence but blaming an absent party, the so-called empty chair defense, is defeated.[82] While it may be possible to get some information from your employing agency's legal counsel or state licensing board in relation to specific aspects of your practice, observing some basic principles will also help to avert problems:

1. Know your licensure law.
2. Don't do what you don't know how to do. (Learn how, if necessary.)
3. Keep your practice updated; CE is essential.
4. Use self-assessment, peer evaluation, audits, and the supervisor's evaluations as guidelines for improving practice, and follow up on criticisms and knowledge/skill gaps.
5. Don't be careless.
6. Be considerate of patients and their significant others.
7. Practice interdependently; communicate with others.
8. Record accurately, objectively, and completely; don't erase.
9. Delegate safely and legally; know the preparation and abilities of those you supervise.
10. Help develop appropriate policies and procedures (in-house law).
11. Carry professional liability insurance.

There are "nurse defenders" who defend their patients from harm and "nurse defendants" whose substandard practices make them a target for litigation.[83] Never forget that licensure is a privilege and a responsibility mandating accountability to the consumer it is intended to protect; therefore, you have a legal and moral obligation to practice safely.

KEY POINTS

1. Malpractice suits of any kind are often stimulated by how the patient and family were treated, as well as by the possible injury.
2. The standard of care by which a nurse is judged in a malpractice case is based on what the "reasonably prudent nurse" of the same background and in the same situation would do.
3. The most common reason for legal suits against nurses is negligence.
4. Negligence frequently occurs in giving medication and treatments because the nurse has inadequate knowledge or is careless.
5. *Darling v. Charleston Community Memorial Hospital* is a landmark case pinpointing the corporate liability of hospitals for the actions of their employees and physicians. For nurses, it underlines the legal

responsibility to follow through and ensure that patients get competent care.

6. Poor communication between doctors and nurses, and among nurses themselves, can endanger patients and result in litigation.

7. To avoid problems in law, be accurate, complete, and objective in charting. Never falsify a record for any reason.

8. When selecting professional liability (malpractice) insurance, among the points to consider is whether it is occurrence based or claims made.

9. When testifying in a court of law, be prepared and calm; give appropriate information without jargon, and be accurate and honest.

10. To avoid malpractice, it is especially important to know your licensure law, stay up-to-date in your practice, communicate with others adequately, be careful, and practice humanistic nursing.

REFERENCES

1. Cohn SD. *Malpractice and liability in clinical obstetrical nursing.* Rockville, MD: Aspen Publishers, 1990.
2. Northrop C, Kelly M. *Legal issues in nursing.* St. Louis: C.V. Mosby Company, 1987, pp. 52–59.
3. Horsley J. Why it's harder to defend nurses now. *RN,* 9:56–59 (November 1986).
4. Trandel-Korenchuk D, Trandel-Korenchuk T. Nursing liability and respondeat superior. *Nurse Practitioner* 7:46–48 (January 1982).
5. Cushing M. Law and orders. *Am J Nurs,* 90:29–32 (May 1990).
6. Creighton H. *Law every nurse should know,* 5th ed. Philadelphia: W.B. Saunders Company, 1986, pp. 165–166.
7. Herrman F. Four kinds of carelessness that can send you to court. *Nurs Life,* 2:63 (May–June 1982).
8. Northrop C. Current case law involving nurses: Lessons for practitioners, managers and educators. *Nurs Outlook,* 37:296 (November–December 1989).
9. Cushing M. Hazards of the infiltrated IV. *Am J Nurs,* 90:31–32 (September 1990).
10. Cushing M. In case of emergency. *Am J Nurs,* 88:1175–1177 (September 1988).
11. Rhodes AM. Carrying out physicians' orders. *MCN,* 15:193 (May–June 1990).
12. Creighton, op. cit., p. 153.
13. Rhodes, op. cit.
14. Regan W. Verbal orders: Invitations to disaster. *RN,* 43:61–62 (July 1980).

15. Greenlaw J. Communication failures: Some case examples. *Law, Med, and Health Care,* 10:77–79 (April 1982).
16. Northrop C. Look and look again. *Nurs 86,* 16:43 (January 1986).
17. Greenlaw, op. cit.
18. Greenlaw J. Nursing negligence in the hospital emergency department. *Law, Med, and Health Care,* 12:118–121 (June 1984).
19. Regan W. How to force that on-call MD to respond. *RN,* 45:77–78 (February 1982).
20. Northrop (1989), op. cit.
21. Northrop and Kelly, op. cit., p. 97.
22. Cushing M. Failure to communicate. *Am J Nurs,* 83:1597–1598 (October 1982).
23. Regan W. When in doubt, check it out. *RN,* 46:87–88 (May 1983).
24. Does the doctor know best? *Nurs 82,* 12:18 (January 1982).
25. Katz B. Reporting and review of patient care: The nurse's responsibility. *Law, Med, and Health Care,* 11:76–79 (April 1983).
26. Tammelleo D. When a phone call is your liability lifeline. *RN,* 12:69–70 (February 1989).
27. Brooke P. When moving fast puts you at risk. *RN,* 11:63–66 (August 1988).
28. Greenlaw J. Documentation of patient care: An often underestimated responsibility. *Law, Med, and Health Care,* 10:172–174 (September 1982).
29. Di Nitto D, et al. After rape: Who should examine rape survivors? *Am J Nurs,* 86:538–540 (May 1986).
30. Aiken MM. Documenting sexual abuse in prepubertal girls. *MCN,* 15:176–177 (May–June 1990).
31. Helberg J. Documentation in child abuse. *Am J Nurs,* 83:234–239 (February 1983).
32. Rhodes AM. Content of nurses' detailed notes. *MCN,* 12:61–62 (January–February 1987).
33. Cushing M. Gaps in documentation. *Am J Nurs,* 82:1899–1900 (December 1982).
34. Killian WH. Nursing students face liability risks, too. *Am Nurse,* 22:13 (October 1990).
35. Greenlaw J. What to do if your supervisor orders a "cover-up." *RN,* 45:81–82 (October 1982).
36. Cushing (May 1990), op. cit.
37. Fink J. Preventing lawsuits: Medication errors to avoid. *Nurs Life,* 3:26–29 (March–April 1983).
38. Rhodes AM. Judging nursing practice. *MCN,* 14:123 (March–April 1989).
39. Cushing C. Two caveats: Listen and use your knowledge of science. *Am J Nurs,* 89:1434 (November 1989).
40. Regan W. The risks of abandoning a patient. *RN,* 46:297–298 (February 1983).
41. Cushing M. First, anticipate the harm. *Am J Nurs,* 85:137–138 (February 1985).

42. Ibid.
43. Tammelleo D. The high cost of not paying attention. *RN*, 10:61–62 (March 1987).
44. Cushing C. Legal lessons on patient teaching. *Am J Nurs*, 84:721–722 (June 1984).
45. Herrman F. Four kinds of carelessness that can send you to court. *Nurs Life*, 2:63 (May–June 1982).
46. Cushing M. Short-staffing on trial. *Am J Nurs*, 88:161–162 (February 1988).
47. Cushing M. Fears of a float nurse. *Am J Nurs*, 83:297–298 (February 1983).
48. Ferrari M. Avoiding legal risks in pediatrics. *Nurs Life*, 6:24–25 (March–April 1986).
49. Rabinow J. Avoiding legal risks in the OR. *Nurs Life*, 5:24–26 (November–December 1985).
50. Cushing M. Perils of home care. *Am J Nurs*, 88:441, 444 (April 1988).
51. Northrop C. Legal responsibilities of public health nurses. *Nurs Outlook*, 33:316 (November–December 1985).
52. Greenlaw J. Nursing negligence in the hospital emergency department. *Law, Med, and Health Care*, 12:118–121 (June 1984).
53. Northrop C. Malpractice crisis and standards of care. *Nurs Outlook*, 34:140 (May–June 1986).
54. Rhodes AM. The expert witness. *MCN*, 14:49 (January–February 1989).
55. Creighton H. Legal value of pharmaceutical inserts. *Sup Nurse*, 11:13–14 (February 1980).
56. Guarriello DL. The legal boobytraps in nursing standards. *RN*, 47:19–21 (June 1984).
57. Rabinow J. Patient injury in the hospital: How to protect yourself. *Nurs Life*, 2:44–48 (January–February 1982).
58. Cushing M. Incident reports: For your eyes only? *Am J Nurs*, 85:873–874 (August 1985).
59. Cournoyer C. Protecting yourself after a patient's injured. *Nurs Life*, 5:18–22 (March–April 1985).
60. Bradford EW. Preventing malpractice suits: What you can do. *Nurs 88*, 18:62–64 (September 1988).
61. Yorker B. Nurses accused of murder. *Am J Nurs*, 88:1327–1328, 1332 (October 1988).
62. Klein C. Assault and battery. *Nurse Practitioner*, 9:47, 50, 52 (July 1984).
63. Klein C. Defamation: Libel and slander. *Nurse Practitioner*, 11:59–60 (January 1986).
64. Creighton (1986), op. cit., pp. 237–238.
65. Northrop C. How good samaritan laws do and don't protect you. *Nurs 90*, 20:50–51 (February 1990).
66. Horsley J. You can't escape the good samaritan role—or its risks. *RN*, 44:87–92 (May 1981).
67. Sandroff R. Why you really ought to have your *own* malpractice policy. *RN*, 46:29–33 (June 1983).

68. Brooke P. Shopping for liability insurance. *Am J Nurs*, 89:171–172 (February 1989).
69. Manta J. Malpractice insurance: Don't get caught without it. *Nurs Life*, 2:44–47 (March–April 1982).
70. Northrop C. 6 questions about malpractice insurance. *Nurs 87*, 17:97–98 (August 1987).
71. Cushing M. Malpractice: Are you covered? *Am J Nurs*, 84:985–986 (August 1984).
72. Rhodes AM. Nursing and the discovery process. *MCN*, 13:53 (January–February 1988).
73. Cushing M. How a suit starts. *Am J Nurs*, 85:655–656 (June 1985).
74. Chenowith S. Tips on giving pre-trial testimony. *RN*, 8:67–68 (February 1985).
75. Rhodes AM. Defining depositions. *MCN*, 13:89 (March–April 1988).
76. Klimon E. Do you swear to tell the truth? *Nurs Economics*, 3:98–102 (March–April 1985).
77. Salmond S. Serving as an expert witness. *Nurs Economics*, 4:236–239 (September–October 1986).
78. Rhodes AM. The expert witness. *MCN*, 14:49 (January–February 1989).
79. Quinley K. Twelve tips for defending yourself in a malpractice suit. *Am J Nurs*, 90:37–38, 40 (January 1990).
80. Mandell M. Ten legal commandments for nurses who get sued. *Nurs Life*, 6:19–21 (May–June 1986).
81. Spaulding JA. Risk management: A hospital-wide approach. *Nurs Mgt*, 13:29–31 (April 1982).
82. Guarriello DL. Can you be sued without cause? RN, 47:19 (February 1984).
83. Alford D. Are you courting disaster? *Nurs Life*, 1:44–48 (November–December 1981).

CHAPTER 13

PATIENTS' RIGHTS; NURSES' RIGHTS

OBJECTIVES

After you have studied this chapter, you will be able to:

1. Identify trends in patients' rights.
2. List the elements of informed consent.
3. Describe the nurse's responsibilities in informed consent.
4. Explain briefly the major legal actions that have affected the patient's right to die.
5. Discuss how a living will can be used.
6. Explain the role of the nurse in protecting a patient's legal rights when research is being carried out.
7. Give two examples of legal problems related to reproduction.
8. Explain what specific kinds of acts can bring about legal action for battery or assault.
9. Describe an employment situation in which an employee might sue and the probable legal outcome.
10. Give the major steps in initiating collective bargaining.
11. Explain the rights of students in relation to their grades.

The growing strength of the consumer movement is having an increasing effect on the health care delivery system. Once health professionals, and especially physicians, were considered unquestionable experts, and patients put themselves in those "expert" hands, grateful if they got minimal information. People were admitted to the hospital after signing general releases and permits for treatment without even reading them because "the doctor knows best." They gave up even basic rights to human dignity and control over their bodies. They may have grumbled quietly but most often did not confront the staff, sometimes because of fear of reprisals. Perhaps their only way to fight back was to file malpractice suits when things went wrong.

However, as people learned more about health and illness, and consumer activists not only told them what their basic rights were but demanded more, the picture changed. *Malpractice,* a 1973 governmental commission report on medical malpractice, was among the first official reports to state bluntly that much of the malpractice crisis of the time was due to violation of patients' rights. In 1982, the President's Commission for the Study of Ethical Problems in Medicine and Biomedical and Behavioral Research (hereafter called the President's Commission) made equally strong statements and recommendations about respecting patients' rights.[1] Anyone following the appellate court decisions could also see the trend toward supporting patients' rights, although various individual decisions seem to flow against that tide.

Obviously, nurses are very much involved in situations concerning patients' rights. Nurses are at the bedside all the time or in the home. They are the ones who must deal with the patient and family in often emotional, always difficult, situations that may indeed be matters of life and death. Patients and families often look to nurses for advice and support. Nurses, besides being conerned about behaving ethically, must now also be aware of the legal implications of their actions. They must know what they can and can't do. Unfortunately, as in other legal situations, the answers are often far from clear. This chapter will highlight the major legal dilemmas with which nurses must deal in relation to people's rights in health care, including those of nurses.

PATIENTS' RIGHTS

Most of the rights about which patients worry are their legal as well as moral rights and have been so established by common law. They are also stated in the codes of ethics of both physicians and nurses (although, to be honest, much is stated by implication and so is open to considerable interpretation). Moreover, they closely resemble the four basic consumer rights President John F. Kennedy listed in his message to Congress in 1962:

Exhibit 13-1

Statement on a Patient's Bill of Rights
American Hospital Association, 1972

The American Hospital Association presents a Patient's Bill of Rights with the expectation that observance of these rights will contribute to more effective patient care and greater satisfaction for the patient, his physician, and the hospital organization. Further, the Association presents these rights in the expectation that they will be supported by the hospital on behalf of its patients, as an integral part of the healing process. It is recognized that a personal relationship between the physician and the patient is essential for the provision of proper medical care. The traditional physician-patient relationship takes on a new dimension when care is rendered within an organizational structure. Legal precedent has established that the institution itself also has a responsibility to the patient. It is in recognition of these factors that these rights are affirmed.

1. The patient has the right to considerate and respectful care.
2. The patient has the right to obtain from his physician complete current information concerning his diagnosis, treatment, and prognosis in terms the patient can be reasonably expected to understand. When it is not medically advisable to give such information to the patient, the information should be made available to an appropriate person in his behalf. He has the right to know by name, the physician responsible for coordinating his care.
3. The patient has the right to receive from his physician information necessary to give informed consent prior to the start of any procedure and/or treatment. Except in emergencies, such information for informed consent should include but not necessarily be limited to the specific procedure and/or treatment, the medically significant risks involved, and the probable duration of incapacitation. Where medically significant alternatives for care or treatment exist, or when the patient requests information concerning medical alternatives, the patient has the right to such information. The patient also has the right to know that name of the person responsible for the procedures and/or treatment.
4. The patient has the right to refuse treatment to the extent permitted by law, and to be informed of the medical consequences of his action.
5. The patient has the right to every consideration of his privacy concerning his own medical care program. Case discussion, consultation, examination, and treatment are confidential and should be con-

ducted discreetly. Those not directly involved in his care must have the permission of the patient to be present.

6. The patient has the right to expect that all communications and records pertaining to his care should be treated as confidential.

7. The patient has the right to expect that within its capacity a hospital must make reasonable response to the request of a patient for services. The hospital must provide evaluation, service, and/or referral as indicated by the urgency of the case. When medically permissible a patient may be transferred to another facility only after he has received complete information and explanation concerning the needs for and alternatives to such a transfer. The institution to which the patient is to be transferred must first have accepted the patient for transfer.

8. The patient has the right to obtain information as to any relationship of his hospital to other health care and educational institutions insofar as his care is concerned. The patient has the right to obtain information as to the existence of any professional relationships among individuals, by name, who are treating him.

9. The patient has the right to be advised if the hospital proposes to engage in or perform human experimentation affecting his care or treatment. The patient has the right to refuse to participate in such research projects.

10. The patient has the right to expect reasonable continuity of care. He has the right to know in advance what appointment times and physicians are available and where. The patient has the right to expect that the hospital will provide a mechanism whereby he is informed by his physician or a delegate of the physician of the patient's continuing health care requirements following discharge.

11. The patient has the right to examine and receive an explanation of his bill regardless of source of payment.

12. The patient has the right to know what hospital rules and regulations apply to his conduct as a patient.

No catalogue of rights can guarantee for the patient the kind of treatment he has a right to expect. A hospital has many functions to perform, including the prevention and treatment of disease, the education of both health professionals and patients, and the conduct of clinical research. All these activities must be conducted with an overriding concern for the patient, and, above all, the recognition of his dignity as a human being. Success in achieving this recognition assures success in the defense of the rights of the patient.

Source: Reprinted with permission of the American Hospital Association. © 1972.

1. The right to safety.
2. The right to be informed.
3. The right to choose.
4. The right to be heard.

Since the well-publicized AHA's "Patient's Bill of Rights" was presented in 1972 (Exhibit 13-1), many rights statements have followed for the disabled, the mentally ill, the retarded, the old, the young, the pregnant, the handicapped, and the dying.

In some cases, these statements have been the basis for new statutory law. By the end of the 1970s, variations of the Patient's Bill of Rights had become law in many states. Some legislatures passed specific laws incorporating either the AHA statement or a similar version; state or municipal hospital codes were similarly changed, sometimes including mental institutions and nursing homes. In 1974, new Medicare regulations for skilled nursing facilities included a section on patients' rights. And, as with other laws, patients must be told what their rights are.

Since that time, the continuing scandals involving violation of patients' and residents' rights in so many LTC facilities have resulted in legislation in various guises, usually requirements under Medicare and Medicaid (see Chapter 3). For the LTC facilities not certified, there is still some control by state regulation. The regulations on rights are enacted and enforced erratically, sometimes depending on the political climate. However, nursing home residents now have the right to talk directly to state surveyors, who ensure that the facilities meet the standards set by the Health Care Financing Administration (HCFA), which include rights statements. Nursing homes also may have a volunteer ombudsman, and teaching nursing homes have students and faculty who observe what goes on. However, such facilities are not usually problem sites. Some states have also given legal attention to the rights of residents in continuing care communities, including such aspects as complete disclosure of costs and other financial data, posting of the last state examination report, freedom to form a residents' organization, and other mechanisms to avoid fraud and deception.

Many rights advocates have little enthusiasm for most of these declarations, particularly the AHA statement, as they tend to hedge about some or many of the rights, voluntary or legal. This is probably because few if any evolved out of some massive "goodness of heart" by the institutions or by government, but rather through consumer pressure.

Some statements are better than others, but Annas's Model Patient Bill of Rights, aimed at all facilities, is indeed a model, covering many of the loopholes in the various institutions' statements. Recognizing that most people are in health care facilities because they have a health problem and therefore are probably not as aggressive about ensuring their rights as they might otherwise be, the final statement in the model recognizes the right to all patients to have 24-hour-a-day access to a patients' rights advocate to assert or protect the rights set out in this document.[2]

It would seem that consumer action has had some ongoing effect on patients' rights. Annas says that the patients' rights movement is "as slow as a glacier, equally relentless in changing the landscape, but ultimately healthy.[3] In addition to the organizations built around specific populations and diseases (children, AIDS), there is one national patient rights organization: The People's Medical Society. These groups generally provide excellent information. A list of addresses is found in Annas's *The Rights of Patients*.

INFORMED CONSENT

For years, when patients were admitted to hospitals, they signed a frequently unread, universal consent form that almost literally gave the physician, his or her associates, and the hospital a free hand in the patient's care. There was some rationale for this because civil suits for battery (unlawful touching) could theoretically be filed as a result of giving routine care such as baths. Patients undergoing surgery or a complex, dangerous treatment were asked to sign a separate form, usually stating something to the effect that permission was granted to the physician and/or his or her colleagues to perform the operation or treatment. Just how much the patient knew about the hows and whys of the surgery, the dangers, and the alternatives, depended on the patient's assertiveness in asking questions and demanding answers and the physician's willingness to provide information. Nurses were taught *never* to answer those questions, or few others, but to suggest, "Ask your doctor." Health professionals, especially physicians, took the attitude that "We know best and will decide for you."

Many patients probably still enter treatment and undergo a variety of tests and even surgery without a clear understanding of the nature of their condition and what can be done about it. Although they may be receiving care that is medically acceptable, they have no real part in deciding what that care should be. Most physicians have believed that anything more than a superficial explanation is unnecessary, for the patient should trust the doctor. Yet patients have always had the right to make decisions about their own bodies. A case was heard as early as 1905 on surgery without consent, and the classic legal decision is that of Judge Benjamin Cardozo (*Schloendorff v. The Society of New York Hospital,* 211 NY. 125, 129–130, 105 NE 92, 93–1914): "Every human being of adult years and sound mind has a right to determine what shall be done with his own body." This principle still stands, and treatment without consent is technically assault and battery.

Annas emphasizes this as he explains that in nonlegal terms, informed consent simply means that a doctor cannot "touch or treat a patient until the doctor has given the patient some basic information about what the doctor proposes to do, and the patient has agreed to the proposed treatment or procedure.[4] In what is still considered the most important study of informed consent, the President's Commission concludes that "ethically valid consent is a process of shared decision-making based upon mutual respect and participation, not a ritual to be equated with reciting the contents of a form that details the risks of particular treatments."[5] For this reason, some lawyers are advocating the use of the term *authorization for treatment,* implying patient control.

The patient's need for and right to this kind of knowledge is highlighted by the increasing number of malpractice suits that involve an element of informed consent. For many years, in such suits, courts have tended to rule that the physician must provide only as much information as is general practice among professional colleagues in the area, as determined by their expert testimony. However, courts are changing this attitude and emphasizing the need for *informed* consent.[6]

Principles of Informed Consent

Consent is defined as a free, rational act that presupposes knowledge of the thing to which consent is given by a person who is legally capable of consent. *Informed consent is* not expected to include the tiniest details but to give the essential nature of the procedure and the consequences. The disclosure is to be "reasonable." The patient may, of course, waive the right to such explanation or any teaching. Consent is *not* needed for emergency care if there is an immediate threat to life and health, if experts agree that it is an emergency, if the patient is unable to consent and a legally authorized person can't be reached, and when the patient submits voluntarily.

Criteria for a valid consent are as follows: It must be written (unless oral consent can be proved in court); it must be signed by the patient or person legally responsible for him or her (a person cannot give consent for a spouse in a nonemergency situation); the procedure performed must be the one consented to; the essential elements of an informed consent must be present, including (a) an explanation of the condition; (b) a fair explanation of the procedures to be used and the consequences; (c) a description of alternative treatments or procedures; (d) a description of the benefits to be expected; (e) an offer to answer the patient's inquiries; and (f) freedom from coercion or unfair persuasions and inducements.[7]

Who Makes the Decision?

The competent patient (someone physically and mentally capable of making a choice) has the right to refuse consent, but a hospital can request, under certain circumstances, a court order to act if the refusal endangers the patient's life. If a patient is considered physically unable, legally incompetent, or a minor, a guardian has the right to give or withhold consent. The trend in court decisions seems to be that the patient, unless proven totally incompetent, has the right to refuse. For example, a Jehovah's Witness may be allowed to refuse a blood transfusion, even though it might mean his or her life, because taking such transfusions are against his or her religious beliefs.[8] In fact, the Witnesses and AMA in 1979 agreed upon a consent form requesting that no blood or blood derivative be administered and releasing medical personnel and the hospital for responsibility for untoward results because of that refusal. (This particular problem has been lessened to some extent as better blood substitutes have become available.) However, in 1990, a Jehovah's Witness sued a major medical center and five physicians because he was given blood after a serious automobile accident. Although he was unconscious and it was an emergency situation, he claimed that his rights were violated. If a minor child of a Witness needs the blood and the parent refuses, a court order requested by the hospital usually permits the transfusion. This is based on a 1944 legal precedent when the Supreme Court ruled that parents had a right to be martyrs, if they wished, but had no right to make martyrs of their children.[9] On the other hand, if the child is deemed a "mature minor," able to make an intelligent decision, regardless of chronological age, the child is allowed to refuse the treatment.

In another type of case, a 79-year-old diabetic refused to consent to a leg amputation. Her daughter petitioned to be her legal guardian so that she (the daughter) could sign the consent. The judge ruled that the woman was old but not senile and had a right to make her own decision. In still another case, a young man on permanent kidney dialysis decided that he did not want to live that way and refused continued treatment. He was allowed to do so and died within a short time.

Other cases can also be cited. The right of a competent patient to refuse treatment seems more firmly established than ever, but when the patient is unconscious or in certain other situations, difficult legal questions arise.

Is Informed Consent Practical?

Some physicians do not believe that it is possible to obtain an informed consent because of such factors as lack of interest or education and high anxiety level, in which case a patient might refuse a "necessary" treatment or operation. On the other hand, the physician may invoke "therapeutic privilege," in which disclosure is not required because it might be detrimental to the patient.[10] Just what that means is not clear. Or information about certain alternatives may be withheld because the physician feels that they are too risky, unproven, or not appropriate. There are physicians and others who believe that despite the increasing number of rulings favoring patients' right to full knowledge, most patients are not given information in such a way that they really understand it (and the courts don't do enough about this problem). Surveys indicate that people *do* want full information even when they trust their doctor completely and will probably go along with his or her recommendations. They may not always remember the details later, but with a full explanation, given in lay terms, and with enough time for questions and answers, they can understand. However, many patients are still reluctant to ask for fear of appearing stupid or "bothering the doctor."

The written consent form that is generally accepted as the legal affirmation that the patient has agreed to a particular test or treatment has undergone a number of changes in the last few years. The catchall admissions consent has already been ruled to be almost completely worthless for anything other than avoiding battery complaints, because it does not designate the nature of the treatment to be given. What has emerged are forms that contain all the required elements for the informed consent process, usually individualized by the physician of each patient and often in an appropriate foreign language. Although many people think of informed consent only in terms of hospitalization, there are already some court cases that indicate that the concept embraces the continuum of health care, such as a clinic or doctor's office. An interesting aspect of one of these cases was that the physician was held to have breached his duty by failing to inform the patient of the risks of *not* consenting to a diagnostic procedure, in this case a Pap smear. The patient died of advanced cervical cancer.[11]

The Nurse's Role in Informed Consent

What is the nurse's role in informed consent? To provide or add information before or after the doctor's explanation has been given? To refer the patient to the doctor? To avoid any participation? The advice given varies. Some suggest that getting involved in informed consent is simply not the nurse's business and is best left to the doctor; others consider it a professional responsibility.

It is generally agreed that nurses do not have the primary responsibility for getting informed consent. However, the President's Commission noted that "nurses as a practical matter typically have a central role in the process of providing patients with information,"[12] and that NPs, including nurse-midwives, have *full* responsibility for informing patients about their conditions, tests, and treatment, and obtaining consent. There was also at least one serious court case in which a patient sued because the physician *and* nurses withheld information about his condition. Both were held liable.[13] Nevertheless, the question asked by most nurses is how much can be told, especially if the physician chooses not to reveal further information. The Tuma case (Chapter 11) did not resolve the nurse's right to supply the missing information, and the nurse may be taking a personal risk. Greenlaw suggests that patients' questions may range over a variety of topics, including what you are doing to the patient and your qualifications (if so, answer honestly) to interpretation of what the doctor said (explain in lay terms) to "What's wrong with me?" (don't answer directly) or "Is my doctor any good?" (tell patients that they have a right to ask their doctor for his or her qualifications and experience or to get a second opinion).[14]

A variety of other opinions are offered, but a point that is always made is that the patient's lack of information should always be discussed with the doctor (tactfully) and, if there is no response, with administrative superiors. There is nothing wrong with questioning the patient to see what he or she really understands and clarifying points, providing that you know what you are talking about. If you decide to give further information, it should be totally accurate and carefully recorded, and the fact that it was given should be shared with the physician and others. Nurses have found ways to make the patient aware of knowledge gaps so that they ask the right questions, but it's unfortunate that many are still employed in situations in which it could be detrimental to them to be the patient's advocate.

Of course, if the patient is coaxed or coerced into signing without such an explanation, the consent is invalid. Moreover, if the patient withdraws consent, even verbally, the nurse is responsible for reporting this and ensuring that the patient is not treated. This is a legal responsibility not only to the patient but also to the hospital, which can be held liable.[15]

Hospitals are beginning to use a clerk to witness the consent form, after the physician provides an explanation, on the theory that only the signature is being witnessed, not the accuracy or depth of the explanation. Other hospitals ask the physician to bring another physician, presumably to validate the explanation. Where nurses still witness the form, it should be clear *what* they are witnessing—the signature or the explanation.[16] Hospital policy can clarify this situation. Usually, nurses' chances of liability in such acts are considered to be minimal.[17]

The nurse's specific responsibility is to explain nursing care, including the whys and hows. An interesting idea to think about is whether you should tell patients about the risks of the *nursing* procedures you do, even though this is not a legal requirement. (Nor does it prevent you from doing so.) The answer seems to be maybe, but carefully.[18] However, as noted in the President's Commission report, nurses who *independently* perform treatments that might put the patient at risk (NPs, nurse-midwives, nurse anesthetists) *are* responsible for giving appropriate information to patients and getting consent.[19]

THE RIGHT TO DIE

Perhaps because improved technology has succeeded in artificially maintaining both respiratory and cardiac functions when a person can no longer do so, the definition of *clinical death* as the irrevocable cessation of heartbeat and breathing is no longer pertinent. What of irreversible coma?

In 1968, faculty of the Harvard Medical School identified certain characteristics of a permanently nonfunctioning brain. In the years since, more than half of the states have passed legislation using variations of those criteria to define *brain death*. Currently, the AMA, the Bar Association, the President's Commission, and others are suggesting that states adopt the following statute:

An individual who has sustained either (1) irreversible cessation of circulatory and respiratory functions, or (2) irreversible cessation of all functions of the entire brain, including the brain stem, is dead. A determination of death must be made in accordance with accepted medical standards.[20]

Not everyone agrees with the concept of brain death, so one of the most disturbing ethical-legal problems today is: what should be done about maintaining artificial life support when someone is in an irreversible coma? Where once the patient would have been allowed to die, now health care institutions and doctors are afraid of legal suits either by family or an outside right-to-life advocate.

The first hurdle is to try to determine what the patient would have wanted. Very often there is evidence that the person would not have wanted to continue to exist in such a state. Assuming that the family, who probably took the case to court, still agrees to discontinuing whatever technology keeps the patient alive, that should end the matter. Often it doesn't. One reason is different opinions about what is treatment or technology and what is ordinary care. Over the years, different aspects of this question have been hammered out in court. There are an increasing number of such cases every day, and there are some classics.

In the Quinlan case, a 22-year-old woman received severe and irreversible brain damage that reduced her to a persistent vegetative state (PVS), and the father petitioned the court to be made her guardian with the intention of having all extraordinary medical procedures sustaining her life removed. The New Jersey Supreme Court ruled that the father could be the guardian and have the life support systems discontinued with the concurrence of her family, the attending physicians, who might be chosen by the father, and the hospital ethics committee. (After disconnection of the respirator, Karen Quinlan continued to live another 10 years, sustained by fluids and other maintenance measures, in a nursing home at the cost of hundreds of thousands of dollars. Health law experts debated the congruity of these and similar cases, and predicted that the other courts faced by other unique circumstances would make separate rulings. This has proven to be an accurate prediction, as in the cases of Brother Fox, Peter Cinque, Earle Spring, and others.[21]

If anything, the issue of the right to die became even more confused in the 1980s. Considering the fact that it is supposed to be a person's basic legal right to make decisions about his or her own body, the proliferation of court cases on that issue may seem surprising. The lack of consistency in the rulings is even more so, as illustrated in these cases. When someone wants to discontinue kidney dialysis today because the quality of life is unacceptable, there is relatively little objection. But that may be because the patient is ambulatory and may simply choose not to come back for treatment. Yet when a competent 77-year-old California man with multiple serious ailments, but not at the point of dying, wanted the right to have his respirator turned off because *he* found the quality of life unbearable, neither the hospital, nor the doctors, nor the court would allow him to do so, and no other hospital or doctor would accept him. (He had signed a living will and other documents.) His arms were restrained to prevent any action on his part; the hospital said that he continued to "live a useful life." His medical and hospital expenses were by then almost $500,000.[22] William Bartling died the day before the state appeals court heard his case. Six weeks later the court ruled that he did have the constitutional right to refuse medical treatment, including the respirator. The family sued the hospital. In New Jersey at the same time, a lower court agreed to removal of a nasogastric tube on an 84-year-old incompetent (but not brain-dead woman), Ms. Conroy, at the request of her nephew. The case was appealed, but the patient died before a final appellate decision was reached.

In the Conroy decision, the New Jersey Supreme Court ruled that termination of any medical treatment, including artificial feeding, on incompetent persons is lawful as long as certain procedures are followed. (Ms. Conroy had indicated, but not in writing, that she would not have wanted to live under those conditions.) It was too late for Ms. Conroy, who died with the feeding tube in place. This case was considered different because the person was in a nursing home, but Annas maintains that the distinction should not have been made.[23] Another problem with the final decision was that although the court articulated the right of competent adults to refuse treatment, it failed to provide any way to require proxies to exercise the right on behalf of incompetent patients. However, in 1987, the New Jersey Supreme Court made three rulings that were expected to influence other states. The court said, first of all, that these life-or-death decisions should be made not by a court, but personally or through a surrogate. The rulings also provided immunity from civil and criminal liability for those making such decisions "in good faith."

Such legal processes can take a long time. The Paul Brophy case in Massachusetts is an example.[25] It took two years and the refusal of the U.S. Supreme Court to review the case (which would have taken even longer) before, after many contrary rules, his wife, a nurse, could have him transferred to a hospital that was willing to do what he would have wished and removed his feeding tube. He died eight days later, kept comfortable but not fed, and cared for by his wife.

The states have created a patchwork of life-and-death laws. There were cases in which a competent person refused food and the court agreed; but with the removal of the respirator much more likely to be agreed to, the next most controversial issue concerning the incompetent PVS patient was discontinuation of artificial (tube) feeding or other means of providing food and hydration.

The idea of having a loved one die of thirst or starvation, as the pro-life group describes it (although there is little evidence that a PVS patient has such sensations), is naturally repugnant to families, and the pressures on them are great. Some advocates with a religious affiliation are strongly opposed to removal, although others are not.[26] Physicians and nurses are likewise divided in their feelings. The nurse who had cared for Ms. Conroy testified in the case, in detail, as to Ms. Conroy's condition; she thought that the tube should not have been removed. Others have stated the opposite point of view. In all such cases, the nurses are the ones in intimate contact with the patient; if the decision is to let the patient die, it is their responsibility to keep the patient as comfortable as possible.

In 1986, the AMA Council of Ethical and Judicial Affairs issued a statement on "Withholding or Withdrawing Life Prolonging Medical Treatment," declaring that "life-prolonging medical treatment and artificially or technologically supplied respiration, including nutrition and hydration, may be withheld from a patient in an irreversible coma even when death is not imminent." In January 1988, the ANA Committee on Ethics issued guidelines on the subject, saying, in essence, that there are few instances in which it is morally permissible for nurses to withhold or withdraw food and/or fluid from persons in their care (see Chapter 9). Fry,[27] a nurse ethicist and philosopher, has done a fine critical analysis of the ANA document in relation to other reports and guidelines issued at that time, among them the Hastings

Center's "Guidelines on the Termination of Life-Sustaining Treatment," which basically views nutrition and hydration as medical treatment that must be evaluated on a case-by-case basis.

It was inevitable that, given the controversy on these issues and the fact that there may be some 10,000 PVS patients, a case would eventually reach the U.S., Supreme Court, probably as a privacy (Fourth Amendment) issue. The first right-to-die case to go before the Court was that of Nancy Cruzan, a 32-year-old woman who was injured in an auto accident in 1983 and reverted to a PVS. In 1988, her case was the first in Missouri to raise the question of whether feeding tubes can be equated with other life-sustaining medical treatments and whether patients in Nancy's condition have any rights regarding their care. The parents, stating that this would have been Nancy's wish, wanted to have the implanted gastrointestinal tube removed. A probate judge ruled that they could do so but was overruled by the Missouri Supreme Court. The case was taken to the U.S. Supreme Court. The five-to-four decision of the Court in June 1990 upheld Missouri, ruling that when a permanently unconscious person has left no clear instructions, a state is free to carry out its interest in "the protection and preservation of human life" by denying a request by family members to terminate treatment. What this means, basically, is that each state must decide how it wants to handle similar situations legally, although almost none have as strict requirements as Missouri. The Court said that the Cruzan family had not shown by "clear and convincing evidence" that Nancy would have wanted to have the treatment stopped."[28]

Although this is considered, legally, as a very narrow decision, since it relates only to Missouri, and is considered by some as embracing form over substance, it is perhaps also indicative of the new conservative bent of the Supreme Court. In his dissenting opinion, Justice William Brennan argued that the Missouri rules are out of touch with reality; that people do not write elaborate documents about how they might die and what interventions physicians might have to prolong life; and that, after all, friends and family are most likely to know what the patient would want, even without written instructions. He added that by ignoring such evidence, the Missouri procedure "transforms [incompetent] human beings into passive subjects of human technology."[29]

One positive aspect of this case is the agreement of almost all the justices that competent people *do* have a constitutional right to refuse life-sustaining treatment, and if there is clear and convincing evidence that the person would refuse further treatment, as demonstrated by a living will or a "duly appointed surrogate," the person's wishes should be upheld. Another important point made by Justice Sandra O'Connor was that "artificial feeding cannot readily be distinguished from other forms of medical treatment" and that, therefore, an individual's decision to reject such treatment is consti-

Exhibit 13-2

Example of a Living Will

To My Family, My Physician, My Lawyer, And All Others Whom It May Concern

Death is as much a reality as birth, growth, and aging—it is the one certainty of life. In anticipation of decisions that may have to be made about my own dying and as an expression of my right to refuse treatment, I, _____,
(print name)

being of sound mind, make this statement of my wishes and instructions concerning treatment.

By means of this document, which I intend to be legally binding, I direct my physician and other care providers, my family, and any surrogate designated by me or appointed by a court, to carry out my wishes. If I become unable, by reason of physical or mental incapacity, to make decisions about my medical care, let this document provide the guidance and authority needed to make any and all such decisions.

If I am permanently unconscious or there is no reasonable expectation of my recovery from a seriously incapacitating or lethal illness or condition, I do not wish to be kept alive by artificial means. I request that I be given all care necessary to keep me comfortable and free of pain, even if pain-relieving medications may hasten my death, and I direct that no life-sustaining treatment be provided except as I or my surrogate specifically authorize.

This request may appear to place a heavy responsibility upon you, but by making this decision according to my strong convictions, I intend to ease that burden. I am acting after careful consideration and with understanding of the consequences of your carrying out my wishes. *List optional specific provisions in the space below.*

_____ **Durable Power of Attorney for Health Care Decisions** _____

(Cross out if you do not wish to use this section)

To effect my wishes, I designate _____,
residing at _____,
(phone #) _____, (or if he or she shall for any reason fail
to act, _____,
residing at _____,
_____, (phone #) _____) as my
health care surrogate—that is, my attorney-in-fact regarding any and all health care decisions to be made for me, including the decision to refuse life-sustaining treatment—if I am unable to make such decisions myself. This power shall remain effective during and not be affected by my subsequent illness, disability or incapacity. My surrogate shall have authority to interpret my Living Will, and shall make decisions about my health care as specified in my instructions or, when my wishes are not clear, as the surrogate believes to be in my best interests. I release and agree to hold harmless my health care surrogate from any and all claims whatsoever arising from decisions made in good faith in the exercise of this power.

I sign this document knowingly, voluntarily, and after careful deliberation, this

_____day of _____, 19_____.

_____
(signature)

Address _____

_____

I do hereby cerfity that the within document was executed and achnowledged before me by the principal this _____day of _____, 19_____.

_____
Notary Public

Witness _____

Printed Name _____

Address _____

_____

Witness _____

Printed Name _____

Address _____

_____

Copies of this document have been given to:

This Living Will expresses my personal treatment preferences. The fact that I may have also executed a declaration in the form recommended by state law should not be construed to limit or contradict this Living Will, which is an expression of my common-law and constitutional rights.

(Optional) my Living Will is registered with
Choice in Dying (Registry No. _____)

Distributed by Choice in Dying, 250 West 57th Street,
New York, NY 10107 (212) 246-6973

tutionally protected. It seems that at least this decision will prevent some of the terrible things that can happen to patients.[30]

As for Nancy Cruzan, after a friend came forward to say that Nancy would not have wanted to be kept alive under the conditions present, the state withdrew its objections and Nancy was allowed to die, with her family at her bedside. An interesting point on this general issue is that a study of court decisions on withdrawing or withholding treatment found that they are affected by gender. Whereas men's treatment preferences, even without a living will, were considered by judges, those of women, even with a living will, were rejected or not considered.[31]

What is a *living will?* A living will, such as that shown in Exhibit 13-2, directs the family, physician, and friends to withhold life-sustaining treatment if there is no reasonable expectation of recovery from a seriously incapacitating or lethal condition. It may also include specific directions about treatments that the individual may refuse, such as "electrical or mechanical resuscitation of my heart when it has stopped beating"; "nasogastric tube feedings when I am paralyzed or unable to take nourishment by mouth"; "mechanical respiration if I am no longer able to sustain my own breathing." Other versions also exist.[32]

The will itself, which can be revoked at any time, has no legal power, although presumably, if the writer's intention were followed, those involved would not be judged guilty of murder. How much the will influences action (legally) when the patient is unconscious has been tested only a few times, with a trend toward its acceptance but also, after a slow start, toward legislation.

In 1977, California enacted a *Natural Death Act,* with carefully delineated and protective living will components. The next year, Arkansas, Idaho, Nevada, New Mexico, North Carolina, Oregon, and Texas followed with similar laws. By 1992, 50 states and the District of Columbia had enacted living will and/or surrogate laws; others were pending. All granted civil and criminal immunity for those carrying out living will requests. Although there were no reported difficulties, some believe that because the right to refuse treatment already exists and each law has its own strict limitations, such legislation only creates problems.[33] In 1984, California also enacted a law entitled the *Durable Power of Attorney for Health Care,* the first of its kind. It allows terminally ill patients to designate another individual (a surrogate) to make life-or-death decisions in the event that the patient is unable to do so.[34] The agreement conveys the authority to consent, refuse, or withdraw consent "to any care, treatment, service or procedure to maintain, diagnose, or treat a mental or physical condition." (This is also an optional statement in the living will.) Perhaps because so many people are still ignorant of their rights in this issue, a federal law, the 1990 Patient Self-Determination Act requires health care institutions to tell patients if their state will let them

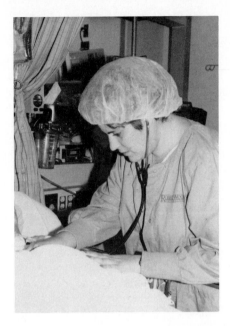

Competent patients have the legal right to decide whether they want complex technology to sustain their lives. *(Courtesy of the Robert Wood Johnson Medical Center.)*

refuse life-prolonging treatment if they become incapacitated, and to record if they do have an "advance directive" (living will).

These right-to-die issues are related to the concept of *euthanasia,* a word of Greek origin meaning painless, easy, gentle, or good death. It is now commonly used to signifiy a killing that is prompted by some humanitarian motive, such as the relief of intolerable pain. There are two major categories of euthanasia: voluntary and involuntary. The first usually involves two parties: the competent adult patient and a doctor, nurse, or both, or an adult friend or relative. (The patient could commit suicide alone.) It is voluntary euthanasia that the natural death laws seek to serve. Involuntary euthanasia, sometimes called *mercy killing,* is performed by someone other than the patient without the patient's consent, possibly because of unconsciousness. There are many pros and cons of euthanasia, with arguments usually falling into secular or religious categories. Nevertheless, according to the law, euthanasia is murder. What may be coming closer to resolution is the problem of resuscitating unconscious patients. (Not to do so is considered by some as passive euthanasia.) Some of the ethical aspects of euthanasia are considered in Chapter 9.

Orders Not to Resuscitate

Patients in irreversible coma may have orders not to resuscitate (*no code, code blue,* or other terms), with or without the consent and knowledge of the family. Are nurses in legal jeopardy if they obey? Are they in trouble if they choose not to? To a great extent, these questions remain unanswered, because families may choose to let the patient die but do not want to say so, and many codes have been carried out with little discussion after the decision was made. Nurses who object on moral or religious grounds cannot be forced to participate (but for some people, it is just as wrong to resuscitate). However, without a specific hospital protocol, *not resuscitating* could be considered malpractice.

Nonwritten orders are a special problem for the nurse. Some physicians believe, wrongly, that their liability is removed by not writing a "do not resuscitate (DNR)" order or cloaking the intent with words such as "comfort nursing measures only." Sometimes a *slow code* is understood or carried out by nurses when a terminally ill patient is not put on DNR. This means that they do not hurry to alert the emergency team. Again, the fear is that the doctor or hospital would be criminally or civilly liable. Even when the family agrees with the decision—and they should always be involved—there are times when both physicians and hospitals are hesitant to act. This does not seem reasonable when cardiopulmonary resuscitation (CPR) procedures were never intended for "cases of terminal irreversible illness where death is not unexpected."[35]

DNR orders are generally the responsibility of the attending physician. If a nurse carries out a verbal DNR or a slow code order, she assumes the risk that it will be disclaimed by the physician. An important AHA publication, "Hospital's Role in Resuscitation Decisions," states that having nurses or other staff solely responsible for making DNR decisions is inappropriate and probably illegal. DNR orders are legally valid, provided that they are in accordance with accepted medical standards. Development of hospital policy on the matter is recommended, including review mechanisms. If there is continuing disagreement about resuscitation, the statement says, the case should be brought to court.

One of the mechanisms mentioned is an ethics committee, similar to what was mandated by the judge in the Quinlan case. An ethics committee, in this context, is a "multidisciplinary group of health professionals within a health care situation that has been specifically established to address the ethical dilemmas that occur within the institution, such as those relating to the treatment or non-treatment of patients who lack decision-making capacities."[37] (Nurses are expected to be part of this group.)

Not many ethics committees had been formed since the Quinlan case (that ruling was binding only in New Jersey), but the case of Infant Doe, discussed later, created a new impetus for their establishment. An AMA official predicted that soon all hospitals would have ethics committees. Suggested functions are education, development of policies and guidelines, consultation, and case review. Some hospitals are following the Massachusetts General Hospital model, in which some critically ill patients are put into four categories ranging from "maximal therapeutic effort" to "all therapy can be discontinued," with definitive protocols for each.[38] The arguments are strong that some policy should be set as a safeguard for all, including the patient.

Greenlaw and other nurse attorneys are all in agreement that nurses should not be involved in slow codes or verbal orders, but there is no doubt that the nurse is intimately involved when a DNR decision must be considered. In some cases, as in LTC facilities, the responsibility for review of DNR orders will fall on the nurse.[39] If there are no policies, nurses can be instrumental in the development of appropriate guidelines and procedures.

RIGHTS OF THE HELPLESS

Children, the mentally ill, the mentally retarded, and certain patients in nursing homes are often seen as relatively helpless, because they have been termed legally incompetent to make decisions about their health care for many years. Often the rights overlap, as when a child or elderly person is mentally retarded. Some of the rights of the elderly are being protected by a legalized bill of rights.

The Mentally Disabled

For mental patients, state laws and some high court decisions have served the same purpose. Both have focused on mental patients' rights in the areas of voluntary and involuntary admissions; kind and length of restraints, including seclusion; informed consent to treatment, especially sterilization and psychosurgery; the rights of citizenship (voting); the right of privacy, especially in relation to records; rights in research; and, especially, the right to treatment. Although rulings have varied, the trend is toward the protection of these rights, even to the point of giving a voluntary mental patient the right to refuse psychiatric medication.[40] In some situations, a structured internal review system in which patients can appeal treatment decisions has seemed to work. On the other hand, follow-up on patients who refused treatment showed a deterioration in their functioning when they were released to the community.[41]

In issues of informed consent, other rulings have determined that if the mentally incompetent cannot understand the benefits or dangers of treatment, the family must be fully informed and allowed to make the decision.[42,43] According to a Supreme Court decision in 1990, prison officials are permitted to treat mentally ill prisoners with psychotropic drugs against their will without first getting permission in a judicial hearing. The prisoners do have some safeguards.

Some legal decisions relate to sterilization of the retarded, an issue that came to a head when it was found that retarded adolescent black girls were being sterilized, with neither the girls nor their mothers apparently having a clear notion of what that meant. Restraints were increasingly put on sterilization until, in 1979, DHEW tightened the regulations for federal participation in funding of sterilization procedures.[44] There is also general concern for the rights of young people in the mental health system, but parents maintain considerable control. In 1979, the Supreme Court upheld the constitutionality of state laws that allow parents to commit their minor children to state mental institutions; several states have such laws.

Rights of Children and Adolescents

The rights of young people and children relate primarily to consent for treatment or research and protection against abuse.[45] It is a general rule that a parent or guardian must give consent for the medical or surgical treatment of a minor except in an emergency when it is imperative to give immediate care to save the minor's life. Legally, however, anyone who is capable of understanding what he or she is doing may give consent, because age is not an exact criterion of maturity or intelligence. Many minors are perfectly capable of deciding for themselves whether to accept or reject recommended therapy. In cases involving simple procedures, the courts have refused to invoke the rule requiring the consent of a parent or guardian for this *mature minor*.[46] If the minor is married or has been otherwise *emancipated* from his or her parents, there is likely to be little question legally.

States cite different ages and situations in which parental permission is needed for medical treatment. The almost universal exception is allowing minors to consent to treatment for venereal disease, drug abuse, and pregnancy-related care. Although it has been understood that health professionals have no legal obligation to report to parents that the minor has sought such treatment, a few states are beginning to add statutes that say that the minor does not need parental permission, but that parents must be notified. In 1983, the Reagan Administration issued a rule that would require parents to be notified whenever children under 18 years of age received any contraceptives from federally funded family planning clinics. After a number of court challenges, this was overruled as infringing on a woman's right to privacy. However, some states continue to set up obstacles, and nurses who counsel teenagers should check the current law.

The entire question of permission for contraception, abortion, and sterilization is in flux. The key appears to be a designation of *mature minor;* emancipated minors are treated as adults. In general, there has been a national trend toward granting minors the right to contraceptive advice and devices, but the political power of conservative groups who oppose this trend is being felt.

An even more dramatic change has occurred in relation to abortion. In 1976, the Supreme Court held that states may not constitutionally require the consent of a girl's parents for an abortion during the first 12 weeks of pregnancy. In addition, it said, parents cannot either prevent or force an abortion on the daughter who, in the eyes of the Court, is now "a competent minor mature enough to have become pregnant."

Since that time, the reproductive rights of teenagers have been gradually eroded by state legislation and federal edicts influenced by conservatives and right-to-life groups. More than half the states have laws requiring teenagers to notify one or both parents, even if divorced, and/or to get permission from them before an abortion. Most of these laws had not been enforced on constitutional grounds. However, that picture changed when the Supreme Court heard two cases requiring parental notification. The justices ruled five to four, in June 1990, that states had a right to make such a requirement of unmarried women under 18 as long as there was an alternative of judicial bypass (speaking to a judge instead) if the law required notice to both parents. This judicial bypass alternative did not apply to the Ohio case, where only one parent had to be noticed. The Minnesota law is so restrictive that it applies even when a parent has never lived with the child or does not have legal custody. (Only one-half of the teenagers in Minnesota live with both natural parents.) The five conservative justices did not allow for the fact that one or both parents might be abusive, alcoholic, or drug-addicted or even that the pregnancy might be due to incest. It is probable that pro-choice forces will now work to overturn these restrictive state laws. Should the young woman decide against an abortion and elect to bear the child, she can receive care related to her pregnancy without parental consent in almost every state. An unwed mature minor may also consent to treatment of her child.

The question of whether parents may make a decision for a child if the child's well-being is their prime consideration, as in giving Laetrile to a leukemic child, has not been decided with any consistency. The legal principles involved are *parental autonomy,* a constitutionally protected right; *parens patriae,* the state's right and duty to protect the child; the *best interest doctrine,* which requires the court to determine what is best for the child; and the *substituted judgment doctrine,* in which the court determines what choice an incompetent individual would make if he or she were competent.[47]

Another unresolved and related issue is whether the grossly deformed neonate should be allowed to die. Few judges will rule to let it die, but often the decision is quietly made by parents and health personnel. These situations are especially difficult for a nurse who cares for the infant. More nurses and others are reporting such situations, but as in the right-to-die issue, ethical and moral considerations weigh strongly.

Several landmark cases occurred in the early 1980s. In Illinois, newborn Siamese twins joined below the waist and sharing an intestinal track and three legs were not expected to live. "Do not feed, in accordance with parents' wishes" was written on the chart. However, several nurses did feed the babies, and someone reported the situation to a government agency. A court order was obtained to gain temporary custody of the children, and a neglect petition was filed. The parents (a doctor and nurse) and the doctor were charged with attempted murder, a charge that was later dismissed. Four months later, they regained custody of the children, whose care had mounted to several hundred thousand dollars. They were also in danger of losing their licenses.[48]

In Indiana, about a year later, a Baby Doe was born with Down's syndrome and a correctable esophageal fistula. The parents refused surgery, and their decision was upheld by the courts. The child was deprived of artificial nutritional life support and died. Although similar action had been taken in other Baby Doe cases, this one came to the attention of President Reagan. It resulted in an HHS regulation that threatened hospitals that neglected such children with loss of funds under Section 504 of the Rehabilitation Act of 1973 (which protects the handicapped). Large signs had to be posted alerting people to a "hot line" number to call to report such incidents. After a series of legal challenges, this regulation was ruled unconstitutional—"arbitrary and capricious," among other things. Eventually, an alternative suggestion by the American Academy of Pediatrics was agreed on: establishment of infant bioethics committees (IBCs) with diverse membership whose responsibility, in part, would be to advise about decisions to withhold or withdraw life-sustaining measures.[49]

Finally, in 1983, a Baby Jane Doe was born in New York with multiple serious congenital conditions, one of which required immediate surgery. The family was told that even if she lived, she would be in a vegetative state, so after consultation with a physician and a religious adviser, they opted for conservative treatment. A right-to-life attorney from Vermont learned of the case and managed to be appointed guardian by a like-minded judge, but this action was overruled by an appeals court. Other right-to-life groups attempted to intervene; so did the federal government, which demanded the child's medical records to see if Section 504 was being violated. After considerable time, effort, and money had been spent, the government finally gave up. The child survived on conservative treatment and went home, where she required constant care for some time because of her paralysis and lack of mental development. Years later, she was reported as slightly retarded but generally all right.

A number of questions are raised by these cases, and all are concerns of nursing. Creighton discusses several similar cases, as well as a Yale study in which some malformed infants were allowed to die with parental and physician consent. She notes how a nurse can influence a family to accept their deformed baby by emphasizing the normal.[50] Such cases will certainly continue, and the issue is not easily resolved; it is not just the rights of the infant that must be considered, but also those of the family and society. However, it appears that the federal government is setting a pattern for intervention. In late 1984, the "Baby Doe" bill, the Child Abuse Amendments of 1984, was signed into law. PL 98-45 made federal funding for a state's child protective services agency contingent on the establishment of procedures for reporting instances of medical neglect of newborns, including "withholding of medically indicated treatment from disabled infants with life threatening conditions." Some exceptions were indicated, and establishment of IBCs was encouraged.

Follow-up on this legislation indicates that many who are concerned about these infants agree that the federal regulations are an ethically inadequate response to the complex needs of the handicapped child, the family, the health care professions, and society as a whole.[51] An ethics committee, if functioning well, can be helpful to the physician and family in making decisions, but the decisions lean toward preserving life.[52] It has also been reported that discriminatory denial of medical treatment has not dramatically changed since enactment of the Child Abuse Amendment of 1984, although others claim that overtreatment is more likely to be the result. One author believes that the fact that treatable infants and children do not receive therapy because state legislation allows parents and religious healers to avoid their obligation to treat is a completely neglected problem that has not been covered by the Child Abuse Act.[53] Several cases have been tried since. Christian Scientist parents have been found guilty of manslaughter because they allowed their child to die without seeking medical treatment. They often received suspended sentences or probation. One major tragedy caused by this law is not easily resolved—that some infants will have their lives prolonged and suffer "a fate worse than death" because the physicians are afraid of the legal consequences of letting them die.[54] Meanwhile, few cases of medical neglect seem to be reported.[55]

A different right-to-die situation involving a minor came to the Maine courts in 1990. Chad Swan, in a PVS and being tube fed after an accident, developed several serious medical complications. With the concurrence of his physician, his family filed for a court order permitting the termination of the feeding. The court ruled that there was clear evidences, based on Chad's statements reported by his family, that he would not want to be maintained in a PVS, but the state attorney general appealed because Chad was only 17 years old. The Maine Supreme Court then expanded a previous right-to-die decision to include minors capable of making a serious decision to forego treatment.

RIGHTS OF PATIENTS IN RESEARCH

The use of new, experimental drugs and treatments in hospitals, nursing homes, and other institutions that have a captive population—for example, prisons or homes for the mentally retarded—has been extensive. Nurses are often involved in giving the treatment or drugs. DHHS regulations require specific informed consent for any human research carried out under DHHS auspices, with strong emphasis on the need for a clear explanation of the experiment, the possible dangers, and the subject's complete freedom to refuse or withdraw at any time.

An interesting trend is toward including very young children in making decisions about research in which they are asked to participate. In the past, as a rule, parents were asked whether they consented to their child's participation in research—medical, educational, psychological, or other. There has always been some concern as to whether the child should be subjected to such research if it was not at least potentially beneficial to him or her (such as the use of a new drug for a leukemic child). The child was seldom given the opportunity to decide whether or not to participate. New knowledge of the potential harm that could be done to the child, however innocuous the experiment, and appreciation of the child as a human being with individual rights have now resulted in recommendations that even a very young child be given a simple explanation of the proposed research and allowed to participate or not, or even to withdraw later, without any form of coercion.[56] Given that choice, some children have decided not to participate. Overall, though, the support for using healthy children in research or being volunteered for procedures not beneficial to themselves is eroding. In 1983, DHHS published rules requiring children's consent to participate in research.

Nurses were in the forefront of the move to protect research subjects, with a statement in the ANA Code of Ethics, "The nurse participates in research activities when assured that the rights of individual subjects are protected," as well as an extensive ANA document on research guidelines. (See Chapter 9). When you are participating in research, at whatever level, ensuring that the rights of patients are honored is both an ethical and a legal responsibility. Know the patients' rights: self-determination to choose to participate; to have full information; to terminate participation without penalty; privacy and dignity; conservation of personal resources; and freedom from arbitrary hurt and intrinsic risk of injury; as well as the special rights of minor and incompetent persons previously discussed.[57] For instance, nurses have been ordered to begin using an experimental drug knowing that the patient has not given an informed consent. The nurse is then obligated to see that that patient does have the appropriate explanation. This is one more case in which institutional policy that sets an administrative protocol for such a situation is helpful.[58]

If you are the investigator, observe all the usual requirements, such as informed consent[59,60] and confidentiality. The quality of research in which human subjects are involved is particularly important. Peer review, such as that offered by a hospital review board, can be helpful. Although sometimes there are no nurses on the board, when they are, they bring a useful perspective to the review.[61]

PATIENT RECORDS: CONFIDENTIALITY AND AVAILABILITY

There is some evidence that, in situations other than the legally required ones, confidentiality of patients' records is frequently violated. From birth certificates to death certificates, the health and medical records of most Americans are part of a system that allows access by insurance companies, student researchers, and governmental agencies, to name a few. The information is often shared illegally with others, such as employers.

One physician, after completing a survey of the number of health professionals and hospital personnel who had access to the chart of one of his patients, called the principle of confidentiality "old, worn-out and useless; it is a decrepit concept." Seventy-five people had a legitimate access to that medical record.[62] Annas also says that it is not realistic for hospital patients to think that medical information about them will be kept confidential, even when staff follow all the basic rules about not discussing patients except in clinical situations. In part, of course, confidentiality is even less likely since the advent of computerized recordkeeping, which has grown tremendously in the last decade.

Nevertheless, maintaining patient confidentiality is a part of both nursing and medical ethical codes, and practitioners have a responsibility to safeguard patients' privacy as much as possible.[63] That includes the privacy of patient records. Many states have enacted laws to protect medical records, and the federal Freedom of Information Act (FOIA) denies access to an individual's medical record without that person's consent. Still, there are practical problems: if certain data are needed, as in following through on occupational health hazards, can exceptions be made for research that would be beneficial to the well-being of people? The problem does not lie in the aggregate figures but occurs when individual records must be scrutinized. The Supreme Court, recognizing the right of privacy, which protects certain personal information from public disclosure, has applied a test that balances

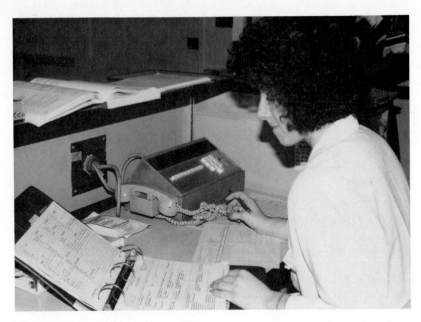

Accurate patient records are important in patient care, and today patients have access to their records. (*Courtesy of the Robert Wood Johnson Medical Center.*)

the individual's constitutional right against the state's interest in maintaining open records. Most states have followed suit.[64]

Physicians and health administrators have historically been hostile to the concept of sharing the record with the patient. Some attorneys serving health care facilities tend to share that feeling, often because they fear that patients may detect errors or personal comments that will result in a legal suit. (Actually, patient access has been mandated in Massachusetts since 1946, without a single reported adverse incident.) Whether or not any person involved in health care still feels that way is immaterial: almost without exception, the patient's medical record is available to him or her upon request—and sometimes without request. Whereas it is legally recognized that the patient's record is the property of the hospital or physician (in his or her office), the information that the record contains is not similarly protected. Both states and the federal government have legislated access— either direct patient access, with or without a right to copy, or indirect access (physician, attorney, or provision of a summary only). The majority of states allow patients direct access to their records. In the others, individuals have a probable legal right to access without going to court.[65] States may differentiate between doctors' and hospital records and have other idiosyncratic qualifications. The Privacy Protection Study Commission, created by the

1974 Privacy Act, also included recommendations on patient access. Of course, one certain way in which the patient can get access is through a malpractice suit in which the record is subpoenaed, a costly process for both provider and consumer. Still, it is interesting to review the literature of simply the last 15 years or so and see the changes in attitudes and legislation, although there were always physicians and others who saw sharing of the record with the patient as not only fair but sensible.

Do you have any legal responsibility to be an intermediary? The answer is more complex than just "yes" or "no." Certainly, you would not hand a patient the chart at request. Most states, as well as health care agencies, that permit access to records have a protocol to be followed. This usually involves providing both privacy and an opportunity for the physician and/or another person to explain the content. However, patients often don't want to see their charts if they feel that they are being given full information and are treated decently. The nurse certainly has a role in giving that open and humane care.

OTHER ASPECTS OF PATIENTS' RIGHTS

Privacy

Nurses and others who work with patients must be especially careful to avoid invading the patient's right to privacy, which is identical to that of any other person.[66] There are a number of special concerns. Consent to treatment does not cover the use of a picture without specific permission, nor does it mean that the patient can be subjected to repeated examinations not necessary to therapy without express consent. Visitors may also violate a patient's privacy. It is especially important that they not read the patient's chart. As it is, with the advent of computerized records, the patient's privacy might easily be violated.

Exceptions to respect for the patient's privacy are related to legal reporting obligations. All states have laws requiring hospitals, doctors, nurses, and sometimes other health workers to report on certain kinds of situations, because the patient may be unwilling or unable to do so. Nurses often have responsibility in these matters because, although it may be the physician's legal obligation, the nurses may be the only ones actually aware of the situation. Even if such reporting is not required by a law per se, regulations of various state agencies may require such a report. Common reporting requirements are for communicable diseases, diseases in newborn babies, gunshot wounds, and criminal acts, including rape. More recently, reporting a physically abused adult[67] or a neglected, battered child has been given legal attention. Every state and the District of Columbia has a child abuse law. Although other kinds of reporting are relatively objective, there are problems in reporting abused children because of the varying definitions of *child* and the question of whether there was abuse or an accident, with the consequent fear of parents suing. Usually, however, the person reporting is protected if good faith exists.[68] In some states, there are penalties for *not* reporting such situations. The nurse may also be obligated to testify about otherwise confidential information in criminal cases.

As the AIDS epidemic grew, new reporting problems arose. By 1987 all states had added AIDS to the list of reportable diseases. About a dozen require reporting of AIDS-related complex (ARC) cases, and even fewer require reporting of AIDS carriers, that is, the reporting of positive test results for the human immunodeficiency virus (HIV). Physicians have been willing to make these reports because of the virulence of the disease and the need to maintain the best possible epidemiological records. However, the problem arises of whether to notify the family, especially a wife or lover, about a person with AIDS. Many patients object to notification and therefore will not come for testing, creating a situation that may be even more serious. The laws on notification are not clear, although in cases related to other infectious diseases, judges have ruled that the physician had a duty to inform the third party. The third party could also sue the physician if infected and not warned. As a rule, this kind of reporting is a public health department's responsibility, it has not yet been determined whether for instance, a home health nurse with information on AIDS-related conditions has a duty to tell the family.[69] What Northrop described as *not* a duty is the action of a nurse, formerly in an AIDS clinic, who passed on an AIDS-infected person's confidential record to the physician in charge of pre-employment physicals when the individual applied for a job in the hospital. Northrop said that the nurse could have been sued for breach of confidentiality and violation of privacy, although in this instance she was not named in the suit. The hospital paid.[70]

Confidential information obtained through professional relationships is not the same as *privileged communication,* which is a legal concept providing that a physician and patient, attorney and client, and priest and penitent have a special privilege. Should any court action arise in which the person (or persons) involved is called to testify, the law (in many states) will not require that such information be divulged. Not all states acknowledge that nurses can be recipients of privileged communication, but there are specific cases in which the nurse-patient privilege has been accepted.[71] A relatively new issue is that psychiatric nurses, like other psychotherapists, have a responsibility to warn potential victims about their homicidal clients.[72] The same may be true of NPs in the case of warnings to the sexual partners of AIDS patients.[73]

Assault and Battery

Assault and battery, although often discussed with emphasis on the criminal interpretation, also has a patients' rights aspect that is related to everyday nursing practice, especially when dealing with certain types of patients. In many cases, where the action taken could come under this legal category, it is particularly important to chart fully and accurately. Grounds for civil action might include the following:

1 Forcing a patient to submit to a treatment for which he or she has not given consent either expressly in writing, orally, or by implication. Whether or not a consent was signed, a patient should not be forced, for resistance implies a withdrawal of consent.
2. Forcefully handling an unconscious patient.
3. Lifting a protesting patient from the bed to a wheelchair or stretcher.
4. Threatening to strike or actually striking an unruly child or adult, except in self-defense.
5. Forcing a patient out of bed to walk postoperatively.
6. In some states, performing alcohol, blood, urine, or health tests for presumed drunken driving without consent. There are some "implied consent" statutes in motor vehicle codes that provide that a person, for the privilege of being allowed to drive, gives an implied consent to furnishing a sample of blood, urine, or breath for chemical analysis when charged with driving while intoxicated. However, if the person objects and is forced, it still might be considered battery. Several states, acknowledging this, have enacted legislation to insulate hospital employees and health professionals from liability.

As a rule, intentional torts, such as assault and battery, are not covered by malpractice insurance.[74]

False Imprisonment

As the term implies, *false imprisonment* means "restraining a person's liberty without the sanction of the law, or imprisonment of a person who is later found to be innocent of the crime for which he was imprisoned." The term also applies to many procedures that actually or conceivably are performed in hospital and nursing situations *if they are performed without the consent of the patient or his or her legal representative.*[75] In most instances, the

nurse or other employee will not be held liable if it can be proved that what
was done was necessary to protect others.

Among the most common nursing situations that might be considered
false imprisonment are the following:

1. Restraining a patient by physical force or using appliances without
    written consent, especially in procedures where the use of restraints is
    not usually necessary. This is, or may be, a delicate situation because
    if you do not use a restraint, such as siderails, to protect a patient, you
    may be accused of negligence, and if you use them without consent,
    you may be accused of false imprisonment. This a typical example of
    the need for prudent and reasonable action that a court of law would
    uphold.
2. Restraining a mentally ill patient who is dangerous neither to himself
    nor to others. For example, patients who wander about the hospital
    division making a nuisance of themselves usually cannot legally be
    locked in a room unless they show signs of violence. If they do, you
    must still be careful.[76]
3. Using arm, leg, or body restraints to keep a patient quiet while admin-
    istering an IV infusion may be considered false imprisonment. If this
    risk is involved—that is, if the patient objects to the treatment and
    refuses to consent to it—the physician should be called. Should the
    doctor order restraints for the patient, make sure that the order is given
    in writing before allowing anyone to proceed with the treatment. It is
    much better to assign someone to stay with the patient throughout a
    procedure than to use restraint without authorization.
4. Detaining an unwilling patient in the hospital. If a patient insists on
    going home, or a parent or guardian insists on taking a minor or other
    dependent person out of the hospital before his or her condition warrants
    it, hospital authorities cannot legally require him or her to remain. In
    such instances, the doctor should write an order permitting the hospital
    to allow the patient to go home "against advice," and the hospital's
    representative should see that the patient or guardian signs an official
    form absolving the hospital, medical staff, and nursing staff of all
    responsibility should the patient's early departure be detrimental to his
    or her health and welfare. If the patient refuses to sign, a record should
    be made on the chart of exactly what occurred, and an incident report
    probably should be filed. Take the patient to the hospital entrance in
    the usual manner.
5. Detaining for an unreasonable period of time a patient who is medically
    ready to be discharged. The delay may be due to the patient's inability
    to pay the bill or to an unnecessarily long wait, at his or her expense,
    for the delivery of an orthopedic appliance or other service. In such
    instances, you may or may not be directly involved, but it is always

wise to know the possibility of legal developments and to exercise sound judgment in order to be completely fair to the patient and avoid trouble.

LEGAL ISSUES RELATED TO REPRODUCTION

Laws permitting abortion have varied greatly from state to state over the years. In early 1973, the Supreme Court ruled that no state can interfere with a woman's right to obtain an abortion during the first trimester (12 weeks) of pregnancy. During the second trimester, the state may interfere only to the extent of imposing regulations to safeguard the health of women seeking abortions. During the last trimester of pregnancy, a state may prohibit abortions except when the mother's life is at stake (*Doe v. Bolton* and *Roe v. Wade*). (Legislation relating to abortion is discussed in Chapter 10; other aspects are covered in Chapter 3).

Twenty years after the *Roe v. Wade* decision, opinions are still strong on abortion issues. The major related court cases have concerned legislation attempting to outlaw or limit abortion. Immediately after *Roe v. Wade,* with a liberal Supreme Court, the rulings were almost consistently directed at freedom of choice, in opposition to restrictions on abortion being enacted by the states and later by the conservative Reagan Administration. The rulings changed dramatically with appointments of conservative judges by President Reagan, until there was a five-to-four conservative majority, with the only woman Justice, Sandra O'Connor, considered the sometime swing vote. (However, she tended to be conservative on abortion issues.)

The case *Webster v. Reproductive Health Services,* in 1989, was considered a turning point,[77,78] the Court provided the states with new authority to limit a woman's right to abortion by upholding a Missouri law that banned abortions in tax-supported facilities except to save the mother's life, even if no public funds are spent; banned any public employee (doctors, nurses, others) from performing or assisting with abortions except to save a woman's life; and required testing of *any* fetus thought to be at least 20 weeks old for viability. Then in 1990, the Court ruled constitutional the Ohio and Minnesota laws requiring parental notification by unmarried teenagers. (Whether the girl was pregnant through incest or if there were other problems to make this difficult were ignored.)[79]

Probably of even more concern to pro-choice advocates and even others who did not necessarily support *Roe v. Wade* was the 1991 decision on *Rust v. Sullivan.*[80] The Court ruled that federal regulations that barred employees of clinics that receive federal funding "from discussing abortion with their patients even if the women ask for the information or if the health care provider believes that an abortion is medically necessary" were constitutional. What shocked health care professionals was not just that poor women who had no other source of family planning would be denied full information, but that physicians, nurses, and other health care workers would be forced to withhold full information from patients, which is not only an ethical but a legal problem. Part of the majority opinion written by Chief Justice William Rehnquist stated that the women's right to have an abortion was not infringed because it was her indigence, not the regulations, that prevented it. Other statements by proponents indicated that, after all, physicians didn't *have* to work in such clinics if this "gag rule" bothered them. Because so many clinics depend on Title X money, some indicated that they would abide by the regulations, others that they would figure out a way around them. A number of Planned Parenthood clinics noted that they would simply have to do without federal funding. People turned to Congress for action, but late in the session, a bill invalidating the regulations was vetoed by President Bush and Congress did not override the veto. Of all the Supreme Court decisions, this one probably affects nurses most, since it prevents nurses working in Title X clinics from giving their patients full and accurate information.

The aim of many of these cases, usually brought by a state, was to force the overturn of *Roe v. Wade*. That did not quite happen, but some state legislatures passed increasingly restrictive laws (even forbidding abortion in cases of incest and rape), in part to try to force the Supreme Court to hear the cases. Governors vetoed some of these laws, but the very fact that they had gotten through two Houses was appalling to many men and women alike. Both pro-choice and pro-life forces concentrated their efforts on legislators and candidates to bring about state laws that supported their particular point of view. The end is not in sight. After particularly restrictive laws were overturned by federal courts in Pennsylvania, Guam, Utah, and Louisiana, their advocates planned to take the cases to the Supreme Court. Because of the clear majority of conservative justices, particularly after the retirement of Justice Thurgood Marshall in 1991, an overturn of *Roe v. Wade* is predicted by some. However, it is important to remember that the U.S. Supreme Court rules only on issues related to the Constitution. In these cases, the Court rules that the state or another petitioner does or does not have a constitutional right to behave in a particular way. The trend now is to give states more freedom to act.

How does this affect nurses? Nurses support both sides of this issue, as was clear by the anger or joy expressed by nurses when ANA took a pro-choice stand. But regardless of their personal feelings, they will care for women and young girls who either made their choices or couldn't. Some girls have already sought back-alley abortionists, with the expected dire results. Theoretically, all hospitals are required to perform abortions within these guidelines, and it is legal to assist with such a procedure; actually, the right to an abortion cannot be withheld unless Roe v. Wade is overturned. However, for religious and moral reasons, some institutions are exempted from complying with the law, and individual doctors and nurses have refused to participate in abortions. Individual professionals or other health workers may make that choice, and there is legal support for them (conscience clause). This does not preclude the right of the hospital to dismiss a nurse for refusing to carry out an assigned responsibility or to transfer her to another unit. There have been some suits by nurses objecting to transfer, but rulings have varied.[81]

Ethically, nurses must give all patients good care, but who gets what care and why, as in the Webster case, may affect nurses professionally as well as personally. As citizens, nurses must stay abreast of such important issues. For instance, many pro-life groups also object to sex education and contraceptive use, yet an astounding number of teenagers get pregnant every year. What should the role of the nurse be in this situation? It is educational to see how other countries handle these issues.[82] It is also important to see how some of these issues interrelate. For instance, groups opposed to abortion are now becoming involved in right-to-die issues, taking a "life-is-sacred" stand.

There are a number of other reproduction-related rights that are also important, such as sterilization, artificial insemination of various kinds, and surrogate parenthood. *Sterilization* means termination of the ability to produce offspring. Both laws and regulations have been in the process of change. Most refer to women. There seems to be little legal concern about male sterilization, *vasectomy,* which is being done with increasing frequency. The legal consequences of unsuccessful sterilization, both male and female, have resulted in suits. Called *wrongful birth,* these suits usually seek to recover the costs of raising an unplanned or unwanted child, normal or abnormal—but usually the latter. Judgments have varied but are more likely to favor the plantiff if the child is abnormal.[83]

Laws on *family planning,* in general, also vary greatly. Some laws appear to be absolute prohibitions against giving information about contraceptive materials, but courts usually allow considerable freedom. Because there are still some state limitations and because, as noted earlier, the federal government is becoming more involved, it is important to keep up-to-date in this area.

Artificial insemination, the injection of seminal fluid by instrument into a female to induce pregnancy, is evolving into an acceptable medical procedure used by childless couples. (Consent by the husband and wife is generally required.) When a woman, for a fee, is artifically inseminated with a man's sperm and bears a child, who is then turned over to the man and his wife, this is termed *surrogate motherhood.* It has already created some legal problems when the woman decided not to give up the child and again when neither wanted a baby born with a birth defect. Even the legality of the process is in doubt.[84,85]

Among the most controversial legal concerns related to reproduction are *in vitro sterilization* and *surrogate embryo transfer,* each of which is intended to enhance the fertility of infertile couples. One of the issues is related to patenting the process, which requires quality control and reproductive privacy.[86]

A relatively new legal aspect of human reproduction concerns the field of *genetics,* with which nurses, physicians, and lay genetic counselors must be concerned. Some of the issues have to do with human genetic disease, genetic screening, in vitro fertilization, and genetic data banks. In addition, legislation, such as the *National Sickle Cell Anemia, Cooley's Anemia, Tay-Sachs, and Genetic Diseases Act,* has encouraged or forced states to expand genetic screening to cover other disorders. Neonatal screening, for instance, will probably be expanded considerably and offers new opportunities and responsibilities for nurses. But with what is still a relatively new science, many legal questions will arise.[87] Confidentiality is of major importance. If a genetic disease is discovered, the counselor should not contact other relatives, even if it would benefit those relatives, without the screenee's consent. One emerging problem is *wrongful life,* which occurs when a deformed baby is born, although abortion was an option, because the physician or other counselor neglected to tell parents of the risk.[88] Informed consent that enables the patient to make such serious decisions as having an abortion, sterilization, or artificial insemination is also very important.

Finally, there are an increasing number of issues that affect the autonomy of women. For instance, over half of the state living will statutes have a clause that suspends activation if the woman is pregnant. Also, some courts have ordered cesarean sections against a woman's wish. One positive action is the 1991 Supreme Court decision that prohibits an employer from excluding a fertile female employee from certain jobs because of concern for the health of a fetus a woman *might* conceive.[89]

TRANSPLANTS AND ARTIFICIAL PARTS

Since Dr. Christiaan Barnard performed the first human heart transplant in 1967, the question of tissue and organ *transplants* has become a point of controversy. Tissue may be obtained from living persons or a dead body. With living persons, the major legal implications relate to negligence and informed consent.[90]

The greatest legal problems arise from getting tissue and organs from a dead body. The big question is: when is an individual dead? When the definition of death as brain death has not been clarified, there have been suits against doctors and hospitals concerning removal of organs before "death," as seen by the family, even if it was a desire of the patient. Lawyers generally advise nurses not to participate if they have doubts about the procedure but to tell their supervisor why.[91]

Common law once prevented the decedent from donating his or her own body or individual organs if the next of kin objected, and statutes prohibited mutilation of bodies. However, now, all 50 states have adopted, in one form or another, the *Uniform Anatomical Gift Act,* approved in 1968 by the National Conference of Commissioners on Uniform State Laws. The basic purposes are to permit an individual to control the disposition of his or her own body after death, to encourage such donations, to eliminate unnecessary and complicated formalities regarding the donation of human tissues and organs, to provide the necessary safeguards to protect the varied interests involved, and to define clearly the rights of all involved.

For almost 20 years, various attempts to get people to donate their organs have generally failed. While the vast majority of people approved of organ transplantation, fewer than 20 percent have executed an organ donation form. Even when a form was signed, physicians would not rely on it to remove organs, even though they could legally do so, without asking permission of the next of kin. As noted earlier, there is a tremendous gap between the need for organs and the supply. Amendments to the law were suggested to simplify donation, but not much changed. The new legal solution in 1987 was *required request,* which mandated that someone ask the next of kin of every potential organ or tissue donor whether or not they want to donate. This, too, has apparently not proved to be very successful.[92] There is some evidence that physicians' and nurses' attitudes also inhibit donation. Some suggestions have been made about what request procedure might work best; these may be helpful to nurses who are hesitant to approach families.[93]

As in so many other situations, ethics and law are closely related here. Because of the scarcity of organs, the criteria are not so limited as they once were, and new scientific findings have opened new frontiers of transplantation. However, ethical concerns, translated into law, have had an impact, both good and bad, on transplantation. For instance, PL 98-507 (1984) prevents the sale of human organs, and court cases have forbidden the transplantation of the organs of anencephalic newborns or fetal tissue transplants.[94] These issues must be resolved, and a better system must be developed to match the available organs with those who need them.

NURSES' RIGHTS

Nurses may have more legal responsibilities because of their RN status, but they have the same rights as any other citizen. Many of the legal rights of nurses are found in the nurse practice acts (Chapter 11), an indication of the power and privilege given nurses by society. Nevertheless, some of the rights nurses may assume they have, such as being patient advocates, may conflict with the rights other professionals see as theirs or what employers see as inappropriate for employees.

Employment Rights

Since most working nurses are employees, knowing their rights in that respect is very important. One common worry is being fired, particularly when positions are hard to find. Can you be fired without reason? The answer is yes, if you have no contract.[95] (This will be discussed later.) However, more suits are being heard charging breach of contract, which may be based on what was said in the interview or written in the employee handbook.[96] The latter is seen to confer contractual rights in a number of states.[97] Due process is always necessary.

Can you be discharged for "blowing the whistle?" A number of nurses have been. Nurses are advised to take all necessary internal steps, such as verification, documentation, and reporting to the appropriate people, but if the result is getting fired, there are legal remedies. These include whistle-blower protection laws (some states); wrongful discharge suits; breach-of-contract suits; and, if a law was violated, consulting with the agency responsible for enforcing that law. (For instance, consult the state board of health if there was a serious safety violation.) In addition, it is possible to invoke the First Amendment (free speech) if you spoke out on a matter of public interest.[98] Still, there's no guarantee that, even with the best case, you'll win. The law is only beginning to develop in this area, and you must be prepared to go to court.[99]

With the nursing shortage, nurses are forced to work in situations of short staffing and sometimes in areas not within their expertise. Can you refuse? As reported in Chapter 12, short staffing is not an excuse if a patient is injured. Nursing administration has the right to assign you where needed (providing you don't have a written contract that says otherwise), but they also have the responsibility to delegate duties *appropriately* and to provide adequate supervision.[100] Some nurses' associations have now negotiated contracts to prevent inappropriate assignment or compulsory overtime. Others have developed a form that says, in essence, that in her or his professional judgment, the nurse's current assignment is unsafe and places the patients at risk, but that he or she will carry it out under protest. A similar form documents the assignment, number, and condition of patients and number and type of staff.[101] The legality of this process has not yet been tested, and there are some other concerns. If a nurse has stated that an assignment is unsafe and then takes it, she or he is vulnerable in case of a later negligence suit. And, of course, the use of the form can be abused.[102]

When refusing an assignment, however, one of the dangers is being accused of abandoning your patients. Just what that means in any specific case is not clear, but it could result in the loss of your license. On the other hand, supervisors use the term loosely to frighten the nurse into staying on the job.[103] Nurses are advised to discuss an inappropriate assignment with the supervisor, putting her or him on notice about your limitations; to identify your options (sharing or trading the assignment); and to document the situation.[104] In the end, it is your decision, and not an easy one, but it is almost inevitable in many institutions. It's best to think it through ahead of time.

Whether you can safely refuse an assignment in other circumstances is not clear. Employers are usually required to offer an alternate position if the refusal is on the basis of a conscience clause. However, if you refuse that assignment, you have little recourse. One situation that has been gaining attention is fair treatment for nurses who cannot work on certain days for religious reasons. As might be expected, rulings have differed, but in 1985, the U.S. Supreme Court ruled that there was no constitutional right involved; that in fact it is unconstitutional for a state to legislate an unqualified right not to work on the sabbath. From a practical point of view, the nurse may be willing to accept alternatives, such as working other holidays or weekend days.

Another point to check in order to see whether you have a case is whether your civil rights were violated, for instance, by discrimination against the handicapped. This approach has also resulted in contradictory judgments, usually because the situation was not clear-cut. In terms of nurses with AIDS, the Office of Civil Rights has established an important precedent: they may work as long as they can perform their assigned duties competently and without endangering the health of others.[105]

Other areas of discrimination are related to racial discrimination[106] and, increasingly, discrimination against male nurses. In a major case, a woman judge in Arkansas upheld a ban on male RNs in the delivery room, ruling that "Due to the intimate touching required in labor and delivery, services of all male nurses are very inappropriate."[107] (What about the services of the male doctor?) Similar cases were lost for a male nurse doing private duty who had never been assigned a woman patient and one in a nursing home who was not permitted to care for women. Here the judge ruled that it might upset the elderly women. However, this situation is changing.

A number of other rights come into play in the job situation. One area is on-the-job safety.[108,109] Another area is sexual harassment, which has become a more visible problem.[110] Action is gradually being taken in support of the victims, with not only the harassers but also the employer considered liable.

Collective Bargaining

Some employment issues are resolved by collective bargaining. Since the enactment of PL 93-360 in 1974, employees of nonprofit institutions have joined the ranks of other workers who have collective bargaining rights. In addition, a Supreme Court ruling in 1991 allowing separate bargaining units for nurses, and in the same year, enactment of a law restoring collective bargaining rights to VA nurses gave further impetus to action. Other labor laws are discussed in Chapters 10 and 14, but nurses' rights in the bargaining process are pertinent here.

The process of collective bargaining, because it is set by law, is similar regardless of who the bargaining agent is, and details can be found in any book on labor relations. In the context of ANA, that is, SNAs as collective bargaining agents, the following is presented as a brief overview.

1. The nurses (or group of nurses) in an institution, discontented with a situation or conditions and having exhausted the usual channels for correction or improvement, ask the SNA for assistance.

2. A meeting is held outside the premises of the institution and always on off-duty time. SNA staff and the nurses explore the problems, and the nurses are given advice about reasonable, negotiable issues and how to form a unit; for instance, they are told who can be included in a unit. Administrative nurses are excluded, but the question of supervisors is still being debated in some places.

3. Authorization cards, which authorize the SNA to act as the nurses' bargaining representative, must be signed by at least 30 percent of the group to be represented. Membership forms are also suggested because the SNA cannot provide services without funds. All collective bargaining activity must be carried out in nonwork areas where the employee is protected from employer interference. (There are a series of NLRB rules governing employee distribution and solicitation.)

4. If sufficient cards are signed, the SNA notifies the employer that organization is going on, calling attention to the fact that the activity is protected. Copies of the notice are distributed to the nurses so that they know they are protected.

5. An informational meeting is held for all nurses and SNA staff. Employers may not interfere; this would be an *unfair labor practice*.

6. If it is agreed that the SNA will represent the nurses, a *bargaining unit* is formed and officers are elected.

7. To seek voluntary recognition of the unit by the employer, a majority of the nurses must sign designation cards; this will probably be checked by a mutually accepted third party.

8. If the employer chooses not to recognize the unit, or if the designation is challenged by another union, a series of actions takes place, including an NLRB-conducted election. To petition for election, any union must have designation cards signed by 30 percent of the nurses in the proposed unit. The election is won or lost by the majority of nurses *voting*. They may vote for a particular union or specify none

at all. The NLRB then certifies the winner as the exclusive bargaining agent. If the majority of nurses vote against *any* bargaining agent, the NLRB certifies this as well.

9.   Assuming that the SNA wins the election, the SNA representative, at the direction of the unit, attempts to settle the problems and complaints of the nurses by negotiating with administration at the *bargaining table*. There are specific rules about what is negotiable and what is not. *Mandatory* subjects include salaries, fringe benefits, and conditions of employment, and both sides must bargain in good faith about these issues. *Voluntary* subjects can be almost anything else that *both* sides want to discuss, except for *prohibited* or illegal subjects such as a requirement that all workers become members of a union before being employed for 30 days. It should be remembered that the nurse executive, both through position and under the law, is an administrator. Even though the director of nursing may be in complete support of the nurses' demands, he or she cannot join them. Quite often the director has previously tried unsuccessfully to help them achieve their goals. Both sides must *bargain in good faith*.

10. If an agreement is not reached in due time, there may be, first of all, *informational picketing* to communicate the issues to the community.

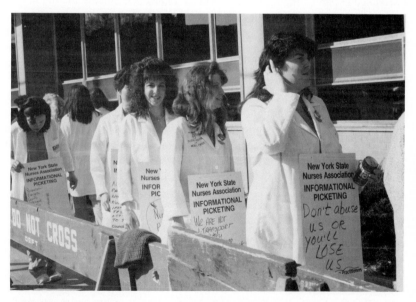

Informational picketing is a means of informing the public about nurses' on-the-job concerns. (*Courtesy of the New York State Nurses' Association; photo by Barry Waldman.*)

Another approach is arbitration. In *mediation-arbitration* (*med-arb*), the arbitrator moves into the situation early and tries to get the two sides to agree. If neither will compromise (*a deadlock*), *binding arbitration* may be called for. In this case, after listening to both sides, the arbitrator makes a decision and both must agree to it. In the *final offer* approach, employers agree on as many points as possible, and submit these and the unresolved issues to an arbitrator who then selects the best package. Then a *contract* is signed. Arbitration is expensive because arbitrators must be paid, but sometimes this is all that will settle a bitter dispute.

The more serious alternative is a *strike*. There are particular NLRB rules in regard to strikes against health care facilities, particularly in relation to giving sufficient notice to allow arrangements to be made for patient care. In most strikes, there is a *picket line,* intended, in part, to discourage other workers or outside services from entering the institution. Even if strikes are successful, there is often a lingering unpleasant feeling between participants and nonparticipants. However, as ANA members agreed when they gradually removed no-strike clauses from ANA and SNA policies, the strike is the ultimate weapon that may be necessary when the employer refuses any attempt to resolve the issues.

Once a strike is settled, the strikers are reinstated if a *reinstatement privilege* is part of the agreement. This assumes that the strikers did not do anything illegal, like preventing others from entering the institution. However, new employees who may have been hired during the strike remain. If strikers return *unconditionally,* some striking nurses may not go back to work immediately. They are placed on a recall list. If those nurses cannot find equivalent employment, they are recalled before new nurses are hired. After a labor contract is in place, there are times when individual nurses are in dispute with the employer. A grievance procedure is generally used to resolve the problem. A grievance may be caused by "an alleged violation of a contract provision, a change in a past practice, or an employer decision that is considered arbitrary, capricious, unreasonable, unfair, or discriminatory."[111] Simple complaints are not considered grievances. If informed discussion does not resolve the issue, a grievance procedure is followed. The steps include the following:

1. Written notice of the grievance is given, with a written response within a set time.
2. If the response is not satisfactory, an appeal to the director of nursing follows.
3. The employee, SNA representative, grievance chairman, and/or delegate, director of nursing, and director of personnel meet.

4. If no resolution occurs, the final step is arbitration by a neutral third
party selected by both parties involved. The technique for carrying out
the process involves interpersonal, adversary, and negotiating skills.

Whether or not a union is the answer to some of the problems of nurse
employees, the right to bargain is a valuable economic tool, as more nurses
are beginning to realize. There are alternatives to collective bargaining, and
some have worked, but sometimes it is the most useful tool for conflict
resolution and controlling professional practice.[112]

Other Contracts

Whether or not nurses are unionized, a good contract is useful in defining
employer-employee and patient-nurse agreements.[113] Fewer problems arise
when both parties understand the rights and responsibilities of each. Although they sometimes do not realize it, nurses are continually making
contracts, whether as employees or as independent practitioners. A *contract*
is defined as a legally enforceable promise between two or more persons to
do or not to do something. The essential elements of a contract are mutual
assent, promises or considerations, two or more parties of competent legal
capacity, and an agreement that is a lawful act and not against public policy.

Several examples of nurse contracts can be given. A nurse seeks employment, and in the interview, employer and employee come to certain
understandings. The nurse will perform the job safely, competently, and in
accordance with the standards and policies of the institution (hours, dress,
behavior). The employer will pay for those services (salary, fringe benefits),
will provide needed equipment to perform the service, and will maintain
the facilities and equipment properly. The contract may be *oral,* but it is
expressed. A written contract has many advantages; it prevents later misunderstandings about such common problems as rotations, shifts, and opportunities for transfer. If the nurse chooses not to come to that institution
after agreeing to do so, that is *breach of contract,* but the employer probably
would not find it worthwhile to seek damages. If the employee had falsified
references or other credentials, the contract would be void, because that is
illegal. If the employee with a *written contract* finds that the employer is
violating it, she or he could seek redress, either damages or the fulfillment
of the clause—for example, transfer to a specialty unit at the next vacancy.

A written employment contract ideally follows a more or less standard
form, setting forth the terms of agreement in understandable language, in
logical sequence, and in readable form. Every written employment contract—both individual and group—should contain the following items: hours,
salary, vacation, sick leave, holidays, Social Security coverage, pension
plan, and duration of contract. Information about rest periods or breaks,

meal hours, and so on may be included, as well as certain additional benefits, such as tuition for education.

Over and above the specific details of the contract and the way it is phrased is the fact that you should be sure you understand it and the terms to which you are agreeing. Also, be sure that the person with whom you make the contract has the authority to do so. If a formal contract is not used, ask for a letter of appointment covering the most important points listed and others of importance in that particular situation. Otherwise, you become an at-will employee and can be dismissed at any time, with or without cause.[114]

RIGHTS AND RESPONSIBILITIES OF STUDENTS

When you began your nursing program, you also in effect, if not in writing, entered into a contract with the school that does not expire until you graduate (or leave). It is understood that both students and the school will assume certain responsibilities, many of which have legal implications. The first legal commitment the school has is to fulfill the minimum requirements for curriculum, faculty, and other resources set by the state board of nursing. Although you are responsible for your own acts in a clinical setting, you are expected to be under the supervision of a qualified teacher. Having your own professional liability insurance is important.

Perhaps you want to work as an aide to earn extra money. You will have to be especially careful because you can legally function only in those capacities not restricted to licensed nursing personnel. State laws governing the practice of nursing vary widely and are subject to misinterpretation by the employing agency. Most laws classify students working part time as employees. In this capacity, if you perform tasks requiring more judgment and skill than the position for which you are employed, you are subject not only to civil suits but also to criminal charges for practicing without a license.

Undesirable student conduct may result in some discipline, including suspension or expulsion, and there has been considerable disagreement on the school's power in such circumstances. Generally, it is expected that the school's rules of conduct are made public and that the student has the right to a public hearing and due process. Legal rulings may be different when applied to private or public universities. Private universities have greater power in many ways.

Constitutional rights are most frequently cited by students in complaints: the First Amendment (freedom of speech, religion, association, expression); the Fourth Amendment (freedom from illegal search and seizure); and the Fifth and Fourteenth amendments (due process of law). The courts recognize the student first as a citizen, so that they will consider possible infringements of these rights. Most commonly, First Amendment rights involve dress codes and personal appearance. Although schools do not possess absolute authority over students in this sense, some lower court rulings have approved the establishment of dress codes necessary for cleanliness, safety, and health.

One case concerning a student's appearance found its way to the U.S. Supreme Court. Sharon Russell was dismissed from her nursing program because she failed to lose weight, as she had agreed to do. Although her grades were good, her weight rose to 303 pounds and she was withdrawn from her senior year. She completed her degree elsewhere but sued for damages, partly because the faculty humiliated her about her obesity. She charged intentional infliction of emotional distress, handicap discrimination, invasion of privacy, and breach of contract. All charges were dismissed except the last. Throughout the various appeals, her award of damages was upheld. The Supreme Court heard the case on narrow procedural grounds, and the case was sent back to the First Circuit Court. It is expected that her award of damages will stand. Nevertheless, still somewhat open are the question of whether obesity is a handicap (to fall under the Rehabilitation Act), whether the way she was treated was "atrocious" in a legal sense, and whether she or the college violated a contract.

Random, unannounced searches that schools had carried out previously are no longer allowed without student permission or a search warrant; otherwise, evidence found is inadmissible in court. If material uncovered is proscribed by *written* institutional policy, it may be used in institutional proceedings.

Due process has been a major issue of legal contention. The rule or law must be examined for fairness and reasonableness. Are the student and faculty understanding of the rule the same? Did the student have the opportunity to know about the rule and its implications? What is the relationship between the rule and the objectives of the school? The National Student Nurses' Association (NSNA) developed grievance procedure guidelines as part of a bill of rights for students. Besides suggesting the makeup of the committee and general procedures, such issues as allowing sufficient time, access to information and appropriate records, presentation of evidence, and use of witnesses were included. The usual steps in any grievance process are also followed for academic grievances: an informal process first, consisting of a written complaint and a suggested remedy by the student grievant, a written reply, a hearing with presentation of evidence on both sides, a decision by the committee within a specific time, right of appeal, and sometimes arbitration. With students, the right to continue with classwork throughout the whole process is considered necessary.

Due process is considered crucial for students who are expelled or suspended for disciplinary reasons or who feel that they are discriminated against in their extracurricular activities because of race, religion, sex, or sexual preference.[115] However, there seem to be an increasing number of grievances filed or legal complaints made because of academic concerns, especially grades. The courts have been reluctant to enter this area of academic freedom. There has yet to be a definitive ruling on curriculum and degree requirements.[116]

Most colleges now have grievance procedures for students who think that they have received unfair grades, and these procedures must be followed first before any lawsuit can be filed.[117] In one case, a nurse who refused to take a predoctoral exam she had failed twice was terminated as a student of the university and not permitted to enter the doctoral program. She sued. The court could find no showing of bad motive or ill will on the part of the faculty, "which would warrant reviewing academic records based upon academic standards that are within the peculiar knowledge, experience, and expertise of the academicians."[118]

Before the student wages an all-out battle, the situation should be considered practically. It must be proved that the grade is arbitrary, capricious, and manifestly unjust, which is generally very difficult (especially when problems have been documented). Furthermore, unless that particular grade is extremely important to a student's career, the cost and time involved are greater than even a favorable result might warrant.

Cases in which the results have been more favorable to the student are related to inadequate program advisement[119] and the school catalog as a written contract.[120] (The school had to deal with the nursing student according to the statements in the catalog the year she or he entered, not the later, more restrictive requirements.) Also, a landmark case was heard by the Supreme Court, which ruled that an all-women's nursing school could not refuse to admit a male student.[121]

Another type of student right involves school records. The types of student records kept by schools vary. They may consist of only the academic transcript, or may include extracurricular activities and problem situations, which are kept in an informal file. The enactment of the Buckley Amendment, described in Chapter 10, has clarified the issue of student access to records. The individual loses the right to confidentiality by waiving the right or by disclosing the information to a third person. A student's academic transcript is the most common document released, particularly to other schools and employers.

As more student activists, most of whom are now voting citizens, request or demand certain rights as part of the academic community, more legal decisions are made such as the "truth in testing" laws. But school rules that were once ironclad have become flexible, even without legal intervention.

The concept of rights need not be seen as an adversary proceeding. Both the student and the school have a new accountability. In the long run, it might be more meaningful to look at certain student rights as freedoms and responsibilities.

HEALTH CARE RIGHTS: WHAT LIES AHEAD?

Optimists will say that the future for people's rights is very bright, that those who demand information, input, and quality in health care will not revert back to the period when their rights were what their providers chose to give them. Though probably true, that statement does not touch on the complexities that must inevitably emerge with new technology, new opportunities, and less money.

The law in all its forms will continue to take over—and change, perhaps almost control, our lives in relation to health care. An enormous area of activity will involve women, their pregnancies, and their rights. And what of the Baby Doe-saved children? Who will be responsible for them? Will the family be forced to care for and pay for a severely deformed child? What of all the issues related to the fetus? Will new technology that has been successful in intrauterine surgery save some of these babies? Cure them? How will new techniques of birth control including the abortion pill, RU 486, change the family planning scene?[122,123] Will they even be permitted in the United States? And on the other side of that coin—infertile couples wanting babies—will the government put restrictions on such techniques as embryo freezing? (There has already been a case where frozen embryos were awarded to a woman in a divorce settlement, somewhat like a child!) There are also already cases of lesbian couples, one of whom has borne a child by artificial insemination, fighting for custody of the child in court when they separate.

An issue that is bringing the threat of legislation is whether health care workers, especially doctors, nurses, and dentists, should be required to be tested for the HIV virus, and, if infected, be required to tell their patients. Generally, the professional organizations object, partly because they see danger to patients as limited. They *would* like to see all patients tested. However, one study of individual doctors and nurses revealed that they felt that *both* health care workers and patients should be tested. Because AIDS is such a deadly epidemic, concerns about the rights of both patients and health care workers will increase, even though the Centers for Disease Control have released guidelines for preventing transmission of HIV between patients and health care workers.

Meanwhile, on both the ethical and the legal fronts, what is expected to be the next big issue is physician-assisted suicide. This subject has been under discussion for some time and is usually brought into open debate after highly publicized physician-assisted suicides like the Debbie case or the suicide device used by a doctor and patient mentioned in Chapter 9. A poll after the latter incident in 1990 found that 53 percent of those polled thought that a doctor should be able to assist a patient who wants to die. Other polls raised the figure to more than 80 percent. However, in 1991, Oregon voters did not approve the first bill legalizing physician-assisted suicide. The issue is further accelerated with the AIDS epidemic, bringing what is almost certain death under painful circumstances. In addition, more cases of family members or friends assisting in suicide are being reported. (These may simply have been unreported before.) Sometimes these people are charged with murder.

One fear of doctor-assisted suicide is the possible abuse of such power. Some people think the possibility would cause patients to fear doctors. Yet, actions are already being taken to legalize euthanasia.[124,125] When a panel of distinguished physicians was brought together to consider the issue, 10 of the 12 members agreed that "if a hopelessly ill patient believes his or her condition is intolerable, it should be permissible for a physician to provide the patient with the medical means and the medical knowledge to commit suicide.[126] In the Netherlands, euthanasia has gained a degree of social acceptance. Since 1984 it is no longer prosecuted in certain approved circumstances, which are said to account for about 1000 to 7000 deaths a year. There is also some evidence that, especially with elderly patients, not all these deaths are voluntary. Other countries have organizations that will assist a person to commit suicide, and the international Hemlock Society, which advocates that people have a right to "die well," is gaining members.

Certainly, physicians are beginning to face the many issues surrounding euthanasia,[127] as well as related concerns such as considering how best to assess the value of modern technology, which can be almost a miracle but is prohibitively expensive. At the same time, it can be a matter of both unwanted life and death for people.[128] Nurses need to do the same. A number of nurses are known to have disconnected life support systems on comatose patients; it has probably happened more often than is known. Legally, they have been charged with everything from murder to practicing medicine without a license. However individual nurses feel about these difficult ethical problems, they are on the firing line; they deal with the patients and families as well as physicians. They simply cannot ignore these matters.

From another point of view, how will the health care needs of the growing number of homeless and prisoners be met? Will they have legislated rights? What of the many issues of privacy? It is true that just about all these issues could be considered ethical concerns. But ethical issues inevitably become legal issues, for better or worse. And there are more unresolved dilemmas. Almost every chapter of this book has discussed some aspect that has involved or does or will involve the law. More often than not, a crisis, not planning, will trigger legal intervention. Yet there are clear indications that some of these issues must be resolved soon, must have priority. Nurses as citizens and professionals should have a hand in determining the what and how.

KEY POINTS

1. Patients are beginning to assert themselves in demanding their legal rights, and generally courts are supporting them.
2. In order to have a legal informed consent, the patient must be competent and not coerced; the process must include an explanation of the condition, the proposed treatment, alternatives, and dangers or benefits.
3. Nurses are not legally responsible for getting consents, but they should try to be sure that the patient knows what he or she consented to.
4. Court decisions, statutory law, and organizational actions seem to be favoring the patient's right to die.
5. The living will is designed to allow individuals to express to their families, health care personnel, and institutions in advance their desires about their care if they are later not able to do so.
6. Legal issues related to abortion, sterilization, family planning, and artificial insemination are becoming more complex as technology offers new options and as advocates for or against certain points of view become more aggressive.
7. The law is changing rapidly in relation to the rights of children and the mentally ill.
8. Even though an action is intended for the patients' own good, forcing them to do something can be considered assault or battery.
9. The steps in collective bargaining and other aspects of the process are set by the NLRB.
10. Employees may be fired for a number of reasons, but in many cases they have legal redress, especially if their civil rights have been violated.
11. The grievance procedure is useful for settling disputes in both the employment and the educational setting.

REFERENCES

1. President's Commission for the Study of Ethical Problems in Medicine and Biomedical and Behavioral Research. *Making health care decisions*. Washington, DC: U.S. Government Printing Office, 1982.
2. Annas G. *The rights of patients: The basic ACLU guide to patient rights,* 2nd ed. Carbondale, IL: Southern Illinois University Press, 1989, pp. 9–12.
3. Ibid., p. 1.

4. Ibid., p. 85.

5. President's Commission, op. cit., pp. 2–3.

6. Creighton H. *Law every nurse should know,* 5th ed. Philadelphia: W.B. Saunders Company, 1986, pp. 34–36.

7. Northrop C, Kelly M. *Legal issues in nursing.* St. Louis: C.V. Mosby Company, 1987, pp. 84–86.

8. Barry M. The life of every creature . . . a case of patients' rights. *Am J Nurse,* 82:1440–1441 (September 1982).

9. Ackerman T. The limits of beneficience: Jehovah's Witnesses and childhood cancer. *Hastings Center Rep,* 4:13–18 (August 1980).

10. Somerville M. Therapeutic privilege: Variation on the theme of informed consent. *Law, Med, and Health Care,* 12:4–12 (February 1984).

11. Creighton H. The right of informed refusal. *Nurs Mgt,* 13:48 (September 1982).

12. President's Commission, op. cit., p. 147.

13. Court case: What went wrong? *Nurs Life,* 2:88 (March–April 1982).

14. Greenlaw J. When patients' questions put you on the spot. *RN,* 46:79–80 (March 1983).

15. Regan W. Informed consent: Must you double-check the MD? *RN,* 46:19–20 (August 1983).

16. Cushing M. Informed consent: An MD responsibility? *Am J Nurs,* 84:437–438 (April 1984).

17. Murphy EK. Informed consent doctrine: Little danger of liability for nurses. *Nurs Outlook,* 39:48 (January–February 1991).

18. Trimberger L, et al. Should you tell your patients about the risks of nursing procedures? *Nurs Life,* 3:26–32 (November–December 1983).

19. Murphy, op. cit.

20. Bernat J, et al. Defining death in theory and practice. *Hastings Center Rep,* 12:5–9 (February 1982).

21. Creighton H. Termination of life-sustaining treatment. *Nurs Mgt,* 14:14–15 (August 1983).

22. Annas GJ. Prisoner in the ICU: The tragedy of William Bartling. *Hastings Center Rep,* 14:28–29 (December 1984).

23. Annas G. When procedures limit rights: From Quinlan to Conroy. *Hastings Center Rep,* 15:24–26 (April 1985).

24. Sullivan J. Rights of patients who wish to die widened in New Jersey. *New York Times* (June 25, 1987), pp. A1, B12.

25. Annas G. Do feeding tubes have more rights than patients? *Hastings Center Rep,* 16:26–27 (February 1986).

26. Meilaender G. On removing food and water: Against the stream. *Hastings Center Rep,* 14:11–13 (December 1984).

27. Fry S. New ANA guidelines on withdrawing or withholding food and fluid from patients. *Nurs Outlook,* 36:122–123; 148–150 (May–June 1988).

28. Aroskar MA. The aftermath of the Cruzan decision: Dying in a twilight zone. *Nurs Outlook,* 38:256–257 (November–December 1990).

29. Annas G. Nancy Cruzan and the right to die. *N Engl J Med,* 323:670–672 (September 6, 1990).
30. Death at a New York hospital. *Law, Med, and Health Care,* 13:261–282 (December 1985). This series of articles was written by the patient's friend and a hospital representative, with additional commentaries.
31. Miles SH, August A. Courts, gender, and the "right to die." *Law, Med, and Health Care* 18:85–95 (Spring–Summer 1990).
32. Cohn S. The living will from the nurse's perspective. *Law, Med, and Health Care,* 11:121–124, 180 (June 1983).
33. Eisendrath S, Jonsen A. The living will: Help or hindrance? *JAMA* 249:2054–2058 (April 1983).
34. Annas GJ. The health care proxy and the living will. *N Engl J Med,* 324:1210–1213 (April 25, 1991).
35. Cushing M. Verbal no-code orders. *Am J Nurs,* 81:1215–1216 (June 1981).
36. Read W. *Hospital's role in resuscitation decisions.* Chicago: Hospital Research and Educational Fund, 1983.
37. Cranford R, Doudera AE. The emergence of institutional ethics committees. *Law, Med, and Health Care,* 12:13–20 (February 1984).
38. Optimum care for hopelessly ill patients. *N Engl J Med,* 295:362–364 (August 12, 1976).
39. Greenlaw J. Orders not to resuscitate: Dilemma for acute care as well as long-term care. *Law, Med, and Health Care,* 10:29–31, 45 (February 1982).
40. Clayton E. From Rogers to Rivers: The rights of the mentally ill to refuse medication. *Am J Law and Med,* 13(1):7–52 (1987).
41. Oriol M, Oriol RD. Involuntary commitment and the right to refuse medication. *J Psychosocial Nurs,* 24:15–20 (November 1986).
42. Trandel-Korenchuck D, Trandel-Korenchuk K. Informed consent and mental incompetency. *Nurs Admin Q,* 7:76–78 (Fall 1983).
43. Weiss FS. The right to refuse: Informed consent and the psychosocial nurse. *J Psychosocial Nurs,* 28:25–30 (August 1990).
44. Annas G. Sterilization of the mentally retarded: A decision for the courts. *Hastings Center Rep,* 11:18–19 (August 1981).
45. Holder A. Disclosure and consent problems in pediatrics. *Law, Med, and Health Care,* 16:219–228 (Fall–Winter 1988).
46. Rhodes AM. A minor's refusal of treatment. *MCN,* 15:261 (July–August 1990).
47. Cushing M. Whose best interest? Parents vs. child rights. *Am J Nurs,* 82:313–314 (February 1982).
48. Cushing M. Do not feed. . . . *Am J Nurs,* 83:602–604 (April 1983).
49. Taub S. Withholding treatment from defective newborns. *Law, Med, and Health Care,* 10:4–10 (February 1982).
50. Creighton H. Shall we choose life or let die? *Nurs Mgt,* 15:16–18 (August 1984).
51. Huefner D. Severely handicapped infants with life-threatening con-

ditions: Federal intrusions into the decision not to treat. *Am J Law and Med*, 12(2):171–205 (1986).

52. Fleischman A. Parental responsibility and the infant bioethics committee. *Hastings Center Rep*, 20:21–22 (March–April 1990).

53. Nolan K. Let's take Baby Doe to Alaska. *Hastings Center Rep*, 20:3 (January–February 1990).

54. Weir R. Pediatric ethics committee: Ethical advisers or legal watchdogs? *Law, Med, and Health Care*, 15:99–109 (Fall 1987).

55. Rhodes AM. Issue update: Baby Doe regulations. *MCN*, 15:379 (November–December 1990).

56. Moore I. Nontherapeutic research using children as subjects. *MCN*, 7:285–289ff (September–October 1982).

57. Shaffer M. Pfeiffer I. Nursing research and patients' rights. *Am J Nurs*, 86:23–24 (January 1986).

58. Marchette L. Experimental drugs: Where do you stand legally? *RN*, 47:23–24 (March 1984).

59. Siantz ML. Defining informed consent. *MCN*, 13:98 (March–April 1988).

60. Floyd J. Research and informed consent. *J Psychosocial Nurs*, 26(3):13–17 (1988).

61. Robb S. Nurse involvement in institutional review boards: The service setting perspective. *Nurs Res*, 39:27–29 (January–February 1981).

62. Annas (1989), op. cit., pp. 178–179.

63. Fry S. Confidentiality in health care: A decrepit concept? *Nurs Econ*, 2:413–418 (November–December 1984).

64. Grad F. *The public health law manual*, 2nd ed. Washington, DC: American Public Health Association, 1990, pp. 282–283.

65. Annas (1989), op. cit., pp. 164–167.

66. Klein C. Invasion of privacy. *Nurse Practitioner*, 10:50, 52 (January 1985).

67. Thobaben M, Anderson L. Reporting elder abuse: It's the law. *Am J Nurs*, 85:371–374 (April 1985).

68. Brass D. Professional and agency liability for negligence in child protection. *Law, Med, and Health Care* 11:71–75 (April 1983).

69. Brent N. Confidentiality and HIV status: A duty to inform third parties? *Home Healthcare Nurse*, 8:27–29 (April 1990).

70. Northrop C. Rights versus regulations: Confidentiality in the age of AIDS. *Nurs Outlook*, 36:208 (July–August 1988).

71. O'Sullivan A. Privileged communication. *Am J Nurs*, 80:947–950 (May 1980).

72. Kjervik D. The psychiatric nurse's duty to warn potential victims of homicidal psychotherapy outpatients. *Law, Med, and Health Care*, 9:11–16, 39 (December 1981).

73. Henry P. Nurse practitioners and the duty to warn. *Nurs Practitioner Forum*, 1:4–5 (June 1990).

74. Creighton H. *Law every nurse should know*, 5th ed. Philadelphia, W.B. Saunders Company, 1981, p. 205.

75. Klein C. False imprisonment. *Nurse Practitioner*, 9:41–44 (September 1984).
76. Jakocki M, Payson A. Out of control. *Am J Nurs*, 85:1335–1336 (December 1985).
77. Rhodes AM. Webster versus reproductive services. *MCN*, 14:423 (November–December 1989).
78. Annas GJ. Four-one-four. *Hastings Center Rep*, 19:27–29 (September–October 1989).
79. High court says states may require girl to notify parents before having abortion. *New York Times* (June 26, 1990) pp. A1, A20.
80. Supreme Court upholds gag rule as constitutional. *Capital Update*, 9:4–5 (June 1991).
81. Regan W. Assisting at abortions: Can you really say no? *RN*, 45:71 (June 1982).
82. Cohen S. Health care policy and abortion: A comparison. *Nurs Outlook*, 38:20–25 (January–February 1990).
83. Northrop and Kelly, op. cit., pp. 161–162.
84. Creighton H. The nurse and the surrogate mother. *Nurs Mgt*, 16:40–43 (June 1985).
85. Andrews L. The aftermath of Baby M: Proposed state laws on surrogate motherhood. *Hastings Center Rep*, 17:31–40 (October–November 1987).
86. Annas G. Surrogate embryo transfer: The perils of patenting. *Hastings Center Rep*, 14:25–26 (June 1984).
87. Nolan K, Swenson S. New tools, new dilemmas: Genetic frontiers. *Hastings Center Rep*, 18:40–42 (October–November 1988).
88. Northrop and Kelly, op. cit., pp. 161–162.
89. Murphy EK. Are pregnant women autonomous decision makers? *Nurs Outlook*, 39:144 (May–June 1991).
90. Creighton (1986), op. cit., p. 280.
91. Simpson H. Understanding the law: Organ donation. *Nurs Life*, 5:24–25 (January–February 1985).
92. Annas G. The paradoxes of organ transplantation. *Am J Pub Health*, 78:621–622 (June 1988).
93. Organ and tissue donation. *Am J Nurs*, 89:1294–1298 (October 1989).
94. Robertson J. Rights, symbolism, and public policy in fetal tissue transplants. *Hastings Center Rep*, 18:5–12 (December 1988).
95. Moskowitz S, Moskowitz L. Protecting your job. *Am J Nurs*, 84:55–58 (January 1984).
96. Kaye G, Burke E. Your grievance procedures alone will not protect you. *Nurs Mgt*, 21:24–27 (February 1990).
97. Horsley J. How your employee handbook protects you. *RN*, 10:58, 60 (June 1987).
98. Feliu A. Thinking of blowing the whistle? *Am J Nurs*, 83:1541–1542 (November 1983).
99. Feliu A. The risks of blowing the whistle. *Am J Nurs*, 83:1387–1389 (October 1983).

100. Feutz S. Nursing work assignments: Rights and responsibilities. *J Nurs Admin*, 18:9–11 (April 1988).

101. Mallison M. Protesting your assignments. *Am J Nursing*, 87:151 (February 1987).

102. Pohlman K. Against nursing advice? *Focus on Critical Care*, 17:57–58 (February 1990).

103. Cushing M. Accepting or rejecting an assignment: Are you abandoning your patients? *Am J Nurs*, 88:1470, 1475 (November 1988).

104. Cushing M. Refusing an unreasonable assignment: Strategies for problem solving. *Am J Nurs*, 88:1635–1637 (December 1988).

105. Northrop C. Nurses with AIDS—On the firing line? *Nurs 87*, 17:64 (August 1987).

106. Creighton H. Hospital guilty of racial discrimination. *Nurs Mgt*, 14:20–21 (March 1983).

107. Greenlaw J. A sexist judgment threatens all of nursing. *RN*, 45:69–70 (July 1982).

108. Regan W. Rape on hospital property: Now you can sue. *RN*, 6:69–70 (April 1983).

109. McGarity T. The new OSHA rules and the workers' right to know. *Hastings Center Rep*, 14:38–45 (August 1984).

110. Duldt B. Sexual harassment in nursing. *Nurs Outlook*, 30:336–343 (June 1982).

111. Beletz E, Meng M. The grievance procedure. *Am J Nurs*, 77:265 (February 1977).

112. Eisenhauer L, Cleland V. Is collective bargaining the solution? *Nurs Outlook*, 31:150–153 (May–June 1983).

113. Wolf G. Negotiating an employment contract. *Nurse Practitioner*, 5:55, 60 (January–February 1980).

114. Murphy E. Professional autonomy v. "at will" employee status. *Nurs Outlook*, 38:248 (September–October 1990).

115. Northrop C. Student nurses and legal accountabilities. *Imprint*, 32:16–20 (November 1985).

116. Niedringhaus L, O'Driscoll D. Staying within the law—Academic probation and dismissal. *Nurs Outlook*, 31:156–159 (May–June 1983).

117. Poteet G, Pollock C. When a student fails clinical. *Am J Nurs*, 81:1889–1890 (October 1981).

118. Creighton H. Right of nursing student to pursue higher degree. *Nurs Mgt*, 14:16–17 (December 1983).

119. Jones J. University liability in program advisement. *Nurs and Health Care*, 4:83–84 (February 1983).

120. Creighton H. Nursing school catalog is written contract. *Nurs Mgt*, 15:68–69 (February 1984).

121. Greenlaw J. *Mississippi University for Women v. Hogan:* The Supreme Court rules on female-only nursing school. *Law, Med, and Health Care*, 10:267–269 (December 1982).

122. Cahill L. "Abortion pill" RU 486: Ethics, rhetoric and social practice. *Hastings Center Rep*, 17:5–8 (October–November 1987).

123. Callahan D. How technology is reforming the abortion debate. *Hastings Center Rep,* 16:33–42 (February 1986).
124. Angell M. Euthanasia. *N Engl J Med,* 319:1348–1350 (November 17, 1988).
125. Risley R. *A humane and dignified death: A new law permitting physician aid-in-dying.* Glendale, CA: Americans Against Human Suffering, 1987.
126. Orentlicher D. Physician participation in assisted suicide. *J Am Med Soc,* 262:1844–1845 (Oct. 6, 1989).
127. Wanzer S, et al. The physicians' responsibility toward hopelessly ill patients: A second look. *N Engl J Med,* 320:844–849 (March 30, 1989).
128. Fuchs VR, Garber AM. The new technology assessment. *N Engl J Med,* 323:673–677 (September 6, 1990).

FROM STUDENT TO PRACTITIONER

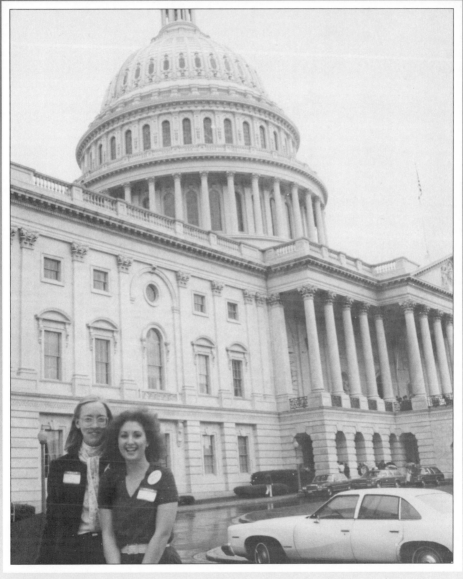

Students, as part of NSNA, visit Capitol Hill to speak with their legislators about support for nursing education. *(Courtesy of the National Student Nurses' Association.)*

CHAPTER 14

NURSING ORGANIZATIONS AND PUBLICATIONS

OBJECTIVES

After studying this chapter, you will be able to:

1. Identify key issues related to nursing organizations.
2. Identify the major activities and programs of ANA.
3. Identify the major activities and programs of NLN.
4. Discuss the key differences between ANA and NLN.
5. Discuss ways in which nursing organizations have sought unity in working together.
6. Identify some of the types of nursing organizations that currently exist.
7. Identify aspects of the nursing literature with which nurses should be familiar.

DIVERSITY AND DIFFERENCES

In 1952, when the six major nursing organizations decided to restructure, the ANA and NLN absorbed the activities of all but the American Association of Industrial Nurses, which stayed separate. The membership interests of most RNs were then focused on these two. (Students became part of the newly formed National Student Nurses' Association, NSNA.) In general, ANA was (and is) considered *the* professional organization, one that every RN can join and in which almost all can find an interest group to participate in. There are several major differences between ANA and NLN. ANA membership is limited to RNs, but NLN includes anyone interested in the purposes of the organization, as well as agency members (health care facilities and programs in nursing). ANA is a lobbying group and is also identified as a union by the NLRB. ANA, in its credentialing center, certifies certain clinical practitioners and nurse managers; it also has an accreditation program for CE programs. NLN is recognized for its accreditation of all kinds of nursing education programs and some health care agencies, primarily home health. Both make policy statements about health and nursing; they also overlap in their public statements about nursing education. Until the last few years, they seemed to cooperate in only a limited way, although often the nursing leaders belonged to both.

The first specialty organization, the American Association of Nurse Anesthetists, began in 1931. In the 1940s and 1950s several others were founded, but beginning in 1968, literally dozens of others were organized. They were usually splinter groups that broke off from ANA and formed their own association as the profession became more specialized. Later, still other organizations formed, as subspecialty groups or groups that felt that they had certain needs that could be best met by uniting with the like-minded. These included ethnic nurses, male nurses, nurses with a certain philosophy of care or social concerns, and gay nurses. Some grew rapidly and acquired staff and headquarters. Others almost literally functioned out of a member's home or office.

Often, nurses who switched membership said that ANA did not meet their needs, particularly after ANA directed more resources to its economic security program. Few held dual membership, either because they could not or would not spare the time or dues money. Special-interest groups seem to have several things in common: they state that they do not intend to get involved in the economic security concerns of their members, and their major concern is to provide a forum for sharing ideas, experiences, and problems related to a particular specialty or interest, including CE and standard setting. Most indicate that they plan to remain autonomous organizations.

COOPERATIVE EFFORTS

The proliferation of nursing organizations, although meeting the special needs of some nurses, has also caused some confusion among nurses, other health workers, and the public. Do these organizations speak for nursing in addition to ANA? In place of ANA? Members of the nursing organizations are also concerned. A lack of unity in common health care interests can hamper the achievement of goals. Therefore, in November 1972, ANA hosted a meeting of 10 specialty groups and NSNA to explore how the organizations could work toward more coordination in areas of common interest. It was found that concerns were similar and that such a meeting was generally considered long overdue.

In its second meeting, hosted by the American Association of Critical-Care Nurses (AACN), the participants accepted the importance of the specialty groups, at the same time recognizing the unique role of ANA. They agreed "in principle" to certain statements. In 1973, the group adopted a name: The Federation of Specialty Nursing Organizations and American Nurses' Association. There were 13 charter members.

Meetings were held on a semiannual basis in the following years, with the member organizations alternating as hosts, responsible for arranging and conducting the meeting and writing the minutes. The nursing press and auditors were permitted to attend meetings. The focus of the meetings was usually on current issues but was often related to CE accreditation procedures and certification, about which ANA and the other organizations seldom agreed. However, the Federation did support ANA on some issues.

In 1981, the title of the organization was changed to National Federation for Specialty Nursing Organizations (NFSNO), which more clearly defined the membership, not all of whom represented clinical specialties. By 1985 NFSNO had changed its requirements for membership, so that general organizations did not fit. ANA, which had been a charter member, moved from member to auditor status. ANA clinical practice councils were given the option to join. The purpose of NFSNO is now "to foster excellence in specialty nursing practice by providing a forum for communication and collaboration and to assume a leadership position in activities that contribute to specialty nursing practice." Regular members must fulfill criteria specifically related to specialty practice. Affiliate members, which must be national in scope and composed primarily of nurses, may enter into debate at NFSNO meetings, but they cannot make motions or vote. (See Appendix 5 for overview of major organizations.)

After years of debate. NFSNO has become a not-for-profit corporation. The mailing address is 875 Kings Highway, West Deptford, New Jersey 08096. Membership continues to grow.[1]

Another cooperative effort aimed at nurse specialists is the National Alliance of Nurse Practitioners (NANP), a coalition of nurse practitioner (NP) organizations formed in 1986. The purpose is to promote the health care of the nation by promoting the visibility, viability, and unity of NPs. Among its major concerns is gaining reimbursement for NP services. Currently, NANP represents some 30,000 NPs.[2] The address is P.O. Box 44707, L'Enfant Plaza SW, Washington, D.C. 20026.

ANA also made an effort to bring together the various nursing organizations. A change in the 1982 bylaws provided for the formation of a Nursing Organization Liaison Forum (NOLF) to promote unified action as an organization on professional and health policy issues. In December 1983, ANA invited 45 nursing organizations to Kansas City to explore the possibilities. The meeting was cordial, but the results were somewhat noncommittal. There was a question of whether NOLF and NFSNO would be duplicative efforts, although ANA indicated that NOLF would focus on broad issues. A particular deterrent to membership was that, since NOLF was an advisory body to ANA, there was no guarantee that any recommendations would be accepted as policy. Some organizations also objected to the fact that representatives had to be members of a state nurses' association (SNA). NOLF's activities and discussions are usually on the same issues as those of NFSNO, but membership is less limited. How they will coexist is still uncertain.

What does appear to be a successful cooperative effort was initiated when, at about the same time that the specialty groups first met, ANA and NLN developed closer working relationships with the relatively new American Association of Colleges of Nursing (AACN). Many of their mutual interests were in the area of federal legislation for health care. From these meetings came the Tri-Council, with the president and executive director of each meeting periodically. Joint policy statements were formulated, with joint action taken when considered appropriate. An example is the decision to support legislation for nursing education and research and to develop a national health plan. In 1985, the American Organization of Nurse Executives (AONE) became a member without a change in name.

Such collaborative activities among nursing organizations show a new maturity in nursing that recognizes the importance of joining together on major health issues. Cooperative action will enable nurses to be a stronger force in the planning and delivery of health care services.

AMERICAN NURSES' ASSOCIATION

The ANA was established in 1897 by a group of nurses who, even then, recognized the need for a membership association within which nurses could work together in concerted action. Its original name was the Nurses' Associated Alumnae of the United States and Canada, but in order to incorporate under the laws of the state of New York, it was necessary to drop the reference to another country in the organization's title. This was done in 1901; however, the name remained Nurses' Associated Alumnae of the

United States until 1911, when it became the American Nurses' Association. The Canadian nurses formed their own membership association.

History shows that ANA's primary concern has always been individual nurses and the public they serve. In its early years ANA worked hard for improved and uniform standards of nursing education, for registration and licensure of all nurses educated according to these standards, and for improvement of the welfare of nurses.[3] Similar efforts continue today.

Since its move to Washington, D.C. in early 1992, as mandated by its membership, ANA headquarters is 600 Maryland Avenue, S.W., Washington, D.C. 20005.

Membership

Members of ANA are the 50 (SNAs) and 3 territorial constituent units. SNAs are made up of district nurses' associations (DNAs). At one time the individual nurse was a member of ANA, but with the adoption of a federation model at the 1982 House of Delegates, the constituent SNA is the member, and individuals join the SNA. SNAs thought that this would give them more power and more opportunity to recruit members independently of ANA, since now nurses no longer need to belong to district, state, and national levels. However, this has not changed the cost, since membership dues are assessed by ANA based on the number of members in a constituent SNA. Members pay SNA dues that include the ANA assessment and DNA dues if they choose to belong to the latter.

Whether or not this reorganization has helped ANA membership is not clear. Only a small percentage of all working nurses belong to ANA. Some belong to specialty or special interest organizations, others to none. Why? Cost may be a factor; dues are more than $150 in most states, considerably more than for other organizations. Some nurses choose to belong to labor unions (where dues are quite high) and find SNA membership a conflict of interest since most SNAs do collective bargaining. Some nurse managers do not belong because they oppose collective bargaining. However, an increasing number of SNA members are part of a collective bargaining unit; membership increase has been primarily from this source. Some nurses are simply not interested in nursing issues and don't know why it is important to be represented in legislation or other policy making. And, of course, others disagree with ANA positions, such as entry into practice.

General Organization

The House of Delegates, which meets yearly, with full conventions in even years, is the policymaking body of ANA. Delegates are elected by each state. Between conventions, decisions based on House policies are made by the board of directors, which has been elected by the House. The board consists of 15 members, including the officers (president, first and second vice president, secretary, and treasurer). Terms are staggered to prevent a complete turnover at any one time and to provide continuity of programs and action.

The ANA staff has a largely RN professional staff, with supporting clerical and secretarial staff. They carry out the day-to-day activities based on policies adopted by the House and ANA's general functions. The executive director, a nurse, is the chief administrative officer and works closely with the board and SNAs.

Like other large organizations, ANA has its *standing committees,* those that are written into the bylaws and that continue from year to year to assist with specific continuing programs and functions of the association. *Special committees* and *task forces* of the House or board are appointed on an ad hoc basis to accomplish special purposes.

Between 1982 and 1990, several other entities were created. A *congress* is an organized, deliberative body that focuses on long-range policy development essential to the mission of the association. There is a *Congress on Nursing Economics* and a *Congress of Nursing Practice,* which came into effect after the 1990 convention. Congresses are accountable to the board of directors and report to the ANA House of Delegates.

According to the bylaws, the major responsibilities of the Congresses are to:

- develop long-range policy essential to the mission of the association.
- establish a plan of operation for carrying out its responsibilities.
- develop and adopt standards.
- develop and evaluate programs.
- address and respond to concerns related to equal opportunity and human rights, ethics, and to nursing education, research, and services.
- recommend policies and positions to the board of directors and the ANA House of Delegates.
- evaluate trends, developments, and issues.

In 1990, the House of Delegates established an *Institute of Constituent Members on Nursing Practice,* which reports directly to the Congress of Nursing Practice. It consists of one representative from each SNA, also called *constituent member (CM).*

The *Institute of Constituent Member Collective Bargaining Programs* was put into place in 1990. It consists of one elected representative from each CM with a collective bargaining program and is autonomous in respect to the development of operational standards, positions, policies, practices, and all other matters related to CM collective bargaining programs. More details about the institutes can be found in the ANA bylaws.[4]

The *Commission on Economic and Professional Security* is an organized,

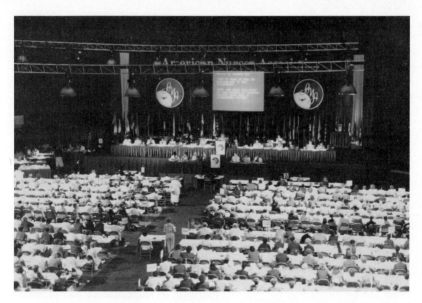

The ANA House of Delegates meets yearly to debate and vote on important issues. (*Courtesy of the American Nurses' Association.*)

deliberative body to which the Congress on Nursing Economics assigns specific responsibilities related to the economic and professional security of individual nurses or groups of nurses. Its major responsibilities are to:

- evaluate trends, developments, and issues related to the economic and professional security of individual nurses or groups of nurses.
- develop standards, positions, and policies for recommendation to the Congress on Nursing Economics.

Councils have a clinical or functional focus and are established by the board. In 1991, they included the Council of Community Health Nurses, Council on Continuing Education, Council on Cultural Diversity in Nursing Practice, Council on Gerontological Nursing, Council on Maternal/Child Nursing, Council on Medical-Surgical Nursing Practice, Council of Nurse Researchers, Council on Nursing Administration, Council of Nurses in Advanced Practice, Council on Psychiatric and Mental Health Nursing, and Council on Computer Applications in Nursing. Their primary purpose relates to providing "a forum for discussion; continuing education; consultation; and promoting adherence to approved standards of nursing through certification and other appropriate means."

The *Constituent Assembly* is made up of the president and chief administrative officer of each CM or their designees. The purpose is to discuss nursing affairs of concern to ANA, CMs, and the profession. *The Nursing Organization Liaison Forum* (NOLF), mentioned earlier, is made up of duly authorized representatives of ANA and other nursing organizations, who meet for the purpose of discussing issues of concern to the profession and promoting concerted action on them.

American Academy of Nursing

A significant action taken by the 1966 House of Delegates was the creation of the American Academy of Nursing (AAN) to provide for recognition of professional achievement and excellence. It was established in 1973. The members, designated as Fellows of the American Academy of Nursing, are entitled to use the initials FAAN following their names. They are selected on the basis of their outstanding contributions to nursing and their potential for continued contributions.[5] Since 1973, the Academy has held a yearly Scientific Session combined with business meetings. Major activities have been the Magnet Hospital Study, described in Appendix 1, the Teaching Nursing Home program,[6] and the Nursing Faculty Practice Symposia to showcase and discuss effective concepts of nursing faculty practice.

The American Nurses' Foundation

The American Nurses' Foundation (ANF) was created by ANA in 1955 to meet the need for an independent, permanent, nonprofit organization devoted to nursing research. The tax-exempt foundation was organized exclusively for charitable, scientific, literary, and educational purposes.

ANF has a Competitive Extramural Grants Program, funded through the contributions of both corporations and individuals, that provides small grants to nurse researchers. In 1983, in collaboration with ANA and AAN, the ANF Distinguished Scholar Program was established. It also administers various study projects and awards.[7] ANF is governed by its bylaws and directed by a nine-member board of trustees. All trustees are RNs. The executive director of ANA is part-time executive director of ANF. There is also a professional headquarters staff involved in carrying out certain research projects. ANF headquarters is the same as ANA.

Major Programs and Services

The programs and services of ANA represent the efforts of members and staff, elected officers, committees, forums, cabinets, and councils. These include meeting with members of other groups and disciplines; planning or attending institutes, workshops, conventions, or committee meetings; developing and writing brochures, manuals, position papers, standards, or testimony to be presented to Congress; and implementing ongoing programs, planning new ones, or trying to solve the problem of how to serve the members best within the limitations of the budget. Every issue of the *American Journal of Nursing* and *The American Nurse* carries reports of these many and varied activities. Presented here are brief descriptions of some (but not all) of the major ANA programs and services.

Certification

Probably the most exciting development in recent years is the ANA certification program. Certification, based on assessment of knowledge, demonstration of current clinical practice (except for administration), and endorsement of colleagues, is a tangible acknowledgement of achievement in a specific area of nursing practice. By 1991 certification examinations were being offered in 21 specialty areas: adult NP, clinical specialist in adult psychiatric and mental health nursing; clinical specialist in child and adolescent psychiatric and mental health nursing; clinical specialist in medical-surgical nursing, in gerontological nursing, and in community health nursing; family NP; college health nursing, gerontological nurse; gerontological NP; medical-surgical nursing; pediatric nurse; perinatal nurse; pediatric NP; psychiatric and mental health nurse; community health nurse; school nurse; school NP; and two levels of nursing administration. There is also an exam in general nursing practice. More programs are planned.

Criteria for certification vary to some extent for the various specialties but may include an examination and evaluation of specified documents submitted by the nurse such as pilot studies, projects, case studies, abstracts representing the candidate's case load, other evidence of continuing growth as a practitioner, statement of a philosophy of practice, references, and biographical data, and a master's for specialist certification. In 1991, the House of Delegates approved a policy requiring the baccalaureate for all *generalist* certification by 1998. Those certified before that time are not affected. Currency in practice beyond the requirements of licensure must always be shown, and the candidate must be licensed in the United States. Past practice experience is no longer required. (There must have been a practice component in the program of study.) Specific details on each certification, including eligibility criteria and cost, are available from ANA. Certification is granted for five years, at the end of which time the individual has the option of submitting evidence and credentials for renewal. As of 1991, over 80,000 nurses had been certified by ANA.

Since 1979, ANA and some of the specialty nursing organizations have been making efforts to cooperate in the certification process. Because certification is intended as a protection of the public, certification of the same type by thirty organizations is confusing. Various alternatives include joint sponsorship of a certification process or endorsement of each other's certification.

Nursing Education

The important ANA function of setting standards and policies for nursing education has been demonstrated in many ways. The 1965 Position Paper was the beginning of a series of specific actions toward implementing the position that education for entry into professional nursing practice should be at the baccalaureate level. (See Chapters 2 and 5.) ANA has made a number of other important educational statements in the last few years; these are available from ANA.

Since 1975, the association has provided a mechanism for voluntary national accreditation of CE in nursing. Through the National Accreditation Board, regional accreditation is granted to various providers of CE in nursing, as well as to specific CE programs and offerings.

Nursing Service and Practice

ANA works continually and in many ways to improve the quality of nursing care available to the public. In its role as the professional association for RNs, it defines and interprets principles and standards of nursing practice. (The first revision since 1973 was developed by the Congress of Nursing Practice in 1991.) These publications are available from ANA, as are the major papers and/or proceedings of conferences and workshops that assist nurses to use the standards, both in general and in specialty nursing practice.

The formation of the Council of Nurse Administrators, increased the ability of ANA to serve the needs of this key group. (Because of ANA's involvement in collective bargaining through the SNAs, some nurse administrators have felt a conflict of interest and have chosen to belong to the NLN or AHA administrator groups.) In 1979, a two-level certification program for nurse administrators was initiated—one for those at the executive level and the other for those in middle management nursing positions.

Legislation and Legal Activities

ANA's legislative program is an important one that often affects, directly and indirectly, the welfare of both nurses and the public (see Chapter 10). ANA's legislative program has three main purposes: (1) to help CMs promote effective nursing practice acts in their states in order to protect the public and the nursing profession from unqualified practitioners; (2) to offer consultation on other legislative and regulatory measures that affect nurses; and

(3) to speak for nursing in relation to federal legislation for health, education, labor, and welfare, and for social programs such as civil rights.

The major responsibility for coordinating legislative information and action lies with the ANA's governmental affairs arm. The Washington staff's responsibilities include lobbying (through its registered lobbyists); development of relationships with congressional members and their staffs and committee staffs; contacts with key figures in the administrative branch of government; maintaining relations with other national organizations; preparing most of the statements and information presented to congressional committees; drafting letters to government officials; presenting testimony; acting as backup for members presenting testimony; and representing ANA in many capacities. Major newspapers and journals have commented on nursing's clout.

Over the years, ANA has represented nursing in the capital on a number of major issues: funds for nursing education, Social Security amendments to cover nurses, national health insurance, quality of care in nursing homes, collective bargaining rights, health hazards, civil rights, Federal Trade Commission authority and regulations, problems of nurses in the federal service, tax revision, higher education, problems of health manpower, prospective reimbursement, and general support for improvement of health care. In addition, ANA lobbies for or against legislation that may affect nursing directly and immediately, such as funding for nursing education, collective bargaining, and reimbursement for nurses. For instance, ANA has always monitored the status of the Nursing Education Act (NEA), which has funded so much of nursing education and research.

ANA has often cooperated and coordinated with other health disciplines, but has also faced areas of disagreement (such as early opposition of AMA and other groups to funding for nurse education). Such philosophical differences still occur, but there has been increasing cooperation with both health and other groups to achieve mutual legislative goals.

Communication about legislative matters is particularly important to help members keep abreast of key legislative issues. Prepared monthly by the legislative staff as a regular part of *The American Nurse,* are various articles that highlight major legislative and related developments. A monthly newsletter *Capital Update,* is sent to over 2000 individuals and groups, including SNAs.

Legislative information is also provided in the *American Journal of Nursing,* and special communications are sent out from the Washington office when membership support is needed for legislative programs. CMs have a vital role in providing information and assistance to members on pertinent legislative issues, and when funds allow, there is often a legislative staff, a lobbyist, and perhaps a separate legislative newsletter at the state level.

In addition to specific legislative action, ANA becomes involved in various legal matters that affect the welfare of nurses. In some cases, ANA acts as a friend of the court, providing information about the issues involved. Since 1973, ANA has filed charges of discrimination in various district offices of the Equal Employment Opportunity Commission (EEOC), some of which it won and some of which are still unsettled. ANA has also presented oral arguments and briefs on various NLRB hearings. The attorneys of CMs also become involved in collective bargaining litigation or, at times, provide support for NPs cited by a medical board for practice of medicine without a license. The number of such services that ANA offers expands yearly.

ANA-PAC, formerly called *N-CAP* (*Coalition for Action in Politics*), is the ANA-related political action group, founded in 1974.[8] Most professional organizations have such groups, which are independent of the organization but related to it. This is because a tax-exempt, incorporated professional organization such as ANA (or AMA) is under definite legal constraints as far as partisan political action is concerned. ANA-PAC operates by providing financial support for candidates and engaging in other political activities, as well as providing political education to nurses. Support may be in the form of endorsement or may include monetary contributions. Endorsements are made in consultation with state PACs whenever possible. State political action coalitions endorse state candidates. To support these activities, ANA-PAC accepts donations from nurses and others. It is headquartered at ANA's new Washington Office.

Economic and General Welfare

The ways in which ANA has worked to promote the welfare of its membership have varied with the times. Although ANA does not serve as bargaining agent for groups of nurses, many SNAs do. ANA helps to develop the principles and techniques for such employer-employee negotiations and advises and assists the SNAs with their economic security activities as much as possible. In addition, a major role of the ANA and the Congress on Nursing Economics (or its related groups) on the national level is to develop policy positions, act as a clearinghouse for information, and take legal actions as appropriate.

The ANA economic security program is often misunderstood by members, nonmembers, and others. Seeing that the economic security of its members is maintained is one of the classic roles of a professional association, and, especially in recent years, economic security has been seen as extending beyond purely monetary matters and conditions of employment to involvement of nurses in the decision-making aspects of nursing care. An example might be that, through an agreed-upon process, perhaps including a formal committee structure, nurses' objections to inadequate staffing or illegal or inappropriate job assignments would be instrumental in bringing about changes that would provide improved care.

In the last few years, the nurse's right to adequate monetary compensation has been recognized almost universally, although in many places, salaries and benefits are still abysmal, and there is still a struggle involved for improvement, with or without CM representation as a bargaining agent. However, there is still employer resistance to allowing nurses a voice in policymaking, both because of the possible financial impact and because of fear of loss of control, as well as on the basis of general philosophic disagreement.

In the years following the 1974 NLRA amendments (see Chapter 10), which allowed employees of nonprofit health care institutions to do collective bargaining, ANA and SNAs were frequently involved in legal actions regarding various aspects of collective bargaining that are unique to nursing: whether nurses could be in separate units, the status of head nurses and supervisors as management, and whether the fact that supervisors and directors of nursing may sit on the board of directors of an SNA means that the collective bargaining agent (the SNA) is controlled by management. Decisions favoring unions have been fluctuating in the last few years as unions have lost ground; this also affects ANA. Such cases are not settled with one ruling, and frequently further action is taken through appeal mechanisms or legislation. One major victory was a 1991 decision by the U.S. Supreme Court to allow nurses to organize in separate (all-RN) bargaining units. The NLRB had made such a ruling, but a suit by AHA had enjoined the NLRB from implementing it.[9] In the same year, President Bush signed legislation restoring collective bargaining rights to health care professionals in VA facilities. Litigation on key issues can be long and expensive, but the carefully structured process of forming a unit also takes knowledge, effort, and sometimes legal consultation. This is described in Chapter 13. Because ANA recognizes that other employed groups also have the right to organize, guidelines have been developed in the event of a dispute between the employer and these groups.

Unions, which have been successful in organizing nonprofessional health workers and a number of professionals, have been giving priority to organizing nurses. There is serious concern that large unions with strong economic backing and single-purpose goals to increase monetary and working benefits may prove competitive, for nurses frequently do not see the professional organization as a strong or even appropriate bargaining agent. Because past experience has shown that unions have taken little action to negotiate contracts involving nurses in decisions that could improve patient care, and because many nurses are not even aware that such participation is possible, one of the most worthwhile purposes of collective bargaining could be lost. Currently, ANA finds itself competing with several powerful unions. Nevertheless, in 1990, ANA represented approximately 139,000 RNs in over 800 bargaining units in 27 states.

Human Rights Activities

ANA works to integrate qualified members of all racial and ethnic groups into the nursing profession and tries to achieve sound human rights practices. Among its activities are human rights conferences and the publication of bibliographies and monographs on historical and contemporary minority/ethnic nursing leaders. In 1974, ANA was awarded a six-year grant by the Center for Minority Group Mental Health Programs of the National Institutes of Mental Health to establish and administer the Registered Nurse Fellowship Program for Ethnic/Racial Minorities. The program was refunded and has continued to support a number of minority nurses in doctoral study in psychiatric mental health nursing or a related behavioral or social science. Later, a clinical fellowship program was awarded, and it, too, educates minority nurses in doctoral work as clinicians in mental health nursing.

ANA's human rights activities, which had been under the aegis of a commission, are now the focus of a newly created staff structure, the Center for Ethics and Human Rights.

Research and Studies

ANA has always been involved in various types of research or data-gathering activities, although funding cuts periodically limit what can be done. However, the staff continually collects data about nurses, nursing, and nursing resources. One result of this effort is *Facts About Nursing,* published periodically, a statistical summary of information about nurses, nursing, and related health services and groups. ANA is also the recipient of contracts to carry out specific programs or projects.

Other Activities and Services

Among other ANA benefits for nurses is insurance of various kinds, available at favorable group rates at national and state levels. A new benefit is a very inexpensive placement center. Many educational programs, seminars, workshops, clinical conferences, scientific sessions, international nursing tours, and so on are available at all levels at reduced rates for SNA members. They are geared to current issues and new developments in health and nursing. Nurses are also becoming increasingly interested in international nursing. ANA was one of the three charter members of the ICN and is an active participant in the work of this international nursing organization.

Cooperation and coordination with other groups is an important part of the function of ANA. Conferences, programs, workshops, task forces, and other meetings to share information and learning or work on mutual problems are ongoing with other nursing, medical, and health organizations, hospital and health professional groups, and many others.[10]

ANA produces many publications, including *The American Nurse* and *Facts About Nursing*; major reports, its *Reports to the ANA House of Delegates* and *Summary Convention Proceedings*; papers presented at meetings; and certain publications of the AAN and ANF. It also publishes position statements, guidelines for practice, bulletins, manuals, and brochures for specialized groups within the organization and sends out news releases and announcements concerning activities of interest to the public. Available from the ANA upon request is its periodically revised *Publications*.

The Individual Nurse and ANA

A classic article by sociologist Robert Merton lists the functions of any professional organization as including social and moral support for individual practitioners to help them perform their role as professionals, to set rigorous standards for the profession and help enforce them, to advance and disseminate research and professional knowledge, to help furnish the social bonds through which society coheres, and to speak for the profession. In carrying out some of these functions, the association is seen as a "kind of organizational gadfly, stinging the profession into new and more demanding formulations of purpose."[11]

Not all members agree with their organization's goals. However, the key to the success of any organization is the participation of its actual and potential members. Even though ANA has only a small percentage of working nurses, it is still the largest nursing organization (Sigma Theta Tau is second in membership). ANA speaks for nurses; nonmembers have no part in that organization and have no right to complain if it does not represent them. The strength in the organization and in nursing lies in thinking, communicating nurses committed to the goal of improving nursing care for the public and working together in an organized fashion to achieve this goal.

INTERNATIONAL COUNCIL OF NURSES

Nursing claims the distinction of having the oldest international association of professional women, the International Council of Nurses (ICN). Antedating by many years the international hospital and medical associations, ICN is the largest international organization primarily made up of professional women in the world. (There are, of course, men in ICN member organizations.) The originator and prime mover of ICN was a distinguished and energetic English nurse, Ethel Gordon Fenwick (Mrs. Bedford Fenwick), who first proposed the idea of an international nursing organization in July 1899.

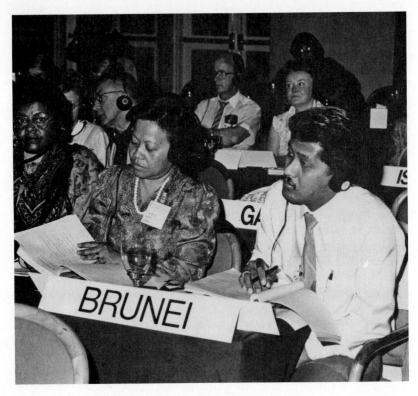

The ICN quadrennial Congress brings together nurses from around the world. (*Courtesy of the American Nurses' Association.*)

ICN today is still a federation of national nurses' associations worldwide. The requirements for membership have been, essentially, that the national association be an autonomous, self-directing, and self-governing body, nonpolitical, nonsectarian, with no form of racial discrimination, whose voting membership is composed exclusively of nurses and is broadly representative of the nurses in that country. Its objectives must be in harmony with ICN's stated objective: to provide a medium through which national nurses' associations may share their common interests, working together to develop the contribution of nursing to the promotion of the health of people and the care of the sick. A majority vote by the ICN's governing body determines the admission of national associations into membership.

Organization

The governing body of ICN, according to a new constitution adopted in 1965, is the Council of National Representatives (CNR), consisting of the presidents of the member associations (104 in 1991). This group, including ICN's board of directors, meets at least every two years to establish ICN policies. Assisting the ICN executive staff, standing committees, and board in their work is an Expert Advisory Panel of nurses expert in various fields of nursing, as well as persons expert in other appropriate fields.[12]

Carrying out ICN's day-to-day activities is its headquarters staff—a group of professional nurses, including ICN's executive director, currently an American nurse. These nurses represent ICN's executive staff, but in their relationships with and services to the member associations, they serve in an advisory and consultative capacity. Staff members are selected from various member countries.

ICN Congresses

Once every four years, the ICN holds its Quadrennial Congress: a meeting of the members of the national nurses' associations in membership with ICN. Nursing students are usually eligible to attend ICN congresses, too, if they are sponsored, and their applications are processed, by their national nurses' association. Students have been meeting as a Student Assembly during the congresses.

During the last several congresses, discussions and resolutions ranged from those focusing specifically on nursing issues to general social concerns. Included, for instance, were career ladders, socioeconomic welfare, educational and practice standards, research, autonomy, the nurse's role in safeguarding human rights, the nurse's role in the care of detainees and prisoners, and nurse participation in national health policy planning and decision making. Related to general health care were such topics as primary care, excision and circumcision of females, increased violence against patients and health personnel, the uncontrolled proliferation of ancillary nursing personnel, environment quality, care for the elderly, and affirmation of the World Health Organization's (WHO's) "Health for all by the year 2000" (HFA/2000) theme. On an even broader scale were the concerns about refugees and displaced persons, nuclear war, poverty, and the status of women.

The activities at ICN congresses are usually reported in the *American Journal of Nursing* (*AJN*) and other nursing journals, including *International Nursing Review*.

Functions and Activities

From the very beginning, ICN has been concerned with three main areas: nursing education, nursing service, and nurses' social and economic welfare. Whenever possible, ICN has sought common denominators in education and practice throughout the world. One such common denominator, for instance, is the international Code of Ethics adopted by ICN and equally applicable to nurses in every country. At the same time, ICN has always recognized the autonomy of its member associations and the principle that each country will develop the systems of education and practice best suited to its individual culture and needs.[13]

In 1983, CNR adopted a blueprint for the long-term future. Fulfilling these objectives will require the same innovative and challenging spirit shown by the founders of ICN. There are clear financial problems with which ICN must cope, reflecting perhaps the financial problems of each country's association, and there are disagreements about policy. However, the blueprint is a good example of cooperative thinking and goal setting, and it is still being worked on.

In the last several years, ICN has added to its accomplishments:

1. Developed definitions of nursing and nursing research.
2. Developed working definitions of *nurse, nursing auxiliary,* and *specialist nurse.*
3. Joined with WHO in developing *WHO/ICN Guidelines for Nursing Management of People Infected with Human Immunodeficiency Virus HIV.*[14]
4. Prepared a statement on torture.
5. Published a book entitled *Nursing and Primary Health Care: A Unified Force.*
6. Accepted a major position paper on regulation.

At the 1989 Congress in Seoul, Korea, ICN celebrated its 90th anniversary and introduced a new book, *ICN: Past and Present,* that brings the history of ICN up-to-date. ICN's history has indeed been illustrious; with its many member countries and close ties with WHO,[15] it has helped to change the health care of the world.

ICN headquarters is located at 3 Place Jean Marteau, 1201, Geneva, Switzerland (mailing address: P.O. Box 42, CH-1201 Geneva 20, Switzerland).

NATIONAL LEAGUE FOR NURSING

The National League for Nursing (usually referred to an NLN or the League) was the first nursing organization in the United States. Established in 1893 under the title of the American Society of Superintendents of Training Schools for Nurses of the United States and Canada, it became the National League of Nursing Education in 1912. Its purpose was to standardize and improve the education of nurses. Originally for nurses only, it broadened its membership policies in 1943 to admit lay members.

In 1989, NLN revised its mission statement as follows:

> The National League for Nursing advances the promotion of health and the provision of quality health care within a changing health care environment by promoting and monitoring effective nursing education and practice through collaborative efforts of nursing leaders, representatives of relevant agencies, and the general public.

As in the past, there remain two major classes of membership within NLN, individual and agency. Individual membership is open to anyone interested in fostering the development and improvement of nursing service, education, and health care. Individual members are eligible to vote in the League's national affairs, constituent (state) league activities, and specialty council elections. Agency membership is for organizations or groups providing various nursing services and for the various schools conducting educational programs in nursing. In 1989, agency membership expanded into two subdivisions, category 1 and category 2. Category 1 membership entitles an agency to 10 votes; category 2, 5 votes. Membership dues and available services vary within each category. There is another category of agency membership (allied) for agencies interested in the work of the NLN but not qualifying within the preceding categories. These agencies do not have voting power.

Individual members join NLN and one of the 48 constituent leagues in the area in which they live or work. If there is no league in that area, they may join NLN directly at the national level. Annual dues for each individual combine the national and constituent league dues. Agency members join NLN directly. As was the case with agency membership, individual membership also underwent restructuring in 1989. Now individual membership includes three avenues for influence and activity: at the national level, within a more local constituent league, and within a council focused on a more particular concern. Individual members may also belong to any number of these membership councils.

General Plan of Organization

Both individual and agency members are concerned with the "further development and improvement of nursing services, education, and the achievement of comprehensive health care." The groups approach the task through membership opportunities in various NLN councils. At NLN business sessions held at the biennial conventions, decisions are made by the individual and agency members present, provided that there are enough to meet the League's quorum requirements.

Membership Councils

Through 11 councils, agency and individual members may influence the policies of the NLN, receive information, attend programs, participate on committees, present ideas, and vote.

The four educational councils are:

1. Council of Associate Degree Programs (CADP).
2. Council of Baccalaureate and Higher Degree Programs (CBHDP).
3. Council of Diploma Programs (CDP).
4. Council of Practical Nursing Programs (CPNP).

The practice and multidisciplinary councils provide opportunities for participants to play key roles in shaping nursing practice and its relationship to nursing education. These are:

1. Council of Community Health Services (CCHS).
2. Council for Nurse Executives (CNE).
3. Council for Nursing Informatics (CNI).
4. Council for Nursing Centers (CNC).
5. Council for Nursing Practice (CNP).
6. Council for the Society for Research in Nursing Education (CSRNE).
7. Council of Constituent Leagues for Nursing (CCLN).

Each council works within its own readily identifiable field of interest, but there are certain activities in which all engage. All are expected to facilitate collaboration among councils and non-NLN groups, ensure consumer involvement in council activities, and develop goals that are not only relevant to individual council activity but are also congruent with those of the NLN. Workshops and programs are held regionally and nationally. The four education councils also have accreditation as part of their programs. Council committees vary according to each council's needs.

Board of Governors, Officers, Committees

The 1989 organizational restructuring process has resulted in a streamlined version of the NLN governing body. Previously known as the *Board of Directors,* the new 18-member NLN Board of Governors consists of three elected officers (president, president elect, and treasurer), the membership council chairs, three governors at large, and the executive director of NLN, who serves as secretary but is not a voting member.

Balloting for national offices is done by mail, with both individuals and agency members entitled to vote. All of these offices and elected positions are open to both nurse and nonnurse NLN members.

Business sessions of the individual councils are held at annual meetings, and the full organization membership meets at a biennial convention. Decisions are made by the individual and agency members present. Each individual membership means one vote, and each member agency has 5 or 10 votes, depending on its membership category.

The NLN has two types of committees, standing and special, which may be elected or appointed. The composition and methods of election or appointment and the term of office of committees are spelled out in the bylaws. The Committee on Nominations is currently the only elected committee of the overall organization. In the appointed category are three standing committees: the Committee on Constitutions and Bylaws, the Committee on Finance, and the Committee on Accreditation. From time to time the League appoints other special committees to deal with matters of general, and often continuing, concern to the organization as a whole.

Services and Programs

More or less permanent components within the League are a variety of services and programs carried out through its organized staff divisions. Among these are CE programs related to issues in education and service, accreditation, and research.

Division of Education and Accreditation

The NLN accrediting service has been a stimulant to the improvement of nursing education since it began in 1949 under the name of the National Nursing Accrediting Service. In nursing education, it is a service that reviews and evaluates nursing education programs of various types such as those preparing PNs, diploma, AD, and baccalaureate degree programs for RNs; and programs leading to a graduate degree in nursing. Those meeting NLN criteria within each category are granted NLN accreditation.

The published criteria for evaluation of each type of program, set by the appropriate council, are basic guides, as is the booklet on policies and procedures of accreditation. Most schools conduct a thorough evaluation of all aspects of their program through committees of faculty and students, use of studies, and review of other data. The results of the evaluation are incorporated in a self-evaluation report, which is sent to NLN (previously notified as to the program's intent to seek evaluation). NLN accreditation is a peer evaluation, and the visitors are faculty and/or faculty administrators of like programs, who have been selected for and specially trained by NLN to review programs. They come to the program to amplify, verify, and clarify the data and explore ramifications of the self-study. Both reports are then studied by a peer member board of review. There is a process of appeal if the Board's decision is not acceptable to the school, and, of course, the opportunity to correct the deficiencies and reapply for accreditation. In recent years, there has been greater flexibility in the acceptance of ways to meet accreditation standards, so that programs of greatly varying educational approaches are being accredited. The common denominator is quality. Increasingly, NLN accreditation is sought and worked toward, because of the significance of this accreditation to the prospective student, the faculty member, and the community. In addition, only NLN-accredited schools are eligible for the nursing education funds made available through the Nurse Training Act of 1964 and later amendments. NLN is officially recognized by the Council on Post-Secondary Accreditation and the U.S. Department of Education as the accrediting agency for master's, baccalaureate, AD, diploma, and PN programs.[16]

Each year, a list of NLN-accredited programs of nursing is published in the NLN journal. There are also pamphlets issued listing all state-approved and accredited nursing programs. By 1991, more than 1550 educational programs held NLN accreditation; over 75 percent of the total of basic RN programs were accredited by the League.

NLN Consultation Network

NLN's newly expanded consultation network offers a wide range of consultation services through a cadre of experts in the fields of nursing education, practice, research, testing and evaluation, and communication/video. Traditionally, nursing schools have utilized NLN consultation services for help with their educational programs. Recent developments in the health care arena, such as spiraling costs and personnel shortages, have increased the demand for assistance from individuals, hospitals, and community health services.

Division of Testing and Evaluation

NLN conducts one of the largest professional testing services in the country. Test batteries have been developed by NLN using experts in tests and educational measurements and in nursing. The tests available through NLN fall into several categories; guidance and placement of students for schools of professional and practical nursing, achievement of professional and practical nursing students while in nursing school, the preimmigration screening examination and nursing tests prepared for the Commission of Graduates of Foreign Nursing Schools, tests designed for nurse practice settings, and certification tests for nursing specialties. The League's testing services are offered on a voluntary basis; no school or state is required to use them. The tests undergo continual evaluation and revision to maintain their validity and ensure appropriateness of content.

Division of Communications

The NLN distributes a wide variety of informative materials. Some of this information is promotional, explaining the nature and purpose of the League, at the same time providing the public with a glimpse of the League's newest products. Other publications are statistical or highly factual, such as school directories and lists of accredited schools of nursing. The bulk of NLN publications are references and texts, written by leading nursing and health care authorities on topics such as administration and management, career guidance, community health care, curriculum, ethics, public policy, research, theory, and long-term care. In addition, videotapes are available on a wide range of subject matters pertinent to the health care arena, with a growing segment developed for the general public.

Each year NLN issues a publications catalog that is available on request from its headquarters office and is also sent to all members. The official journal, *Nursing and Health Care,* is published 10 times a year. A subscription to this journal is included with NLN membership. Periodic bulletins help members keep informed of current federal and state legislation, important health care issues, and League positions on major issues.

Division of Research

Activities of the Division of Research include data collection (as well as development of the data-gathering instruments), research studies, and special projects. Annually, for instance, NLN collects information on admissions, graduations, and enrollments in programs of practical and professional nursing education. Aspects of these data are reported in various NLN publications. The *NLN Nursing Data Review* is a compilation of statistical information on nursing education and newly licensed nurses. Also published are booklets and directories on state-approved programs preparing students for licensure as RNs or LPNs. The directories indicate types of programs, accreditation status, administrative control, financial support, and data on admissions, enrollments, and graduation. The Nursing Student Census and a Nurse-Faculty Census are also published.

NLN, as need and resources permit, surveys or studies other selected aspects of nursing education or nursing service programs. In addition, it carries on both short-term and long-term research projects. Some of these projects are financed by the League itself; some are financed through grants from other agencies. (NLN, unlike ANA, enjoys tax-exempt status, and funds granted to it are not considered taxable income.)

Other Services and Activities

Because of its tax-exempt status as an educational and charitable organization, the League (and its constituent leagues) is prohibited from participating in any political campaign on behalf of or in opposition to any particular candidate, and no substantial part of its activities may consist of influencing legislation. However, this prohibition does not extend to dealing with administrative agencies or the executive branch of the government. The League is also permitted to inform members fully of proposed legislation, engage in nonpartisan analysis or study and disseminate results, and give factual testimony and information. Preferably these presentations are made on request of the legislators. Within this framework, NLN has been involved in legislation affecting nursing and has been helpful in its implementation. NLN works closely with ANA, AACN, and AONE (especially as part of the Tri-Council) on these and other issues. However, throughout its entire program, NLN also maintains active liaison with many other national agencies, both governmental and voluntary.

In 1973, the NLN chose the National Library of Medicine in Bethesda, Maryland, home of the world's largest collection of health sciences literature, as the official repository of NLN's historical documents and records. These include the history of NLN, old photographs of American nurses, correspondence by Florence Nightingale and other nursing leaders, and the history of NOPHN.

The impact of NLN on nursing does not lie only in the services and activities of the organization and its component groups. It is equally important to look at some of the major pronouncements made by NLN in taking stands on nursing issues. Many are on education and practice. These were discussed earlier. Other position papers are on a national health plan and on nursing's responsibility to minorities and disadvantaged groups.

NATIONAL LEAGUE FOR HEALTH CARE

Over the course of several years, the National League for Nursing, through its Long Range Planning Committee, investigated how to best approach an organizational restructuring. It became apparent that a more flexible structure was needed to accommodate the growth and diversity of activities of the League. A proposal of restructuring was fashioned along those lines in the spring of 1987.

The formation of the National League for Health Care (NLHC, Inc.) as a parent organization was recommended to provide a structure that could easily adapt as new ventures and possibilities presented themselves. The NLN Board endorsed this recommendation during the 1989 biennium, when it voted to establish NLHC, Inc. NLHC provides support and coordination of the activities of its subsidiaries, NLN and the Community Health Accreditation Program (CHAP).

In 1987, CHAP became a fully independent subsidiary of the NLN. CHAP's purpose is to employ accreditation to elevate the quality of home care in this country and to counter public fears about a quality crisis in this increasingly crucial health care arena. CHAP accreditation certifies to the public that CHAP-accredited organizations have voluntarily met the highest standards for home care and community health care in the nation. Agencies seeking CHAP accreditation perform an extensive self-study, which is submitted to CHAP offices for preliminary analysis of specific areas. A site visit is then performed by visitors selected to ensure a range of expertise, including both management and service delivery areas, who come from an agency similar to that of the applicant organization. Site-visit findings along with the agency's self-report are then studied by a peer-member board of review. There is a process of appeal if the Board's decision is not acceptable to the agency. Organizations are accredited for a three-year cycle, during which additional site visits occur, focusing on specific standards. In 1991, DHHS granted CHAP *deemed status,* meaning that CHAP is given authority to determine whether home health agencies are eligible for Medicare reimbursement.

The NLN headquarters is located at 350 Hudson Street, New York, New York 10014.

NATIONAL STUDENT NURSES' ASSOCIATION

The National Student Nurses' Association, Inc. (NSNA), established in 1953, is the national organization for nursing students in the United States and its territories, possessions, and dependencies. According to its bylaws, NSNA's purpose is

> to assume responsibility for contributing to nursing education in order to provide for the highest quality health care; to provide programs representative of fundamental and current professional interests and concerns; and to aid in the development of the whole person, his/her professional role, and his/her responsibility for the health care of people in all walks of life.

The NSNA is autonomous, student financed, and student run. It is the voice of all nursing students speaking out on issues of concern to nursing students and nursing.

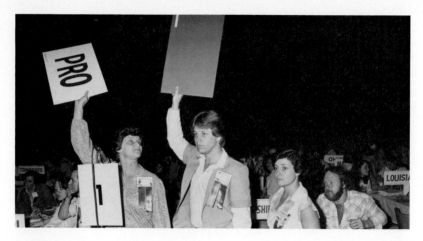

Student nurses at an NSNA convention are serious about the issues they vote on. (*Courtesy of the National Student Nurses' Association.*)

In its first few years, NSNA had little money, a small membership, no real headquarters of its own, and no headquarters staff. It did have financial and moral support from ANA and NLN. Today the association pays for headquarters offices, a staff, and all the other expenses incidental to running the business of a large association. It holds and finances its own annual convention. And, at the same time, it has initiated and financed several important projects in the interest not only of its members but of the nursing profession as a whole.

Membership

Students are eligible for active membership in NSNA if they are enrolled in state-approved programs leading to licensure as an RN or are RNs enrolled in programs leading to a baccalaureate degree in nursing. Students are eligible for associate membership if they are prenursing students enrolled in college or university programs designed to prepare them for programs leading to a degree in nursing. Associate members have all of the privileges of membership except the right to hold office as president and vice president at state and national levels. Application for membership is made directly to NSNA. Dues paid to NSNA are a combination of national and state association dues.

Organization

The policies and programs of NSNA are determined by its House of Delegates, whose membership consists of elected representatives from school and state associations. The delegates at each annual convention elect NSNA's three officers; six directors, one of whom will become editor of *Imprint,* the official journal of NSNA; and a four-member nominating committee. Officers serve for one year or until their respective successors are elected. The board of directors manages the affairs of the association between the annual meetings of the membership. There is only one standing committee (nominating), but the board has the authority to establish other committees as needed. Two consultants are appointed, one each by the ANA and NLN, in consultation with the NSNA board of directors. Their role is to act as resource people and to provide an interchange of information between NSNA and their respective organizations. Constituent organizations may or may not function in a similar manner; their bylaws must be submitted to NSNA for review.

Projects, Activities, Services

NSNA has a wide variety of activities, services, and projects to carry out its purpose and functions. Even in its early years, the association sought participation in ANA and NLN committees and sent representatives to the ICN. Today, NSNA representatives sit on committees of ANA and other health organizations. It is a leading participant in the student assembly of the ICN. NSNA members are involved in community health activities such as hypertension screening, health fairs, child abuse, teenage pregnancy, and education on death and dying. Some of these activities are carried out in cooperation with other student health groups.

In addition to health- and nursing-related issues, social, women's, and human rights issues are supported by NSNA. A major project was Breakthrough to Nursing, aimed at recruiting minority group members into nursing and helping them financially, morally, and educationally to undertake such a career.[17] Their participation in legislative activities at the state and national level has also been impressive.

NSNA has shown a forward-looking interest in the health and social problems of society, often combined with like interest in interdisciplinary cooperation. With the American Medical Student Association (AMSA), Student American Pharmaceutical Association (SAPhA), and American Student Dental Association (ASDA), nursing students have participated in a variety of activities.

Scholarship Funds

The Foundation of the National Student Nurses' Association administers its own scholarship program. The fund is incorporated and has obtained federal tax exemption. Scholarship monies are obtained from various organizations, and contributors have included both commercial enterprises and professional organizations as well as individuals.

Publications

Imprint, the official NSNA magazine, came into existence in 1968, and a subscription is given to members.[18] Subscriptions are also available to other interest groups, schools, and individuals. *Imprint,* published five times during the academic year, is the only publication of its kind specifically for students. It is the only nursing magazine written by and for nursing students, and students are encouraged to contribute articles and letters. There are also various newsletters and handbooks.

Other Professional Activities

At the tenth anniversary of its founding, NSNA had accomplished a great deal. Before its thirtieth, it had become an involved group whose activities demonstrated committed professionalism. Gone are the stunt nights and uniform nights of the early days. Now students are involved in many of the same issues as ANA and NLN and often seem to show more foresight. Resolutions have addressed such issues as nuclear war, abortion, licensure, patients' rights, environmental hazards, collective bargaining, quality of care, nursing education and practice.[19]

As in other fields, nursing students have also fought for their own rights, and NSNA has maintained a commitment to students' rights. In 1970, a guideline for a student bill of rights was distributed to all constituents, a mandate of the 1969 delegates. In 1975, a comprehensive bill of rights, responsibilities, and grievance procedures was accepted and published. The statement was adopted in schools throughout the country.

NSNA offers the opportunity for nursing students to be heard, becomes a forum for debates on health and social issues as well as nursing issues, provides opportunities for interdisciplinary contacts, and is a testing ground for leadership skills. Participation and involvement can be a meaningful and valuable part of the nursing student's education.[20]

NSNA headquarters is at 555 West 57th Street, New York, New York 10019.

HEALTH-RELATED ORGANIZATIONS

Many health-related organizations, both governmental and nongovernmental, frequently provide opportunities for participation by nurses through some form of membership, consultation, or inclusion on committees or programs.

A number provide services specifically for nurses, such as workshops, conferences, publications, and audiovisual materials. Nurses may be invited to attend other program sessions, present papers, or serve on panels. Some examples include the American Cancer Society, the American Heart Association, the American Medical Association, and the Catholic Hospital Association.

There are also organizations in which there are large, active nursing components, such as the American Hospital Association and, particularly, the American Public Health Association (see Appendix 5). The American Red Cross, particularly, has many activities in which nurses are involved, including their disaster health services and educational programs. Nurses may give volunteer service and apply for enrollment as a Red Cross Nurse.[21]

Especially important is the Division of Nursing, which is the one unit in the federal government concerned exclusively with nursing. It is responsible for grant programs (program grants and nurse traineeships) that assist nurses to prepare themselves for research, teaching, supervision, administration, and clinical specialization on a graduate level. All of these and their major reports (Chapters 2 and 5) have had a significant impact on nursing.[22]

Further information may be obtained by writing to the Division of Nursing, Bureau of Health Professions, Public Health Service, Health Resources and Services Administration, U.S. Department of Health and Human Services, 5600 Fishers Lane, Rockville, Maryland 20857.

THE NURSING LITERATURE

Not long ago, text or reference books in nursing were generally limited to the major clinical fields. Now there is scarcely any area relating to nursing that does not have books on the subject. New titles show the extremely diverse nature of the subjects that nurses must read and write about today. Many of these books (this one, for instance) must be frequently revised and published in new, updated editions to keep up with new knowledge and expanding concepts.

Reading the book advertisements in the nursing magazines is almost an education in itself; by doing this, you are reminded of the "hot" topics of the day—or of tomorrow. Even more important is reading the reviews of these books, also published in the nursing journals. That way, you get a better knowledge of their content and the reviewer's estimate (and he or she is usually an expert in the field) of their value. Then it is easier to decide whether to buy it, borrow it from the library, glance through it there, or forget about it. It is impossible to read all the books published in the nursing field today, so you will want to select those that are most worthwhile for you.

It is the nursing journals, however, that will keep you up-to-date and well informed. Usually at least six months pass between the writing of a book and its appearance in print, and a few more months may pass before it is reviewed. But the nursing journals, especially those that are published monthly, make available news, reviews, and information promptly. Within the past 15 years alone, there has been a remarkable increase in the numbers and kinds of nursing magazines (over 100 in 1991). Some you will want to subscribe to and keep for reference, others to look at each month in the library. It is helpful to have at least an idea of the content, purpose, and approach of all of them,[23] whether for reading purposes or sometime to publish yourself. Writing for publication is becoming more important as changes in nursing and health care occur; therefore, learning how to write and publish is worth considering.[24]

It is not feasible to review the content of all these periodicals; some are listed in Appendix 5, if they are associated with a professional organization. There are also other general and clinical journals, published by the non-profit American Journal of Nursing Company, owned by ANA, journals owned by commercial publishers, journals of the SNAs, and national journals

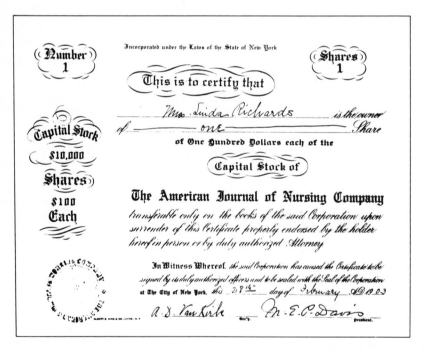

Nurses bought the stock of the American Journal of Nursing Company and then donated it to ANA. (*Courtesy of the American Journal of Nursing Company.*)

of other countries. It is worthwhile to review these journals sometimes if possible (they are not subscribed to by many libraries), as well as the other health-related journals, because they contain useful information. All nursing journals and serials are listed in *INI,* the *International Nursing Index.* A listing of nursing and allied health periodicals, with addresses, is given in the *Cumulative Index to Nursing and Allied Health Literature (CINAHL).* Other health-related journals are found in *Index Medicus.*

Other Reference Sources

Most schools of nursing today do not have a collection adequate enough to meet the needs of a serious scholar or even of someone who wants to go beyond the major nursing journals and books. Nevertheless, nurses who learn how to use the library, the interlibrary loan service, and the various computer information retrieval services will find a new world of reference sources. For instance, CINAHL indexing from 1983 to the present is available electronically as an on-line database and on CD-ROM. In these formats, abstracts from many of the journal articles are also available. The online database is updated monthly; the CD-ROM, every two months.

As noted elsewhere, INI is published by the American Journal of Nursing Company in cooperation with the National Library of Medicine (NLM), a federal agency. All of the citations appearing in INI are part of MEDLINE, the massive, world-renowned biomedical database produced by NLM and updated twice a month. Some 360,000 citations from 3500 journals are added each year to MEDLINE. A selected number of nursing journals appear in *Index Medicus,* its print counterpart.

Although an excellent source for general biomedical information, MEDLINE is not as efficient as CINAHL for retrieving nursing literature.[25] However, because it is federally supported, MEDLINE is extremely inexpensive and is widely available in online, locally mounted, and CD-ROM formats. An advantage for the researcher is that it contains data as far back as 1966.

NLM provides access to a number of related databases of interest to nurses. Among some 30 NLM databases are AIDSLINE, which consists of citations on acquired immunodeficiency syndrome; BIOETHICSLINE, a database containing citations covering ethics and public policy in health care and biomedical research; several cancer databases; DIRLINE, a directory of organizations; and HEALTH, a database developed in cooperation with the AHA, on nonclinical aspects of health care delivery.

Located in Sigma Theta Tau's Center for Nursing Scholarship in Indianapolis, Indiana, the International Nursing Library serves as a comprehensive focal point for information relating to nursing research. This electronic library is designed to assist nurses with the development, utilization, and dissemination of nursing information and to provide the public with information about breakthroughs in nursing research.

There are a number of ways to become knowledgeable about appropriate reference sources. One that is readily available is the "Selected List of Nursing Books and Journals" published in *Nursing Outlook,* until 1992, which provides necessary or helpful sources that all libraries serving nurses should have, and informs nurses and others of what is potentially available. Included are listings of books considered essential in the clinical specialties, administration, communication, education, ethics, nursing law, science, nutrition, nursing trends, issues, and theories, transcultural nursing, and practical nursing. Also included are dictionaries and nursing reviews, as well as a basic list of nursing journals. References are made to other sources of information, including audiovisual materials. Both U.S. and Canadian listings are given. A more extensive compilation, also published until 1992 in *Nursing Outlook,* is "Reference Sources for Nursing," which includes both nursing and biomedical reference works.

Other reference sources of interest to nurses, such as directories, handbooks, review texts, and manuals, are too numerous to list in these pages. A number of guides regularly provide libraries and nurses with lists of recommended journals, books, and other materials. For specific needs, it is advisable to consult a professional librarian.

You will not want to confine yourself to the limits of nursing's literature. The publications of medical and hospital groups, allied professions, education, administration, the social services, and other related fields frequently contain useful and interesting material. Understanding social, economic, educational, and other issues is as important to understanding current and future changes in nursing as knowledge of medical and scientific progress.

Of course, all the reference sources in the world are of little value if you can't use them properly. Experts offer some good advice.[26,27] What follows are some of the ways students and professionals can maximize the benefit they receive from the library's services:

- Establish personal contact with a professional librarian in the institution's library. Information management is the librarian's expertise, and he or she can provide valuable support in meeting educational and clinical goals. Librarians want to meet information needs, but they can do so only if they know their patrons and their specific needs.
- Take advantage of library orientations and tours, and keep up with regular library newsletters. Internal library operations are fast becoming totally computerized, and knowing how to retrieve needed data quickly from online catalogs and other systems will prove advantageous. Some training is also needed to use the library's electronic systems for searching the databases mentioned previously. It's also valuable to know how to request copies of articles or books from other libraries.

KEY POINTS

1. The rapid increase in various specialty nursing organizations resulted in some lack of coordination in advancing nursing goals.
2. NFSNO, NOLF, and the Tri-Council are examples of the way in which nursing organizations have established relationships that allow them to communicate and, at times, collaborate in areas of mutual interest.
3. Key differences between ANA and NLN are in the areas of size, membership, collective bargaining, credentialing, and legislative activity.
4. ANA focuses considerable attention on nurses' economic and general welfare, lobbying, standard setting, certification, accreditation of CE programs, and relationship with other groups. ANA sees itself as speaking for nurses.
5. NLN's major activities are in accreditation of educational programs, consulting, and testing.
6. Specialty organizations include those that are clinical, have special interests in ethnic or other minority concerns, or maintain a scholarly, educational, or socially oriented focus.
7. Health-related organizations, such as AHA, APHA, and the Red Cross often have activities in which nurses participate.
8. There are a number of aids for nurses that will help them find the kinds of references they need; nurses should seek them out and become familiar with the use of computers for this purpose.

REFERENCES

1. Kelly LY. *Dimensions of professional nursing*. Elmsford, NY: Pergamon Press, 1991, pp. 598–600.
2. Ibid., p. 600.
3. Flanagan L. *One strong voice: The story of the American Nurses' Association*. Kansas City, MO.: American Nurses' Association, 1976.
4. American Nurses' Association. *Bylaws*. Kansas City, MO: The Association, 1990, pp. 20–23.
5. Kelly, op. cit., pp. 573–574.
6. Mezey M, et al. The teaching nursing home program. *Nurs Outlook,* 32:146–150 (May–June 1984).
7. Kelly, op. cit., pp. 582–584.
8. Rothberg J. The growth of political action in nursing. *Nurs Outlook,* 33:133–135 (May–June 1985).
9. Unanimous Supreme Court vote for all-RN units ignites a major campaign to organize nurses. *Am J Nurs,* 91:95, 103–104 (June 1991).
10. Kelly, op. cit., p. 584.

11. Merton R. The functions of the professional association. *Am J Nurs,* 58:50–54 (January 1958).
12. Kelly, op. cit., p. 630.
13. Ibid., p. 634.
14. ICN/WHO joint declaration on AIDS. *Int Nurs Rev,* 35:41 (March–April 1988).
15. Almost the entire May–June 1988 issue of *International Nursing Review* focuses on ICN–WHO relationships.
16. Millard R. The accrediting community: Its members and their interrelationships. *Nurs and Health Care,* 5:451–454 (October 1984).
17. Kelly, op. cit., pp. 562–563.
18. Byrne M. *Imprint,* the NSNA journal, 1968–1973: A profession's messages to its students in turbulent times. *Imprint,* 37:97–105 (April–May 1990).
19. Nayer D. NSNA: How it grew. *Imprint,* 34:80–86 (April–May 1987).
20. Fitzpatrick ML. NSNA: Path to professional identity. *Imprint,* 34:63–66 (April–May 1987).
21. Little C. At risk with the Red Cross. *Nurs and Health Care,* 12:124–129 (March 1991).
22. Kalisch P, Kalisch B. Nurturer of nurses: A history of the Division of Nursing of the U.S. Public Health Service and its antecedents—1798–1977—Summary Review, unpublished report to the Division of Nursing, March 1977.
23. Swanson EA, et al. Publishing opportunities for nurses: A comparison of 92 U.S. journals. *Image,* 22:33–38 (Winter 1990).
24. Kelly, op. cit., pp. 649–655.
25. Fried A, et al. Computerized databases in nursing. *Computers in Nursing,* 6:244–252 (December 1988).
26. Kilby S, et al. Access to nursing information resources. *Image,* 21:26–30 (Spring 1989).
27. Saba V, et al. How to use nursing information sources. *Nurs Outlook,* 37:189–195 (July–August 1989).

CHAPTER 15

TRANSITION INTO PRACTICE

OBJECTIVES

After you have studied this chapter you will be able to:

1. Describe the stages of socialization through which you may go in moving from student to graduate status.
2. Definite biculturalism.
3. Last five symptoms of burnout.
4. Identify four things you can do to combat burnout.
5. Explain what strategies you can use to adjust successfully to the work world.
6. Describe the major kinds of CE.
7. List funding sources for continuing your formal education.
8. Identify ways in which you can enhance your professional and personal lives as a nurse.

ADJUSTING TO A NEW ROLE

By the time you are ready to graduate, you probably think that you have gained a pretty good idea about what nursing is and what you can expect on your first job. Most nurses do. Then how does it happen that new graduates seem to go through stages of frustration that they never expected? Some of this, of course, is due to the euphoria that most of us feel when we finish a demanding job (in this case, school) and look forward to a different world, a new challenge. It is not cynical to say that seldom is anything as wonderful as we might have anticipated, especially a new job. It *is* different to be a student in a somewhat protected environment one day and, almost the next, be subject to the pressures of new relationships, little time, and enormous responsibility. But you probably guessed that that might be a problem. One thing most students don't recognize is that when they become graduates, they have a more subtle adjustment to make: resocialization into the work world after years of being socialized into nursing in the educational setting.

Socialization has been described as a "chain of events, a set of phases." It begins with anticipatory expectations of a role and is expected to end with adaptation to and acceptance of the role as defined by the group.[1] One interesting model of this conversion as related to student nurses, describes the process.

Stage 1. Initial innocence: students enter the profession with an image of what they expect to become and how they should behave, often based on public stereotypes. Most have had some degree of a "serving humanity" mentality, with emphasis on touching and doing. In the educational system, they are praised for presenting an analysis of the action more than the action itself.

Stage 2. Recognition of incongruity: students sharing their concerns can begin to recognize what is different from their expectations.

Stages 3 and 4. "Psyching out" and role simulation: those who want to continue in nursing must identify appropriate behaviors and role model them. Soon those behaviors become part of their own repertoire of how to act.

Stages 5 and 6. Provisional and stable internalization. First, nurses vacillate between behaviors now attached to the new professional imagery and those reflecting previous lay images. But as they become more comfortable in practicing those behaviors and have increasing identification with nurse-teacher role models, they move to stage 6, in which the imagery and behavior of the newly socialized nurse-student reflect the professionally, educationally approved model.[2]

So, now you are socialized into the nursing role as seen by your teachers. What happens in the work setting? For all but a few new graduates, the first job is as an employee in some bureaucratic setting, the opposite of professionalism. A comparison of the characteristics of a profession and a bureaucracy clearly shows the differences. One emphasizes hierarchy and task specialization, the other classic professional interests.[3]

DEALING WITH REALITY SHOCK

Kramer identified the problems of new graduates in resolving their role in a bureaucratic-professional conflict and called it *reality shock,* "the specific shocklike reactions of new workers when they find themselves in a work situation for which they have spent several years preparing and for which they thought they were going to be prepared, and then suddenly find that they are not."[4] Reality shock is different from, but related to, both culture shock and future shock.[5]

Thus, when the new nurse, who has been *in* the work setting but not *of* it, embarks on the first professional work experience, there is not an easy adaptation of school-learned attitudes and behaviors, but the necessity for an entirely new socialization. Kramer has categorized and described these as follows:

1. *Skills and routine mastery:* The expectations are those of the employment setting. A major value is competent, efficient delivery of procedures and techniques to clients, not necessarily including psychological support. New graduates immediately concentrate on skill and routine mastery.
2. *Social integration:* This involves getting along with the group and being taught by them how to work and behave: the "backstage" reality behaviors. New graduates who stay at stage 1 may not be seen as competent peers. Those who try to incorporate some of the professional concepts of the educational setting and adhere to those values may alienate the group.
3. *Moral outrage:* Given the differences between what was taught and what is identified and labeled, new graduates feel angry and betrayed by both their teachers and their employers. They weren't told how it would be, and they aren't allowed to practice as they were taught.
4. *Conflict resolution:* The graduates may and do change their behavior but maintain their values; change both values and behaviors to match the work setting; change neither values nor behavior; or work out a relationship that allows them to keep their values but begin to integrate them into the new setting.[6]

In the last stage, the individuals who make the first choice may be the group with potential for making changes, but they simply slide into the bureaucratic mold or, more likely, they withdraw from nursing practice altogether. Those who choose bureaucracy take on an "it's a job" attitude, or they may eventually reject the values of both. Others become organization men and women, who move rapidly into the administrative ranks and totally absorb the bureaucratic values. Those who will change neither values nor behavior, what might be called "going it alone," either look for a place to practice where professional values are accepted or try the "academic lateral arabesque" (also used by the first group), going on to advanced education with the hope of finding new horizons or escaping. The most desirable choice, says Kramer, is the last, which she calls *biculturalism*.

It has been documented that new graduates do indeed go through variations of the socialization process described. That there has been little change in the adjustment process for decades can be seen by reviewing journals in the interim and by the nomadic patterns of nursing that must reflect deepseated job dissatisfaction. Turnover and absenteeism are signs of boredom, lack of involvement, and apathy.

Why is this still happening? Some say that the gap in communication between educators and nursing service administrators is part of the problem; no matter how fine the students' education is, not enough schools have prepared students for evolving needs such as specialization.[7] Educators answer that in no other professional field is the new practitioner expected to be a finished product; all have periods of training and support. In fact, the attitude of the administration is too often echoed by the staff, who may be only critical, not helpful, and do not provide the kinds of role models new graduates need.[8] Not all behave in this way, of course, and seasoned nurses talk about how their first job was horrible or great, often depending on the kind of support they got. (They also counsel patience; but if things don't work out, they try another unit or even another place.)[9] One author, recognizing the pressure confronting staff nurses, has offered suggestions for making the new graduate more comfortable,[10] and still another suggests that nurses take responsibility for creating a developmental environment, guiding, supporting, teaching, and doing for new nurses when necessary, recognizing and rewarding strengths and contributions.[11] (The nursing shortage, for all the serious problems it has created, has also made the institution more receptive to these ideas.)

In addition, as the concept of reality shock became accepted, both teachers and employers have recognized their responsibility to ease the transition from student to graduate and have adopted or adapted Kramer's suggestions on ways to do it. *Anticipatory socialization* helps guide the student toward biculturalism while still in school through lectures, exposure to reality situations, discussion, and constant reinforcement and support in meeting and resolving reality shock issues.[12] A second aspect is to develop a postgraduate socialization process on the job as part of the orientation. Here new graduates are given an opportunity to meet together in order to share experiences and to support one another. These approaches have been shown to work well. New graduates overwhelmingly agree that they have been helped to adjust.[13]

Others, recognizing that some of the problems are related to the new graduate's need to hone skills, have developed innovative orientation programs, internships, or internship-type experiences planned cooperatively by the school and the service agency (see Chapters 5 and 7). Apparently, awareness that there *are* stresses and making these supportive efforts have improved the situation for new graduates. However, there are continued work pressures that cause other problems.

DEALING WITH BURNOUT AND STRESS

Burnout, considered by some as an occupational hazard for those in service occupations, has been described as a debilitating psychological condition resulting from work-related frustrations. Some of the symptoms and effects are lack of motivation, cynicism, negativism, and overwhelming sense of hurt, rejection, failure, and severe loss of self-esteem.[14] Among the early symptoms is emotional and physical exhaustion—not feeling good, not sleeping well, reluctance to go to work, and being prone to all kinds of minor illnesses. Then the burned-out professional becomes negative and just wants to be left alone.[15] A final phase, terminal burnout, is total disgust with everyone and everything.

Burnout is caused by various situations. Sometimes it happens because of the emotionally charged, stressful environment found in clinical units where death and pain are constant companions, added to understaffing and interpersonal staff tensions. It has also been found that when there are personal or home problems, the situation is aggravated. Prevention or cure may start with simply being good to yourself, taking time for yourself and a break when necessary, and taking care of physical problems. A "decompression routine" is also helpful—perhaps some physical activity such as swimming, walking, jogging (not competitive sports), or even doing some form of meditation. Sharing feelings and problems with others is also important. Sometimes a change of job is necessary, but lateral job transfers or spending a period of time in another type of unit often provides the necessary change.

Your own attitude about life and work can make a difference in how you respond to pressures. Those who do well have a good self/professional image, are risk takers, and have self-direction, hopeful attitudes, networks, and support systems. They are able to use stress for growth, and can decompress at home and at work.[16] This profile is almost the direct opposite of that of a burned-out nurse who is sure that nothing will change.

An interesting approach to avoid or overcome burnout recognizes the importance of inner determination and suggests an analysis of your own feelings:

> What can I do to help myself?
> Who will support me?
> Whom can I support?
> What is the potential outcome?
> How will I benefit or be affected?
> How much of myself and my time am I willing to give?

The author notes, "The term *burnout* is a label for feelings. It is something all of us could use as an excuse for giving up control of our lives—or just plain copping out. It's the only life you'll ever have. Why not take charge, instead?"[17]

Stress

Today stress appears to be the universal condition. A number of psychologists have listed stresses and developed scales so that people can determine if they are likely to be stressed and can prepare. Stress can have both a positive and a negative side. In a positive sense, it can be, and often is, a great motivator. However, when the energy released by the stress response is turned inward, the result is negative. "The body turns on itself, so to speak, and in doing so, may cause serious physical or emotional disturbances."[18] Physiological indications of stress include anorexia, uncontrolled eating, urinary frequency, insomnia, lethargy, muscular tension and aches, rashes, diarrhea, headaches, tachycardia, palpitations, tightness in the chest, increased blood pressure, blushing, twitching or trembling, nausea, increased perspiration, and hyperactivity. Psychologically the person may feel disoriented and disorganized, angry, frustrated, depressed, apathetic, helpless, indecisive, afraid, irritable, withdrawn, or unable to concentrate. If nothing is done about it, these symptoms or "cues" may develop into such physical disorders as colitis, ulcers, myocardial infarctions, or asthmatic attacks, or such emotional disorders as depression, addiction, or psychosis.

An unusual amount of stress by any one individual or subgroup can cause pressure in the work situation. Group indicators of stress are interpersonal and include such behaviors as snapping at and arguing with others; scapegoating staff members (for example, blaming another shift or the administration for unit tension); or responding to others with sullenness and silence, harried and "busy" behavior, defensiveness, and intolerance of others' ideas or behavior. Trends toward tardiness, absenteeism, errors, inefficiency, and rapid staff turnover may also indicate the presence of stress in the group. If stress is not recognized and dealt with, poor morale and uncooperative behavior may progress to vindictive behavior, to apathy, and then to paranoia. The end result is a totally dysfunctional system.[19]

Some of the sources of stress can be related to the type of nursing done, such as intensive care or oncology, where part of nursing consists of dealing with the emotional concerns of very sick patients and their families. On the other hand, people react to stress differently and handle it differently. One small study comparing ICU nurses with other staff nurses found that the nurses in the high-stress ICU did not feel as stressed as other staff nurses, perhaps because of personality factors or simply having learned to cope with stress.[20] Other problems causing stress may be understaffing, the fear of not doing what is right or even safe, and dealing with difficult physicians and nonsupportive administration. Most experts feel that one factor is having unrealistic expectations. That is one of the "games nurses play," which also include avoiding accountability, winning at any cost, never trying to resolve recurring problems, and never making waves.[21-23] These "games" add stress to the workplace until they are faced and discontinued.

Nurses appear to progress in stages from stress to adaptation. First, they are defensive, quick-tempered, anxious, and irritable, while denying that job-related stress exists. Second, they become angry, which eventually becomes depression. Third, less stress is experienced and new relationships formed. Peer support seems to help move people out of the helpless/hopeless stage. Fourth, they become change agents, although if they don't succeed in doing this, they may fall back into stages one and two.[24]

Much advice has been given on dealing with stress. A noted cardiologist says, "Rule No. 1 is, don't sweat the small stuff. Rule 2 is, it's all small stuff. And if you can't fight and you can't flee, flow.[25] A yoga "scientist" says, "By understanding that *you* are the main source of your own stress, you can begin to alter and conquer it. The solutions to stress are amazingly simple. They aren't easy, but they're available. You need to experiment personally and try to see which ones work for you. The first is to gain self-knowledge."[26] He focuses on the individual's habits and gives suggestions for breaking or controlling poor eating habits, physiological habits, and tension habits. (Biofeedback and yoga are approaches suggested by a number of people). Some psychologists have demonstrated that the interpretation of an event, not the event itself, produces emotions. They suggest controlling stress by understanding how you label an event, and give advice on gaining control over irrational thoughts and combating distortions.[27]

Another interesting concept is the personality characteristic labeled *hardiness,* which the psychologist Kobasa viewed as "an inherent health-promoting factor in a stress-laden human environment."[28] Hardiness is seen as a composite of commitment, control, and challenge; various studies have shown that an individual with hardiness is much less likely to be subject to burnout.[29]

Many other suggestions have been made about how to ease (or survive) stress, including exercise, relaxation techniques, and what one author calls *self-care.* She lists five self-strategies, with a number of subcategories that nurses have used to relieve stress. The major categories are acting assertively; cultivating (encouraging good will); catharsis (discharging pent-up emotions); withdrawing (getting away by yourself); and humor.[30] As expected, not all of these techniques work for everyone,[31] so much advice continues to be given on dealing with stress.

Job dissatisfaction, discussed in Chapter 8, is one outcome of stress and burnout in the workplace, or perhaps vice versa. Testing whether you and your job belong together has been suggested as a way to clarify values, identify needs, and analyze job compatability. A tool that was developed for that purpose is a useful way to do this.[32] At the least, it makes you think about the job and yourself in a different way.

One nurse suggests that you can't accomplish any of your goals if you don't care for *yourself.* Her "tips that will help you take better care of yourself—and others"—are as follows:

- Check your immediate work setting and ask for it to be upgraded if necessary.
- Find a quiet place to retreat when you are overstressed.
- Examine the peer support you give and get.
- Let go of routine tasks.
- Take some time away from the patient-care area.
- Start a mentor system.
- Don't be satisfied with easy answers.
- Help your coworkers and your students to grow.
- Check the messages you are sending.
- Trust your instincts.[33]

There is no pat answer to the problems in today's work environment anywhere, but self-management efforts are a key to overcoming them. Self-pity is foolish. It's quite possible to bring about change, to develop a network[34] and a peer support system, and to achieve autonomy, as described in Chapter 8. It does take commitment, effort, and caring.

STRATEGIES FOR SUCCESS

Dealing with Realities

Students who have survived what might have been a reality shock in nursing education can adopt the strategies learned and use them to meet the challenges of the work world.

Gortner makes some useful suggestions:

1. Become competent in what you do.
2. Know well the organization in which you work.
3. Be a master of the art of the possible.
4. Recognize and seize the opportunity for doing more.
5. Consider few problems to be original. Hence, the solution is somewhere and that is the challenge.
6. Recognize the value of support systems. Build and use some for yourself.
7. Know yourself well.[35]

Probably the first thing that you, as a new graduate, must realize is that you may not have chosen or been able to choose an institution that wants to or knows how to help an entering employee to adjust. An early problem could arise from your belief in a printed job description. Too often, having one does not rule out the possibility of being asked (or assigned) to responsibilities not included in the job description. The first consideration should be the safety of the patient, and you will have to decide whether you are prepared and able to carry out this function and are legally permitted to do so. If not, what will you do about it? There are legal considerations, described in Chapter 13, as well as ethical problems, and a good nurse administrator will recognize the importance of having you trained in that area. Should this not be so, you have another decision to make. The decision to refuse may cost you the job but will also be only the first of many ethical decisions to be made. (Needless to say, this does not refer to learning new techniques of nursing care that are developed with advances in medical and nursing care.)

It is also not unusual for new graduates to be put temporarily in the position of charge nurse or team leader, for which they may not be prepared. This is especially likely to occur on the evening or night shift. In a good orientation or in-service program, this possibility is foreseen, and you will be given the appropriate learning experiences in such situations under supervision or guidance. When this kind of preparation is not included, you should at least be assigned with a more experienced nurse to share the responsibilities. (In anticipation of such assignments, you might have asked the prospective employer about the availability of such training and supervision and might have indicated a willingness to learn and practice such responsibilities before assignments using them are made. The response of the employer could well be one means of judging the working environment.)

It may be necessary to learn new techniques to cope with unexpected assignments, such as learning to manage time and people,[36,37] and to activate beginning leadership skills. In some cases, assertiveness training, consciousness-raising groups, and internal support systems make the difference between disillusionment and challenge.[38,39]

Getting Along with Others

Nursing students are usually taught to respect the individuality of the patient/client and family and to maintain therapeutically effective relationships with them. Not as much attention is given to human relationships with coworkers. However, conflict in a work situation where you must relate to everyone is not easy to ignore. Anyone who has worked in a situation with tensions and pressures caused by personality conflicts and lack of respect for others knows how destructive such an atmosphere can be. It doesn't matter whether it is caused by a sense of competition, disenchantment with the job, personal, mental, physical, or social problems, or whether it comes from authority groups or peer groups, the end result is not only an unhappy atmosphere but often a poorer quality of nursing care.[40] On the other hand the stimulation of controversy can help you grow, provided, of course, that the controversies are not based on petty, personal disagreements, and stubborn behavior, but rather are the outgrowth of objective and constructive thought. You can develop in your profession through healthy interpersonal relationships with your colleagues.[41] Today's nurse is being educated to be a change agent; to be successful in this role requires the ability to relate well to others[42–44] but to avoid codependency.[45]

Continuing Your Education

Life without the stimulation of continued learning would be pretty dull. In a general way, you can continue to grow through reading, travel, community activities, and home study. Maintaining professional competence, however, takes a little more effort.[46]

The term *continuing education* (*CE*) has been interpreted in many ways. Most agree that it includes any learning activity after the basic educational program. However, most often those programs leading to an academic degree are separated out. There is still much confusion among nurses who are sure that the renewed social and legal pressures for CE mean that they must enroll in a baccalaureate program. This is not so.

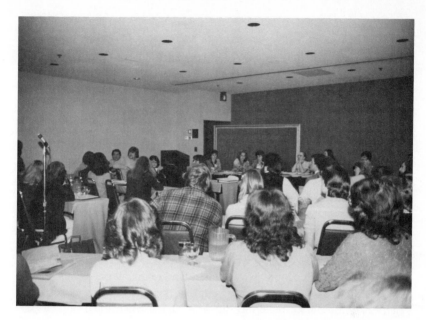

Continuing your education after graduation, either formally or informally, is an important part of professional growth. (*Courtesy of the National Student Nurses' Association.*)

The basic and overriding purpose of CE in nursing is maintaining competence so that the care of the patient is safe and effective. The rapid changes in society, the emergence of new knowledge and technologies, make it impossible to function effectively with only the knowledge and skills gained in your basic program, no matter how outstanding the program. Some nurses maintain that working with patients is CE. Of course, it can be, depending on the setting, the opportunity for learning, and the nurse's inclination to use these opportunities. There are also nurses who merely repeat past experiences and do not recognize or choose to use available learning experiences.

Who should bear the cost of the nurse's CE is a controversial issue. Formalized programs in CE are offered as in-service education on the job; through conferences, workshops, institutes, and other program meetings of professional or other health organizations, or in CE programs offered by colleges and universities. Only in-service education is always free. The other programs frequently charge at least a token fee of some kind because the cost of providing quality programs is high. (See Chapter 5 for additional information on CE.)

You should expect to assume at least part of the cost. There are those who feel that because the employers ultimately benefit from the employee's improved performance, they should provide such support as partial or full tuition payment, sabbaticals, or short-term leaves. On the other hand, hospitals and like institutions often maintain that these additional costs must be passed on unfairly to the patient, and that they have a right to expect competent practitioners. With current tight money restrictions, that philosophy is bound to prevail, although some employers do offer opportunities for CE as a fringe benefit.

With CE programs proliferating (and getting more expensive), you should give some thought to what is worth spending time and money on. A good idea is to figure out what you must know to be competent, diagnose whether you are, and if not, what the gaps are. Some of this preliminary testing can be done by taking some of the tests in journals, and by carefully evaluating your own practice and getting feedback from peers and supervisors as well.

Other methods of CE learning, besides formal classes or conferences, are well worth investigating, although, of course, there is often an added value in interaction with other nurses in group activities. One expert in CE suggests some useful ways of weighing the choices offered, including figuring the costs (registration, travel, time off); looking at objectives, intent, and learning methods in relation to your own specific needs; evaluating the quality of the program regarding speakers and sponsors; and finding programs that are suitable.[47]

With or without formal CE, nurses (and other professionals) must make a commitment to lifelong learning. Therefore, knowing how to locate needed information is essential. Judith Shockley, editor of a guide to information sources for nursing, emphasizes that "quality professional nursing care depends on timely access to existing information and the development of information skills.[48]

But how can a nurse keep up with what's being published, given the virtual explosion of biomedical information? Fortunately, technological developments over the past 20 years have made it possible for massive bodies of data to be stored, processed, retrieved, analyzed, and transmitted electronically. To search for and obtain information in this form, a searcher needs only a computer terminal and a modem, a device to communicate over phone lines. Thus a library or nursing department, no matter how small or how limited its physical collection of journals and books or indexes, has access to most of the world's published literature. In some sites, tapes of databases are mounted on institutional mainframe computers for in-house searching. Today, through developments in laser technology, databases on small compact discs can be searched directly. Once needed data are identified, electronic networks can be tapped to request materials not in the library from other cooperating institutions. In some cases, the full copy can be retrieved from an electronic database. (See Chapter 14 for specific details on database searching.)

For nurses, the institution's library can serve as an important vehicle for keeping up with changes in health care and in a particular specialty. In addition to literature searches, the library frequently offers valuable services for staying current. You might also begin to write yourself.[49]

Formal Higher Education

Besides participating in CE programs, you may want to give serious consideration to formal education leading to another degree (or a first one, if you have none). Educational standards for all positions in nursing are growing steadily higher. If you really want to advance professionally to positions of greater scope and challenge, you will, in the very near future, need an advanced degree, at least a baccalaureate. Advanced education is not a substitute for clinical skill, teaching ability, or administrative expertise. However, it is unlikely that anyone makes it to the top or to a good mid-level position without higher education. Besides, it will add considerably to personal life and interests. In fact, these are the reasons given most often by nurses.[50]

Suppose that you're thinking of a baccalaureate of some kind. First, give some thought to your future goals. It's fun to explore new fields and study whatever you wish without the pressure of time or the need to fulfill requirements for a program. But if these interests are in any of the liberal arts or the social or physical sciences, they can probably be used as electives in many nursing programs, and you will also be started toward a degree.

Because baccalaureate programs with a nursing major are not always available (or affordable) in a particular geographic area, a number of programs have sprung up offering a degree in nursing or another field, giving credit for the lower-division nursing courses and offering no upper-division nursing courses. Evaluate them in relation to your career goals. This type of program is *not* usually acceptable for future graduate studies in nursing, and you may not be able to enroll in a graduate program without having taken upper-division nursing courses. Some nurses have found it necessary to complete a second baccalaureate program, this time with a nursing major, in order to continue into a master's program. If you are interested in a baccalaureate degree for personal development, any accredited baccalaureate program might, of course, meet these objectives. In some cases, individual courses would also enhance your understanding of nursing. The crucial question is whether you wish to enhance, deepen, and broaden the *nursing* knowledge you've already acquired and/or advance in newer nursing fields. If so, an accredited (or equivalent) nursing baccalaureate program is essential.

As noted in Chapter 5, RNs receive varying amounts of recognition or credit for their basic nursing courses and may perhaps need to take challenge examinations. Nursing baccalaureate programs vary a great deal in this respect, but more and more nursing programs are offering some form of educational articulation or outreach program.[51] NLN publications listing baccalaureate, master's and doctoral programs are helpful.

Many of the same points apply to graduate education. There are still some limitations in available nursing master's programs—limitations in their very existence or in the major within nursing that is available. Consider carefully what you want from a program, and prepare yourself for this more competitive admission procedure.[52] Some nurses complete graduate programs in the various sciences or education, with or without any nursing input. Again, you must consider your specific career goals. Someone with a nursing major or at least a minor may be given preference in a position requiring a graduate degree, particularly in educational positions. Or if you are hired now, there is no guarantee that later, when there are more nurses with graduate nursing degrees, you may not be bypassed for promotion or may be required to take a second graduate degree in nursing in order to hold the current position.

Suppose that you don't want any degree? Or suppose that you enroll in an accredited nursing program but then, in time, drop out? That's your decision. There is no reason why you can't function at an acceptable level of competence, maintaining and improving that competence through CE. If, however, you withdrew because of disappointment or lack of interest in that particular program, it may well be that the program is just not right for you. Consider a second try, taking time to find out whether a program's philosophy, objectives, approaches to teaching, and attitudes are what you want. Some of this information can be obtained from the catalog, the faculty or advisor interviews, informal contact with students or *recent* graduates (programs do change). Sometimes, if some courses may be taken without need for full matriculation, a sampling of courses will prove especially informative.

These are practical considerations presented here for information. You must still make the educational choices you wish, but with as complete a knowledge of the pros and cons as possible. For RNs, going back to school is not easy, particularly if you have a family. One nurse who did it (and has a sense of humor) suggests the following:

1. Begin the course only if you're 100 percent committed.
2. Prepare yourself financially.
3. Unless you can afford days off without pay, start accumulating vacation days; you may need them for a clinical rotation.
4. If you don't type, learn; there are lots of papers to write.
5. Invest in a computer early; it saves time and effort.
6. Use your hospital library; that saves time, too.
7. Decide before beginning that you don't really need a 4.0 average to be successful; you don't need the extra stress.

8. Enlist the support of your coworkers and manager.
9. Refuse extra assignments at work.
10. Schedule something fun every week.
11. Cross off each week on a calendar.
12. Remind yourself that others completed the course and you can, too.
13. Delegate everything possible to your children.
14. Have regular study times.
15. Give yourself a mental health break by skipping a routine class occasionally.
16. Frequently visualize what you'll feel like when it's over.
17. Nourish yourself physically, spiritually, and socially, enough to feel healthy and supported.
18. When it's over, celebrate with everyone who made your dream come true.[53]

That's not bad advice for any nontraditional student!

Sources of Financial Aid

The problem of finances is one of the most common blocks to advanced education for able nurses. Review your financial resources realistically. If you are going to request financial aid, you will need to estimate as accurately as possible your expected income and expenses. Major educational expenses will include tuition, books, educational fees, and perhaps travel. Related personal expenses depend on where and how you live. Economizing may mean enrolling in a community college for the liberal arts and later transferring to a local or state college. Economy should not include enrolling in a poor program. Graduating from a nonaccredited nursing program may create difficulties in advancing to the next higher degree. Not all nonaccredited programs are poor, but this risk does exist.

The major sources of income for a self-supporting graduate nurse in an advanced educational program are savings or other personal resources, part-time work, scholarships, and loans. If you plan to do part-time work while attending college, make reasonably sure that a position is available at a satisfactory salary and that it seems to be professionally suitable, including offering enough flexibility to make it possible to take courses. Consider also your mental and physical health under this double load. Can you manage? One answer is cooperative education, which is part work and part school; some higher education programs function in this mode.

There are a number of scholarships, fellowships, and loans earmarked for educational purposes for which nurses are eligible. Some sources of financial assistance are well known and are used regularly; others are not used simply because people do not know about them. The financial aid officer at the institution where you plan to enroll is an excellent source of information.

The National League for Nursing, 350 Hudson Street, New York, New York 10014, sells a publication entitled *Scholarships and Loans for Nursing Education*. It contains a great deal of information that may help you decide where to apply first for financial assistance, thus saving valuable time in making applications.

The professional nursing journals frequently carry news items and articles about such funds, which can be found through the annual and cumulative indexes. Most college catalogs also list sources of student financial support. Exhibit 15-1 lists some of the possible sources of funds. Some give relatively small amounts of money, but these sums do add up. Check also for special funding for ethnic and minority students.

How you apply for financial assistance may have considerable bearing on whether or not you obtain it. Correspondence, personal interviews, application forms, and references should all show the same meticulous attention that is given to an application for a new position.

Exhibit 15-1

Sources of Financial Aid for Education

Local
School alumni associations
District and state SNAs
District and regional Leagues
Other local or state nursing
   organizations
State government
Chapters of national
   fraternities/sororities
Fraternal organizations (Elks,
   Amvets)
Local foundations
Hospital associations
Your place of employment
College or university loans or
   scholarships
Bank loans
Local companies
Women's groups

National/international
Federal government—DHHS;
   Dept. of Education
Nurses Educational Funds
American Nurses' Foundation
Sigma Theta Tau
Other national nursing
   organizations
National Student Nurses'
   Association Foundation
Veterans Administration
Private foundations
Military
International Council for Nursing
World Health Organization
Large corporations

Professional and Community Activities

Active participation in community activities is very rewarding. Some activities are directly related to nursing, such as attending alumni and nurses' association meetings and accepting appointments to committees and offices. Others include volunteer work on a regular or special basis, such as participating in student nurse recruitment programs or career days, soliciting donations for various health organizations, helping with the Red Cross blood program, assisting with inoculation sessions for children, acting as adviser to a Future Nurse Club, or volunteering time at a free clinic.

The importance of nursing input into the various community, state, and national joint provider-consumer groups that study means of improving the health care delivery system is discussed in Chapter 8. Although participation at the state or national level may not be immediately feasible for a nurse who has not yet achieved professional recognition, just showing interest and volunteering your services will often open doors at a local level. That's an important foot in the door!

Consumer activism has resulted in the formation of other groups concerned with health delivery, and nurses offering their expertise and understanding of health care services problems can make valuable contributions. Sometimes you need to convince these groups that you have a sincere interest in improved health care services and are willing to work cooperatively. In some areas, ethnic and minority groups are especially suspicious of professional health workers outside of their own group, because unfortunate experiences have shown some of them to be more concerned with defending their own interests than the consumer's well-being, as the consumer sees it. In these groups, it is even more important to listen than to talk. Participation can lead to development of free clinics, health fairs, health teaching classes, recruitment of minority students for nursing programs, tutoring sessions for students, liaison activities with health care institutions, programs for the aged, and legislative activities directed toward better health care. The opportunities, challenges, and satisfactions are unlimited.

Consumer health education is being stressed more and more today, and in what better area can nurses offer their expertise? Classes can be held under the auspices of health care institutions, public health organizations, and public and private community groups, and include teaching for wellness as well as teaching those with chronic or long-term illnesses. Nurses who like to teach and are skilled and enthusiastic can participate in programs already set up and, equally important, can work to develop other programs and involve others on the health team.

Keeping the public informed about nursing and the changes that have occurred in recent years in both education and practice is a contribution to the community. Offers to present programs about nursing are often welcome in the many community, social, business, professional, and service groups that meet frequently and are interested in community service. And yes, you *can* become a good speaker.[54]

Activities such as these involve you in the community and are stimulating and satisfying. They also require time, effort, and often patience. But besides having the satisfaction of being useful, you'll gain in self-development and growth as a nurse and as an individual, a double reward that can't be bought.

A LOOK AT YOUR FUTURE

Nursing is an exciting field that offers people an important life role and social status, a job, or a career—and many choices. For some, dedication to the job may be limited by other interests, such as commitments to family, school, or personal interests. For others, nursing is a career—the work of their lives. Preparation, advancement, and concern with professional issues are important to nurse careerists.[55] Identifying with careerists in nursing opens up interesting professional and personal opportunities. It certainly places nurse careerists on the path with other men and women who plan to move up corporate hierarchies to positions of leadership and influence.

This does not mean that women nurses cannot lead a full family life as well. For years, nurses have balanced multiple and competing demands, often feeling that they never do anything as well as they could. Now that women are an active presence in the workplace, more attention and support are being given to families and working women.[56] No longer is the nurse the only woman in her neighborhood who works. New social support systems make careerism a real choice for the nurse who wants a family. But it's up to you—one of your many choices.

The relatively brief accounts of movement in civic and political spheres and nursing have been presented in this book to expand your awareness that being a career nurse means that you are committed to more than bedside nursing. It is not enough to say: "I am a good nurse; I take care of my patients." The changing political, social, and economic environments require nurses interested in their profession to be politically sophisticated as well as clinically competent.

Chances are that you will have a career in nursing; the opportunities, salaries, and satisfaction in nursing are increasing every day. Some will follow the old pattern, taking opportunities as they come but not "orchestrating" a career. That procedure can still bring an added fillip to your life because you may explore areas you never thought of before. However, give some thought to managing your career. Some suggestions on beginning are as follows:

- Size up your present situation.
- Think big.
- Network.
- Set a goal.
- *Seek out* career opportunities.
- Become assertive.[57]

McBride describes what she calls *career stages,* an interesting and provocative way of looking at a career. In the first stage, you prepare to contribute: with your educational program or programs, CE, perhaps certification, experience, and some sort of mentor. Next, you begin to make professional contributions, which tend to be discipline specific. Then you may become so proficient that you move on to something else, perhaps administration. In this third stage, you represent your institution and your profession at meetings, write more, and become involved in policymaking.

Finally, in the fourth phase of your career, you are asked for advice. You may or may not still be expert in your area of specialization, but you have the broad experience, talent, and reputation to be a valuable consultant.[58]

That may not be the path you follow, but there's much to look forward to. You are in a field of service that is indispensable, a caring art as well as one of knowledge and expertise. Things may not always be easy; they seldom are in any career, but there's no reason to be either burned out or "bored out." You can be creative and innovative and perform at your personal peak potential if the concept of "work excitement" is part of your philosophy.[59]

Today, more than ever before in modern history, your constructive talents and abilities are needed. Nursing, with its unlimited frontiers and exciting future, needs the full and unstinting output of its practitioners. The rewards promise to be many.

KEY POINTS

1. The stages of socialization begin with an image you hold about the group you are becoming a part of, and then advances to recognizing the incongruities and trying to "psych out" the appropriate behavior before arriving at some stage of adjustment.
2. Accepting that you hold different values from those in a bureaucracy and working out a relationship that accommodates both values and the reality of the workplace is a healthy way to adjust to "reality shock."

3. Burnout occurs when the various pressures of a job and dissatisfaction with the work situation seem to be impossible to cope with.

4. Being good to yourself, allowing for personal activities, as well as working with a support group, can relieve some aspects of stress and burnout.

5. CE for nurses may include in-service programs, self-learning, and programs offered by educational institutions and professional organizations.

6. The primary purpose of CE for nurses is to ensure competence in practice.

7. You should take time and care in selecting the right educational program, whether for CE or for a degree, so that you don't waste your time or money.

8. Funding for formal nursing education is available from a variety of sources, but it saves time to consult first with the financial officer of the school in which you are interested.

9. Participating in nursing and community organizations is a way to enrich your life as a nurse and as a person.

10. More nurses are successfully combining family life and a nursing career, including formal education.

REFERENCES

1. Hinshaw AS. Socialization and resocialization of nurses for professional nursing practice. In: *Socialization and resocialization of nurses for professional nursing practice*. New York: National League for Nursing, 1977.

2. Kramer M. *Reality shock*. St. Louis: C.V. Mosby Company, 1974, pp. 5–6.

3. Ibid., p. 15.

4. Ibid., pp. vii–viii.

5. Ibid., pp. 3–10.

6. Ibid., pp. 155–162.

7. O'Leary J. What employers will expect from tomorrow's nurses. *Nurs and Health Care*, 7:207–209 (April 1986).

8. Meissner J. Nurses, are we eating our young? *Nurs 86*, 6:51–53 (March 1986).

9. Huey F. Your first job: Great news or giant nightmare? *Am J Nurs*, 88:452–457 (April 1988).

10. Madden T. From classroom to hospital: Bridging the gap for new nurses. *Nurs 89*, 19:44–45 (June 1989).

11. Valiga T. It's time for nurses to begin nursing nurses. *Nurs and Health Care*, 5:331–335 (June 1984).
12. Kramer, op. cit., pp. 67–77.
13. Holleran S, et al. Bicultural training for new graduates. *Nurse Educator*, 5:8–14 (January–February 1984).
14. Maslack C. Burned out. *Hum Behavior*, 5:16–22 (September 1976).
15. McConnell E. How close are you to burn-out? *RN*, 44:29–33 (May 1981).
16. Magill K. Burnin, burnout, and the brightly burning. *Nurs Mgt*, 13:17–21 (July 1982).
17. Brown DL. Burnout—or cop-out? *Am J Nurs*, 83:1110 (July 1983).
18. Selye H. *Stress without distress*. Philadelphia: J.B. Lippincott Company, 1974.
19. Scully R. Stress in the nurse. *Am J Nurs*, 80:912 (May 1980).
20. Maloney J. Job stress and its consequences on a group of intensive care and nonintensive care nurses. *Adv Nurs Science*, 4:31–41 (January 1982).
21. Roberts J. Games nurses play: Merry-go-round and catch. *Am J Nurs*, 86:848–849 (July 1986).
22. Roberts J. Games nurses play: Monopoly and make a wish. *Am J Nurs*, 86:1041–1042 (September 1986).
23. Roberts J. Games nurses play: Pin the tail on the donkey and war. *Am J Nurs*, 86:1101–1102 (October 1986).
24. Nicholson L. Stress management in nursing. *Nurs Mgt*, 21:53–55 (April 1990).
25. Stress: Can we cope? *Time*. 123:48–54 (June 6, 1983).
26. Nuernberger P. Freedom from stress: A holistic approach. *Nurs Life*, 1:61–68 (November–December 1981).
27. McKay M, et al. Are you listening to yourself? *Nurs Life*, 3:57–64 (January–February 1983).
28. Lambert C, Lambert V. Hardiness: Its development and relevance to nursing. *Image*, 19:92–95 (Summer 1987).
29. Rich V, Rich A. Personality hardiness and burnout in female staff nurses. *Image*, 19:63–66 (Summer 1987).
30. Hutchison S. Self-care and job stress. *Image*, 19:192–196 (Winter 1987).
31. Albrecht T. What job stress means for the staff nurse. *Nurs Admin Q*, 7:1–19 (Fall 1982).
32. Billings C, Quick M. Does your job work for you? *Am J Nurs*, 85:407–409 (April 1985).
33. Haddad A. Caring for yourself comes first. *RN*, 47:77–78 (June 1984).
34. Havens D. Networking. In Nowak J, Grindel C, eds. *Career planning in nursing*. Philadelphia: J.B. Lippincott Company, 1984, pp. 41–86.
35. Gortner S. Strategies for survival in the practice world. *Am J Nurs*, 77:618–619 (April 1977).
36. Johnson M, Gallagher D. Making every minute count: Effective time management. *Imprint*, 36:75–76, 83 (September–October 1989).

37. Davidhizar R. The best approach is doing "nothing." *Nurs Mgt*, 21:42–44 (March 1990).
38. Tofias L. Expert practice: Trading examples over pizza. *Am J Nurs*, 89:1193–1194 (September 1989).
39. Chinn P, et al. Friends on friendship. *Am J Nurs*, 88:1094–1096 (August 1988).
40. Green C. How to recognize hostility and what to do about it. *Am J Nurs*, 86:1230–1234 (November 1986).
41. Storlie F. Surviving on-the-job conflict. *RN*, 45:51–53, 96 (October 1982).
42. Laser R. I win–you win negotiating. *J Nurs Admin*, 11:24–29 (November–December 1981).
43. Manthey M. Effective problem solving: You gotta believe. *Nurs 86*, 16:60–61 (November 1986).
44. Keenan M, Hurst J. Conflict management, problem solving through collaboration. *Nurs Success Today*, 2:8–14 (December 1985).
45. Hall S, Wray L. Codependency: Nurses who give too much. *Am J Nurs*, 89:1456–1460 (November 1989).
46. Millonig VL. Motivational orientation toward learning after graduation. *Nurs Admin Q*, 9(4):79–86 (1985).
47. del Bueno D. How to get your money's worth out of continuing education. *RN*, 41:37–42 (April 1978).
48. Shockley J, ed. *Information sources for nursing: A guide*. New York: National League for Nursing, Publication No. 41-2200, 1988, p. 1.
49. Kelly LY. *Dimensions of professional nursing*, 6th ed. Elmsford, NY: Pergamon Press, 1991, pp. 649–654.
50. Millonig, op. cit.
51. Rich J. In pursuit of a BSN. *Nurs 90*, 9:118, 120 (February 1990).
52. Williams RA. Applying to graduate school. *Am J Nurs*, 87:517–518, 520 (April 1987).
53. Le Roy A. How to survive as a nontraditional nursing student. *Imprint*, 35:73–74, 79–86 (April–May 1988).
54. Winslow EH. Overcome the fear of speaking in public. *Am J Nurs*, 91:51–53 (May 1991).
55. Smith M. Career development in nursing: An individual and professional responsibility. *Nurs Outlook*, 30:128–131 (February 1982).
56. Sandroff R. Nurse/mother: How to cope with a double career. *RN*, 43:53–57 (July 1980).
57. Sharkey C. Decide to manage your career. *Am J Nurs*, 88:105–106 (January 1988).
58. McBride A. Orchestrating a career. *Nurs Outlook*, 33:244–247 (September–October 1985).
59. Simms L, et al. Breaking the burnout barrier: Resurrecting work excitement in nursing. *Nurs Economics*, 8:177–186 (May–June 1990).

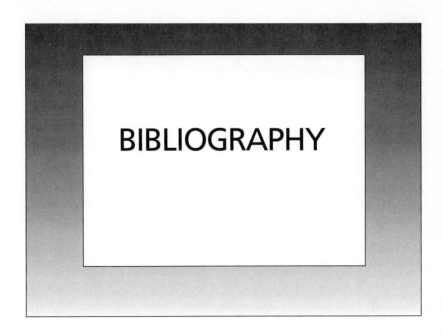

BIBLIOGRAPHY

CHAPTER 1 Care of the Sick: How Nursing Began

Berges F, Berges C. A visit to Scutari. *Am J Nurs,* 86:811–813 (July 1986).

Bullough VL. Nightingale, nursing and harassment, *Image,* 22:4–7 (Spring 1990).

Bullough V, et al. *Florence Nightingale and her era: A collection of new scholarship.* New York: Garland Publishing, Inc., 1990.

Hays J. Florence Nightingale and the India sanitary reforms. *Pub Health Nurs,* 6:152–154 (September 1989).

Henry B, et al. Nightingale's perspective of nursing administration. *Nurs and Health Care,* 11:200–206 (April 1990).

Monteiro L. Florence Nightingale and public health nursing. *Am J Pub Health,* 75:181–186 (February 1985).

Nuttal P. The passionate statistician. *Int Nurs Rev,* 31:24–25 (January–February 1984).

Vicinus M, Nergaard B, eds. *Ever yours, Florence Nightingale: Selected letters.* Cambridge, MA: Harvard University Press, 1990.

Woodham-Smith C. *Florence Nightingale.* New York: McGraw-Hill Book Company, 1951.

See also the sections on Nightingale in the Bullough and Bullough, Dolan, and Kalisch and Kalisch books. An outstanding collection of Nightingale's writings can be found in the Adelaide Nutting Historical Nursing collection at Teachers College, Columbia University, New York. Some of her most noted works are listed in *Dimensions of professional nursing,* 6th ed.

CHAPTER 2 Nursing in the United States: American Revolution to Nursing Revolution

Baer E. Nursing's divided loyalties: An historical study. *Nurs Res,* 38:166–171 (May–June 1989).

Benson E. Nursing and the world's Columbian exposition. *Nurs Outlook,* 34:88–90 (March–April 1986).

Bullough B, et al. *Nursing: A historical bibliography.* New York: Garland Publishing, Inc., 1981.

Bullough V, et al. *American nursing: A biographical dictionary.* New York: Garland Publishing, Inc., 1988.

Dammann N. *A social history of the Frontier Nursing Service.* Sun City, AZ: Social Change Press, 1982.

Donahue MP. Isabel Maitland Stewart's philosophy of education. *Nurs Res,* 32:140–146 (May–June 1983).

Dreves KD. Nurses in American history: Vassar training camp for nurses. *Am J Nurs,* 75:2000–2002 (November 1975).

Focus: Nursing's proud history. Entire issue, *Imprint* (April–May 1990).

Hamilton D. Faith and finance. *Image,* 20:124–127 (Fall 1988).

Heinrich J. Historical perspectives on public health nursing. *Nurs Outlook,* 31:317–320 (November–December 1983).

Kalisch P, et al. Louise Bourgeois and the emergence of modern midwifery. *J Nurse-Midwifery,* 26:3–17 (July–August 1981).

Lagemann E. *Nursing history: New perspectives, new possibilities.* New York: Teachers College Press, 1983.

Maker MD. *To bind up the wounds.* New York: Greenwood Press, 1989.

Moments in American history. *Nurs Res,* 39:126–127 (March–April 1990).

Parsons M. Mothers and matrons. *Nurs Outlook,* 31:274–278 (September–October 1983).

Progress and promise 1900–1990. *Am J Nurs,* anniversary issue (October 1990).

Rawnsky M. The Goldmark report: Midpoint in nursing history. *Nurs Outlook,* 21:380–383 (June 1973).

Wuthrow S. Our mothers' stories. *Nurs Outlook,* 38:218–222 (September–October 1990).

In the text of Chapter 5, in *Dimensions of professional nursing,* 6th ed. (ref. 7), the publisher and date of publication are cited for older studies that were widely available. Many of these reports are now out of print. However, some libraries have photocopies, and microfilmed editions of most of them are also available. All of Christy's historical biographies are also listed in the bibliography of *Dimensions.* These and others are available in *Pages from nursing history* (New York: American Journal of Nursing Company, 1984).

CHAPTER 3 The Health Care Setting

Aaron HJ. *Serious and unstable condition: Financing America's health care.* Washington DC: The Brookings Institute, 1991.

Abel E, Nelson M. *Circles of care: Work and identity in women's lives*. Albany, NY: State University of New York Press, 1990.

Applebaum R, Phillips P. Assuring the quality of in-home care: The "other" challenge for long-term care. *Gerontologist*, 30(4):444–450 (1990).

Baker E, ed. *Surveillance in occupational health and safety*. Atlanta: Centers for Disease Control, 1989.

Barsky A. The paradox of health. *N Engl J Med*, 318:414–418 (February 18, 1988).

Braunstein J. National health care: Necessary but not sufficient. *Nurs Outlook*, 39:54–55 (March–April 1991).

Chavkin W. Drug addiction and pregnancy: Policy crossroads. *Am J Pub Health*, 80:483–487 (April 1990).

Dimond M. Health care and the aging population. *Nurs Outlook*, 37:76–77 (March–April 1989).

Downie RS, et al. *Health promotion: Models and values*. New York: Oxford University Press, 1990.

Ehrlich P, Ehrlich A. *The population explosion*. New York: Simon & Schuster, 1990.

Freedman S. Megacorporate health care: A choice for the future. *N Engl J Med*, 312:579–582 (February 28, 1985).

Friedson E. *Medical work in America*. New Haven, CT: Yale University Press, 1989.

Ginzberg E. *The medical triangle: Physicians, politicians and the public*. Cambridge, MA: Harvard University Press, 1990.

Glanty K, et al. *Health behavior and health education: Theory, research, and practice*. San Francisco: Jossey-Bass Publishers, 1990.

Gold R. *Abortion and women's health: A turning point for America?* New York: Alan Guttmacher Institute, 1990.

Grace H. Can health care costs be contained? *Nurs and Health Care*, 2:124–131 (March 1990).

Hendrickson G, Kovner C. Effects of computers on nursing resource use. *Computers in Nurs*, 8:16–22 (February 1990).

Hynes HP, ed. *Reconstructing Babylon: Essays on women and technology*. Bloomington, IN: Indiana University Press, 1991.

Kelly LS. Another look at the future of health care. *Nurs Outlook*, 39:150–151 (July–August 1991).

Kent V, Hanley B. Home health care. *Nurs and Health Care*, 11:234–240 (May 1990).

McKenzie N, ed. *The crisis in health care*. New York: Penguin Books, 1990.

Osborn J. AIDS, politics and science. *N Engl J Med* 318:444–447 (February 18, 1988).

Powderly K, Smith E. The impact of DRGs on health care workers and their clients. *Hastings Center Rep*, 19:16–18 (January–February 1989).

Roemer M. *An introduction to the U.S. health care system*, 2nd ed. New York: Springer Publishing Company, 1986.

Saba VK, et al. *Nursing and computers: An anthology*. New York: Springer-Verlag, 1989.

Schwartz WB, Mendelson DV. Hospital cost containment in the 1980s: Hard lessons learned and prospects for the 1990s. *N Engl J Med*, 324:1037–1042 (April 11, 1991).

Siendwall D, Tavani C. The role of public health in providing primary care for the medically underserved. *Pub Health Rep*, 106:2–4 (January–February 1991).

Stanfield P. *Introduction to the health professions*. Boston: Jones and Bartlett Publishers, 1990.

Starck PL. Health care under siege: Challenge for change. *Nurs and Health care*, 12:26–31 (January 1991).

Strumpf N. A new age for elderly care. *Nurs and Health Care*, 8:444–448 (October 1987).

Williamson K, et al. Occupational health hazards for nurses. *Image*, 20:162–168 (Fall 1988).

The Chronicle of Higher Education is a weekly newspaper that presents reports and discussions of the trends and issues in the field. Both the *American Journal of Public Health* and *The Nation's Health*, publications of the American Public Health Association, publish numerous articles and reports on population, environmental hazards, and other aspects of public health.

The *American Journal of Nursing* has articles on nurses' health hazards periodically; see February and April 1990 issues. There is also a computer column in the *American Journal of Nursing*, and an increasing number of such articles are found in many other nursing journals. Nursing and other health care journals have many articles on AIDS, and the February–March 1989 issue of *Imprint* is devoted to the topic.

Other good reference sources for current issues, problems, and trends in institutions are *Hospitals*, the AHA journal; *Health Progress*, the Catholic Hospital Association (CHA) journal, and other journals in the field, which always include nontechnical articles.

The best source of current, comprehensive data on health resources, although usually several years old; is the U.S. Department of Health and Human Services.

CHAPTER 4 Nursing in Theory and Practice

Aaronson L. A challenge for nursing: Re-viewing a historic competition. *Nurs Outlook*, 37:274–279 (November–December 1989).

Alfano G. A different kind of nursing. *Nurs Outlook*, 36:34–37 (January–February 1988).

Barnum B. Nursing's image and the future. *Nurs and Health Care*, 10:18–21 (January 1989).

Barnum B. *Nursing theory: Analysis, application, evaluation*, 3rd ed. Philadelphia: J.B. Lippincott Company, 1990.

Benner P, Tanner C. Clinical judgment: How expert nurses use intuition. *Am J Nurs*, 87:23–31 (January 1987).

Benner P. Wrubel J. *The primacy of caring*. Menlo Park, CA: Addison Wesley Publishing Company, 1989.

Brider P. Who killed the nursing care plan? *Am J Nurs*, 91:35–39 (May 1991).

Buresh B, et al. Who counts in coverage of health care? *Nurs Outlook*, 39:204–208 (September–October 1991).

Carnegie ME. *The path we tread: Blacks in nursing, 1854–1984*. Philadelphia: J.B. Lippincott Company, 1986.

Christman L. A view of the future. *Nurs Outlook*, 35:216–228 (September–October 1987).

Christman L. Perspectives on role socialization of nurses. *Nurs Outlook*, 39:209–212 (September–October 1991).

Diers D. Learning the art and craft of nursing. *Am J Nurs*, 90:65–66 (January 1990).

Donahue P. *Nursing, the finest art: An illustrated history*. St. Louis: C.V. Mosby Company, 1985.

Donley R. Spiritual dimensions of health care. *Nurse and Health Care*, 12:178–183 (April 1991).

Franzoi S. A picture of competence. *Am J Nurse*, 88:1109–1112 (August 1988).

Gortner S. Nursing values and science: Toward a science philosophy. *Image*, 22:101–105 (Summer 1990).

Henderson V. The essence of nursing in high technology. *Nurs Admin Q*, 9(4):1–9 (1984).

Hine D. *Black women in white: Racial conflict and cooperation in the nursing profession, 1890–1950*. Bloomington, IN: Indiana University Press, 1989.

Jones A. *Images of nurses: Perspectives from history, art, and literature*. Philadelphia: University of Pennsylvania Press, 1988.

Kalisch P, Kalisch B. *The changing image of the nurse*. Menlo Park, CA: Addison-Wesley Publishing Company, 1987.

Kidd P, Morrison E. The progression of knowledge in nursing: A search for meaning. *Image*, 20:222–224 (Winter 1988).

Kohler P, Edwards T. High school students' perception of nursing as a career choice. *J Nurs Ed*, 29:26–30 (January 1990).

Kraegel J, Kachoyeanos M. *"Just a nurse."* New York: E.P. Dutton, 1989.

Leininger M, ed. *Caring, an essential human need: Proceedings of the three national caring conferences*. Detroit: Wayne State University Press, 1988.

Lippman D, Ponton K. Nursing's image on the university campus. *Nurs Outlook*, 37:24–27 (January–February 1989).

Lundh U, et al. Nursing theories: A critical view. *Image*, 20:36–40 (Spring 1988).

Lynaugh J, Fagin C. Nursing comes of age. *Image*, 20:184–190 (Winter 1988).

Mangum, et al. Perceptions of nurses' uniforms. *Image*, 23:127–130 (Summer 1991).

Mitchell G. Nursing diagnosis: An ethical analysis. *Image*, 23:99–104 (Summer 1991).

Stephany TM. Lesbian nurse. *Nurs Outlook,* 36:295 (November–December 1988).

Turkoski B. Nursing diagnosis in print, 1950–1985. *Nurs Outlook,* 36:142–144 (May–June 1988).

Walsh M, Ford P. *Nursing rituals: Research and rational actions.* London: Heinemann Nursing, 1989.

Wiley K, et al. Care of AIDS patients; Student attitudes. *Nurs Outlook,* 36:244–245 (September–October 1988).

Wolf Z. Uncovering the hidden work of nursing. *Nurs and Health Care,* 10:463–467 (October 1989).

Note also the "Microcosmos" column by Veneta Masson in every issue of *Nursing Outlook* since 1988 for a fascinating glimpse of a nurse's reflections on everyday nursing issues. Look for the new emphasis on caring, as in the September 1990 issue for *Advances in Nursing Science.* Surveys in various journals such as the *American Journal of Nursing, Nursing,* and *RN* often present provocative, although limited, looks at nurses' views on various topics.

CHAPTER 5   Education and Research in Nursing

Betz C, et al. Nursing research productivity in clinical settings. *Nurs Outlook,* 38:180–183 (July–August 1990).

Blaney D. An historical review of positions on baccalaureate education in nursing as basic preparation for professional nursing practice, 1960–1984. *J Prof Nurs,* 25:182–185 (May 1986).

Bloch D. Strategies for setting and implementing the national center for nursing research priorities. *App Nurs Res,* 3:2–6 (February 1990).

Crissman S, Betz L. Education and image: Critical issues confronting the nursing profession. *J Contemp Health Law and Policy,* 3:179–184 (Spring 1987).

Deering-Flory R, Neighbors M. NLN competencies for the associate degree nurses: Are the new graduates meeting them? *Nurs and Health Care,* 12:474–479 (November 1991).

Downs F. Differences between the professional doctorate and the academic/research doctorate. *J Prof Nurs,* 5:261–265 (September–October 1989).

Duffy M. The research process in baccalaureate nursing education: A ten-year review. *Image,* 19:87–91 (Summer 1987).

Flaherty MJ. Advocacy and nursing education in the twentieth century. *J Contemp Health Law and Policy,* 3:169–178 (Spring 1987).

Free T, Mills B. Faculty practice in primary care. *Nurs Outlook,* 33:192–197 (July–August 1985).

Grace H. Issues in doctoral education in nursing. *J Prof Nurs,* 5:266–270 (September–October 1989).

Hart S. Single purpose institutions for nursing programs: To be or not to be. *J Prof Nurs,* 6:55–58 (January–February 1990).

Hinshaw AS. Using research to shape public policy. *Nurs Outlook,* 36:21–24 (January–February 1988).

Kelly L. Nursing, nothing but nursing. *Nurs Outlook,* 36:227 (September–October 1988).

Pullen C. Are we easing the transition from LPN to ADN? *Am J Nurs,* 88:1129 (August 1988).

Pyle S. The business of nursing: Managing our future through continuing education. *Imprint,* 35:95–97 (November 1988).

Seidle A, Sauter D. The new non-traditional student in nursing. *J Nurs Ed,* 29:13–19 (January 1990).

Smith MC. Forces guiding the future of nursing research. *Nurs and Health Care,* 8:23–25 (January 1987).

Styles M, et al. Entry: A new approach. *Nurs Outlook,* 39:200–203 (September–October 1991).

Williamson N, et al. Nurse faculty practice: From theory to reality. *J Prof Nurs,* 6:11–20 (January–February 1990).

Woolley A. Defining the product of baccalaureate education. *Nurs and Health Care,* 7:199–201 (April 1986).

Various nursing journals carry a large number of articles on nursing education and research: *Journal of Nursing Education, Nurse Educator, Journal of Continuing Education, Journal of Professional Nursing, Nursing Outlook,* and *Nursing and Health Care.*

CHAPTER 6   Employment Guidelines

Campbell L. Fired! What to do if it happens to you. *RN,* 47:58–60 (June 1984).

Kiely M. The résumé writer's task. *Focus on Crit Care,* 10:10–11 (June 1988).

La Rocco S. Interviewing: A necessary skill in today's shrinking job market. *Imprint,* 32:5–7 (December 1985–January 1986).

Manley MJ, et al. The bilateral job interview. *Am J Nurs,* 84:1237–1241 (October 1984).

O'Connor P. Résumés: Opening the door. *Nurs Econ,* 5:428–431 (November–December 1986).

Sosin J. What you need to pin down a job offer. *RN,* 48:75–76 (May 1985).

Nursing journals and the yearly *Career Guide,* published by some, periodically carry articles on career guidance and employment guidelines. Business journals, and especially career women's magazines, have also been emphasizing these topics. Any bookstore has a section devoted to career development; some of the books are best-sellers and may be found in paperback.

CHAPTER 7   The Practice of Nursing

Aiken L. Charting the future of hospital nursing. *Image,* 22:72–78 (Summer 1990).

Boyar DC, Marteson DJ. Intrapreneurial group practice. *Nurs and Health Care*, 11:28–33 (January 1990).

Buerhaus P. Not just another nursing shortage. *Nurs Econ*, 5:267–279 (November–December 1987).

Burge S, et al. Clinical nurse specialist role development: Quantifying actual practice over three years. *Clinical Nurs Spec*, 3(1):33–36 (1989).

Clark L, Quinn J. The new entrepreneurs. *Nurs and Health Care*, 9:7–15 (January 1988).

Collins H. How much would you earn as an office nurse? *RN*, 12:26–29 (February 1989).

Deckard G, et al. Long term nursing: How satisfying is it? *Nurs Econ*, 4:194–200 (July–August 1986).

Diehl D. Private practice: Out on a limb and loving it. *Am J Nurs*, 86:907–909 (August 1986).

Flaherty MJ, De Moya D. An entrepreneurial role for the nurse consultant. *Nurs and Health Care*, 10:258–263 (May 1989).

Hamilton C, Neubauer B. Hospice nursing: Serving ambivalent clients. *Nurs and Health Care*, 10:320–322 (June 1989).

Hamric A, Sprosa J. *The clinical nurse specialist in theory and practice*, 2nd ed. Philadelphia: W.B. Saunders Company, 1989.

Hendrickson G, Doddato T. Setting priorities during the shortage. *Nurs Outlook*, 37:280–284 (November–December 1989).

Hospital best practices in nurse recruitment and retention. *Nurs Econ*, 7:98–106 (March–April 1989).

Kester-Beaver P. Tales from travelers. *Am J Nurs*, 91:50–56 (April 1991).

Krugman ME. Nurse executive role socialization and occupational image. *Nurse and Health Care*, 11:526–531 (December 1990).

Manion J. Nurse intrapreneurs: Heroes of health care's future. *Nurs Outlook*, 39:18–21 (January–February 1991).

Martin EJ. A specialty in decline? Psychiatric mental health nursing, past, present, and future. *J Prof Nurs*, 1:48–53 (January 1985).

Masters F, et al. Role development: The nursing quality assurance coordinator. *J Nurs Qual Assur*, 4(2):51–62 (1990).

McElreath BJ. Why I'm an agency nurse. *Am J Nurs*, 89:678–679 (May 1989).

Menard S, ed. *The clinical nurse specialist: Perspectives on practice*. New York: John Wiley and Sons, 1987.

Mezey M, McGivern D. *Nurses, nurse practitioners: The evolution of primary care*. Boston: Little, Brown and Company, 1986.

Once a nurse . . . always a nurse? *Imprint*, 33:38–41 (February–March 1989).

Pierce S, et al. Nurses employed in nonnursing fields. *J Nurs Admin*, 21:29–34 (June 1991).

Prescott P. Another round of nurse shortage. *Image*, 19:204–209 (Winter 1987).

Prescott PA, et al. Changing how nurses spend their time. *Image*, 23:23–27 (Spring 1991).

Raumen K, et al. *The nurse intrapreneur: Opportunities and benefits for nursing*. Philadelphia: J.B. Lippincott Company, 1988.

Rogers B. Occupational health nursing practice, education, and research. *AAOHN J*, 38:536–543 (November 1990).

Rogers B, et al. Employment and salary characteristics of nurse practitioners. *Nurse Practitioner*, 9:56–66 (September 1989).

Rooks JP. Nurse-midwifery: The window is wide open. *Am J Nurs*, 90:30–36 (December 1990).

Salmon M. Public health nursing: The neglected specialty. *Nurs Outlook*, 37:226–229 (September–October 1989).

Sandrick K. Other options: Great opportunities outside the hospital. *Nurs Life*, 7:33–37 (July–August 1987).

Schimmenti C, Dormody M. Taking flight. *Am J Nurs*, 87:1420–1423 (November 1987).

Vogel G, Dolyesh N. *Enterpreneuring: A nurse's guide to entrepreneuring and consulting*. New York: National League for Nursing, 1988.

Werner J, et al. Clinical nurse specialization: An annotated bibliography—Evaluation and impact. *Cl Nurse Spec*, 3(1):20–23 (1989).

Wilbur J, et al. Career trends of master's prepared family nurse practitioners. *J Am Acad of Nurse Practitioners*, 2:79–82 (April–June 1990).

Willard MM. How to take nursing skills on the road. *RN*, 52:32–34 (January 1989).

Almost all the nursing journals publish articles on careers periodically. Articles about nursing in other countries also appear periodically. In addition, the NP and specialty journals, such as the *Journal of Nurse Midwifery*, carry articles on the role of their practitioners. See also *Imprint* (September–October 1991) and *Clin Nurse Specialist*, Vol. 4, No. 3, 1990.

CHAPTER 8   Power, Autonomy, Influence

Aaronson L. A challenge for nursing: Re-viewing a historic competition. *Nurs Outlook*, 37:274–279 (November–December 1989).

Bernhard L, Walsh M. *Leadership, the key to professionalism of nursing*, 2nd ed. St. Louis: C.V. Mosby Company, 1990.

Bidwell AS, Brasker ML. Role modeling versus mentoring in nursing education. *Image*, 21:23–25 (Spring 1989).

Campbell-Heider N. Do nurses need mentors? *Image*, 18:110–113 (Fall 1986).

Collins S, Henderson M. Autonomy: Part of the nursing role? *Nurs Forum* 26(2):23–29 (1991).

Contemporary minority leaders in nursing: Afro-American, Hispanic, Native American perspectives. Kansas City, MO: American Nurses' Association, 1983.

Davis G. Nursing values and health care policy. *Nursing Outlook*, 36:289–292 (November–December 1988).

del Bueno D. Power and politics in organizations. *Nurs Outlook*, 34:124–128 (May–June 1986).

Fain J, Viau P. Networking: A strategy for strengthening the role of the clinical nurse specialist. *Cl Nurse Spec*, 3(1):29–31 (1989).

Hamilton E, et al. Effects of mentoring on job satisfaction, leadership behaviors, and job retention of new graduate nurses. *J Nurs Staff Dev*, 5:159–165 (July–August 1989).

Harrison J, Roth P. Empowering nursing in multihospital systems. *Nurs Econ*, 5:70–76 (March–April 1987).

Harter C, et al. Networking to implement effective health care. *MCN*, 14:387, 390, 392 (November–December 1989).

Henry B, Ives S. Language, leadership and power. *J Nurs Admin*, 17:19–24 (January 1987).

Johnson P. Normative power of chief executive nurses. *Image*, 21:162–167 (Fall 1989).

Joston LV. Wanted: Leaders for public health. *Nurs Outlook*, 37:230–232 (September–October 1989).

Kelly L. The grass is not greener. *Nurs Outlook*, 37:115 (May–June 1989).

Kilkus S. Self-assertion and nurses: A different voice. *Nurs Outlook*, 38:143–145, 135 (May–June 1990).

Mackay H. *Swim with the sharks without being eaten alive*. New York: William Morrow and Company, 1988.

Mason D, et al. Toward a feminist model for the political empowerment of nurses. *Image*, 23:72–77 (Summer 1991).

Maternal Child Nursing. Entire issue (January–February 1991).

Moccia P. The nurse as policymaker: Toward a free and equal health care system. *Nurs and Health Care*, 5:481–485 (November 1984).

O'Connor K. For want of a mentor . . . *Nurs Outlook*, 36:38–39 (January–February 1988).

Perlman D, Takacs G. The 10 stages of change. *Nurs Mgt* 21:33–38 (April 1990).

Pillar B, et al. Technology, its assessment and nursing. *Nurs Outlook*, 38:16–19 (January–February 1990).

Poulin M. Leadership and the caring role. *Imprint*, 34:51, 53–54 (April–May 1987).

Sampselle CM. The influence of feminist philosophy on nursing practice. *Image*, 22:243–247 (Winter 1990).

Sovie M. Exceptional executive leadership shapes nursing's future. *Nurs Econ*, 5:13–20 (January–February 1987).

Stivers C. Why can't a woman be less like a man; Women's leadership dilemma. *J Nurs Admin*, 21:47–51 (May 1991).

Warner DC. Nursing and public policy: What is the high ground? *J Nurs Admin*, 21:52–57 (May 1991).

Weekes DP. Mentor-protege relationships: A critical element in affirmative action. *Nurs Outlook*, 37:156–157 (July–August 1989).

Biographies or interviews with living nursing leaders and their perceptions of nursing appear periodically in a number of nursing journals. See *Nurs-*

ing Outlook (September–October 1987, May–June 1990, and May–June 1991), as well as various issues of *Nursing and Health Care, Nursing Economics,* and *Nursing Success Today.*

CHAPTER 9   Ethical Issues in Nursing and Health Care

Anderson G, Glesnes-Anderson V. *Health care ethics: A guide for decision makers.* Rockville, MD: Aspen Publishers, 1987.

Annas GJ. Ethics committees: From ethical comfort to ethical cover. *Hastings Center Rep,* 21:18–21 (May–June 1991).

Baruch E, et al, eds. *Embryos, ethics and women's rights: Exploring the new reproductive technologies.* New York: Haworth Press, 1988.

Brecht MC. Nursing's role in assuring access to care. *Nurs Outlook,* 38:6–7 (January–February 1990).

Callahan D. Allocating health resources. *Hastings Center Rep,* 18:14–20 (April–May 1988).

Capron AM. The burden of decision. *Hastings Center Rep,* 20:36–41 (May–June 1990).

Cassel C, Meier D. Morals and moralism in the debate over euthanasia and assisted suicide. *N Engl J Med,* 323:750–752 (September 13, 1990).

Chervenack FA, McCullough LB. Justified limits on refusing intervention. *Hastings Center Rep,* 21:12–18 (March–April 1991).

Davis AJ, Slater PV. U.S. and Australian nurses' attitudes and beliefs about the good death. *Image,* 21:34–39 (Spring 1989).

Edwards B, Haddad A. Establishing a nursing bioethics committee. *J Nurs Admin,* 18:30–33 (March 1988).

Fries E. The ethical issues of transplanting organs for anencephalic newborns. *MCN,* 14:412–414 (November–December 1989).

Fry S. Ethical issues in research: Scientific misconduct and fraud. *Nurs Outlook,* 38:296 (November–December 1990).

Fry S. Moral values and ethical decisions in a constrained economic environment. *Nurs Econ,* 4:160–164 (July–August 1986).

Fry S. New ANA guidelines on withdrawing or withholding food and fluids from patients. *Nurs Outlook,* 36:122–123, 148–150 (May–June 1988).

Fry S. New proposals to increase organ donations: Are they ethical? *Nurs Outlook,* 39:192 (September–October 1991).

Fry S. Rationing health care to the elderly: A challenge to professional ethics. *Nurs Outlook,* 36:256 (September–October 1988).

Fry S. Research on ethics in nursing: The state of the art. *Nurs Outlook,* 35:246 (September–October 1987).

Gillian C, et al, eds. *Mapping the moral domain: A contribution of women's thinking to psychological theory and education.* Cambridge, MA: Harvard University Press, 1989.

Haack MR, Hughes TL. *Addiction in the nursing profession.* New York: Springer Publishing Company, 1990.

Hadorn DC. The Oregon priority-setting exercise: Quality of life and public policy. Conference report. *Hastings Center Rep*, 21:11–16 (May–June 1991).

Hoyer PJ, et al. Clinical cheating and moral development. *Nurs Outlook*, 39:170–173 (July–August 1991).

Human rights guidelines for nurses in clinical and other research. Kansas City, MO: American Nurses' Association, 1985.

Kapp M. Medical empowerment of the elderly. *Hastings Center Rep*, 19:5–7 (July–August 1989).

Lund M. Stopping treatment: Who decides? *Ger Nurs*, 12:147–148, 151 (May–June 1991).

Pence T, Cantrall J, eds. *Ethics in nursing: An anthology*. New York: National League for Nursing, 1990.

Porter-O'Grady T. Credentialing, privileging, and nursing bylaws: Assuring accountability. *J Nur Admin*, 15:23–27 (December 1985).

Reilly D. Ethics and values in nursing: Are we opening Pandora's box? *Nurs and Health Care*, 37:91–93 (February 1989).

Roemer R. The right to health care—Gains and gaps. *Am J Pub Health*, 78:241–247 (March 1988).

Rogers B. Ethical dilemmas in occupational health nursing. *AAOHN J*, 36:100–105 (March 1988).

Trinkoff AM, et al. The prevalence of substance abuse among registered nurses. *Nurs Res*, 40:172–174 (May–June 1991).

Viens D. A history of nursing's code of ethics. *Nurs Outlook*, 37:45–49 (January–February 1989).

The *American Journal of Nursing, Nursing Outlook,* and various other nursing journals have monthly or periodic columns on ethics. The October 1988 issue of *RN* is devoted to the topic of ethics. The *Hastings Center Report* consists totally of articles on ethics.

The April 1989 issue of *Advances in Nursing Science* and much of the Winter 1990 issue of *Image* also have a number of articles on ethics.

The November–December 1990 issue of *American Nurse* has a number of articles about nurses and AIDS patients.

Publications by the President's Commission for the Study of Ethical Problems in Medicine and Biomedical and Behavioral Research can be obtained from the Superintendent of Documents, U.S. Government Printing Office, Washington, DC 20402. These are *Defining death; Implementing human research regulations; Deciding to forego life-sustaining treatment; Protecting human subjects; Making health care decisions; Screening and counseling for genetic conditions; Splicing life; Securing access to health care; Whistleblowing in biomedical research;* and *Summing up*.

CHAPTER 10   Law and Legislation

Abdellah F. The federal role in nursing education. *Nurs Outlook*, 35:224–227 (September–October 1987).

Brown L. *Health policy in the United States: Issues and options*. New York: Ford Foundation, 1988.

Clark L. The advice of an expert: Making a difference on Capitol Hill. *Nurs and Health Care*, 9:289–294 (June 1988).

Cohen S. Health care policy and abortion: A comparison. *Nurs Outlook*, 38:20–25 (January–February 1990).

Cohen W, Milburn L. What every nurse should know about political action. *Nurs and Health Care*, 9:295–297 (June 1988).

Congress and health: An introduction to the legislative process and its key participants. New York: National Health Council, revised periodically, sometimes with each Congress.

Cushing M. Safeguarding the spirit of competition. *Am J Nurs*, 89:1035–1036, 1038 (August 1989).

Gallagher D. The student's role in legislation. *Imprint*, 35:44–46 (September–October 1988).

Goldwater M, Zusy MJL. *Prescription for nurses: Effective political action*. St. Louis: C.V. Mosby, 1990.

Harrington C, Lempert L. Medicaid: A program in distress. *Nurs Outlook*, 36:6–8 (January–February 1988).

Harrington C. Policy options for a national health care plan. *Nurs Outlook*, 37:223–228 (September–October 1990).

Mason D, et al. *Politics and Policy of Nursing*. Philadelphia: W.B. Saunders Company, 1991.

Milburn L, et al. The information seeker's guide to health policy news. *Nurs and Health Care*, 9:307–309 (June 1988).

Natapoff J, Weiczorek R, eds. *Maternal-child health policy*. New York: Springer Publishing Company, 1990.

Statham A, et al. *The worth of women's work: A qualitative synthesis*. Albany, NY: State University of New York Press, 1988.

Wakefield M. Influencing the legislative process. *Nurs Econ*, 8:188–190 (May–June 1990).

Will G. For the handicapped, rights but no welcome. *Hastings Center Rep*, 16:5–8 (June 1986).

Wold J. Workers' compensation and the occupational health nurse. *AAOHN J*, 8:385–387, August 1990.

Most of the January 1991 issue of *Nurs and Health Care* is devoted to nurses and health policy. Many publications of ANA and NLN relate to legislation and politics, as do those of most other large health associations and the National Health Council. Useful government publications include *Congressional Record* (verbatim transcript of the proceedings of the Senate and House (*Congressional Record Office*, H-112, Capitol, Washington, DC 20515) and an annual subscription from the Superintendent of Documents, Government Printing Office, Washington, DC 20401; *Digest of Public General Bills*, also from the Superintendent of Documents; *Committee Prints and Hearing Records*, available about two months after the close of hearings, is free but requires a self-addressed label sent to the publications clerk of the committee from which the document is issued.

CHAPTER 11   Health Care Credentialing and Nursing Licensure

Allen A. Specialty nursing organizations support development of a national board of nursing specialties. *J Post Anesth Nurs,* 4:187–190 (June 1989).

Barnum B. Interview with Jeanette C. Hartshorn, project director, Committee for the National Board of Nursing Specialties. *Nurs and Health Care,* 10:276–279 (May 1989).

del Bueno D. The promise and reality of certification. *Image,* 20:208–211 (Winter 1988).

Greenlaw J. Definition and regulation of nursing practice: An historical survey. *Law, Med and Health Care,* 13:117–121 (June 1985).

Hadley E. Nurses and prescriptive authority: A legal and economic analysis. *Am J Law and Med,* 15(2):245–299 (1989).

Maroun V, Serota C. Demanding quality when foreign nurses are in demand. *Nurs and Health Care,* 9:361–363 (September 1988).

Massaro T. Continuing competency–regulatory alternatives. *Issues,* 7(4):8–10 (1986).

Kelly L. Institutional licensure. *Nurs Outlook,* 21:566–572 (September 1973).

Kelley R. The path to addiction—and recovery. *Am J Nurs,* 87:176–179 (February 1987).

Northrop C. The nursing shortage and nursing's legal scope of practice. *Nurs Outlook,* 37:104 (March–April 1989).

Peplau H. Is nursing's self-regulating power being eroded? *Am J Nurs,* 85:141–143 (February 1985).

Tammeleo A. Don't be afraid to blow the whistle on incompetence. *RN,* 53:61–65 (June 1990).

News items on changes in licensure and appropriate articles appear in almost all nursing journals. ANA, NLN, and the National Council of State Boards of Nursing all have materials about licensure in their publication lists. *Issues,* a NCSBN news publication, is very useful.

CHAPTER 12   Legal Aspects of Nursing Practice

Anderson BJ. Serving justice: How to give a deposition. *Am J Nurs,* 91:32, 35 (March 1991).

Annas G. Not saints, but healers: The legal duties of health care professionals in the AIDS epidemic. *Am J Pub Health,* 78:844–849 (July 1988).

Bradford E. Preventing malpractice suits: What you can do. *Nurs 88,* 18:63–64 (September 1988).

Braun A, Mainardi P. Before you act as a witness . . . *Nurs 86,* 16:32L–32M (February 1986).

Brent N. Legal issues in health education: Focus on diabetes. *Home Healthcare Nurse,* 6(5):35–36 (1986).

Brent N. Right drug, wrong route. *Nurs Life,* 6:72 (March–April 1986).

Cerrato P. What to do when you suspect incompetence. *RN,* 13:36–41 (October 1988).

Chagnon L, Easterwood B. Managing the risks of obstetrical nursing. *MCN,* 11:303, 306–310 (September–October 1986).

Cushing M. Drug errors can be bitter pills. *Am J Nurs,* 86:895, 899 (August 1986).

Cushing M. Who transcribed that order? *Am J Nurs,* 86:1107–1108 (October 1986).

Cushing M. Million-dollar errors. *Am J Nurs,* 87:435–436, 420 (April 1987).

Cushing M. When the courts define nursing: What it is, what it does. *Am J Nurs,* 87:773–774 (June 1987).

Cushing M. A strong defense. *Am J Nurs,* 87:1278–1280 (October 1987).

Cushing M. First, anticipate the harm . . . *Am J Nurs,* 87:1278–1280 (October 1987).

Cushing M. When hospitals don't listen to nurses' complaints. *Am J Nurs,* 87:1547–1548 (December 1987).

Cushing M. Dealing with details. *Am J Nurs,* 88:955–956 (July 1988).

Cushing M. *Nursing jurisprudence.* Norwalk: Appleton and Lange, 1988.

Cushing M. Finding fault when patients fall. *Am J Nurs,* 89:809 (June 1989).

Dirschel K. A mandate for standards of care. *Nurs and Health Care,* 7:27–29 (January 1986).

Feutz S. Testifying in legal actions. *J Nurs Admin,* 18:5–7, 42 (July–August 1988).

Fiesta J. The nursing shortage: Whose liability problem? Part I. *Nurs Mgt,* 21:24–25 (January 1990).

Fiesta J. The nursing shortage: Whose liability problem? Part II. *Nurs Mgt,* 21:22–23 (February 1990).

Fiesta J. Agency nurses: Whose liability? *Nurs Mgt,* 21:16–17 (March 1990).

Good intentions gone awry. *Nurs Life,* 6:55–56 (March–April 1986).

Hogue E. 5 lessons you can learn from court decisions. *Nurs 86,* 16:45–47 (April 1986).

Klein C. Malicious prosecution. *Nurse Practitioner,* 10:42 (June 1985).

Klimon E. Nursing professional liability insurance: An analysis. *Nurs Econ,* 3:132–159 (May–June 1985).

Law and aging. Entire issue. *Law, Medicine, and Health Care.* Fall 1990.

Mahoney D. Under oath: Testifying against a physician. *Am J Nurs,* 90:23, 26 (February 1990).

Mandell M. How to defend yourself against lawyers' attack. *Nurs Life,* 7:25–29 (May–June 1987).

Northrop C. Malpractice and standards of care. *Nurs Outlook,* 34:160 (May–June 1986).

Northrop C. Home health care: Changing legal perspectives. *Nurs Outlook,* 34:256 (September–October 1986).

Quigley F. Responsibilities of the consultant and expert witness. *Focus on Crit Care,* 18:238–239 (June 1991).

Rabinow J. Where you stand in the eyes of the law. *Nurs 89*, 19:34–42 (February 1989).

Rhodes AM. Malpractice suits: Implications for obstetric nurses. *MCN*, 11:203 (May–June 1986).

Rhodes AM. Liability for the actions of others. *MCN*, 11:315 (September–October 1986).

Rhodes AM. Content of nurses' detailed notes. *MCN*, 12:61–62 (January–February 1987).

Rhodes AM. Wrongful birth and wrongful life. *MCN*, 14:171 (May–June 1989).

Segal E, Sherry C. You too can be an expert witness. *Nurs Life*, 7:39–40 (July–August 1987).

Especially useful in keeping abreast of legal issues are *Law, Medicine and Health Care* and the *American Journal of Law and Medicine*. See also columns on legal aspects of nursing in various journals such as the *American Journal of Nursing, RN, Nursing Management,* and *Nursing Outlook*.

CHAPTER 13   Patients' Rights: Nurses' Rights

AIDS: Public health and civil liberties. *Hastings Center Rep*, 16 (Spec. Supplement):1–36 (December 1986).

Annas GJ. Webster and the politics of abortion. *Hastings Center Rep*, 19:36–38 (March–April 1989).

Annas GJ. One flew over the Supreme Court. *Hastings Center Rep*, 20:28–30 (May–June 1990).

Annas GJ. Foreclosing the use of force: A.C. reversed. *Hastings Center Rep*, 20:27–29 (July–August 1990).

Annas GJ. Crazy-making: Embryos and gestational mothers. *Hastings Center Rep*, 21:35–38 (January–February 1991).

Arbeiter J. Can a nurse be fired for having AIDS? *RN*, 10:53–54 (February 1987).

Backus L, Inlander C. Consumer rights in health care. *Nurs Econ*, 4:314–317, 324 (November–December 1986).

Barnes M, et al. The HIV-infected health care professional: Employment policies and public health. *Law, Med, and Health Care*, 18:311–330 (Winter 1990).

Bellocq J. Student dismissal: Part I. How much documentation is enough? *J Prof Nurs*, 4:147, 230 (May–June 1988). Part II 4:236, 308 (July–August 1988).

Cantor N. The permanently unconscious patient, non-feeding and euthanasia. *Am J Law and Med*, 14(4):381–438 (1989).

Cushing M. Nurses have rights, too. *Am J Nurs*, 87:167–170 (February 1987).

Cruzan: Clear and convincing? Commentaries. *Hastings Center Rep*, 20:5–11 (September–October 1990).

Danis M, et al. A prospective study of advance directives for life-sustaining care. *N Engl J Med*, 324:882–895 (March 28, 1991).

Devettere R. Reconceptualizing the euthanasia debate. *Law, Med, and Health Care*, 17:145–155 (Summer 1989).

Ethics committees: How are they doing? *Hastings Center Rep*, 16:9–24 (June 1986).

Fiesta J. Whistleblowers: Heroes or stool pigeons? Part I. *Nurs Mgt*, 21:16–17 (June 1990).

Fiesta J. Whistleblowers: Retaliation or protection? Part II. *Nurs Mgt*, 21:38 (July 1990).

Four easy ways to lose a job in nursing. *Am J Nurs*, 90:27–28 (June 1990).

Grandstrom D. Calling a code: Your role in helping a family decide. *RN*, 50:24–29 (June 1987).

Helms LB, Weiler K. Suing programs of nursing education. *Nurs Outlook*, 39:158–161 (July–August 1991).

Hogue E. What you should know about informed consent. *Nurs 86*, 16:47–48 (June 1986).

Kellmer D. No code orders: Guidelines for policy. *Nurs Outlook*, 34:179–183 (July–August 1986).

Murphy E. Celebrating the Bill of Rights in the year of Rust v. Sullivan. *Nurs Outlook*, 39:238–239 (September–October 1991).

Northrop C. Nursing practice and the legal presumption of competency. *Nurs Outlook*, 36:112 (March–April 1988).

Northrop C. Refusing unsafe work assignments. *Imprint*, 36:20 (February–March 1989).

O'Neill E. Treatment decisions with the terminally ill incompetent patient. *Nurs Econ*, 5:37–41 (January–February 1987).

Pavalon E. *Human rights and health care law*. New York: American Journal of Nursing Company, 1990.

Refusal of treatment legislation. New York: Society for the Right to Die, 1991.

Rhodes AM. A minor's refusal of treatment. *MCN*, 15:261 (July–August 1990).

Rhodes AM. Major legal initiatives in MCH (1975–1990). *MCN*, 16:45 (January–February 1991).

Rhodes AM. Refusing nutrition and hydration: The Cruzan case. *MCN*, 16:141 (May–June 1991).

Rhodes AM. Treatment decisions. *MCN*, 16:225 (July–August 1991).

Ruark J, et al. Initiating and withdrawing life support: Principles and practice in adult medicine. *N Engl J Med*, 318:25–30 (January 7, 1988).

Saunders J, Valente S. Code no code?: The question that won't go away. *Nurs 86*, 16:60–64 (March 1986).

Steinbock B. Baby Jane Doe in the courts. *Hastings Center Rep* 14:13–19 (February 1984).

Steinbock B. The logical case of "wrongful life." *Hastings Center Rep*, 16:15–20 (April 1986).

Tamborlane T. Rights of employees with AIDS. *Caring*, 3:36–40 (February 1990).

Wakefield-Fisher M. Balancing wishes with wisdom: Sustaining infant life. *Nurs and Health Care,* 8:517–520 (November 1987).

Weiss F. The right to refuse: Informed consent and the psychosocial nurse. *J Psychosocial Nurs,* 28(8):25–30 (1990).

The fall 1989 issue of *Law, Medicine and Health Care* focuses on "Life and Death Choices." This journal also has other theme issues. The articles in the *American Journal of Law and Medicine* are very detailed and give perspectives not available in the other journals cited here.

CHAPTER 14   Nursing Organizations and Publications

Haller K. Conducting a literature review. *MCN,* 13:148 (March–April 1988).

Hanson S. Write on. *Am J Nurs,* 88:482–483 (April 1988).

Kalisch B, Kalisch P. *Nurturer of nurses: A history of the Division of Nursing of the U.S. Public Health Service and its antecedents, 1798–1977.* Summary report of a study for the Division of Nursing, March 1977.

Kilby SA, et al. Access to nursing information resources. *Image,* 21:26–30 (Spring 1989).

Little C. Inside ICN headquarters with Constance Holleran. *Nurs and Health Care,* 11:406–410 (October 1990).

Mullen F. *Plague and politics: The story of the U.S. Public Health Service.* New York: Basic Books, 1989.

Swanson EA, et al. Publishing opportunities for nurses: A comparison of 92 U.S. journals. *Image,* 23:33–38 (Spring 1991).

CHAPTER 15   Transition into Practice

Abrams A, et al. Going through channels and getting results. *Nurs 87,* 17:121–122 (September 1987).

Anastas L. *Your career in nursing,* 2nd ed. New York: National League for Nursing, 1988.

Bailey B. How to float safely and effectively. *Nurs 90,* 20:113–116 (February 1990).

Barone-Amenduri P. How to give better presentations. *Nurse 90,* 90:32Y–32BB (June 1990).

Batra C. Socializing nurses for nursing entrepreneurship roles. *Nurs and Health Care,* 11:34–37 (January 1990).

Bilderback B. Surviving the stages of peer consultation. *Am J Nurs,* 80:113–114 (January 1989).

Breakwell G. Are you stressed out? *Am J Nurs,* 90:31–33 (August 1990).

Culture in a nursing organization. *Nurs Mgt,* 21:14–15, 17 (January 1990).

del Bueno D. How well do you use power? *Am J Nurs,* 87:1495–1498 (November 1987).

Diers D. Learning the art and craft of nursing. *Am J Nurs,* 90:65–66 (January 1990).

Fiedor G, Keys M. Coping with nights. *Am J Nurs,* 87:1166–1168 (September 1987).

Forté PS. Prospering nurse: Overcoming oxymoron. *Nurs Econ,* 7:87–90 (March–April 1989).

Grainger RD. Anxiety interrupters. *Am J Nurs,* 90:14 (February 1990).

Grainger RD. Managing fatigue. *Am J Nurs,* 90:13 (March 1990).

Grainger RD. Self-confidence: A feeling you can create. *Am J Nurs,* 90:12 (October 1990).

Greipp M. Nursing preceptors: Looking back—looking ahead. *J Nurs Staff Dev,* 5:183–186 (July–August 1989).

Guidera M, Gilmore C. In defense of fellowship. *Am J Nurs,* 88:1017 (July 1988).

Hamilton J. You're not an angel; You're a nurse. *Nurs 86,* 16:113–115 (May 1986).

Kang R, et al. Life without burnout: Using consultation in community health nursing. *MCN,* 12:301–304, 306 (September–October 1987).

Kramer M, Hafner L. Shared values: Impact in staff nurse job satisfaction and perceived productivity. *Nurs Res,* 38:174–177 (May–June 1989).

Laff E, Leff H. If you're having another bad day. *Am J Nurs,* 87:1362–1363 (October 1987).

Lartin J. Scapegoating: Identifying and reversing the process. *J Nurs Admin,* 18:25–31 (September 1988).

McGonigle D. Making self-talk positive. *Am J Nurs,* 88:725–727 (May 1988).

McVeigh D, et al. Career mobility for all RNs. *Nurs Outlook,* 39:30–31 (January–February 1991).

Nurse intern programs. *Nurs and Health Care,* 7:270–271 (May 1986).

Ramirez D. Culture in a nursing service organization. *Nurs Mgt,* 21:14–15, 17 (January 1990).

Rukall L, Layton S. BSN completion: Achievement with style. *Imprint,* 36:86–91 (September–October 1989).

Wilson L. High gear nursing: How it can run you down and what you can do about it. *Nurs Life,* 6:44–47 (May–June 1986).

Wilting J. *Nurses, colleagues, and patients: Achieving congenial interpersonal relationships.* Edmonton, Canada: University of Alberta Press, 1990.

Winstead-Fry P. *Career planning: A nurse's guide to career advancement.* New York: National League for Nursing, 1990.

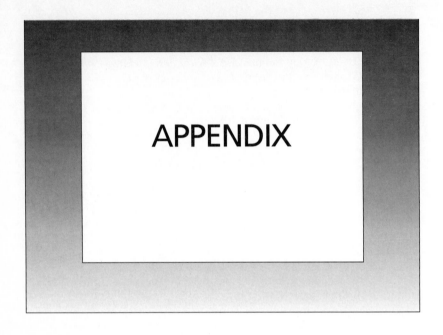

APPENDIX

Appendix

Appendix 1   Major Studies of the Nursing Profession

Study	Year	Sponsor; Project Director	Key Points, Recommendations, Impact
The Educational Status of Nursing	1912	American Society of Superintendents of Training Schools for Nurses; M. Adelaide Nutting, RN	Revealed many appalling working and living conditions of students; limited and poor teaching. No real action taken, but set precedent for later studies. Highlighted need for nursing schools to be independent of hospitals.
Nursing and Nursing Education in the United States	1923	Rockefeller Foundation; Josephine Goldmark (nonnurse researcher)	Found poor educational practices and often poor quality of teachers and students. Education for public health nurses should include postgraduate courses in public health nursing. High educational standards should be maintained. The average hospital school does not adequately prepare high-grade nurses; university schools should be developed and strengthened. Resulted in founding of Yale School of Nursing.
Nurses, Patients, and Pocketbooks (first study)	1928	Committee on Grading of Nursing Schools, with members from major nursing and health care organizations; partly funded by nurses; Dr. May Ayres Burgess (statistician)	Showed oversupply of nurses; serious unemployment and maldistribution; low salaries and poor working conditions; some serious incompetence, but both the public and physicians generally satisfied with nurses' services (primarily private duty). Should secure public support for nursing education; replace student nurses with graduates in hospitals.
An Activity Analysis of Nursing (second study)	1934	Committee on Grading of Nursing Schools; Ethel Johns and Blanche Pfefferkorn (lay persons)	First large-scale attempt to find out what nurses were actually doing on the job. Included an explanation of what constitutes good nursing care and a description of basic conditions calling for the services of a nurse.
Nursing Schools Today and Tomorrow (third study)	1934	Committee on Grading of Nursing Schools; Ethel Johns	Proposed characteristics of what a "professional" nurse should know and be able to do. Set forth conditions essential for growth and functioning of a professional school, including types of control, funding, and qualifications of faculty.

Appendix 1   (Continued)

Study	Year	Sponsor; Project Director	Key Points, Recommendations, Impact
Study of Incomes, Salaries and Employment Conditions Affecting Nurses (Exclusive of Those Engaged in Public Health Nursing)	1938	American Nurses' Association (ANA)	Data from 11,000 questionnaires returned by private-duty, institutional, and office nurses. Had considerable bearing on the development of the ANA economic security program.
Administrative Cost Analysis for Nursing Service and Nursing Education	1940	National League of Nursing Education (NLNE); American Hospital Association (AHA); ANA	Provided data on the cost of a school of nursing to the hospital and the economic value of services rendered by students. No real action taken.
The General Staff Nurse	1941	ANA, NLNE, AHA, Catholic Hospital Association (CHA) (joint committee)	Indicated that staff nurses had little status, as reflected by their hours of duty (often split shifts), salaries, and personnel policies. Gave impetus to the movement to upgrade staff nurses' status.
Nursing for the Future	1948	Carnegie Foundation; Russell Sage Foundation; National Nursing Council (representatives of various health organizations); Esther Lucile Brown, Ph.D. (social anthropologist)	Pointed out continued inadequacies of schools of nursing; emphasized need for official examination of all, with publication of names of accredited schools and pressure to eliminate those not accredited. Found nursing education "not professional." Nursing education should be part of the mainstream of education. Nurses could be divided into "professional" and "practical" categories. Mixed reviews. Similar recommendations given in other reports 20 years later.

Study	Year	Sponsor; Project Director	Key Points, Recommendations, Impact
Nursing Schools at the Mid-Century	1950	National Committee for the Improvement of Nursing Services (committee of members of all six national nursing organizations); Russell Sage Foundation; Margaret Bridgman, RN EdD (former Academic Dean)	Reported on practices of over 1000 schools of nursing (organization, cost, curriculum content, clinical resources, student heatlh). Gave schools the opporotunity to evaluate their performance. stimulated improvement in baccalaureate schools.
Twenty Thousand Nurses Tell Their Story	1958	ANA and American Nurses' Foundation (ANF); Dr. Everett C. Hughes (professor of sociology)	Part of a five-year sequence of 34 studies of nursing functions. Funded in part by individual nurses. Intended to produce better patient care; revealed what nurses actually did, their attitudes about the job, and job satisfaction. Formed basis for development of ANA nursing functions, standards, and qualifications.
Community College Education for Nursing	1959	Institute of Research and Service in Nursing Education Teachers College, Columbia University; Mildred Montag, RN EdD	Report of five-year Cooperative Research Project in Junior and Community College Education for Nursing, based on Montag's doctoral study. Included evaluation of seven two-year nursing programs leading to an associate degree (AD) in nursing. A second part presented data from 811 graduates. Influenced establishment of more AD programs.
Toward Quality in Nursing: Needs and Goals	1963	Consultant Group on Nursing—panel of nurses, others in the health field and the public; Apollinia Adams, RN (special assistant to Division of Nursing Chief)	Report to U.S. Surgeon General to advise him on nursing needs and to identify the role of the federal government in ensuring adequate nursing service for the nation. Noted qualitative and quantitative shortages of nursing personnel, problems in recruiting and retaining nurses, need for more nursing research, and improvement of nursing education and administration. Recommended study of nursing education and federal funding for nursing.

Appendix 1   (Continued)

Study	Year	Sponsor; Project Director	Key Points, Recommendations, Impact
An Abstract for Action (Report of the National Commission on Nursing and Nursing Education)	1970	ANA, ANF, National League for Nursing (NLN), Avalon (Mellon) and Kellogg Foundations; Jerome Lysaught, EdD	Analyzed current practices and patterns of nursing and assessed future needs. Included observations and analysis of findings from other studies; feedback from various groups reiterated many of Brown's findings and recommendations from 1948. Recommended joint practice committees of physicians and nurses; state master planning committees for nursing education; federal funding for nursing research and education; different approaches to nursing curriculum; degree programs in diploma schools. Got mixed reviews. Followed by new federal funding (for a short time), short term joint practice committees. Later follow-up showed little lasting impact.
Extending the Scope of Nursing Practice: A Report of the Secretary's Committee to Study Extended Roles	1971	U.S. Department of Health Education and Welfare (DHEW); Faye Abdellah, RN, EdD, Assistant Surgeon General	Appointed by Secretary Elliott Richardson. Reviewed current responsibilities of nurses; noted nurses' role on the health team. Recommended: curricular innovations demonstrating physician-nurse concept in health care delivery; financial support for educating nurses in extended role; economic studies to assess impact of extended nursing practice on health care system. Resulted in federal funding and growth of nurse practitioner programs.
The Study of Credentialing in Nursing: A New Approach	1979	ANA; Inez Hinsvark, RN, EdD (nursing professor)	Consisted of a comprehensive review of credentialing, especially health care and nursing. (Contains excellent information.) Followed by appointment of a Task Force to implement recommendations. Reaffirmed earlier recommendation to establish free-standing credentialing center for nursing. Not accepted by nursing organizations.

Study	Year	Sponsor; Project Director	Key Points, Recommendations, Impact
Magnet Hospitals: Attraction and Retention of Nurses	1983	American Academy of Nursing (AAN), AAN Task Force on Nursing Practice; Margaret McClure, RN, EdD, chair (nurse executive)	Identified U.S. hospitals able to attract and retain RNs. Studied 41 (questionnaires, interviews). Findings included the importance of well-prepared nurse managers and chief nurse executive; good nurse executives (seen as strong, supportive, visible); clearly enunciated high standards; participatory management; good personnel policies and competitive salaries; career development opportunities.
Nursing and Nursing Education; Public Policies and Private Actions	1983	DHHS contracted to the Institute of Medicine (IOM) Study Committee included some nurses; Dr. Katharine Bauer (nonnurse)	Mandated by PL 96-76, the Nurse Training Act Amendments of 1979, to determine whether further substantial outlays of federal monies for nursing education were needed to ensure an adequate supply of nurses. Recommended in part that various combinations of public and private support be applied to financial aid for nursing students in basic programs; graduate programs and students and NPs; programs to upgrade skills of RNs, LPNs, and aides in LTC facilities; improvement of supply and job tenure by addressing employment conditions; continued support for collection and analysis of nursing data; establishment of a federal organizational entity for nursing research. Seen as influential in establishment of National Center for Nursing Research (NCNR).

Appendix 1 (Continued)

Study	Year	Sponsor; Project Director	Key Points, Recommendations, Impact
National Commission on Nursing Study	1983	American Hospital Association (AHA); Hospital Research and Educational Trust; American Hospital Supply Corporation. Independent Commission; members from various fields, including nursing; Marjorie Beyers, RN, PhD	Primarily initiated in response to the nursing shortage. Final report much weaker than initial report, probably due to need for compromise to further implementation. Stated need for all types of nursing programs with baccalaureate education as an "achievable goal"; promoted educational mobility. Omitted statement urging utilization of nurses according to educational background. Other recommendations: high priority for nursing research; strong affiliations between academic institutions and practice settings; involvement of nursing in hospital policymaking; recognition of nursing as a clinical practice; salaries and benefits commensurate with nurse education, experience, and performance.
Secretary's Commission on Nursing	1988	DHHS; Lillian Gibbons, RN, PhD	Established in response to widespread nursing shortage; to advise the DHHS Secretary, Dr. Otis Bowen. Documented pervasive and serious nursing shortage and reinforced themes of previous nursing shortage studies concerning need for improvement of status and working conditions of nurses. Demand for nurses seen as increasing. To increase supply, saw need for increased financial support for education, improved program accessibility, promoting nursing as a career.
Nursings' Vital Signs: Shaping the Profession for the 1990s Report of the National Commission on Nursing Implementation Project (NCNIP)	1989	Tri Council, made up of ANA, NLN, American Association of Colleges of Nursing (AACN), American Organization of Nurse Executives (AONE); Vivien De Back, RN, PhD	NCNIP was launched in 1984 with Kellogg Foundation funding to implement selected recommendations of the IOM and the National Commission on Nursing Reports. Described innovative approaches and strategies developed by the work groups on education, management and practice, research, and development. Distributed a number of brochures and documents offering recommendations for the future of nursing.

Study	Year	Sponsor; Project Director	Key Points, Recommendations, Impact
			Also noted that NPs and CNMs not used to fullest, in part due to lack of reimbursement. Held number of conferences on differentiated practice (nursing assignments according to competence, experience, and educational background); nursing information systems; and nurses' contribution to health care. Developed proposal for Advertising Council to clarify image of nursing. Successful National Nursing Image Campaign seen as partially responsible for increasing nursing school enrollments. Project concluded in 1991; seen as fostering coalitions between nursing and other groups.
Secretary's Commission on the National Nursing Shortage	1991	DHHS; Caroline Burnett, RN, ScD	Appointed for one year by DHHS Secretary, Dr. Louis Sullivan, to advise federal officials on projects to implement the recommendations of the 1988 report. Focus: recruitment, retention; restructuring nursing services; data collection and analysis; information system in nursing.

Appendix 2 Major Health Care Services Personnel

Occupation/ profession	Estimated active supply[a] (if available)	One year or less	Associate degree, or 2- or 3- year program	Baccalaureate	Clinical[e]
			Basic education[b]		
Primary Care					
Chiropractor (DC)	30,000			2 years min.	4 years
Clinical psychologist	NA				4 years
Dentist (DD)	147,000			3 years min.	3–4 years +
Doctor of Medicine (MD)	587,500			3 years min.	5 years +
Doctor of Optometry (OD)	26,000		X	2 years min.	4 years
Doctor of Osteopathy (DO)	26,500			3 years min.	4 years
Doctor of Podiatric Medicine (DPM) (Podiatrist)	11,500			3 years min.	4 years
Nurse-midwife (NM)[g]	4,500		X	X	X
Nurse practitioner (NP)[g]	25,000–35,000		X	X	X
Nursing (all areas except primary care)					
Registered nurse (RN)	Approximately 2 million		X	2 years min.	1–2 years
Licensed practical nurse (LPN)	781,406	X			

Graduate	State regulation:[c] licensure, certification, registration	Major issues and trends[d]
	X[f]	Not accepted as legitimate by some health care providers, especially MDs. After battle, recognized in all states as primary care providers, with reimbursement, including Medicare and Medicaid.
Usually PhD	X[f]	Competing with psychiatrists and others in mental health for patients. Seeking prescriptive authority.
	X[f]	Oversupply. Some dental schools closing or admitting fewer. Looking for new areas of practice.
	X[f]	Oversupply predicted by 2000, especially specialists. Others encroaching on their practice. Less control. More becoming employees. More are marketing services.
	X[f]	Education expanding to prepare better for expanded diagnosis and treatment; MDs object. Growth in pediatric, rehabilitative, and geriatric optometry.
	X[f]	Still growing; oversupply not reported, perhaps because fewer in specialties (although increasing).
	X[f]	Struggling with MDs to expand practice. Residency programs (advanced training) expanding, although not required. Want more liberal hospital privileges. Concern about wages, autonomy, federal funding.
X	X[f]	More middle-class women want their services; more MDs trying to limit their practice. Major insurance crisis with soaring rates resulted in first nurse self-insurance. Only half employed in practices that include deliveries. Lay midwives are seeking legal recognition.
X	X[f]	More states allowing for expanded practice, prescriptive authority and reimbursement. Still difficult to have independent practice. MD opposition continues.
X	X[f]	Greater movement to higher education. New opportunities outside of hospitals. Possible change in licensure. Major shortages.
	X[f]	Fewer being employed, except in some shortage areas. Longer educational program being suggested. More continuing to RN.

Appendix 2   (Continued)

Occupation/ profession	Estimated active supply[a] (if available)	Basic education[b]			
		One year or less	Associate degree, or 2- or 3- year program	Baccalaureate	Clinical[e]
Nurse anesthetist	21,000		X	X	X
Nursing assistant (NA) Home health aid (not including mental health)	850,000 +	X			

Others providing direct services or therapy					
Art, music, dance therapists[h]	NA			X	
Dental assistant[b]	197,000	X	X		
Dental hygienist[h]	61,000		X		
Dietitians[b]	40,000			X	1 year
Dietetic technician Assistant[h]	5,000	X	X		
Emergency medical technician (EMT)[h]	NA	X	X		
Pharmacist	158,000	X		5 years	1–2 years (PharmD)
Physician's assistant (PA)[h]	21,000		X	X	
Psychiatric mental health technician[h]	NA	X	X		
Respiratory therapist[h]	65,000	X	X	X	
Surgical technologist (OR technician)[h]	NA	X	X		
Therapeutic recreational specialist[h]	NA			X	

Graduate	State regulation:[c] licensure, certification, registration	Major issues and trends[d]
X	X	Major shortage.
	X	Many in nursing homes. Low salaries continue. Some increase in hospital employment to relieve nursing shortage. Being encouraged to continue education to LPN; RN level. New requirements for some kind of state regulation, including training, for some types of aides.
		Limited use.
	X	
	X[f]	More seeking independent practice, not controlled by dentist, and role expansion; dentists objecting. Some giving anesthesia.
		Some see need for licensure; achieved in few states. Concern about image, third-party reimbursement.
		More delegation from dietitian in management and routine diet instruction; assistants suggested for broader role in nursing home.
	X[f]	Some struggle with nursing because of their use as nurse substitutes, especially in emergency rooms.
	X[f]	Looking for ways to expand role. Some as clinical pharmacists, some in primary care (like the NP). PharmD wanted as entry-level degree. External degree programs for pharmacists who want PharmD.
X	X[f]	Programs expected to grow. Being used in hospitals instead of residents. Must work under direction of MD. A few states permit prescribing. Some competition with NPs. Some going on to nursing or public health. Now equal number of women and men.
	X	Much used in state, local government hospitals. RN concern about overuse, competence. Low salary.
	X	Disagreement as to whether nurses should reassume some of these responsibilities. Increased demand in hospitals.
		Disagreement as to whether OR nurses should include this role; report to nurse or MD. Low salary.
X		Limited use.

Appendix 2   (Continued)

Occupation/ profession	Estimated active supply[a] (if available)	Basic education[b]			
		One year or less	Associate degree, or 2- or 3- year program	Baccalaureate	Clinical[e]
Diagnostic Services					
Clinical laboratory technicians[h]			X		
Technologists[h]	264,000[i]			X	
EEG technician[h]	NA	X	X		
EKG technician[h]	NA	X	X		
Nuclear medicine technologist[h]	NA		X		
Radiologic technologist (x-ray technician)[h]	125,000[i]	X	X	X	
Administration, Business, Record Keeping					
Hospital administrator[i]	NA			X	Nonclinical residency sometimes
Assistant[i]	NA				
Middle manager	NA			X	
Nursing home administrator	18,000+	X	X	X	Possible residency
Medical records administrator (RRA)[h]	56,000		X	1–2 years	
Technician (HRT)[h]			X		
Medical secretary-unit clerk	NA	X	X		
Unit (ward) manager	NA	X	X	X	
Rehabilitation, Counseling, and Social Support					
Denturist (dental technician)	66,700		X (or apprenticeship)		

Graduate	State regulation:[c] licensure, certification, registration	Major issues and trends[d]
	X	More complex technology and computers being used. Some leaving because of fear of AIDS.
	X	Low salaries at technician and assistant level.
		Low salaries.
		Low salaries.
		More complex technology.
	X[f]	Becoming more complex with subspecialization in field. Major shortage.
X		Oversupply for hospitals predicted. Need for strategic planners, financially astute people cited.
		May be entry-level for higher administration. Competition in hospitals greater; opportunities in free-standing clinics; may compete there with nurse managers.
X	X[f]	More sophisticated, educated managers needed as small faciltities are taken over; cost pressures.
	X	Great need predicted, especially because of importance of records for reimbursement; more computer use.
		Computer affecting how a job is done.
		May be entering position for management career ladder.
	X	Looking for independent practice, free of dentists.

Appendix 2 (Continued)

Occupation/ profession	Estimated active supply[a] (if available)	Basic education[b]			
		One year or less	Associate degree, or 2- or 3- year program	Baccalaureate	Clinical[e]
Occupational therapist (OT)	31,600			X	X
Assistant	NA	X	X		
Optician	NA	X	X (or apprenticeship)		
Physical Therapist (PT)[a]	66,000		X	X	X
Technician[h]		X			
Rehabilitation counselor[h]	NA				
Speech pathologist/[h]	83,000			X	X
Audiologist				X	X
Medical social worker (SW)[h]	NA			X	X
Vocational rehabilitation therapist[h]	NA				

Public/community health; environment

Occupation/ profession	Estimated active supply[a] (if available)	One year or less	Associate degree, or 2- or 3- year program	Baccalaureate	Clinical[e]
Community/school health educator	NA			X	X
Environmentalist (sanitarian)	NA				
Industrial hygienists and safety technicians	NA		X	X	

[a]Most figures are cited from seventh *Report to the President and Congress on the Status of Health personnel in the United States,* Department of Health and Human Services, Bureau of Health Professions, 1990. Estimated *active* number only recorded.

[b]Specialization, teaching, or supervision generally require higher credentials beyond this basic education. When technician and technologist are in the same field, technician education is usually at associate degree, technologist at baccalaureate. Some educational programs require only 2 years of college, followed by a clinical program, but often students already have or choose a baccalaureate first. When more than one X is present, student has a choice of basic education.

[c]Available, not necessarily required, in at least one state. Often inconsistent from state to state.

[d]Almost all share the concern of diminishing federal support and need for ensuring continued competence.

[e]Usually assumes liberal arts or other baccalaureate that does not include clinical work; usually a separate school or program such as medicine or optometry, sometimes followed by specialization training.

Graduate	State regulation:[c] licensure, certification, registration	Major issues and trends[d]
X	X	More needed in home care. Major shortage now.
X	X X	Great demand; many have private practices; more needed in home care. Set entry at master's. Major shortage.
X		Some competition with other rehabilitation groups.
X X	X[f] X[f]	Growing fields; more with graduate education.
X	X[f]	Looking for ways to expand role. Overlap with others. Competing with nurses in case management. Move toward doctorates. More needed.
X		Some competition with social workers; governmental positions may decrease with budget cuts.
X		Expanding role as prevention/health promotion is funded; some competition with nurses.
X		More complex problems to deal with because of new discoveries of environmental dangers.
X		May be under pressure in work situations because of pressures from employers vs. labor.

[f]Mandatory CE (if known).

[g]Have basic licensure as RN, but may also be licensed as CNM or NP. Basic nursing education could be from AD to baccalaureate. Specialty program could be nondegree or graduate.

[h]Designated as allied health by federal government. Estimate of total employed allied health personnel is 1,400,000. Where numbers are not reported in this chart, federal government does not have figures. One general concern is lack of minorities and women entering programs and some trend by administrators to want general-purpose, not specialized worker. Career ladder is lacking for most nonprofessionals.

[i]Includes other allied health workers in that field.

[j]Administrators/managers of community health agencies, group practices, and other free-standing facilities are not included.

Appendix 3   Educational Options in Nursing

Types	Approximate number of programs (1990)	Program sites	Program length	Admission requirements[a]	Cost per year tuition and fees (1990)
Practical/ vocational nursing education	1154	Vocational/ technical school; junior college; hospital; high school/independent agency/college (rarely)	12–18 months[d]	High school or equivalent unless program is in high school.	$1585 public; $3344 private
Associate degree (AD) education	829	Junior/ community, technical college; senior college; hospital (rarely)	2 academic years (12–18 months) to 2 calendar years	College requirements. High school or equivalent. Specific courses may be required to enter nursing program.	$967 public; $5227 private

Curriculum	Credential[b]	Educational Mobility	Competencies at Graduation[c]
Basic theory on illness and health. Introductory biological and social sciences. About two-thirds of time in clinical settings.	Certificate; diploma; associate degree[d], LPH/LVN license after NCLEX-PN.	Career ladder usually with testing into RN programs. External AD or BSN degrees available.	1. Practices primarily in hospitals and nursing homes, functioning under the guidance and supervision of an RN, physician, or dentist, to provide basic therapeutic rehabilitative and preventive care to patients with well-defined health problems. 2. Assesses basic physical, emotional, spiritual, and sociocultural needs of the health care client and provides appropriate nursing care. 3. Collects data within established protocols and guidelines from various sources. 4. Utilizes knowledge of normal values to identify deviations in health status. 5. Documents data collection. 6. Communicates findings to appropriate health care personnel, recording accurately. 7. Contributes to the development of nursing care plans utilizing established nursing diagnoses for clients with common, well-defined health problems. 8. Prioritizes nursing care needs of clients. 9. Assists in the review and revision of nursing care plans to meet the changing needs of clients. 10. Establishes and maintains therapeutic relationships with clients, families, and significant others.

Adapted from K. Beaver et al., *Entry-level competencies of graduates of educational programs in practical nursing,* 2nd ed. (New York: National League for Nursing, 1989).

Basic natural and social sciences, humanities; nursing courses; supervised experiences in hospital and other agencies. About $1/2$ program is general education.	Associate degree. Licensure after passing NCLEX-RN. Some certification later if exams passed.[g]	Most of nonnursing courses transfer to baccalaureate. May need to test for advanced standing in nursing. Some programs have direct articulation. External BSN degree available	1. Functions as a generalist in a structured setting where policies, procedures, and protocols for health care are established. 2. Develops, implements, and evaluates a nursing plan, using established nursing diagnoses and data related to the client's cultural, spiritual, psychosocial, and physical needs, to promote, maintain, and restore health; revises plan as needed.

Appendix 3   (Continued)

Types	Approximate number of programs (1990)	Program sites	Program length	Admission require-ments[a]	Cost per year tuition and fees (1990)
Associate degree *(Continued)*					
Diploma education	139	Hospital	Usually 24–30 months; could be three years	High school or equivalent. Good academic achievement. Prerequisite courses.	$2826 public; $3094 private

Curriculum	Credential[b]	Educational Mobility	Competencies at Graduation[c]
			3. Provides direct care for clients with common well-defined diagnoses, using the nursing process; establishes priorities for care.
			4. Administers and monitors the medical regimen for clients undergoing therapeutic and/or diagnostic procedures.
			5. Communicates effectively, verbally and in writing, concerning client's response to treatment, and uses communication techniques that assist client and significant others to cope with and resolve problems.
			6. Modifies and implements teaching plan as needed, collaborating with other health care workers.
			7. Recognizes need for referral, confers with other appropriate personnel, and makes referral.
			8. Delegates aspects of care appropriately to LPNs and ancillary personnel, and is accountable for care delegated.
			9. Provides for continuity of care in management of chronic health care needs.
			10. Recognizes the importance of nursing research.

Adapted from *Educational outcomes of associate degree nursing programs: Roles and competencies.* (New York: National League for Nursing 1990 and *Defining and differentiating ADN and BSN Competencies* (MAIN, 1985).

Curriculum	Credential[b]	Educational Mobility	Competencies at Graduation[c]
Natural and social sciences, sometimes from a college. Nursing courses, early clinical experience focused on hospital nursing.	Diploma; AD; BS[e] Licensing after passing NCLEX-RN.[d] Some certification later if pass exam.[g]	College courses may transfer. May need to test for advanced standing in nursing, BSN external degree available.	1. Provides nursing care for individuals, families, and groups by utilizing the nursing process. 2. Provides for the promotion, maintenance, and restoration of health, and support and comfort to the suffering and dying. 3. Utilizes management skills including collaboration, coordination, and communication with individuals, families, groups, and other members of the health care team. 4. Assumes a leadership role within the health care system. 5. Teaches individuals, families, and groups based on identified health needs.

Appendix 3 (Continued)

Types	Approximate number of programs (1990)	Program sites	Program length	Admission require-ments[a]	Cost per year tuition and fees (1990)
Diploma education (*Continued*)					
Baccalaureate education	489 (generic) 139 (BRN)	College; university; hospital[e]	4 academic years	Admission requirement for institution and program. Good academic standing.	$1626 public; $7414 private

Curriculum	Credential[b]	Educational Mobility	Competencies at Graduation[c]
			6. Functions as an advocate for the consumer and the health care system to improve the quality and delivery of care.
			7. Practices nursing based on a theoretical body of knowledge, ethical principles, and legal standards.
			8. Evaluates nursing practice for improvement of nursing care.
			9. Accepts responsibility and accountability for professional practice.
			10. Utilizes opportunities for continuing personal and professional development.
			11. Participates in health-related community services.
			12. Utilizes critical thinking in professional practice.

Adapted from *Role and competencies of graduates of diploma programs in nursing,* 2nd ed. (New York: National League for Nursing, 1989).

Curriculum	Credential[b]	Educational Mobility	Competencies at Graduation[c]
About one-half liberal arts and sciences. Nursing theory and practice last 2 years. Clinical experience in many settings, including public health.	Bachelor of Science. Other baccalaureate. Licensing after passing NCLEX-RN. Some certification later if exam is passed.[g]	Can advance directly to graduate work if other qualifications met.	AD competencies plus: 1. Practices as a generalist in all settings. Provides comprehensive services of assessing, promoting, and maintaining physical and mental health of individuals, families, groups, and aggregates (populations with shared characteristics of environment).
			2. Plans, implements evaluates, and directs care for clients, including those with complex health care needs, assuming a leadership role.
			3. Interprets medical plan of care into nursing activities.
			4. Evaluates nursing research for applicability to nursing actions and incorporates appropriate findings after consulting with nurse researcher.
			5. Collaborates with colleagues and citizens in identifying and effecting needed changes in health care.
			6. Synthesizes theoretical and empirical knowledge from nursing, scientific, and humanistic disciplines with practice.

Appendix 3   (Continued)

Types	Approximate number of programs (1990)	Program sites	Program length	Admission requirements[a]	Cost per year tuition and fees (1990)
Baccalaureate education (*Continued*)					
Graduate education (basic)	Under 10 (master's) 2 doctorate	University University	2–3 academic years 3 academic years	Baccalaureate in any field. May require prerequisite courses. Mature; high academic standing or other achievements.	(Relates to all) Graduate education tuition varies greatly according to type of program and region. Mean annual tuition $3,438 (may go to $19,000) Part-time $247 per credit mean. Can be much higher.
Master's (advanced)	231	University	1–3 academic years	Nursing baccalaureate usually necessary;[f] good academic standing.	
Doctorate	50	University	1–2 academic years beyond master's plus dissertation	Same as master's, but have good grades standing in graduate study and research capabilities. Other special requirements.	

Curriculum	Credential[b]	Educational Mobility	Competencies at Graduation[c]
			7. Enhances the quality of nursing and health practices within practice settings through the use of leadership skills and a knowledge of the political system. 8. Evaluates research for the applicability of its findings to nursing practice.

Adapted from *Characteristics of baccalaureate education* in nursing (National League for Nursing, 1987) and *Defining and differentiating ADN and BSN competencies* (MAIN, 1985.)

Curriculum	Credential[b]	Educational Mobility	Competencies at Graduation[c]
Nursing theory and practice. Nursing sciences if not prerequisite. Clinical experience in diverse settings.	Master in Science or other master's. Doctor of Nursing (ND). Certification later if pass exam.	Master's graduates advance directly to doctorate if other requirements met. NDs continue to specialization master's and doctorates.	Similar to baccalaureate, but in master's program, some of the time may be devoted to specialization. ND particularly geared to scientific inquiry.
Nursing theory and practice in clinical specialization, administration, or education. Usually research courses. Research, advanced theory, and practice in selected field.	Master of science. Other Master's. Certification if pass test.[g] DNS, PhD, other doctorates.	Same as above. Postdoctoral study available.	Builds on baccalaureate plus: 1. Practices in all health care settings as clinical specialist/nurse practitioner or clinician with specialized clinical knowledge and skills caring for individuals, family, groups, or aggregates. Nurse administrators or nurse educators may have and use some or all of these clinical skills in performing their functions. 2. Acts as consultant to colleagues in nursing, other health disciplines, agencies, and organizations. 3. As clinician, provides additional insight in coordinating medical and nursing care plans. 4 Collaborates as equal with other disciplines. 5. Initiates nursing research and collaborates in research with nursing and other colleagues.

Appendix 3   (Continued)

Curriculum	Credential[b]	Educational Mobility	Competencies at Graduation[c]
Graduate study (*Continued*)			6. Improves nursing and health care through expert practice and through the advancement of theory in practice. 7. Assumes leadership role in development of nursing as profession and as influential part of health care delivery and policy making. 8. Collaborates with colleagues and citizens in identifying and effecting needed changes in health care.

[a]Most programs require references and some indication of motivation to succeed in a field. This becomes very important in acceptance for advanced education. Some require admissions test.

[b]All nursing programs have the option of seeking accreditation by the National League for Nursing.

[c]All speak to ethical and legal practice and accountability.

[d]North Dakota requires AD for LPN and BSN for RN. Other states may follow.

[e]A few states have permitted some hospital based schools to give degrees.

[f]Some programs accept nurses with nonnursing baccalaureates, usually with prerequisite courses and/or experience.

[g]Some specialty certification is available after testing and specialty experiences or education without advanced degrees. Trend toward requiring degree for specialities.

Appendix 4   State Boards of Nursing (1991)

Alabama Board of Nursing
500 Eastern Blvd., Suite #203
Montgomery, AL 36117

Alaska Board of Nursing Licensing
Dept. of Commerce and Economic
  Development, Division of
  Occupational Licensing
P.O. Box D-LIC
Juneau, AK 99811-0800

Arizona Board of Nursing
2001 W. Camelback Rd., #350
Phoenix, AZ 85015

Arkansas Board of Nursing
University Tower Bldg.
1123 S. University Ave., Suite 800
Little Rock, AR 77205

California Board of Registered Nursing
P.O. Box 944210
1030 13th St., Suite 200
Sacramento, CA 94244-2100

Colorado Board of Nursing
1560 Broadway, Suite 670
Denver, CO 80203

Connecticut Board of Examiners for
  Nursing
150 Washington St.
Hartford, CT 06106

Delaware Board of Nursing
Margaret O'Neill Bldg.
Federal and Court Sts.
Dover, DE 19901

District of Columbia Board of Nursing
614 H St., N.W.
Washington, DC 20001

Florida Board of Nursing
111 E. Coastline Dr., Suite 504
Jacksonville, FL 32202

Georgia Board of Nursing
166 Pryor St., S.W., Suite 400
Atlanta, GA 30303

Guam Board of Nurse Examiners
Box 2816
Agana, Guam 96910

Hawaii Board of Nursing
Box 3469
Honolulu, HI 96801

Idaho Board of Nursing
2800 N. 8th St., Suite 210
Boise, ID 83720

Illinois Department of Professional
  Regulation
320 W. Washington St.
Springfield, IL 62786

Indiana State Board of Nursing
Health Professions Bureau
One American Square,
  Suite 1020
P.O. Box 82067
Indianapolis, IN 46282-0004

Iowa Board of Nursing
1223 E. Court
Des Moines, IA 50319

Kansas State Board of Nursing
Landon State Office Bldg.
900 SW Jackson, Rm. 551
Topeka, KS 66612-1256

Kentucky Board of Nursing
4010 Dupont Circle, Suite 430
Louisville, KY 40207

Louisiana Board of Nursing
150 Baronne St., Rm. 907
New Orleans, LA 70112

Maine Board of Nursing
State House Station 158
Augusta, ME 04333

Maryland Board of Nursing
Metro Executive Center
4201 Patterson Ave.
Baltimore, MD 21215-2299

Appendix 4 (Continued)

Massachusetts Board of
  Registration in Nursing
R. 1519, 100 Cambridge St.
Boston, MA 02202

Michigan Board of Nursing
P.O. Box 30018
Lansing, MI 48909

Minnesota Board of Nursing
2700 University Ave. W., #108
St. Paul, MN 55414

Mississippi Board of Nursing
239 N. Lamar St.
Suite 401
Jackson, MS 39201

Missouri Board of Nursing
3605 Missouri Blvd.
P.O. Box 656
Jefferson City, MO 65102

Montana Board of Nursing
Dept. of Commerce
Arcade Bldg. Lower Level
111 N. Jackson
Helena, MT 59620-0407

Nebraska Board of Nursing
Box 95007
Lincoln, NE 68509

Nevada Board of Nursing
1281 Terminal Way, Suite 116
Reno, NV 89502

New Hampshire Board of Nursing
Div. of Public Health Services
Health and Welfare Bldg.
6 Hazen Dr.
Concord, NH 03301-6527

New Jersey Board of Nursing
1100 Raymond Blvd., Rm. 508
Newark, NJ 07102

New Mexico Board of Nursing
4253 Montgomery NE, Suite 130
Albuquerque, NM 87108

New York Board of Nursing
State Education Dept.
Cultural Education Center
Albany, NY 12230

North Carolina Board of Nursing
Box 2129
Raleigh, NC 27602

North Dakota Board of Nursing
919 S 7th St., Suite 504
Bismark, ND 58504-5881

Ohio Board of Nursing
77 S. High St., 17th Floor
Columbus, OH 43266-0316

Oklahoma Board of Nurse Registration
  and Nursing Education
2915 N. Classen Blvd., Suite 524
Oklahoma City, OK 73106

Oregon Board of Nursing
10445 SW Canyon Rd., Suite 200
Beaverto, OR 97005

Pennsylvania Board of Nursing
P.O. Box 2649
Harrisburg, PA 17105-2649

Puerto Rico Board of Nurse Examiners
Call Box 10200
Santurce, PR 00908

Rhode Island Board of Nurse
  Registration and Nursing Education
Cannon Health Building
75 Davis St.
Providence, RI 02908

South Carolina Board of Nursing
220 Executive Center Dr., Suite 220
Columbia, SC 29210

South Dakota Board of Nursing
304 S. Phillips Ave., Suite 205
Sioux Falls, SD 57102

Tennessee Board of Nursing
Bureau of Manpower and Facilities
283 Plus Park Blvd.
Nashville, TN 37219-5401

Texas Board of Nurse Examiners
9101 Burnet Rd., Suite 104
Austin, TX 78758

Utah Division of Occupational and
  Professional Licensing of Nursing
Heber M. Wells Bldg., 4th floor
160 East 300 South
P.O. Box 45802
Salt Lake City, UT 84145

Vermont Board of Nursing
Redstone Bldg.
26 Terrace St.
Montpelier, VT 05602

Virgin Islands Board of Nurse Licensure
Medical Arts Complex
P.O. Box 7309, Suite 13
Harwood Highway, Contant
Charlotte Amalie
St. Thomas, VI 00801

Virginia Board of Nursing
1601 Rolling Hills Dr.
Richmond, VA 23229

Washington Board of Nursing
Licensing Information
Division of Professional Licensing
Box 9649
Olympia, WA 98504

West Virginia Board of Examiners for
  Registered Nurses
Embleton Bldg., Rm 309
922 Quarrier St.
Charleston, WV 25301

Wisconsin Board of Nursing
Rm 174, P. O. Box 8935
Madison, WI 53708

Wyoming Board of Nursing
Barrett Bldg., 3rd Floor
2301 Central Ave.
Cheyenne, WY 82002

Note: See the April directory of the *American Journal of Nursing* for changes.

Appendix 5   Major Nursing and Related Organizations

Organization	Year established[a]	Membership eligibility[b]	Primary purpose
General Nursing Organizations			
American Nurses' Association (ANA) 600 Maryland Ave. S.W., Washington, DC 20005	1897	Only state and territorial nurses' organizations (SNA) are members. RN licensure for individual membership in SNA	Work for improvement of health standards and availability of care for all; foster high standards of nursing; stimulate and promote professional development of nurses and advance their economic and general welfare.
International Council of Nurses (ICN) 3, Place Jean-Marteau 1201, Geneva, Switzerland	1900	National nurses' organizations.	Share knowledge so nursing practice throughout the world is improved; provide a medium through which national nurses' associations may share common interests to promote health of the people and care of the sick.
National League for Nursing (NLN) 350 Hudson St., New York, NY 10014	1893	(1) Anyone interested in fostering development and improvement of nursing service and education, and (2) nursing service and education agencies.	Foster development and improvement of nursing services and nursing education through coordinated action of nursing and others, so that nursing needs of the people are met. Accredit nursing education and service agencies.[g]
National Student Nurses' Association (NSNA) 555 W. 57th St., New York, NY 10019	1953	Students in state approved programs leading to RN licensure or RNs enrolled in baccalaureate nursing programs.	Contribute to nursing education to provide for highest quality health care; CE; aid in development of student.

Activities[c]							
Certifi-cation[d]	CE	Standards set and published	Legislative activities[e]	Research activities[f]	Members of NFSNO	NOLF	Publications (monthly unless otherwise indicated)
X	X	X	X	X		X	*American Nurse; American Journal of Nursing; Capital Update;* Other[h]
	X	X		X			*International Nursing Review;* other[h]
	X	X	X	X		X	*Nursing and Health Care;* other[h]
	X		X	X		X	*Imprint;* other[h]

Appendix 5   (Continued)

Organization	Year established[a]	Membership eligibility[b]	Primary purpose
Speciality Nursing Organizations			
American Association of Critical-Care Nurses (AACN) 101 Columbia, Aliso Viejo, CA 92656	1969	Any RN who provides specialized care to critically ill patients or is interested in the specialty; includes faculty and nurse administrators.	Improve practice; provide CE for critical-care nurses; promote environments that facilitate comprehensive nursing practice for people with critical illness or injury.
American Association of Neuroscience Nurses (AANN) 218 N. Jefferson, Suite 204, Chicago, IL 60606 (related to World Federation of Neurosurgical Nursing)	1968	RNs active or interested in neurological, neurosurgical nursing.	Foster and promote interest, education, research, and high standards in neurosurgical nursing and promote growth of nursing.
American Association of Nurse Anesthetists (AANA) 216 W. Higgins Park Ridge, IL 60068	1931	RNs qualified by training and experience to give anesthesia.	Advance science and art of anesthesia; promote cooperation with other disciplines; CE; develop standards.
American Association of Occupational Health Nurses (AAOHN) 50 Lenox Point Atlanta, GA 30324	1942	RNs employed in occupational health	Maintain professional excellence in OHN through education and research programs; promote OHN; stimulate interest and provide forum for issues in field.

Activities[c]							
Certifi-cation[d]	CE	Standards set and published	Legislative activities[e]	Research activities[f]	Members of NFSNO	NOLF	Publications (monthly unless otherwise indicated)
X	X	X	X	X	X	X	*AACN News; Heart and Lung: The Journal of Critical Care; Focus on Critical Care;* other[h]
X	X	X	X	X	X	X	*Journal of Neuroscience Nursing; Synapse* (both bimonthly); other[h]
X[g]	X	X	X	X	X	X	*J. Am. Ass'n of Nurse Anesth.* (bimonthly); *AANA News-bulletin;* other[h]
X	X	X	X	X	X	X	*AAOHN Journal; AAOHN News;* other[h]

Appendix 5   (Continued)

Organization	Year established[a]	Membership eligibility[b]	Primary purpose
American Association of Spinal Cord Injury Nurses (AASCIN) 75-20 Astoria Blvd. Jackson Heights, NY 11370-1178	1983	RNs engaged in care of patients with spinal cord injury	Promote excellence in meeting needs of those with spinal cord injury; disseminate information; promote education and research.
American College of Nurse Midwives (ACNM) 1522 K Street NW, Suite 1120, Washington, DC 20005	1955	Certified nurse-midwives or RN students in accredited nurse-midwifery programs.	Set standards for education and practice and evaluate these. Facilitate efforts of CNMs who provide quality service to individuals and child-bearing families. Promote research.
American Nephrology Nurses Association (ANNA) North Woodbury Rd., Box 56, Pitman, NJ 08071	1969	RNs interested in care of patients with renal disease	Develop and update standards of practice in this field; to promote individual growth, promote research and development in field; CE.
American Public Health Association (APHA) Public Health Nursing Section, 1015 15th St. N.W., Washington, DC 20005	APHA 1872; PHN section 1923	RNs practicing or interested in PH nursing.	Improve nursing service and education in broad perspective of public health.
American Society of Ophthalmic Registered Nurses (ASORN) P.O. Box 193030, San Francisco, CA 94119	1976	RNs engaged in ophthalmic nursing.	Unite RNs in field to promote excellence in ophthalmic nursing; CE
American Society of Plastic and Reconstructive Surgical Nurses (ASPRSN) North Woodbury Rd., Box 56, Pitman, NJ 08071	1975	LPNs, RNs engaged in field of plastic and reconstructive surgery.	Promote highest professional standards for better and safer care; CE.

Activities[c]

Certifi-cation[d]	CE	Standards set and published	Legislative activities[e]	Research activities[f]	Members of NFSNO	NOLF	Publications (monthly unless otherwise indicated)
	X	X	X	X	X	X	*SCI Nursing* (quarterly) other[h]
X[g]	X	X	X	X	X	X	*Journal of Nurse Midwifery; Quickening* (bimonthly); other[h]
X	X	X	X	X	X	X	*ANNA Journal; ANNA Update;* other[h]
	X	X	X	X	X	X	*American Journal of Public Health; Nation's Health;* other[h]
	X				X	X	*Insight* (bimonthly); other[h]
	X	X			X	X	*Journal of Plastic and Reconstructive Surgical Nursing;* other[h]

Appendix 5   (Continued)

Organization	Year established[a]	Membership eligibility[b]	Primary purpose
American Society of Post Anesthesia Nurses (ASPAN) 11512 Allecingie Pkwy, Richmond, VA 23235	1980	RNs with primary practice in post anesthesia care.	CE. Upgrade standards of care; promote professional growth; facilitate cooperation with others in field; encourage specialization and research.
American Urological Association, Allied (AUAA) 11512 Allecingie Pkwy, Richmond, VA 23235	1972	Persons in health care profession engaged in care of urologic patient.	Serve as vehicle for distribution of all available information in field; point way to advanced nursing technique and equipment; help nurses to become specialists.
Association of Operating Room Nurses (AORN) 10170 E. Mississippi Ave., Denver, CO 80231	1954	Nurses employed in perioperative practice, education, research	Enhance professionalism of perioperative nurses; improve their performance; provide a forum for interaction and idea exchange.
Association of Pediatric Oncology Nurses (APON) 11512 Allecingie Pkwy, Richmond, VA 23235.	1974	RNs interested in or engaged in pediatrics, oncology, pediatric oncology.	Promote optimal care of children with cancer and their families.
Association for Practictioners in Infection Control (APIC) 505 E. Hawley, Mundelein, IL 60060	1972	All individuals involved in infection control activities.	Improve patient care, support development of effective and rational infection control programs, promote quality research in field.
Association of Rehabilitation Nurses (ARN) 5100 Old Orchard Rd., Skokie, IL 60077	1974	RNs in rehabilitation nursing.	Advance quality of rehabilitation nursing; CE.

Activities[c]

Certifi-cation[d]	CE	Standards set and published	Legislative activities[e]	Research activities[f]	Members of NFSNO	NOLF	Publications (monthly unless otherwise indicated)
X	X	X			X	X	*Breathline* (bimonthly); *Journal of Post Anesthesia Nursing*; other[h]
X	X	X	X	X	X	X	*Urologic Nursing, Urogram* (both quarterly); other[h]
X	X	X	X	X	X	X	*AORN Journal;* other[h]
	X	X		X	X		*Journal of Pediatric Oncology* (quarterly); other[h]
X	X	X	X		X	X	*American Journal of Infection Control;* newsletter; other[h]
X	X	X	X		X	X	*Rehabilitation Nursing* (bimonthly); other[h]

Appendix 5   (Continued)

Organization	Year established[a]	Membership eligibility[b]	Primary purpose
Dermatology Nurses' Association (DNA) North Woodbury Rd., Box 56, Pitman, NJ 08071	1982	RNs, LPNs and techicians in dermatology nursing.	Develop and foster highest standards of dermatologic nursing care; enhance professional growth through education and research; promote interdisciplinary collaboration; enhance communication.
Emergency Nurses' Association (ENA) 230 E. Ohio, Chicago, IL 60611	1970	RNs in emergency care with special skills or knowledge in emergency nursing.	Provide optimum care to patients in emergency departments; CE.
International Association for Enterostomal Therapy (IAET) 2081 Business Center Dr., Suite 290, Irvine, CA 92715	1968	RNs who are enterostomal therapists; RNs specializing in incontinence rehabilitiation.	Promote highest standards of education, research, and practice in field.
Intravenous Nurses Society (INS) Two Brighton St., Belmont, MA 02178	1973	RNs in specialty practice of IV therapy.	Enhance the practice of an IV nurse through research, education, and standards.
National Association of Orthopaedic Nurses (NAON) North Woodbury Rd., Box 56, Pitman, NJ 08071	1980	RNs/LPNs involved in orthopedic nursing.	Enhance personal and professional growth of members through continuing education.
National Association of Pediatric Nurse Associates and Practitioners (NAP-NAP) 1101 Kings Hwy Rd., Suite 206, Cherry Hill, NJ 08034	1973	RNs who are primary care specialists in pediatrics.	Support legislation to improve the quality of health care to children and adolescents; CE.

Activities[c]

Certifi-cation[d]	CE	Standards set and published	Legislative activities[e]	Research activities[f]	Members of NFSNO	Members of NOLF	Publications (monthly unless otherwise indicated)
	X				X	X	*Focus* (bimonthly newsletter); *DNA Nursing Journal*
X	X	X	X	X	X	X	*Journal of Emergency Nursing;* other[h]
X	X	X	X	X	X	X	*Journal of Enterostomal Therapy;* newsletter; other[h]
X	X	X	X	X	X	X	*NITA Journal; NITA Update;* newsletter (both bi-monthly); other[h]
X	X	X	X	X	X	X	*Orthopaedic Nursing;* other[h]
X	X	X	X	X	X	X	*Journal of Pediatric Health Care;* newsletter (bimonthly); other[h]

Appendix 5   (Continued)

Organization	Year established[a]	Membership eligibility[b]	Primary purpose
National Association of School Nurses (NASN) Box 1300, Lamplighter Lane, Scarborough, ME 04074	1969	School nurses employed by boards of education, institutions of higher learning and state departments of education.	Strengthen education of children by providing leadership in promotion and delivery of adequate health services by qualified school nurses.
National Nurses' Society on Addictions (NNSA) 5700 Old Orchard Rd., Skokie, IL 60077	1975	RNs; senior nursing students interested in chemical dependency problems.	Extend knowledge, disseminate information; promote quality care for the addicted patients and their families; become involved in social issues and public policy concerning addiction.
NAACOG: The Organization for Obstetric, Gynecologic, and Neonatal Nurses 409 12th St. SW, Washington, DC 20024	1969	RNs engaged in or interested in Ob/Gyn, or neonatal nursing.	Promote highest standards in Ob/Gyn and neonatal nursing practice, education and research; stimulate interest in field.
Oncology Nursing Society (ONS) 1016 Greentree Rd., Pittsburgh, PA 15220	1975	RNs engaged in or interested in oncology.	Develop new knowledge in cancer detection and improvement of care; CE; encourge nurses to specialize in cancer nursing.

Organizations Related to Leadership and Scholarship

Alpha Tau Delta, National Fraternity for Professional Nurses 5207 Mesada St., Alta Loma, CA 91701	1921	Students in accredited baccalaureate or higher degree programs; based on scholarship, personality, and character. Also alumnae chapters.	Further professional and education standards, develop leadership, encourage excellence.

					Members of		Publications

Certifi-cation[d]	CE	Standards set and published	Legislative activities[e]	Research activities[f]	NFSNO	NOLF	Publications (monthly unless otherwise indicated)
X	X	X	X		X		*School Nurse* (newsletter quarterly); other[h]
X	X	X	X		X	X	*NSA* newsletter (quarterly)
X	X	X	X	X	X	X	*Journal of Obstetrics, Gynecologic and Neonatal Nursing;* newsletter; other[h]
X	X	X	X		X	X	*Oncology Nursing Forum* (6 times a year); other[h]
						X	*Cap'tions of Alpha Tau Delta* (2 times a year)

Activities[c]

Appendix 5 (Continued)

Organization	Year established[a]	Membership eligibility[b]	Primary purpose
American Academy of Nursing (AAN) 600 Maryland Ave. SW, Washington, DC 20005	1973	Elected by current members, based on contributions to nursing; members are called fellows (FAAN).	Advance role of nursing in health care delivery; identify and explore issues in health care, the professions and society; and propose resolutions; disseminate scholarly concepts; formulate strategies to improve health care.
Sigma Theta Tau International Honor Society of Nursing 550 W. North St., Indianapolis, IN 46202	1922	High academic achievement and leadership qualitities as student in baccalaureate and higher degree programs. Also community leaders.	Recognize superior achievement, leadership qualities, foster high professional standards, encourage creative work; support scholarliness in nursing.
Chi Eta Phi Society 3029 13th St. N. W., Washington, DC 20029	1932	Interested RNs and students in U.S. and Africa; focus is on black nurses.	Encourage CE; recruit into nursing, identify corps of nursing leaders who will be agents of social change.

Organizations with Ethnic, Racial, Religious Interests

American Assembly for Men in Nursing (AAMN) P.O. Box 31753, Independence, OH 44131	1971	Men nurses.	Provide support to men nurses; encourage men into nursing.
National Association of Hispanic Nurses (NAHN) 6905 Alamo Downs Pkwy, San Antonio, TX 78238	1976	Hispanic nurses, any RN interested.	Improve care of Hispanic patients; educate about health care needs; recruitment and retention of Hispanic students; assure equal opportunities for Hispanic nurses.

Activities[c]

Certifi-cation[d]	CE	Standards set and published	Legislative activities[e]	Research activities[f]	Members of NFSNO	NOLF	Publications (monthly unless otherwise indicated)
	X		X	X			Newsletter; other[h]
	X			X		X	*Image: The Journal of Nursing Scholarship* (4–6 times annually); *Reflections* (5 times annually); other[h]
	X					X	Newsletter (periodic)
	X					X	
	X		X	X		X	*El Faro* (newsletter) quarterly

Appendix 5   (Continued)

Organization	Year established[a]	Membership eligibility[b]	Primary purpose
National Black Nurses' Association (NBNA) 1012 Tenth St. NW, Washington, DC 20001	1970	RNs, LPNs, students.	Improve care for black consumers; influence legislation about blacks; recruit blacks into nursing; unify black nurses.
Nurses Christian Fellowship (NCF) P.O. Box 7895, 6400 Schroeder Rd., Madison, WI 53707	1948	Christian nurses and students.	Help students and nurses grow spiritually; focus on ministering to whole person.

Job-Related Special Interest Groups

Organization	Year established[a]	Membership eligibility[b]	Primary purpose
American Academy of Ambulatory Nursing Administration (AAANA) N. Woodbury Rd., Box 56, Pitman, NJ 08071	1978	Any RN interested in ambulatory nursing care.	Promote high standards of ambulatory care nursing administration and practice through education, exchange of information, and scientific investigation.
American Association of Colleges of Nursing (AACN) One Dupont Circle, Suite 530, Washington, DC 20036	1969	Heads of baccalaureate or higher degree nursing programs.	Promote academic leadership in nursing; disseminate information about higher education in nursing; advance the quality of baccalaureate and higher nursing education; promote research.
American Association of Nurse Attorneys (AANA) 720 Light St., Baltimore, MD 21230	1982	Nurse attorneys, nurses in law school.	Facilitate information sharing; develop the profession; educate nurses about law; influence health policy.
American Organization of Nurse Executives (AONE) 840 North Lake Shore Dr., 10E, Chicago, IL 60622	1967	Nurse executives; nurse managers; graduate faculty in nursing administration.	Provide leadership for advancement of nursing practice and patient care in organized health care systems, through achievement in excellence in nurse executive practice; shape policy in health care.

Activities[c]

Certifi-cation[d]	CE	Standards set and published	Legislative activities[e]	Research activities[f]	Members of NFSNO	NOLF	Publications (monthly unless otherwise indicated)
X			X			X	
							Journal of Christian Nursing (quarterly); other[h]
X	X			X	X		*Viewpoint* (bimonthly)
X			X	X			*Journal of Professional Nursing* (bimonthly); *AACN Newsletter;* other[h]
X			X	X		X	Inside TAANA (semiannual newsletter)
X			X	X			*Nurse Executive* (newsletter); other[h]

Appendix 5 (Continued)

Organization	Year established[a]	Membership eligibility[b]	Primary purpose
National Association for Health Care Recruitment (NAHCR) P.O. Box 5769 Akron, OH 44372	1975	Those working in hospitals or health care agencies actively involved in health care recruiting.	Promote and exchange principles of professional health care recruitment.
National Council of State Boards of Nursing 676 N. St. Clair, Suite 550 Chicago, IL 60611	1978	Boards of nursing in states and territories.	Develop licensing exams; assist boards in administering them; develop model licensure laws and regulations; disseminate information.

Other Special Interest Groups

Organization	Year established[a]	Membership eligibility[b]	Primary purpose
American Association for the History of Nursing (AAHN) P.O. Box 90803 Washington, D.C. 20090	1982	Anyone interested in purpose of the association.	Educate public about history and heritage of nursing; support historical research; promote development of centers for preservation of historical materials; disseminate information on nursing history.
American Holistic Nurses Association (AHNA) 4101 Lake Boon Trail, Suite 201, Raleigh, NC 27607	1980	Nurses and others interested in holistically oriented health care.	Promote the education of nurses in concepts and practice of the health of the whole person; serve as advocate of wellness.
North American Nursing Diagnosis Association (NANDA) 3525 Caroline St. St. Louis, MO 63104	1982	Any RN interested in nursing diagnosis.	Develop a taxonomy of nursing diagnosis.
Nurses Environmental Health Watch (NEHW) 33 Columbus Ave., Somerville, MA 02143	1979	Nurses interested in environmental health concerns.	Provide education about actual and potential health hazards.

Activities[c]

Certifi-cation[d]	CE	Standards set and published	Legislative activities[e]	Research activities[f]	Members of NFSNO	NOLF	Publications (monthly unless otherwise indicated)
	X			X			Recruitment directions (10 per year); other[h]
	X		X	X			*Issues* (quarterly newsletter); other[h]
	X			X			*Bulletin* (quarterly)
	X		X	X		X	*Journal of Holistic Nursing* (annually); *Beginnings* (10 times a year)
	X			X		X	*Nursing Diagnosis* (other)[b]
	X		X				*Health Watch* (quarterly newsletter)

Appendix 5 (Continued)

Organization	Year established[a]	Membership eligibility[b]	Primary purpose
Regional Nursing Organizations			
Midwest Alliance in Nursing (MAIN) 2511 E 46th St., Suite E-3 Indianapolis, IN 46205 (Midwest Nursing Research Society is independent affiliate)	1979	Nursing education programs and health care institutions/ agencies providing nursing care in 13-state Midwest region.	Facilitate regional investigation, planning, communication; collaborate to obtain shared goals and resolve issues in order to achieve maximum utilization of resources for cost-effective care.
New England Organization for Nursing (NEON), (joined by Mid-Atlantic Regional Nursing Association in 1991). Hewitt Hall University of N.H. Durham, NH 03824	1983	Nursing education programs and health care agencies with identifiable nursing department in 6-state New England region and Mid-Atlantic region.	Bring about cooperative planning and collaboration between nursing education and service to improve health care of the region.
Southern Council on Collegiate Education for Nursing, affiliated with Southern Regional Board (SREB) 1340 Spring St. NW, Atlanta, GA 30309	SREB 1948; Council 1962	AD, Baccalaureate and higher degree programs in nursing in SREB 14-state region.	Generate and implement projects related to improvement of nursing education; provide forum for college-based programs to receive information and conduct regional planning.
Western Institute of Nursing (WIN) P.O. Box Drawer P, Boulder, CO 80301	1986	Individual RN nursing education programs and nursing service agencies in 13 Western states, including Alaska and Hawaii.	Influence the quality of health care in the West through monitoring issues and trends and designing, implementing, evaluating regional, action-oriented, nursing strategies in education, practice, research.

<table>
<tr><td colspan="8" align="center">**Activities**[c]</td></tr>
<tr>
<td>Certifi-cation[d]</td>
<td>CE</td>
<td>Standards set and published</td>
<td>Legislative activities[e]</td>
<td>Research activities[f]</td>
<td colspan="2" align="center">Members of
NFSNO   NOLF</td>
<td>Publications (monthly unless otherwise indicated)</td>
</tr>
<tr>
<td>X</td>
<td></td>
<td></td>
<td>X</td>
<td>X</td>
<td></td>
<td></td>
<td>*Mainlines* (quarterly); other[h]</td>
</tr>
<tr>
<td>X</td>
<td></td>
<td></td>
<td>X</td>
<td></td>
<td></td>
<td></td>
<td>Newsletter (periodic)</td>
</tr>
<tr>
<td>X</td>
<td>X</td>
<td></td>
<td>X</td>
<td>X</td>
<td></td>
<td></td>
<td>Newsletter (periodic); other[h]</td>
</tr>
<tr>
<td>X</td>
<td>X</td>
<td></td>
<td>X</td>
<td>X</td>
<td></td>
<td></td>
<td>Newsletter (periodic); *Western Journal of Nursing Research;* other[h]</td>
</tr>
</table>

Appendix 5   (Continued)

| | Year | Membership | |
Organization	established[a]	eligibility[b]	Primary purpose
Health-Related Organizations			
National Association for Practical Nurse Education and Service (NAPNES) 1400 Spring St., Suite 310, Silver Spring, MD 20910	1941	LPNs/LVNs, RNs, nurse educators, physicians, administators and consumers interested in practical nursing; agency; members.	Improve and extend PN education to meet public needs.
National Federation of Licensed Practical Nurses (NFLPN) 3948 Browning Pl., Suite 205, P.O. Box 18088, Raleigh, NC 27619	1949	State organizations made up of LPNs/LVNs and individual LPNs.	Secure recognition and effective utilization of LPNs; promote LPN welfare; improve standards of practice and education.

[a]The organization may have been established under another name.

[b]Some organizations have associate membership for students and interested LPNs or others.

[c]All organizations have some type of meetings or conventions and carry out public relations activities of some sort to educate or influence the public about themselves. Many offer other benefits such as insurance and travel discounts.

[d]Certification may be done by a separately incorporated organization.

[e]Legislative activities include staying on top of legislative and governmental issues and actions, alerting members to these, providing information to legislators, and lobbying.

Activities^c

Certifi-cation^d	CE	Standards set and published	Legislative activities^e	Research activities^f	Members of NFSNO	NOLF	Publications (monthly unless otherwise indicated)
	X	X	X	X			*Journal of Practical Nursing;* other^h
	X	X	X	X			*Licensed Practical Nurse;* other^h

^{f}Research activities include data collection and/or dissemination, research projects, funding for research, and educating on research.

^{g}Accreditation is also done. (In organizations other than NLN, this is done by a separate corporation.)

^{h}Write to the organization for a list.

Note: *The American Journal of Nursing* lists the addresses of most nursing organizations in each April issue; addresses change frequently.

Appendix 6   Basics of Parliamentary Procedure

By-laws. An organization's by-laws are the basis on which it functions. It includes:

Name
Purposes
Functions
Requirements for membership
Dues
The officers
Governing body
Committees
Other organizational units and their responsibilities
How elected or appointed
How amendments are made
The parliamentary authority used to conduct business (often *Robert's Rules of Order Newly Revised*)

Usual order of business at a meeting (may have additional parts at a convention).

1. Call to order
2. Minutes of previous meetings
3 Reports of officers, boards, standing committees
   Executive reports
   Executive announcements
   Reports of:
      President
      Vice President
      Secretary
      Treasurer
      Board of Directors
      Standing committees
4. Reports of special committees
5. Announcements
6. Unfinished business
7. New business
8. Adjournment

Motions are proposals or suggestions that initiate action or enable the assembly to express itself. To make a motion:

1. Stand or raise your hand or go to a microphone when indicated.
2. Wait for the chair's signal to go ahead.
3. Address the presiding officer as "Madame (or Mister) Chairman," "Chairperson," "President," or "Speaker."
4. Identify yourself by name and whatever else is customary in that organization, such as office, affiliation, city, or state.

5. State the motion clearly and as briefly as possible. Write out a motion if time permits, for accuracy and the record. Frequently a written motion is given to the secretary for the minutes.
6. Ask to speak to the motion after making it. Don't speak first and then make the motion.
7. The chair will call for a second. (Not required if it is a committee motion.)
8. For seconding, rise, identify yourself and say "I second the motion."
9. If no one seconds, the motion is automatically lost and not recorded.
10. If the motion is seconded, the chair says, "It has been moved and seconded that . . . Is there any discussion?"
11. If there is a discussion, it may take the form of comments and/or a motion suggesting an amendment.
12. The amendment is voted on first, then the original motion with the amendment, if it was accepted.
13. Discussion may be stopped by saying, "I move to close debate" or "I call for the question." This is not debatable and if carried, the motion on the floor is voted on immediately.
14. There may be motions to table a motion (set it aside temporarily—sometimes permanently), to postpone action, or to refer it to a committee. All avoid further action at that time.
15. If an action is taken, that, for whatever reason, people regret, someone on the *prevailing* side may ask to bring it before the assembly again. Anyone can second. This takes precedence and is acted on at once, following the usual procedure. The result may be the same or different, usually different.

Resolutions are indications of the organization's position on key issues.

1. Resolutions are submitted to a resolutions committee by any member, committee, or other organizational entity.
2. The format usually begins with: Whereas (giving one or more reasons) and ends with Therefore be it resolved: (stating one or more resolutions related to the "whereas").
3. Resolutions are reviewed by the committee, and sometimes edited or combined with a similar resolution, with permission of the originators.
4. Resolutions usually go to the board, but do not necessarily have to be approved by them, depending on policy.
5. A rejected resolution can usually be presented from the floor.
6. At conventions, there may be an open resolutions committee hearing in which resolutions are discussed and debated without formal parliamentary procedure. They may then be changed before formal presentation at the business meeting, saving time and confusion.
7. Resolutions are voted on like motions.
8. Courtesy resolutions at the end of the meeting are usually formalities, showing appreciation to various people or groups.

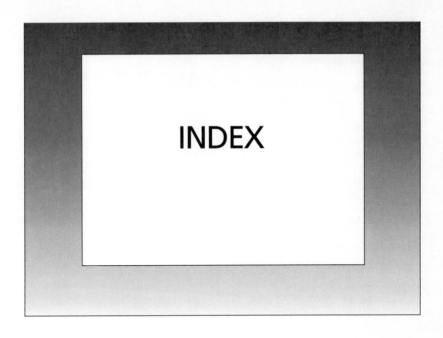

INDEX

Page numbers followed by "f" designate figures or displays; numbers followed by "t" designate tables.